Tiziano Tealdo - Marco Bevilacqua - Paolo Pera

COLUMBUS BRIDGE PROTOCOL

SURGICAL AND PROSTHETIC GUIDELINES FOR AN IMMEDIATELY LOADED, IMPLANT-SUPPORTED PROSTHESIS IN THE EDENTULOUS MAXILLA

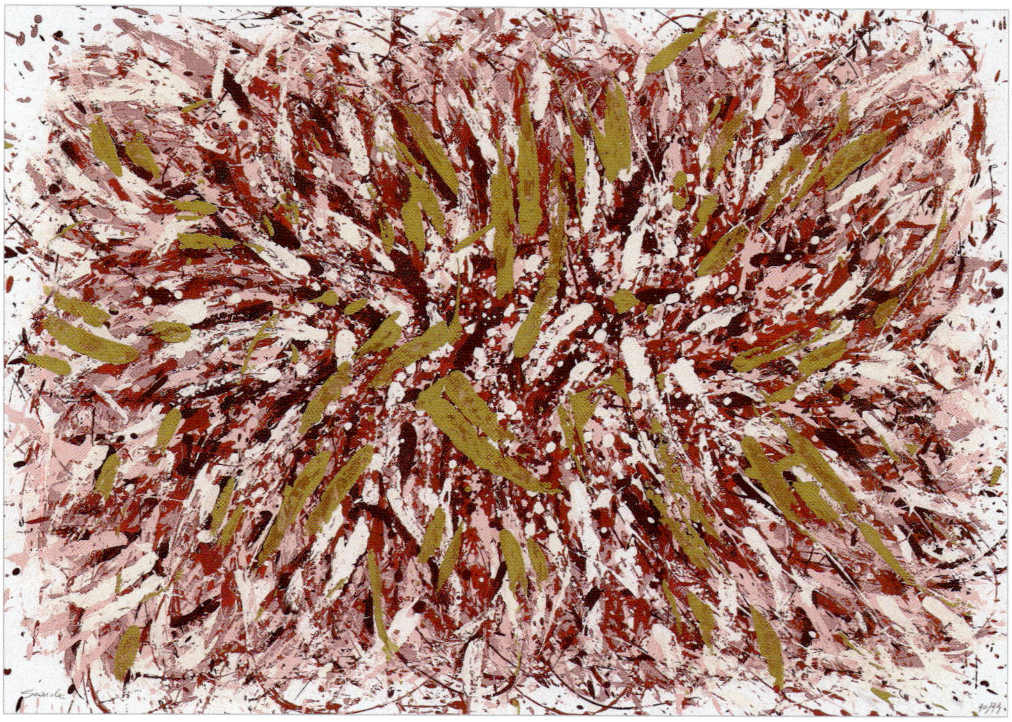

Preface by George Zarb and Giulio Preti

Translation by Genni Anna Genobbio, Cuneo

Milan, Berlin, Chicago, Tokyo, Barcelona, Bombay, Istanbul,
London, Moscow, Paris, Prague, Saõ Paolo, Warsaw

The translation of this work has been funded by SEPS
Segretariato Europeo per le Pubblicazioni Scientifiche

SEGRETARIATO EUROPEO PER LE PUBBLICAZIONI SCIENTIFICHE

Via Val d'Aposa, 7 - 40123 Bologna - Italy
seps@seps.it - www.seps.it

Quintessenza Edizioni S.r.l.
via Ciro Menotti, 65 - 20017 Rho, Milan (Italy)
Tel.: +39.02.93.18.08.21 - Fax: +39.02.93.18.61.59
E-mail: info@quintessenzaedizioni.it

ISBN 88-7492-154-3
978-88-7492-154-6

Columbus Bridge Protocol Patent Pending.

Front cover illustration: *Terra d'oro,* acrylic/canvas by Giuseppe Scaiola, Bergeggi, Italy.

Printed in Italy

AUTHORS

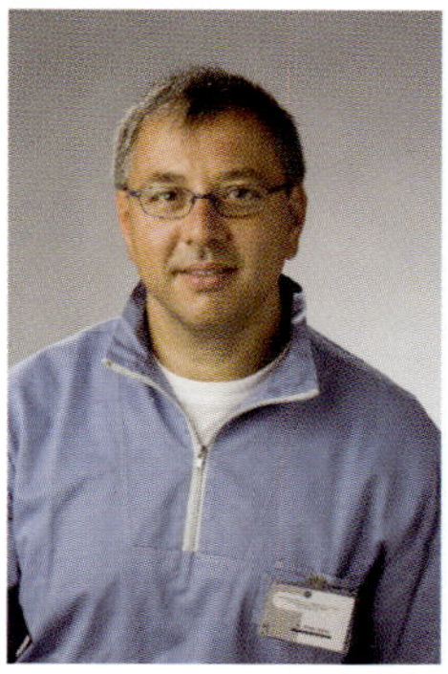

Tiziano Tealdo, *DDS, MS, CDT,* obtained his certificate in dental laboratory technology in 1984. Dr Tealdo graduated in dentistry at the University of Turin, Italy in 1991.
At the same university, he earned his postgraduate degree in oral surgery in 1993.
Dr Tealdo obtained the university certificate in implantology at the University of Aix-Marseille, France, in 1998.
From 1998 to 2000 he completed Dr Carlo Tinti's postgraduate periodontal program, which focused on reconstruction of hard and soft tissue in conjunction with implant surgery.
Dr Tealdo's interest in implant-prosthetic therapy led him to attend the Brånemarkkliniken and the Brånemark Osseointegration Center, Gothenburg, Sweden; the Department of Oral and Maxillofacial Surgery at the University of Ümea, Sweden; and the Malo Clinic in Lisbon, Portugal.
Since 1997 he has been in charge of the Implant Division in the Department of Implant and Prosthetic Dentistry of Genoa University, Italy.
Currently, at the same university, he is professor of Prosthodontics.
Dr Tealdo is a member of the International College of Prosthodontists.

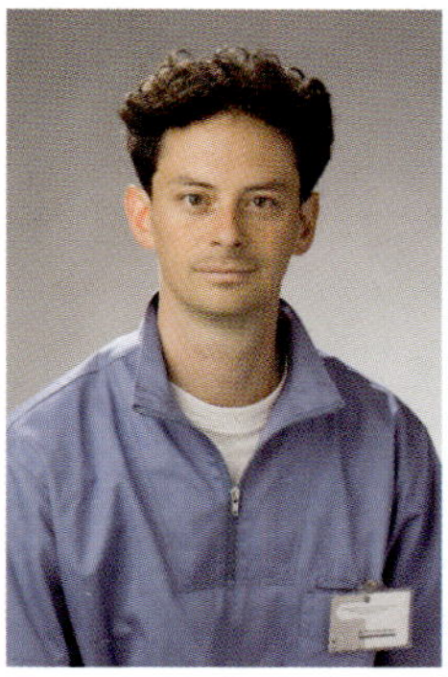

Marco Bevilacqua, *DDS,* graduated with honors in dentistry from the University of Turin, Italy in 1998.
Dr Bevilacqua began his studies in implantology while attending an International Training Course at the Brånemark Clinic of Gothenburg, Sweden, in 2002.
In 2004 he specialized in oral implantology at the University of Genoa, Italy.
Currently Dr Bevilacqua is working and lecturing at the University of Genoa teaching predoctoral and postdoctoral students in the Department of Implant and Prosthetic Dentistry, directed by Professor Paolo Pera.
Since 2009 he has been a reviewer for the *Journal of Prosthodontics.*

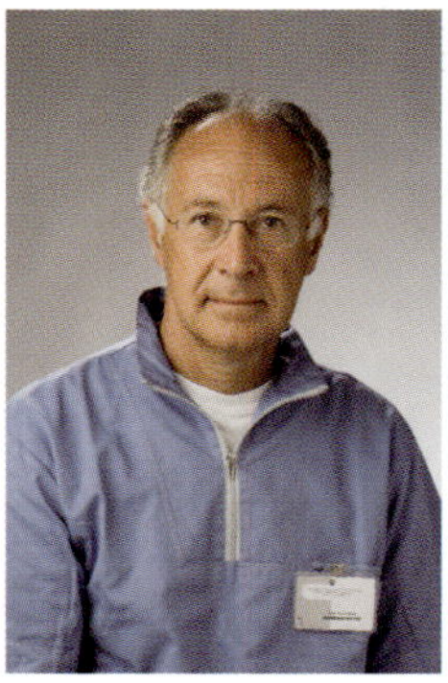

Paolo Pera, *MD, DDS, PhD,* graduated in medicine from the University of Turin, Italy in 1975.
Professor Pera was a former postgraduate student of Professor Giulio Preti and specialized in dentistry in the University of Turin in 1979.
Since 1980, he collaborated with the clinical, teaching, and research activity of the Prosthodontics Department of Turin University.
He lectured as assistant professor at many Universities in Italy and abroad.
In 1997 Professor Pera became a full professor of prosthodontics at the University of Genoa, Italy.
Past president of the Italian Society of Prosthetic and Implant-Prosthetic Dentistry and of the Dental Hygiene School of the University of Genoa.
Professor Pera currently heads the Department of Implant and Prosthetic Dentistry of Genoa University.
He has published many papers in Italian and international journals and university books text.
Since 2004 Professor Pera has been a reviewer for the *International Journal of Prosthodontics.*

COAUTHORS

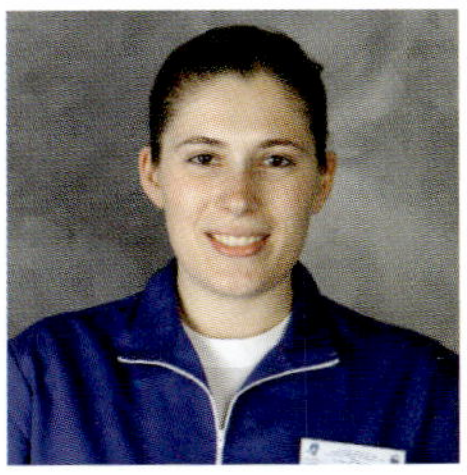

Maria Menini, *DDS*
Assistant Professor, Faculty of Medicine, University of Genoa, Italy

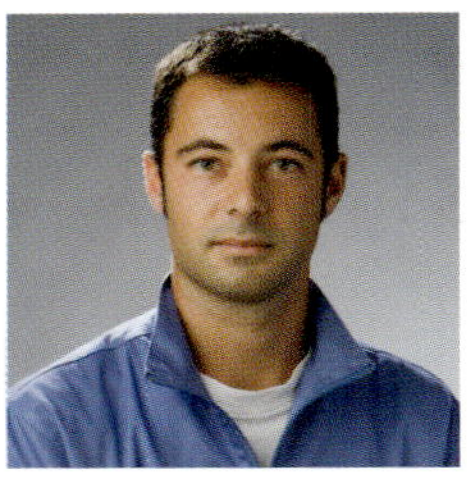

Francesco Pera, *DDS*
PhD student, Faculty of Medicine, University of Turin, Italy

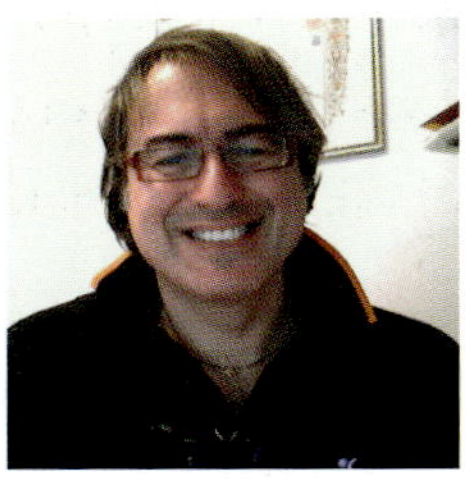

Enrico Conserva, *DDS*
Professor, Faculty of Medicine, University of Genoa, Italy

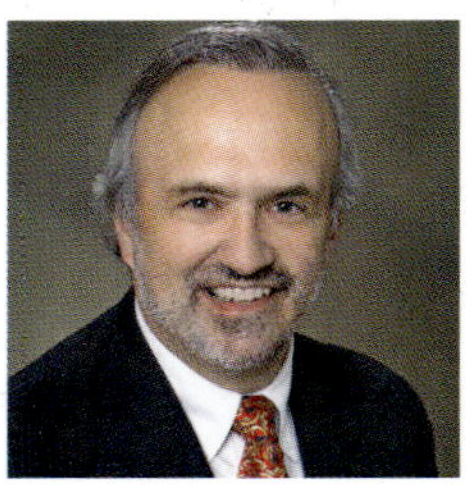

Carl Drago, *DDS, MS*
Associate Professor, The Ohio State University College of Dentistry, Columbus, Ohio

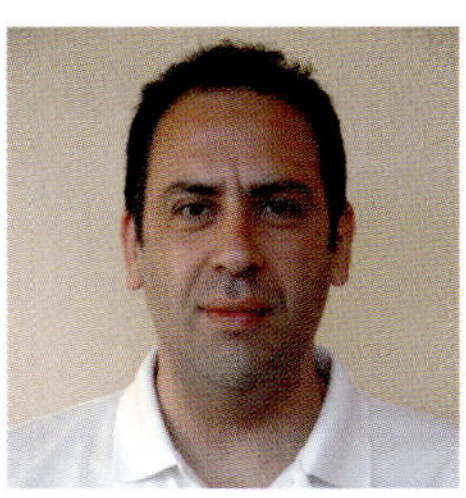

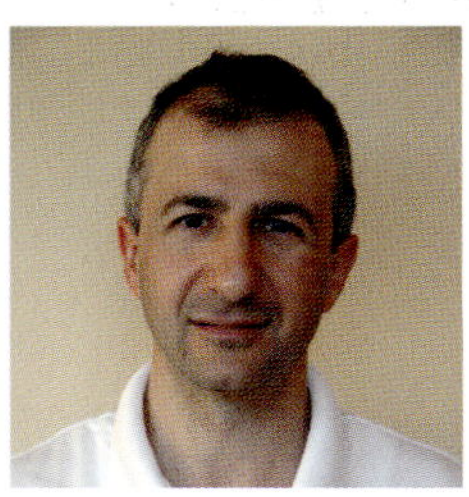

Luca Scaglione, *CDT and* **Piercarlo Seghesio,** *CDT*
Dental technicians in Santo Stefano Belbo, Italy

FOREWORD

The invitation to write a foreword to this exceptional text reminds me that we, as clinical academics and practitioners, are at a crossroads in our joint efforts to manage problems of mutual professional concern. We recognize that most of our universities are funded by the commercial manufacturing giants, somewhat like the pharmaceutical industry, and that this may not be particularly controversial. However, there is a familiar risk here, and that is the inadvertent and sometimes even deliberate blurring of the line between disinterested advice and sales pitches, which underscores what is happening in the current populist approach to dental implant treatment. The most disturbing thing is not so much the marketing methods per se, but the goals that are implied and even articulated.

In medicine, it has been frequently observed that it is not in the economic interests of a corporation who sells pills to unhealthy people for those folks to be actually healthy. Or to be more precise, for the people to perceive themselves as being healthy. Their actual physical state then becomes irrelevant since what really matters is whether someone believes there is something wrong that can be rectified with pills. If so, the company has a new potential customer. Critics call this *disease mongering* – a stark reminder that "health condition branding" shifts the line between the healthy and the diseased states. We risk a comparable emerging predicament in dentistry where any number of missing or diseased teeth is marketed as an ominous case of *partial edentulism* or worse still a *terminal dentition*. No wonder general dentists are tempted to flock to weekend courses when there is such a pandemic around, waiting to be diagnosed and treated both surgically and prosthodontically.

Professional judgment and integrity remain the key determinants that make our profession special, with a bottom line that must continue to engage us scrupulously and unremittingly. It is therefore both a privilege and a delight to encounter scientifically based treatment concepts developed and applied in the manner that our Genoan colleagues have systematically sought to present. They applied their ideas with intellectual rigor and in the context of well-argued and scrupulously designed protocols.

Their results speak for themselves and already offer enormous promise for those patients whose dental disease outcomes necessitate this text's described interventions. Above all, the authors' judgment reflects integrity of purpose and interpretation that is indeed noteworthy. This book offers a clean line of demarcation between commercial interests and professional ones. It recognizes the indispensable role of quality standards from different manufacturers without attributing documented successes to product specification. And in so doing, the primacy of clinical judgment and skills is underscored – a rare but desirable approach in today's era of implant and technique material brands. This text encourages all of us to seek to match, and perhaps even hope to emulate, the authors' outstanding treatment outcomes by recognizing that scientifically based rigor in patient management remains the major determinant of time-dependent success.

George Zarb
Professor Emeritus, University of Toronto, Canada
Editor-in-Chief, *International Journal of Prosthodontics*

The original surgical-prosthetic protocol designed by Per-Ingvar Brånemark for long-term, predictable osseointegration of endosseous implants has undergone important changes and modifications secondary to continued basic science and clinical research and improved clinical experiences. Modifications in the protocol have occurred in both surgical and prosthetic aspects.

A protocol that was originally designed to treat mandibular edentulism has evolved to treat edentulous and partially edentulous patients, including the most difficult situations. These changes, together with unprecedented commercial pressures, led the entire dental community to focus their interests on implant techniques independent from levels of specialist competencies. In the many-sided panorama created by this phenomenon, basic principles of prosthetic treatment, the definitive goal for osseointegrated implants treatments, were not always taken into account.

Disappointing results, similar to those obtained in the beginning of osseointegrated implant treatment, were recorded. Brånemark himself in the article "On looking back with Per-Ingvar Brånemark" (Int J Prosthod 2004;17:395-396) stigmatized this situation. Long-term predictable surgical and prosthetic results described by the international scientific community validated the concept of osseointegration. Published results and findings should not disregard the competence and precision of those involved with clinical research and treatment; competence and precision are the specific characteristics of this work I am pleased to introduce.

The authors describe solutions to maxillary edentulism with immediately loaded fixed prostheses based on obtaining primary implant stability and controlling masticatory loads. The treatments illustrated in this text have been applied with a rigorous approach in the scope of a protocol following basic principles of oral treatment: assessment of the local and functional systemic conditions of the stomatognathic system. The most appropriate treatment solutions were chosen on the basis of preoperative conditions and the characteristics of edentulism for each specific patient. The surgical treatment phase was accomplished with the use of surgical templates precisely and specifically fabricated for each patient.

All essential prosthodontic parameters were identified for fabrication of the prostheses: sophisticated precision of master casts; measurements of jaw relationships; passive; accurate fit of the prostheses; optimal esthetics; and phonetics.

In conclusion, this is an exceptional textbook resulting from the varied clinical experiences of the authors, acquired over many years of treating patients with implant prosthodontics and developed in the academic environment by the Department of Prosthodontics, University of Genoa. Readers and clinicians who apply the protocol described in this work will embark on a sure path, without the uncertainties of the first voyage to America of the great explorer from Genoa, who inspired the authors in choosing the title of their work.

Giulio Preti
Professor Emeritus, University of Turin, Italy
Director of the Italian National Observatory of Oral Health of Disadvantaged Communities

AUTHORS' NOTE

The use of dental implants inserted into alveolar bone as substitutes for lost or nonrestorable teeth has radically modified prosthodontic treatment planning. Before osseointegration of dental implants provided predictable results to treat edentulism with fixed implant prostheses, dentists were compelled to use prosthetic treatments supported and retained by edentulous ridges and natural teeth.
The studies conducted and reported by Brånemark and his colleagues at the University of Göteborg introduced the use of endosseous implants in clinical dentistry. Implants of various materials and shapes had been proposed and used for years previous to the discovery of osseointegration. Brånemark did not invent dental implants; through in-depth clinical trials and studies on bone repair, Brånemark proposed a strict protocol for dentists relative to using commercially pure titanium dental implants and a precise surgical protocol with scientifically-documented predictability. Over time, the applied principles of osseointegration and implant prosthetics have been modified. The scientific method has been used to simplify the original protocols proposed by Brånemark.

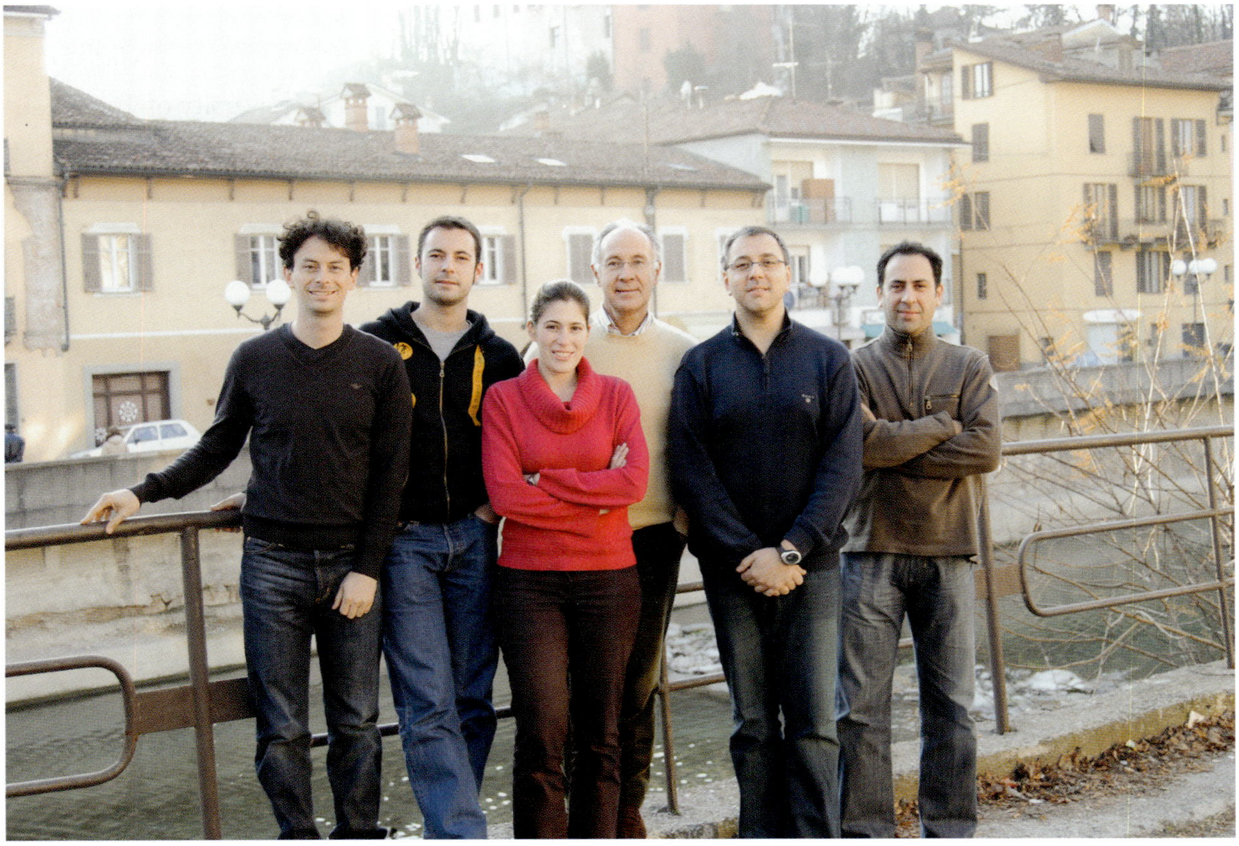

Columbus Bridge Team, Ceva, Northern Italy, December 2007.

In recent years, immediate occlusal loading in edentulous jaws has become an accepted treatment option in implant protocols. Increased knowledge and reported experiences by numerous researchers and clinicians modified the original principles proposed by Brånemark, especially regarding the optimal times to load implants. Reductions in the times relative to loading dental implants were proposed, researched, and studied; reduced loading times were still cognizant of patient needs and scientific principles. In fact, the use of new protocols with immediate functional loading of dental implants also reduced patient discomfort and facilitated treatment by decreasing the amount of time patients may have needed to continue to wear removable prostheses. Clinical visits were also decreased. In order for the profession to accept the new protocols, the protocols had to achieve implant survival and prosthesis success consistent with the results obtained with traditional, unloaded healing protocols.
The Columbus Bridge Protocol was developed consistent with the above goals: maintenance of predictable implant/prosthetic treatment specifically designed for edentulous maxillae, fixed prostheses, and immediate occlusal loading.

Why Columbus? The great navigator did not invent the Americas. The Americas existed well before Columbus indicated the route that allowed his society to reach them and develop their huge natural resources. In the same way, the Columbus Bridge Protocol indicated a path that, when observed, describes treatment of edentulous maxillae with immediately loaded implants to obtain predictable therapeutic, functional, and esthetic results.
In the field of implants/prosthodontics, where new treatments without sufficient scientific documentation have too often been presented, the authors in the Department of Prosthodontics at the University of Genoa think that dedication of the protocol described in this text to Columbus is appropriate, as Columbus was moved by great curiosity in his quest for the route to the West Indies. Columbus meticulously prepared for his voyage, which was considered indispensable for him and his crew to reach new horizons. The authors believe that clinicians should possess the same curiosity and skill in preparing to treat their patients as Columbus exhibited in his desire to explore the New World.

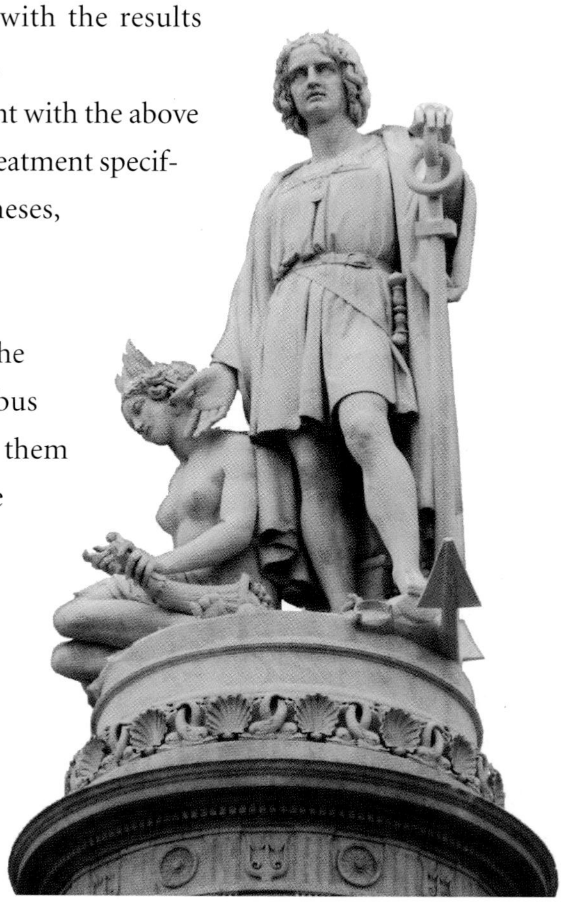
Christopher Columbus

ACKNOWLEDGMENTS

The authors would like to thank all those who have contributed to creating this book.

- Dr Giulio Preti and Dr George Zarb for their invaluable teaching.
- Genni Anna Genobbio for the translation of the English version of the book.
- Dr Domenico Baldi from the Department of Implant and Prosthetic Dentistry, Genoa, Italy, for his scientific contribution to chapter 4.
- Dr Paola Zunino, Dr Paola Gavoglio, Dr Simona Lavagnino, Dr Emilia D'Agostino, and Dr Marta Defferrari from the Department of Implant and Prosthetic Dentistry, Genoa, Italy, for their scientific contribution to chapter 15.
- Dr Sergio Caputi, Dr Tonino Traini, and Dr Giovanna Orsini from the Prosthodontics Department at Chieti University, Italy, for the visual images in chapter 2.
- Dr Antonio Zicca and Dr Ranieri Cancedda from Genoa University, Italy, for their reviews in chapter 2.
- Dr Giambattista Ravera from Genoa University, Italy, for the statistical analysis.
- Dr Stefano Carossa, Dr Francesco Bassi, Dr Gianmario Schierano, Dr Gianfranco Gassino, and Dr Marco Mozzati from the Prosthodontics Department at Turin University, Italy, for the visual images in chapters 1, 3, and 6.
- Dr Clara Cassinelli and Dr Marco Morra, chief executives at Nobil Bio Ricerche, Italy, for the implant surface analysis in chapter 4.
- Dr Giuseppe Casalino and Dr Fabio Giorgi from the Engineering Department at Genoa University, Italy, for the masticatory robot construction and data in chapter 10.
- Dr Alexei Mossolov, chief executive at ITERA Srl, Italy, for the finite element analysis in chapter 6.
- Dr Paolo Ronchi, Dr Paolo Nicoli, Dr Paolo Canepa, Dr Alessandro Caputo, Dr Angelo Gamalero, Dr Marco Porcella, Dr Alessandra Evangelisti, Dr Ivan Calimodio, Dr Alberto Coccalotto, Dr Andrea Giannattasio, Dr Arianna Ottonello, Dr Paolo Pesce, Dr Bruno Musante, Dr Eugenio Patrone, Dr Federico Parodi, Dr José Tubino, Dr Elena Dellepiane, Dr Corrado Cameroni, Dr Luca Bruzzone, Dr Sandra Nobili, Dr Paolo Benedetto, Dr Giuseppe Berlingueri, Dr Salvatore Cunsolo, Mrs Sabrina Oppedisano, and Mrs Silvana Gullifa from the Department of Implant and Prosthetic Dentistry, Genoa, Italy, for their contribution in treating patients.
- Aldo Porotti, Mario Notari, Canio Summa, Arcangelo Traversi, Luca Fernandez, Roberto Olla, Fabio Gondolo, Roberto Ceretto, and Andrea De Benedetto, dental technicians in Italy, for their laboratory collaboration.
- Ugo Giletta, chief executive at San Firmino Film, Italy, for shooting the Columbus Bridge Protocol short film.
- Mrs Jani Kahukiwa, Mrs Deborah Dawson, and Mrs Lina Saracino, English teachers, for their contribution to the English version of this book.
- Artist Giuseppe Scaiola, Italy, for the cover image.
- Ernesto Valdesolo, Antonio Coppola, Roberto Ferrari, Filippo Trisolino, Michele Micheletti, and Fabrizio Costa from Biomax Spa for their support.
- Janson Lars, Danielle Young, Kate Mendillo, Berta Torrens, and Jürg Probst, from Biomet 3i for their endorsement.

CONTENTS

CHAPTER 1
PRINCIPLES AND GUIDELINES OF IMPLANT-PROSTHETIC REHABILITATION

HISTORICAL PERSPECTIVE

Preosseointegration Implantology

Implant dentistry involves the replacement of missing teeth with alloplastic materials (dental implants). This practice dates back to about AD 600 as evidenced by the 1931 discovery of a human jaw of Mayan origin in which three incisive teeth were replaced by shell fragments inserted into bone.[1] In the early years of the 19th century, the introduction of alloplastic materials such as gold, silver, and ceramics as substitutes for natural tooth roots helped minimize the risk of infectious diseases previously noted in tooth transplants. However, the first detailed description of dental implants was not published until 1910 when Greenfield[2] reported his experiments with platinum-iridium implants.

The start of modern dental implantology in the 1950s was marked by the publication of various empirical techniques. These techniques were supported by very little refereed scientific documentation. Most of the so-called documentation on dental implants reported one or two cases as a case series. These studies did not report on the survival of dental implants inserted later and did not define "successful" implants with scientific criteria. Nevertheless, a number of dentists referenced the cases that they regarded as successful and began applying the techniques in their own practices.

Though a variety of implants existed, two types were commonly used: subperiosteal implants and blade implants. Subperiosteal implants consisted of metal frameworks made directly on the residual edentulous ridges of the jaws and positioned beneath the periosteum. Some published reports of the long-term duration of subperiosteal implants are available,[3] but they record numerous soft tissue problems and fractures of the metal frameworks. Blade implants also had little follow-up that justified their use, especially in regard to long-term survival, and although they had been used for more than 25 years, only two controlled clinical trials for blade implants were published.[4,5] Out of the two trials, Kapur's study[4] was the more notable due to number of treated patients. He reported on the results of 173 blade implants after 5 years of follow-up. Of these, 35 had negative results, and an additional 43 showed bone loss over one-third of the length of the implant. The use of blade implants could hardly be justified by these meager reports, especially given their long-term survival rates.

To promote their products, however, clinicians asserted that implants were anchored to bone with a "pseudoperiodontal ligament" that imitated the ligamentous anchoring of natural teeth; clinicians initially referred to this anchorage as *fibrointegration*. The pseudoperiodontal ligament was later determined to be histologically undifferentiated cicatricial tissue with weak mechanical characteristics. Therefore, these tissues were under constant risk of overload with physiologic masticatory loads.

Osseointegration

During the 1960s, Brånemark and his collaborators at the University of Göteborg conducted animal experiments indicating that direct contact could be established between bone and endosseous implants[6] if precise guidelines were followed. They used these data to develop a new dental implant protocol for obtaining direct bone-implant anchorage, which they termed *osseointegration*. A clinical report published several years later showed that osseointegration could also be achieved in humans.[7]

The concept behind osseointegration is based on research that began in 1952.[8] Surgical trauma was induced in rabbit fibula, and wound healing was then observed in situ with a microscope attached to a titanium camera. The camera was inserted into the surgical sites and included an optical system that transilluminated them. With this system, the researchers were able to observe microscopic elements of wound healing in the bone and marrow, including the growth of a layer of new bone tissue. They found that both induced and controlled conditions led to bone formation during osseous healing.

These experiments helped reveal the osseointegration process that occurs between living bone tissue and the load-carrying surfaces of titanium endosseous dental implants. In fact, osseointegration was so successful that Brånemark's team could not remove the optical cameras from the surrounding bone after the initial experiments were completed. The titanium optical chambers had "bonded" with the bone, and the mineralized tissue had become firmly inserted into the microirregularities of the titanium surfaces. This experimental observation suggested that missing dental elements could be substituted with titanium implants that were intentionally anchored into bone. Brånemark's team then took the next step of developing clinical procedures using screw-shaped, cylindric fixtures made of commercially pure titanium that were 3.75 mm in diameter and 10 mm in length. Brånemark reported that an unloaded healing period of 3 to 6 months was necessary for osseointegration to predictably occur, after which, the implants were surrounded by compact bone. Tantalum had previously been used for vital microscopic observations. However, the Brånemark group used commercially pure titanium because its mechanical and surface characteristics were better suited for use in biologic tissues.

Histologic and radiographic analysis proved that osseointegration and implant stability could be maintained for 10 years in dogs without any significant unfavorable reactions on the hard or soft tissues when oral hygiene procedures were performed once or twice a year. Single fixtures had a load capacity of about 1,000 N in the mandible and from 300 to 500 N in the maxilla. After the animals were put down, the titanium fixtures could not be removed from the experimental sites without fracturing the surrounding bone. The bone-titanium interfaces remained intact. Integration of titanium devices at the level of soft tissues did not show any collateral effect when titanium chambers for bone marrow observation were used.

Brånemark's team was the first to recommend direct anchorage into bone and promote the clinical advantages of such osseointegration, but the scientific community was not persuaded of its benefits. This reluctance partly resulted from 1970s dental culture and partly from a lack of direct histologic evidence due to researchers' inability to section intact samples of bone in contact with metal.

Schroeder et al[9–11] were the first researchers to give clear evidence of osseointegration. Starting in the mid 1970s, in full autonomy from Brånemark's researchers, Schroeder's team devoted themselves to the study of implants with direct anchorage to bone. Using high-quality microtopographic images, they succeeded in showing that direct contact exists between bone and implants, and their work led to the development of the Straumann oral implant system.

A few years later, Albrektsson and colleagues[12] reported a list of factors that were extremely important and needed to be controlled for osseointegration of dental implants to occur. These included *(1)* biocompatibility, shape, and surface treatment of the implant; *(2)* state of the implant site; *(3)* surgical technique at the time of insertion; and *(4)* load conditions applied after implant placement. Subsequently, Albrektsson's team studied these variables, and their doctoral dissertations reported on the biocompatibility of metals,[13,14] bone cement[15] and hydroxyapatite,[16] macroscopic implant designs,[17] implant surfaces,[18] conditions of the implant site,[19,20] and surgical technique.[21]

Two-Stage, One-Stage, and Immediate Loading Protocols

After establishing the long-term success of bone-titanium anchorage experiments and the behavior of soft tissues adjacent to it, Brånemark treated the first patient according to the principles of osseointegration in 1965. The patient was treated with a two-stage, unloaded healing protocol, and the bone was prepared with a relatively atraumatic technique to encourage osseointegration. The crucial factor in determining clinical success was for the bone and marrow to heal as highly differentiated tissues without transforming into undifferentiated connective tissue. The implants were cylindric screws made from commercially pure titanium. They had an external diameter of 3.75 mm, and they ranged in length from 7 to 18 mm. The implants were connected to the standard abutments with abutment screws. The prosthesis was directly fixed onto the abutment with retaining screws. This system allowed all restorative components to be removed for repairs and replacements if needed. On the basis of experimental and clinical studies, Brånemark and his colleagues developed a protocol that enabled clinicians to achieve osseointegration with high predictability. Brånemark et al[12] defined four factors essential to the success of all implant-prosthetic therapies:

1. Preparation of the implant site not to exceed 2,000 rpm
2. Detailed studies of the bone-titanium relationship
3. Unloaded healing of submerged implants
4. Avoidance of bone overheating

In 1977, Brånemark, in his continuing work in the field of dental implants, defined *osseointegration* as "a direct structural and functional connection between ordered living bone and the surface of a load-carrying implant".[7] Over the next several decades, the results of surgical and prosthetic treatments were published in numerous multicenter prospective and retrospective studies. These studies,[22] with up to 9-year follow-up periods, confirmed the high cumulative survival rates of titanium implants: about 91% in the edentulous mandible and about 81% in the edentulous maxilla. These results were consistent with the first results published by Brånemark et al.

The 1982 Toronto Conference (Fig 1.1) presented a large number of research papers on the surgical and prosthetic implant treatment of edentulous patients. Participants at the conference

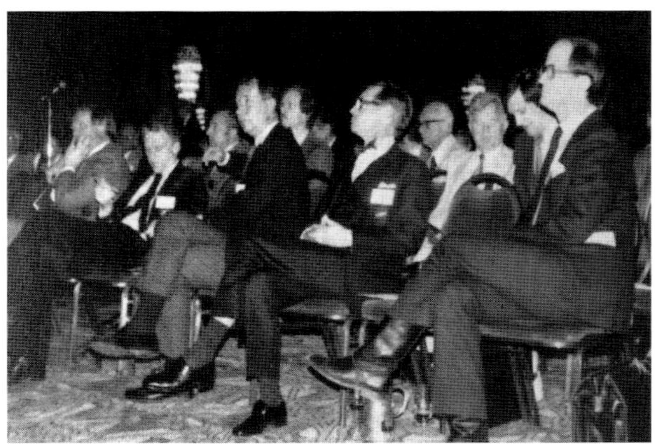

Fig 1.1 - Toronto Conference, May 1982. *(Courtesy of Dr George A. Zarb, Toronto, Canada).*

proposed that osseointegration was applicable on a large scale with high predictability and that these conclusions were consistent with the principles of evidence-based medicine. This protocol is still being used today and has been defined as the classic two-stage, unloaded healing protocol. It involves the following steps:

- Inserting implants into bone
- Placing cover screws on the implants
- Suturing the tissues over the implants and cover screws
- Unloaded healing over a period ranging from 3 to 6 months (Fig 1.2)
- uncovering the implants in a second surgery.

Subsequent appointments are then made for fabrication of the implant-supported prostheses.

During the 1980s and 1990s, the research of Buser et al,[23] Becker et al,[24] and Ericsson et al[25] led to a modification of the surgical protocol from a two-stage to a successful one-stage protocol. Their work demonstrated that there was no significant difference in the osseointegration rate of implants placed with either of these two protocols.

Unlike the original protocol, implants inserted according to the one-stage protocol emerge through the soft tissues into the oral cavity rather than being covered. A major benefit of this change was the reduced number of surgical appointments. However, this protocol did not modify the healing times between implant placement and prosthetic loading of the implants (Fig 1.3).

At the beginning of the 1980s, Ledermann[26] made an additional change to implant surgical protocols by immediately loading the implants with bar-supported overdentures.

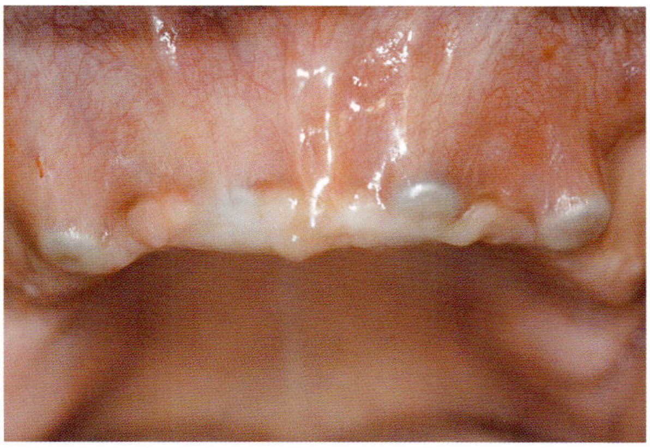

Fig 1.2 - Clinical intraoral image of edentulous maxilla approximately 3 months after implant placement with the classic two-stage surgical protocol. This protocol requires a period of unloaded healing with implants that were submerged after the first surgical appointment.

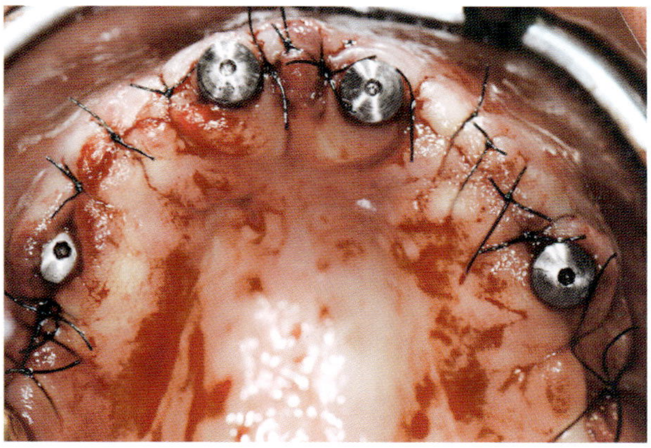

Fig 1.3 - Clinical intraoral image of edentulous maxilla immediately after placement of implants in a single-stage surgical protocol. This protocol is designed to let the implants emerge through the peri-implant soft tissues, with loading occurring approximately 3 to 6 months after implant placement (delayed loading).

In this protocol, the implants were placed under masticatory loads at the time of implant placement when they were only mechanically stable and osseointegration had not yet occurred. The possibility of functionally loading implants with fixed prostheses within 24 to 48 hours after implant placement (Fig 1.4) was hypothesized in the 1990s. Gapski and colleagues,[27] in a critical review of the literature published over the previous 20 years, analyzed the advantages and disadvantages of immediate loading and described the factors that affect success. These include patient selection; bone quality at the implant sites; implant length and macro- and microstructural characteristics; ability of the operator or surgeon; implant primary stability; and occlusal loading. Among the factors that Gapski listed, implant primary stability seems to be the most important prerequisite for successful immediate loading.

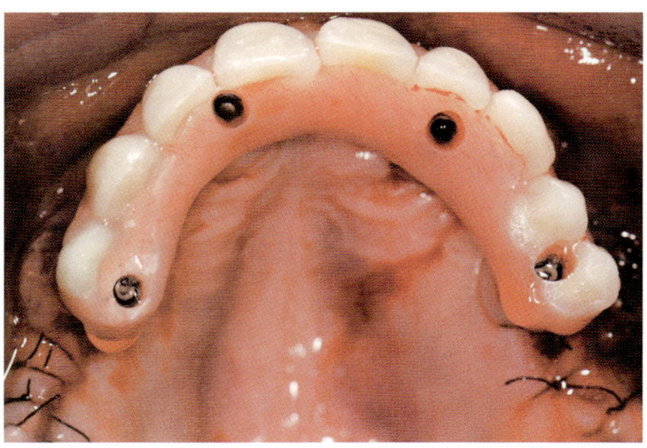

Fig 1.4 - Clinical intraoral occlusal image of a maxilla treated with a fixed full-arch provisional prosthesis using an immediate-loading protocol.

In fact, implant immobility, or high primary stability, is so essential in achieving osseointegration that if it is not obtained at the time of implant placement, conventional protocols with delayed, unloaded healing should be followed instead.

Attard et al[28] highlighted how other factors such as bone quality, prosthetic factors, and ability of the operator or surgeon can affect cumulative survival rates. Therefore, factors other than implant primary stability also must be evaluated before immediate loading can be considered a realistic treatment alternative for a patient.

Recently, a systematic literature review was published about the effect of loading time on fixed or removable prostheses and the treatment results. Jokstad and Carr[29] selected 187 of 1,882 articles published before May 2005 on the subject of implants. After extrapolating only the publications that strictly related to loading times associated with implant prosthetic treatments, they eventually examined 22 articles published from 1990 to 2005. The authors' conclusions were cautious; they maintained, however, that even if the average of the results recorded in the literature were in favor of delayed loading, some indications should be considered for immediate or early loading protocols. In conclusion, Jokstad and Carr asserted that further studies regarding implant loading protocols were necessary.

ADVANTAGES OF IMMEDIATE LOADING

The immediate occlusal loading protocol offers numerous advantages. These include *(1)* shorter treatment times; *(2)* elimination of provisional removable prostheses and consequent psychologic benefits; *(3)* fewer surgical appointments and, as a result, less tissue damage; and *(4)* the possibility of decreased direct costs for the patient and less time away from work.

Shorter treatment times are an indisputable advantage for both patients and clinicians. The delivery of a single-tooth, partial, or full-arch prosthesis on the same day as implant placement restores function and esthetics without the discomfort sometimes associated with wearing provisional removable prostheses.

Elimination of provisional removable prostheses yields psychologic benefits that also merit consideration. With life expectancies increasing around the world, there has been an increase in pathologies associated with aging, including edentulism and an overall decline in oral health. While the psychologic effects of tooth loss are not completely known, the negative impact of edentulism on a person's quality of life has been well documented. Edentulism may be perceived as a particularly stressful loss of the integrity of one's body to which it may be difficult to adapt.

In a study by Blomberg and Lindquist,[30] 44% of patients wearing removable dental prostheses reported that this condition had worsened their quality of life. Similarly, Kronström et al[31] reported that patients with complete dentures canceled social engagements because they feared their prostheses might fall out. In this study, a follow-up of the rehabilitated patients with fixed, implant-retained prostheses generated positive results. Patients reported that they felt like were their old selves again and that their implant prostheses felt like their own natural teeth. Treatment with full-arch immediate loading eliminates clinical problems associated with complete dentures as reported by patients and allows them to move directly from a condition with compromised dentitions to one with efficient, stable, implant-supported prostheses.

Another advantage of immediate occlusal loading is that it eliminates the second surgical appointment. The prosthetic phase begins immediately after implant placement, often before suturing begins. In this way, the time between surgery and prosthesis insertion is decreased. A direct consequence of the decreased number of surgical sessions is reduced surgical trauma to the soft and hard tissues. With immediate occlusal loading, the transmucosal tissues surrounding implants heal without the pressure and discomfort associated with removable prostheses. Healing occurs more quickly, and patients are much more comfortable. And because the contours of the provisional fixed prosthesis have been established in the laboratory, healing of the peri-implant soft tissues is optimized (Fig 1.5).

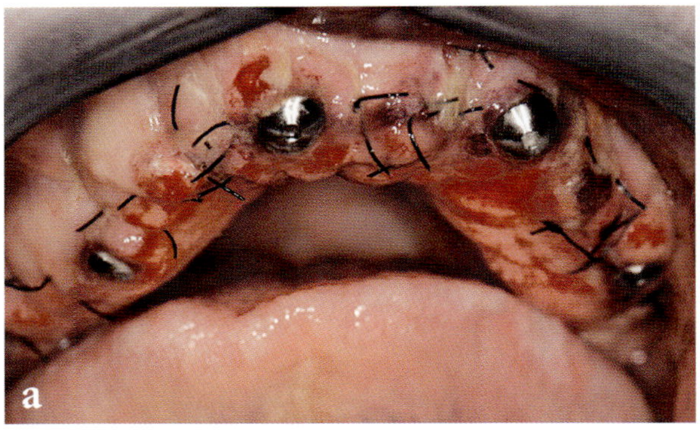

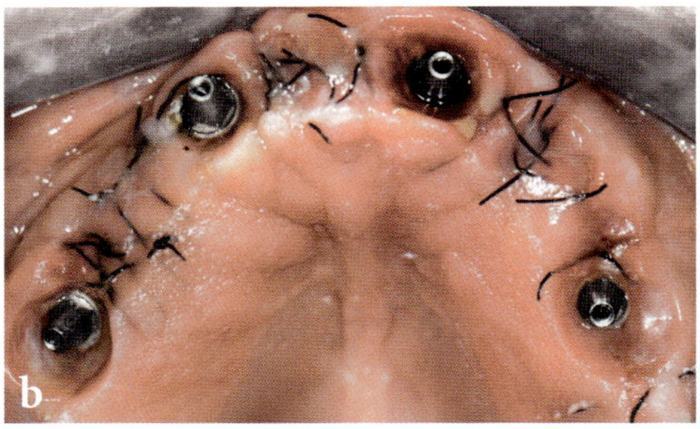

Fig 1.5 - (*a*) Full-arch immediate loading. Intraoral post-surgical view with the conical abutments protected by the healing caps. (*b*) Intraoral postoperative view 1 week after implant placement. The patient presented for suture removal. The prosthesis was removed, and the conical abutments are visible. During this week, the peri-implant soft tissues have adapted to the prosthetic profiles of the provisional prosthesis.

Furthermore, concentrating the surgical and prosthetic stages into a short period of time may enable the dental staff to perform the treatment at a reduced cost for patients, and the shorter treatment time allows patients to return to work more quickly.

CHARACTERISTICS OF THE IMMEDIATE FUNCTIONAL LOADING IMPLANT PROTOCOL

With rare exceptions,[32] the immediate-loading protocols reported in the literature are not supported by the long follow-up periods that accompanied the early research on osseointegration. As a rule, only the immediate-loading protocol that involves cases of total maxillary and/or mandibular rehabilitation should be regarded as immediate loading. The case illustrated in Fig 1.6 demonstrates immediate functional loading. In contrast, rehabilitation with fixed partial dentures or single crowns are considered immediate *nonfunctional* rehabilitations. In such cases, the implant-retained crown has a predominantly esthetic function since it is usually made without occlusal contacts (Fig 1.7).

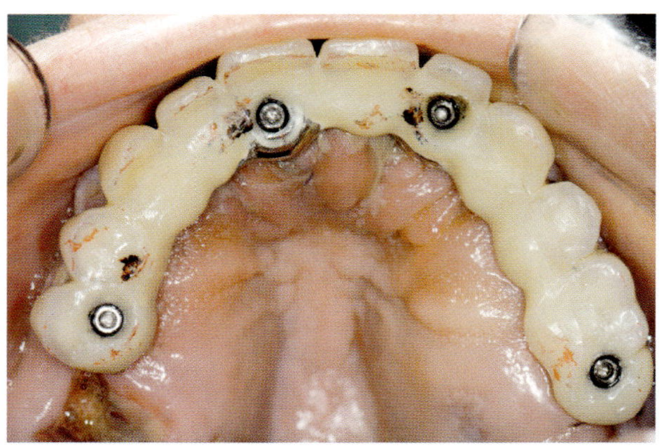

Fig 1.6 - Occlusal view of the fixed full-arch maxillary prosthesis. The articulating paper highlights the masticatory load in centric occlusion.

The last point to be made concerns the remarkable heterogeneity of protocols regarding the timing and laboratory steps in the prosthetic phase of treatment. In some protocols, the prosthetic phases are relegated to incidental, marginal roles in the overall scope of the implant rehabilitations. After reviewing the data available in the current literature regarding immediate loading, the Prosthetic Department of the University of Genoa has developed its own surgical and prosthetic protocol for the treatment of total edentulism with implants and have called it the *Columbus Bridge Protocol.*[33]

Surgical Protocol

The surgical technique for the Columbus Bridge Protocol was developed to attain and enhance implant primary stability, which, as stated previously, many authors regard as the key factor in successful immediate loading. *Primary stability* is defined as being mechanical in nature; it is affected by bone quality, site preparation, and the macrostructure of the implants. Currently, the implants in common use present a modified, or "roughened," surface. This surface microtopography does not affect implant primary stability. It does, however, improve the level and the rapidity of attainment of *secondary stability*, also defined as *biologic stability*.

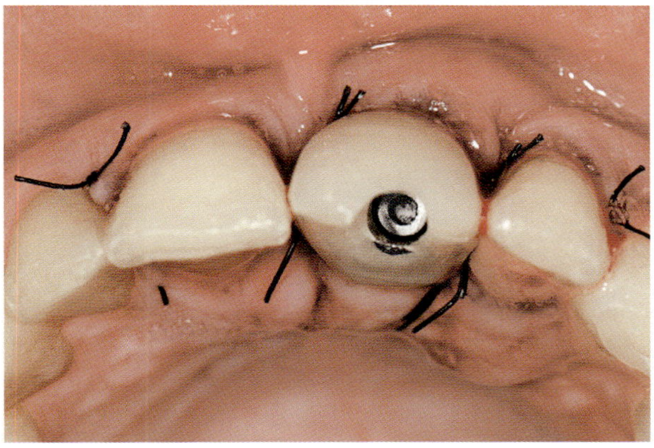

Fig 1.7 - Clinical intraoral occlusal image of an implant-retained crown that was fabricated out of occlusal function. This is an example of nonocclusal loading since the restoration was a single unit and was not splinted to other implants. This restoration was designed for esthetics and phonetics, not for occlusal function.

It is difficult to obtain high primary stability in areas with poor bone quality. Where bone quality or quantity of a residual ridge makes it unsuitable for implant placement, guided bone regeneration techniques and block (bone) grafts should be accomplished prior to implant placement. Grafting procedures should be avoided in conjunction with immediate occlusal loading protocols.

In the Columbus Bridge Protocol, underpreparation of the osteotomies (consistent with the type of bone that a patient presents with) is essential to obtain high implant insertion torques and a high level of implant primary stability. The osteotomies are accomplished by using a given company's implant surgical kit and following the manufacturer's instructions. Although some protocols suggest that torque values of around 30 Ncm are sufficient, this protocol requires torque values of at least 40 Ncm when possible; implants equal to or greater than 13 mm in length seem to be the most suitable for achieving this value. In addition to following the surgical kit manufacturer's suggestions, the authors make the following recommendations for underpreparation of the osteotomies:

- Into dense bone, for a cylindric-shaped implant 4 mm in diameter, the last drill used should be 0.25 to 1 mm narrower than the implant diameter while the osteotomy depth equal to the implant length
- Into an area of poor bone quality, for a tapered implant 4 mm in diameter, the last drill used should be up to 2 mm narrower than the implant diameter and, in addition, the osteotomy depth should be shorter in length according to bone mineralization

Generally, patients treated with the Columbus Bridge Protocol need 4 to 6 implants for the construction of the immediate provisional prosthesis. The bridge typically consists of 10 to 12 masticatory units. It must also be remembered that the emergence of the implants should be consistent with the locations of strategic abutments as in a traditional fixed prosthesis design. The canine and first molar areas provide optimal quadrilateral support (Fig 1.8). In many maxillary situations, implants are not inserted in parallel, vertical positions as in the original Brånemark protocol principles (Fig 1.9).[34] In some instances, implants may be inclined as much as 45 degrees from the true vertical position (Fig 1.10); however, high levels of insertion torque are still required to obtain the requisite implant primary stability.

Anatomical limitations such as the maxillary sinus and inferior alveolar nerve may preclude the use of

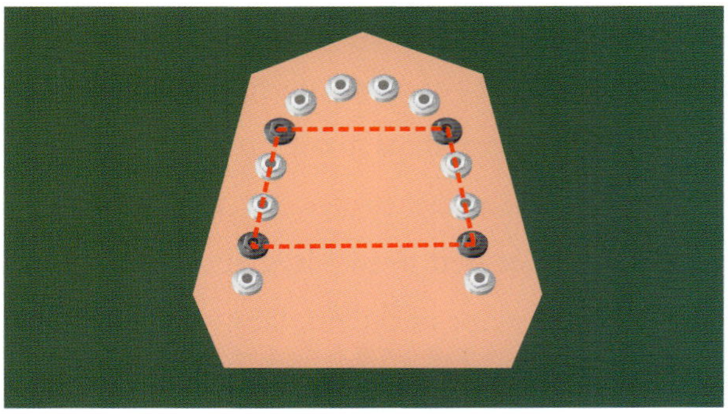

Fig 1.8 - Prosthetic quadrilateral support concept in an edentulous jaw. Implants in the canine and the first molar zones are considered to be strategic abutments for the optimal distribution of functional loads.

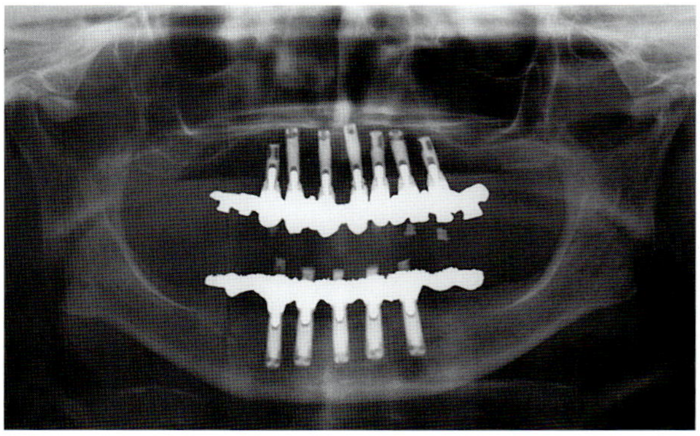

Fig 1.9 - Panoramic radiograph shows fixed, full-arch treatment in the edentulous maxilla and mandible. The implants were inserted upright, consistent with the original Brånemark protocol.

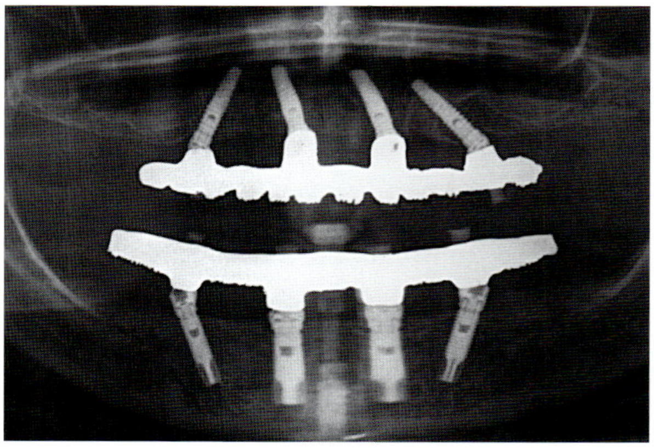

Fig 1.10 - Panoramic radiograph demonstrates that in the maxilla and mandible distal implants were placed with tilts to avoid critical anatomical structures.

long implants, especially in the premolar and molar areas. However, long implants (equal to or greater than 13 mm) may be used if placed parallel to the anterior wall of the maxillary sinus or with an inclination over the mental foramen in the mandible. These implants will demonstrate an inclination in the sagittal plane and also in the frontal one. Certain maxillary tilted implants are called *pterygoid* or *zygomatic* implants[35] (Zygoma Dental Implants, Nobel Biocare). These implants may be used in severely atrophic maxillae when patients do not wish to undergo any type of bone grafting procedures. Zygomatic implants have longer dimensions than do traditional implants and may be manufactured with lengths of up to 52.5 mm. Zygomatic implants are inserted with a significant inclination so that they can be stabilized in the zygomatic processes of maxillae. The inclinations of these implants can be corrected by means of angled abutments. The prosthetic emergence for zygomatic implants is always palatal with respect to the ideal position of the missing teeth (Fig 1.11). The surgical phases for zygomatic implants are complex and carry some risks. To prepare the osteotomies for these implants, the surgeon must operate near delicate and important anatomical areas, such as the orbital floor and the arteries, veins, and nerves associated with it. Injury to one of these structures can lead to massive hemorrhages or severe neurologic damage. It follows that the technique should not be performed in an outpatient setting but in a surgical center where appropriate professionals can be summoned in case of an emergency. This technique is limited in that it can be applied only to the maxilla.

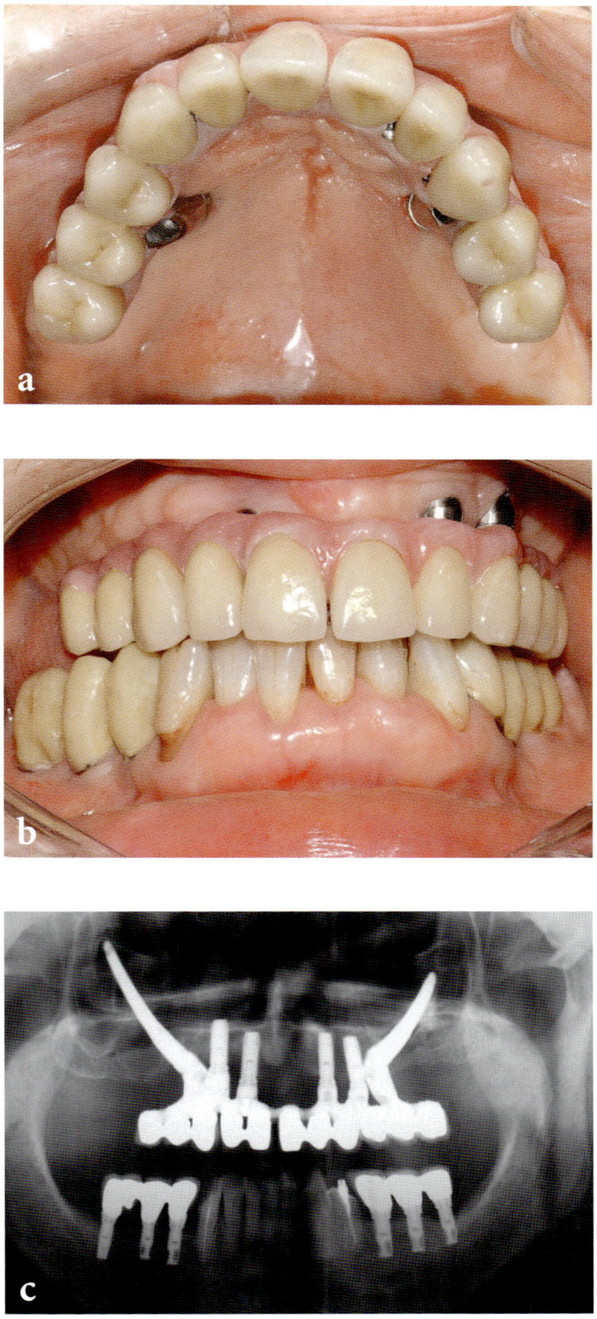

Fig 1.11 - (*a*) Occlusal view of a full-arch prosthesis supported, in part, by zygomatic implants. (*b*) Front view of a full-arch prosthesis supported, in part, by zygomatic implants, with the patient in centric occlusion. (*c*) Panoramic radiograph that demonstrates the inclination of the zygomatic implants (*Courtesy of Dr Francesco Bassi and Dr Marco Mozzati, Turin, Italy.*)

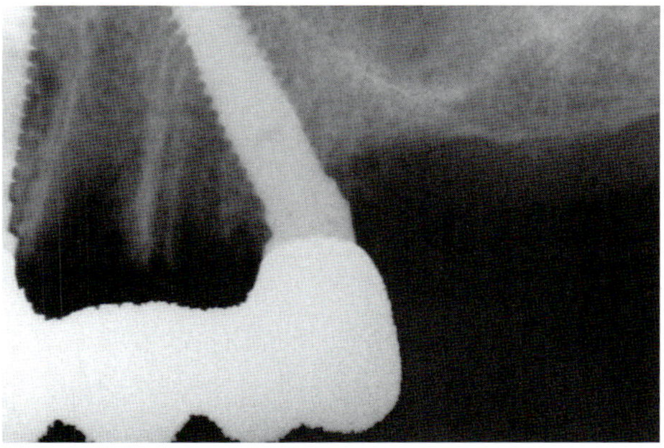

Fig 1.12 - Intraoral radiograph of a tilted implant in a left maxillary posterior quadrant that provides the distal support for an immediate, full-arch prosthesis. Note the proximity to the anterior wall of the maxillary sinus.

On the contrary, 13 to 20 mm tilted implants can be used in both the maxilla and the mandible and can be performed with more routine surgical procedures (Fig 1.12). The use of inclined implants in the Columbus Bridge Protocol is described in detail in chapter 6.

Prosthetic Protocol

The concept of an immediate full-arch prosthetic rehabilitation protocol had its beginnings in the 2000s with the Brånemark Novum Protocol.[36–39] The Brånemark Novum was the first integrated protocol developed that accounted for surgical, prosthetic and laboratory considerations in the immediate rehabilitation of edentulous mandi-

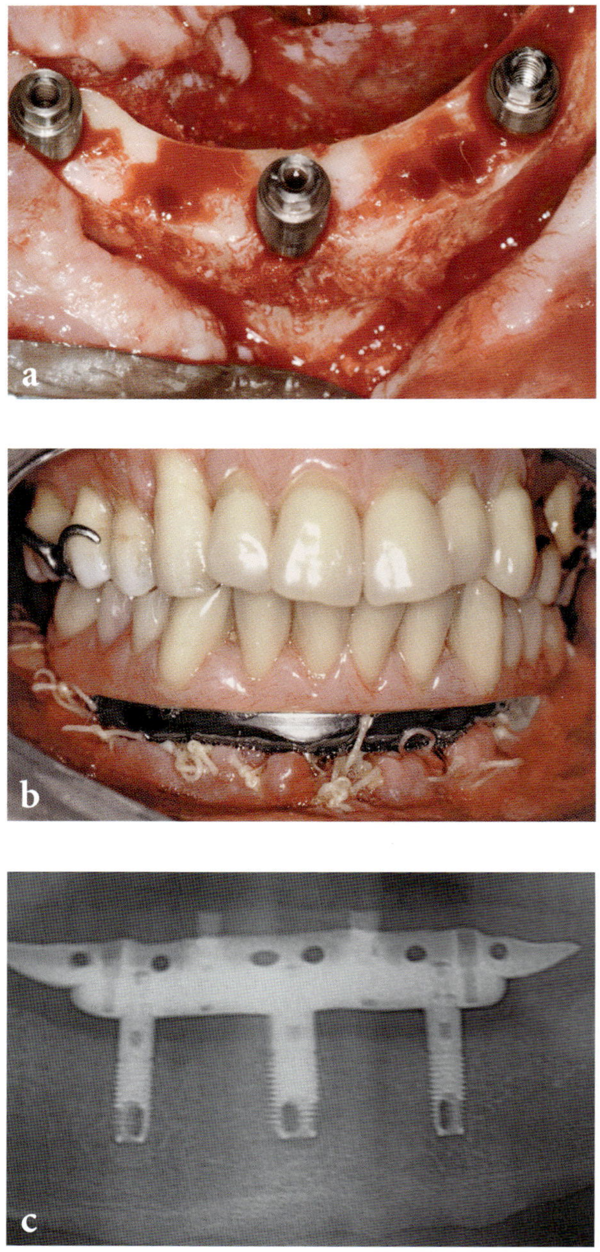

Fig 1.13 - These three photographs illustrate the treatment of an edentulous mandible with an immediate fixed prosthesis according to the Brånemark Novum Protocol. (*a*) Clinical intraoral image of three implants placed between the mandibular foramen in the anterior mandible. (*b*) Clinical image immediately after the prosthesis was placed into the implants. (*c*) Radiograph 4 months postoperatively. Excellent bone-implant contact among all of the implants and the surrounding bone is achieved.

bles. This system makes use of prefabricated surgical guides to insert three implants into mandibular interforaminal areas. Prosthetic treatment was accomplished by fabricating a fixed prosthesis on premanufactured metal frameworks retained to the implants with titanium screws (Fig 1.13). The key factors for the Columbus Bridge Protocol with a provisional screw-retained prosthesis for immediate loading were extrapolated from the characteristics of this system.

The Columbus Bridge Protocol provides for the realization of a full-arch, screw-retained provisional prosthesis within 24 hours from implant placement surgery (Figs 1.14 to 1.20).

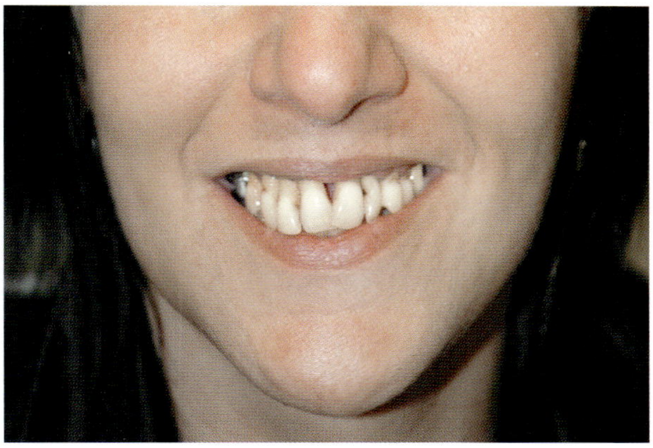

Fig 1.14 - Preoperative clinical full-facial image of a patient about to be treated per the Columbus Bridge Protocol.

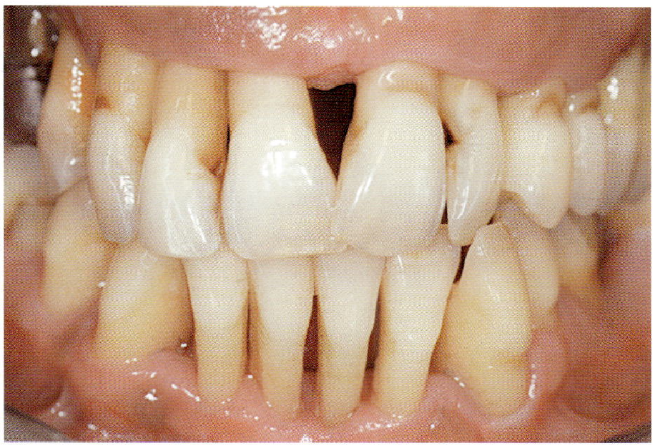

Fig 1.15 - Clinical intraoral anterior image. The patient had significant preexisting bone loss secondary to periodontal disease.

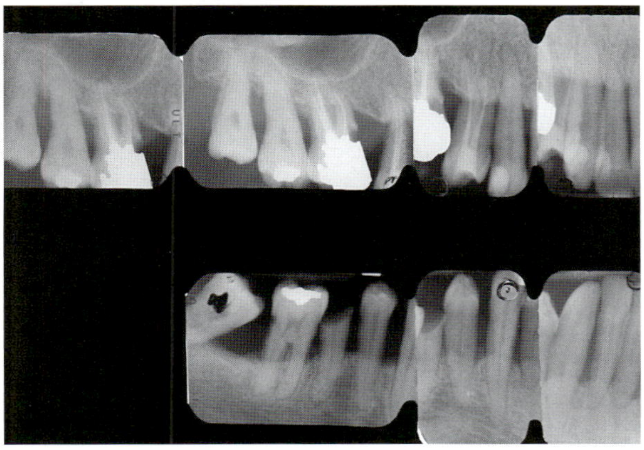

Fig 1.16 - Full-mouth radiographs (right side).

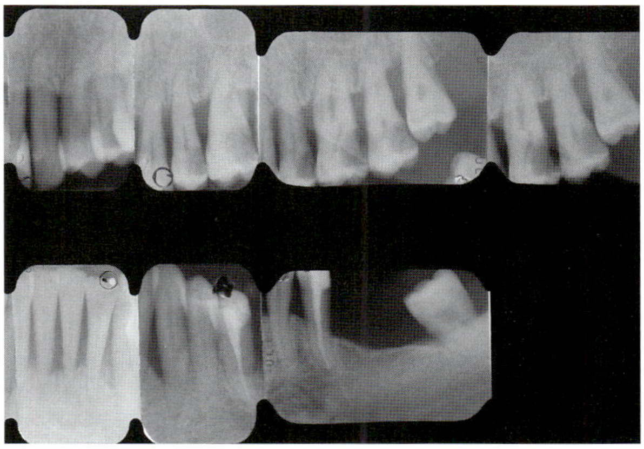

Fig 1.17 - Full-mouth radiographs (left side) demonstrating significant bone loss around the remaining teeth. The maxillary teeth were considered to have a hopeless prognosis and were scheduled to be extracted.

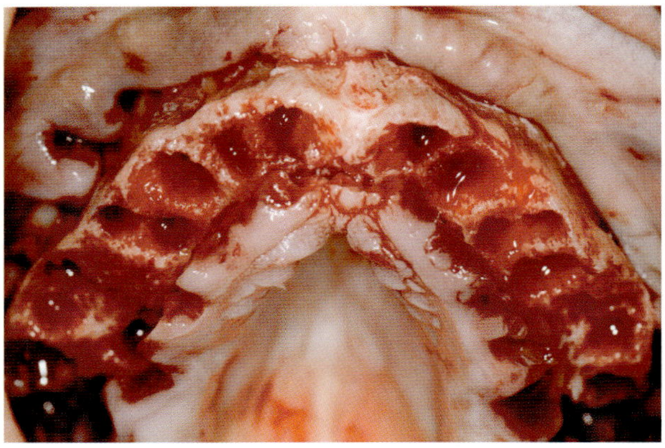

Fig 1.18 - Surgical intraoral maxillary occlusal image immediately after extraction of the maxillary teeth.

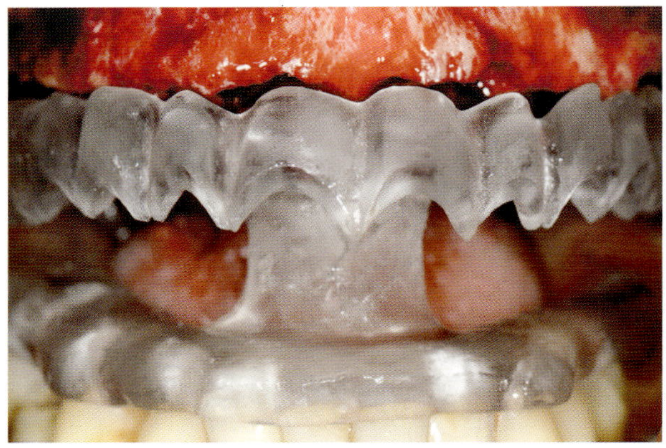

Fig 1.19 - Surgical image of the surgical-prosthetic template in place after extraction of the maxillary teeth. The lower part of the template was retained by the mandibular teeth.

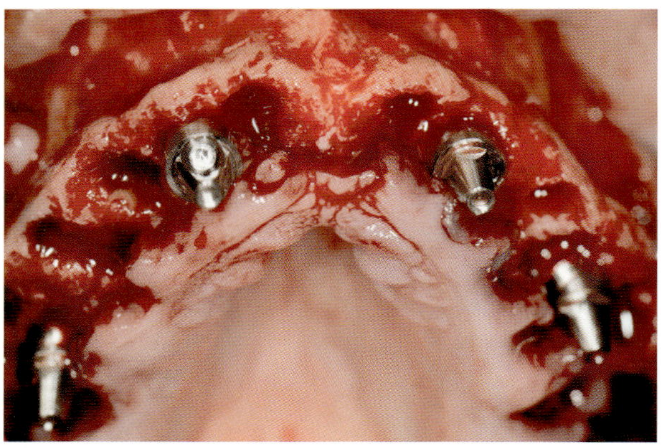

Fig 1.20 - Surgical image of the edentulous maxilla immediately after insertion of four implants. The conical abutments were in place at the time of this photograph and are routinely placed prior to suturing.

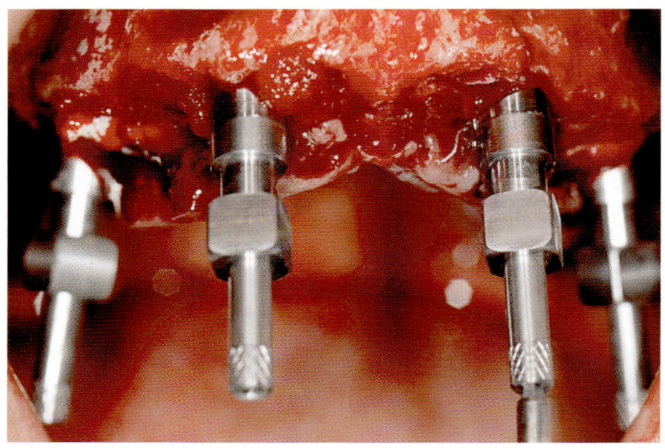

Fig 1.21 - Clinical intraoral image of the screw-retained, pickup abutment impression copings in place on the conical abutments prior to the impression. Note that the soft tissues have not been sutured yet.

Heckmann et al[40] reported that in implant-prosthetic treatment, 50% of errors are caused by the impression technique and fabrication of the master casts. The other 50% of errors are caused by incorrect laboratory procedures. In the Columbus Bridge Protocol, the impression technique includes the use of abutment pickup impression copings.

Abutments are placed directly onto the implants prior to flap closure, and immediately thereafter, abutment impression copings are seated directly onto the abutments, which allows clinicians to confirm that the abutments and impression copings are accurately and completely seated (Fig 1.21). Impression plaster is used as the impression material (Fig 1.22).

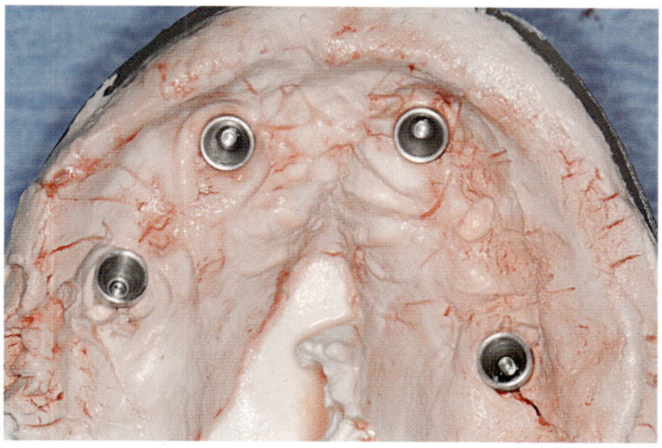

Fig 1.22 - Laboratory intaglio view of the impression that was made with impression plaster in a perforated plastic stock impression tray.

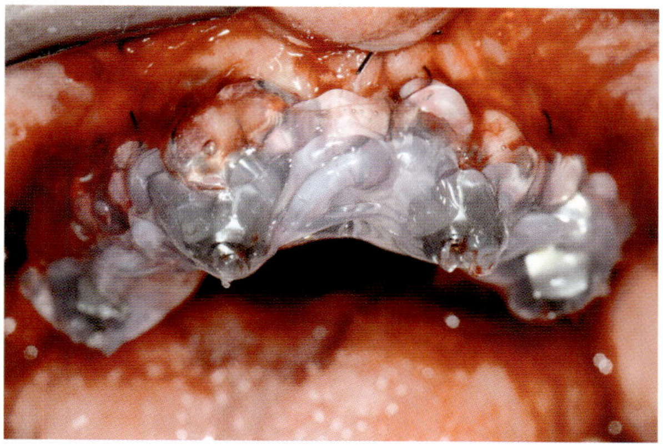

Fig 1.23 - Postsurgical silicone dressing for edema control.

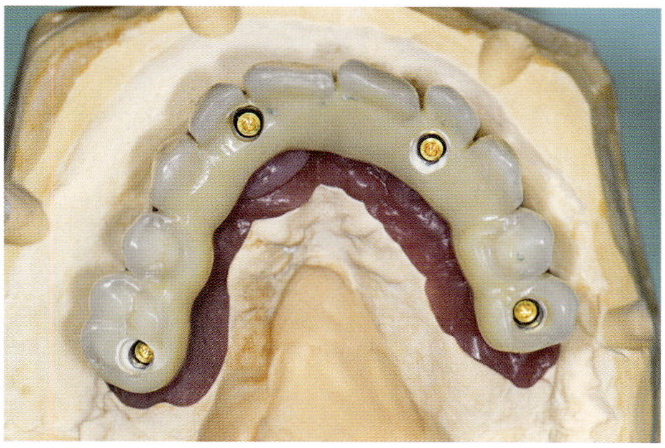

Fig 1.24 - Laboratory occlusal image of the screw-retained provisional prosthesis after processing and polishing. Note the absence of distal cantilevers.

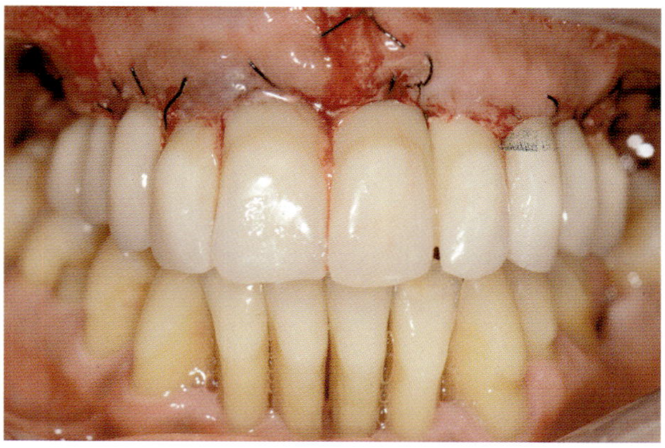

Fig 1.25 - Anterior clinical image of the immediate fixed provisional prosthesis in place 24 hours after implant placement.

The provisional prosthesis is made with a rigid, cast-metal framework that splints the implants together. This also provides for cross-arch stabilization for the implants and prosthesis. The masticatory surface is made of acrylic resin. The provisional prosthesis is inserted within 24 to 48 hours of implant surgery and must have a passive fit.[41] The immediate, provisional prostheses made with the Columbus Bridge Protocol are made without cantilevered extensions. This design prevents overloading of the distal implants (Figs 1.23 to 1.27).

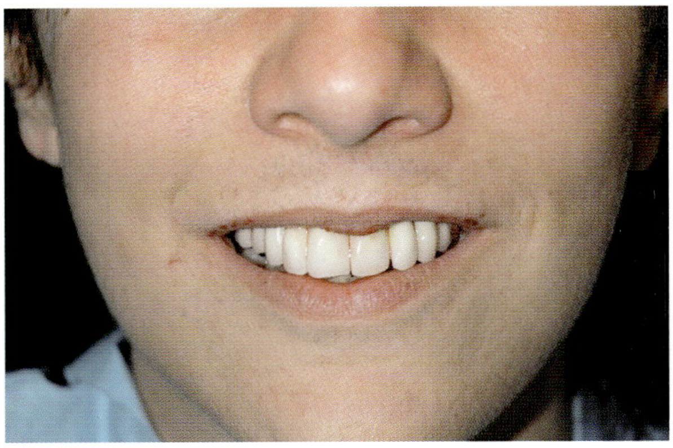

Fig 1.26 - Clinical image of the patient smiling, with the maxillary immediate fixed provisional prosthesis in place 24 hours after extraction and implant placement. Note the absence of extraoral ecchymosis and the presence of minimal swelling.

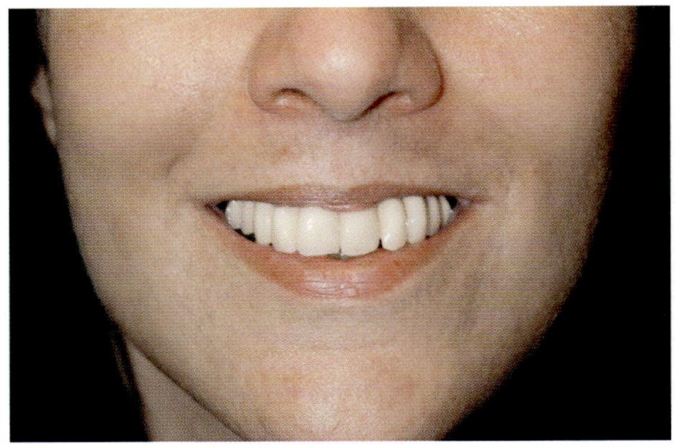

Fig 1.27 - Clinical image of the patient smiling 1 week postsurgery. Note the significant improvement in overall esthetics from the preoperative condition in Fig 1.14.

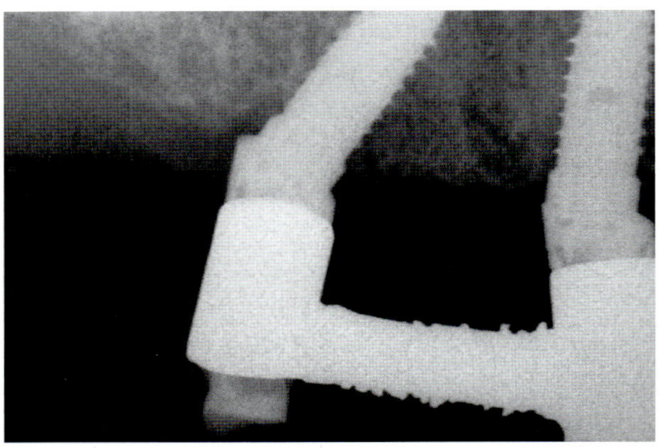

Fig 1.28 - Intraoral radiograph of the right distal implant 4 months postsurgery. Note the metal framework contained within the prosthesis and the absence of a cantilever distal to the implant.

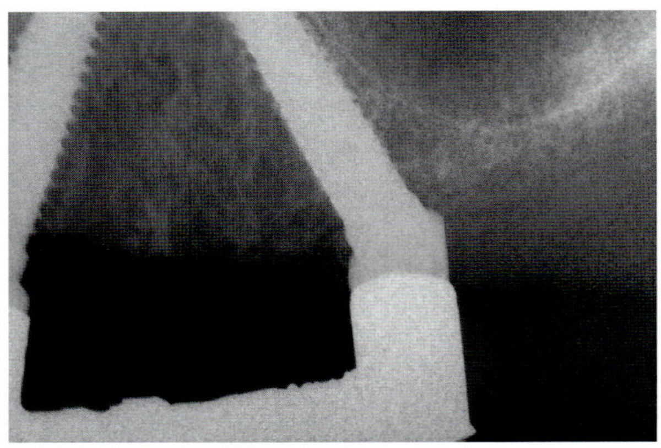

Fig 1.29 - Intraoral radiograph of the left distal implant 4 months postoperatively. There was excellent bone-implant contact and minimal crestal bone loss.

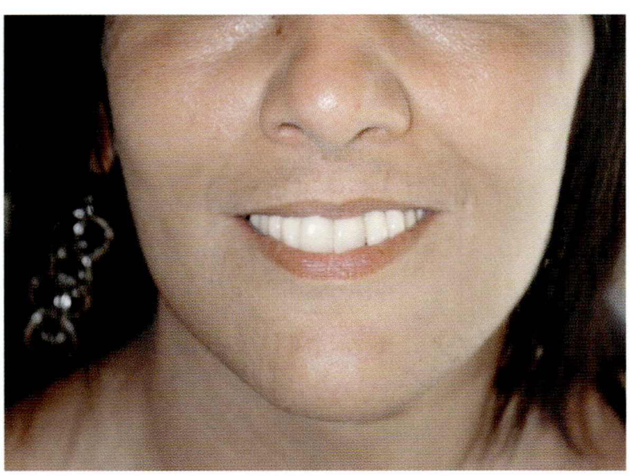

Fig 1.30- Clinical image of the patient smiling with the definitive prosthesis in place. The esthetic results are similar to the results obtained with the immediate provisional prosthesis.

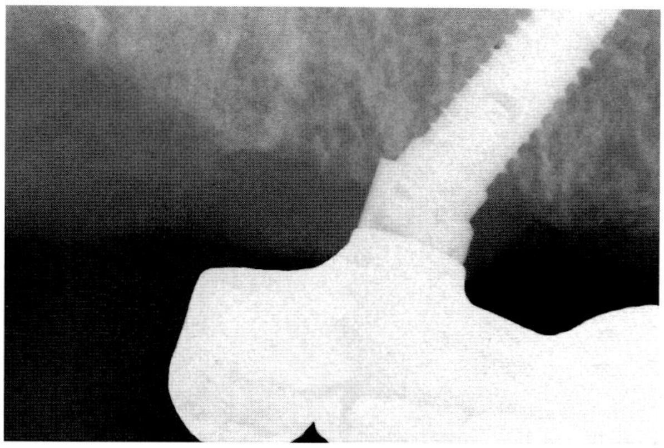

Fig 1.31 - Intraoral radiograph of the right distal implant approximately 12 months after implant insertion. Note that a distal cantilever was fabricated within the definitive prosthesis, which contained 12 masticatory units.

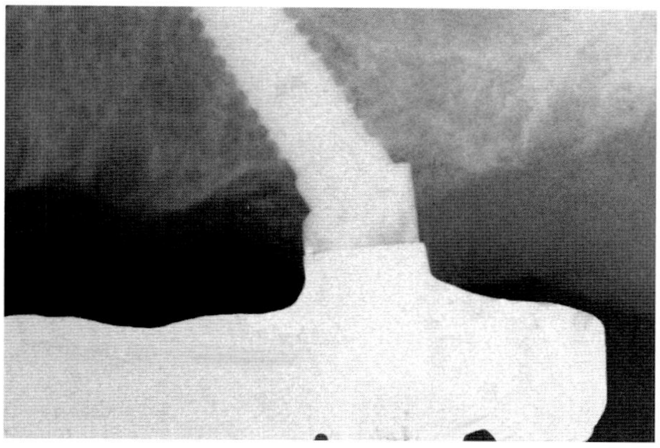

Fig 1.32 - Intraoral radiograph of the left distal implant approximately 12 months after implant insertion.

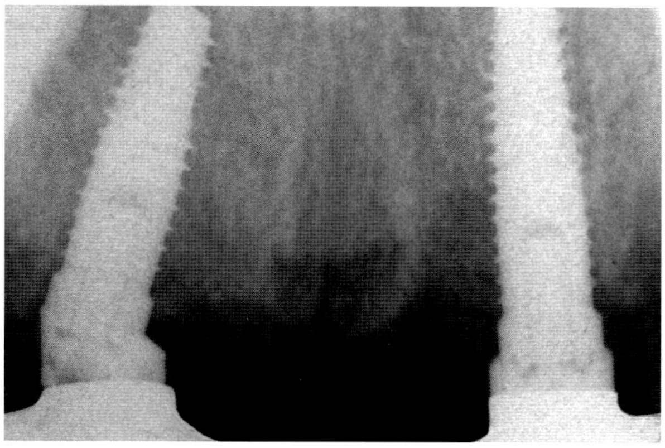

Fig 1.33 - Intraoral anterior radiograph taken 12 months after implant placement and immediate occlusal loading demonstrated excellent bone-implant contact and no radiolucencies and was considered to be confirmation of osseointegration.

The prosthetic reevaluation is made approximately 4 months after implant placement and immediate occlusal loading. If necessary, the use of different angled abutments could improve the emergence profiles and thus the esthetic result. The definitive prostheses may be fabricated with distal extensions if needed to restore the entire dentition (Figs 1.28 - 1.33).

The following chapters describe and illustrate, in detail, the operational phases for the Columbus Bridge Protocol, its biologic principles, and the experimental evaluations that led to its use. The table on the following page (Table 1.1) shows key points associated with the Columbus Bridge Protocol.

COLUMBUS BRIDGE PROTOCOL	
SURGICAL PROTOCOL	**PROSTHETIC PROTOCOL**
External hex rough-surface implants	Screw-retained fixed prosthesis
Implant length ≥ 13 mm, Ø 4 mm	Plaster impression with pickup technique
Underprepared osteotomy	Rigid splinting with metal framework
Implant insertion torque ≥ 40 Ncm	Passive fit with the luting technique
Angled implants in native bone	Acrylic resin occlusal surfaces
Angled conical abutments	No distal cantilevers
No bone regenerative techniques	Immediate functional load 24–48 h after surgery

Table 1.1 - Columbus Bridge Protocol: main characteristics of the surgical and prosthetic protocols for full-arch treatment of edentulous maxillae with immediate loading.

REFERENCES

1. Ring ME. Dentistry: an Illustrated History. New York: Abrams, 1992.
2. Greenfield EJ. An artificial root. Dent Brief 1910;15:837–839.
3. Bodine R, Yanase R, Bodine A. Forty years of experience with subperiosteal implant dentures in 41 edentulous patients. J Prosthet Dent 1996;75:33–44.
4. Kapur KK. Veterans Administration Cooperative Dental Implant Study–Comparisons between fixed partial dentures supported by blade-vent implants and removable partial dentures. Part II. Comparisons of success rates and periodontal health between two treatment modalities. J Prosthet Dent 1989;62:685–703.
5. Spiekermann H. Clinical and animal experiences with endosseous metal implants. In: Heimke G (ed). Dental Implants, Materials and Systems. Vienna: Hanser Verlag, 1980:49–54.
6. Brånemark PI, Adell R, Breine U, Hansson BO, Lindstrom J, Ohlsson A. Intra-osseous anchorage of dental prostheses. I. Experimental studies. Scand J Plast Reconstr Surg 1969;3:81–100.
7. Brånemark PI, Hansson BO, Adell R, et al. Osseointegrated implants in the treatment of the edentulous jaw. Experience from a 10-year period. Scand J Plast Reconstr Surg Suppl 1977;16:1–132.
8. McClarence E (ed). Close to the Edge: Brånemark and the Development of Osseointegration. Chicago: Quintessence, 2003.
9. Schroeder A, Pohler O, Sutter F. Tissue reaction to an implant of a titanium hollow cylinder with a titanium surface spray layer. SSO Schweiz Monatsschr Zahnheilkd 1976;86:713–727.
10. Schroeder A, Stich H, Straumann F, Sutter F. The accumulation of osteocementum around a dental implant under physical loading. SSO Schweiz Monatsschr Zahnheilkd 1978;88:1051–1058.
11. Schroeder A, van der Zypen E, Stich H, Sutter F. The reactions of bone, connective tissue, and epithelium to endosteal implants with titanium-sprayed surfaces. J Maxillofac Surg 1981;9:15–25.
12. Albrektsson T, Brånemark PI, Hansson HA, Lindstrom J. Osseointegrated titanium implants. Requirements for ensuring a long-lasting, direct bone-to-implant anchorage in man. Acta Orthop Scand 1981;52:155–170.
13. Johansson C. On Tissue Reaction to Metal Implants [thesis]. Gothenburg: University of Gothenburg, 1991.
14. Sennerby L. On Bone Tissue Response to Titanium Implants [thesis]. Gothenburg: University of Gothenburg, 1991.
15. Morberg P. On Bone Tissue Reaction to Acrylic Cement [thesis]. Gothenburg: University of Gothenburg, 1991.
16. Gottlander M. On Hard Tissues Reaction to Hydroxyapatite-Coated Titanium Implants [thesis]. Gothenburg: University of Gothenburg, 1994.
17. Carlsson LV. On the Development of a New Concept for Orthopaedic Implant Fixation [thesis]. Gothenburg: University of Gothenburg, 1989.
18. Wenneberg B. On Surface Roughness and Implant Incorporation [thesis]. Gothenburg: University of Gothenburg, 1996.
19. Jacobsson M. On Bone Behaviour After Irradiation [thesis]. Gothenburg: University of Gothenburg, 1985.
20. Buch D. On Electrical Stimulation of Bone Tissue [thesis]. Gothenburg: University of Gothenburg, 1985.
21. Ericsson I. Heat Induced Bone Tissue Injury [thesis]. Gothenburg: University of Gothenburg, 1984.
22. Adell R, Lekholm U, Rockler B, Brånemark P-I. A 15-year study of osseointegrated implants in the treatment of the edentulous jaw. Int J Oral Surg 1981;10:387–416.
23. Buser D, Weber HP, Lang NP. Tissue integration of non-submerged implants. 1-year results of a prospective study with 100 ITI hollow-cylinder and hollow-screw implants. Clin Oral Implants Res 1990;1:33–40.
24. Becker W, Becker BE, Israelson H, et al. One-step surgical placement of Brånemark implants: A prospective multicenter clinical study. Int J Oral Maxillofac Implants 1997;12:454–462.

25. Ericsson I, Randow K, Glantz PO, Lindhe J, Nilner K. Clinical and radiographical features of submerged and nonsubmerged titanium implants. Clin Oral Implants Res 1994;5:185–189.
26. Ledermann PD. Improved retention of a mandibular complete denture with four plasma-coated screw implants. Quintessenz 1981;32:465–473.
27. Gapski R, Wang HL, Mascarenhas P, Lang NP. Critical review of immediate implant loading. Clin Oral Implants Res 2003;14:515–527.
28. Attard NJ, David LA, Zarb GA. Immediate loading of implants with mandibular overdentures: One-year clinical results of a prospective study. Int J Prosthodont 2005;18:463–470.
29. Jokstad A, Carr AB. What is the effect on outcomes of time-to-loading of a fixed or removable prosthesis placed on implant(s)? Int J Oral Maxillofac Implants 2007;22(suppl):19–48.
30. Blomberg S, Lindquist LW. Psychological reactions to edentulousness and treatment with jawbone-anchored bridges. Acta Psychiatr Scand 1983; 68:251–262.
31. Kronström M, Trulsson M, Söderfeldt B. Patient evaluation of treatment with fixed prostheses supported by implants or a combination of teeth and implants. J Prosthodont 2004;13:160–165.
32. Engstrand P, Gröndahl K, Ohrnell LO, Nilsson P, Nannmark U, Brånemark PI. Prospective follow-up study of 95 patients with edentulous mandibles treated according to the Brånemark Novum Concept. Clin Implant Dent Relat Res 2003;5:3–10.
33. Attard N, Zarb GA. Early-loading protocols. In: Zarb GA, Albrektsson T, Baker G, et al (eds). Osseointegration. Chicago: Quintessence, 2008; 10:151–152.
34. Brånemark P-I, Zarb GA, Albrektsson T (eds). Tissue-Integrated Prostheses: Osseointegration in Clinical Dentistry. Chicago: Quintessence, 1985.
35. Brånemark PI, Grondahl K, Ohrnell LO, et al. Zygoma fixture in the management of advanced atrophy of the maxilla: Technique and long-term results. Scand J Plast Reconstr Surg Hand Surg 2004;38:70–85.
36. Brånemark PI, Engstrand P, Öhrnell LO, et al. Brånemark Novum: A new treatment concept for rehabilitation of the edentulous mandible. Preliminary results from a prospective clinical follow-up study. Clin Implant Dent Relat Res 1999;1:2–16.
37. Engstrand P, Nannmark U, Martensson L, Galeus I, Brånemark PI. Brånemark Novum: Prosthodontic and dental laboratory procedures for fabrication of a fixed prosthesis on the day of surgery. Int J Prosthodont 2001;14:303–309.
38. Henry PJ, van Steenberghe D, Blombäck U, et al. Prospective multicenter study on immediate rehabilitation of edentulous lower jaws according to the Brånemark Novum Protocol. Clin Implant Dent Relat Res 2003;5:137–142.
39. Parel SM, Triplett RG. Rescue procedure for the Brånemark Novum protocol. Int J Oral Maxillofac Implants 2004;19:421–424.
40. Heckmann SM, Karl M, Wichmann MG, Winter W, Graef F, Taylor TD. Cement fixation and screw retention: Parameters of passive fit. An in vitro study of three-unit implant-supported fixed partial dentures. Clin Oral Implants Res 2004;15:466–473.
41. Wee AG, Aquilino SA, Schneider RL. Strategies to achieve fit in implant prosthodontics: A review of the literature. Int J Prosthodont 1999; 12:167–178.

CHAPTER 2
BONE TISSUE REPAIR

COLUMBUS BRIDGE PROTOCOL	
SURGICAL PROTOCOL	**PROSTHETIC PROTOCOL**
External hex rough-surface implants	Screw-retained fixed prosthesis
Implant length ≥ 13 mm, Ø 4 mm	Plaster impression with pickup technique
Underprepared osteotomy	Rigid splinting with metal framework
Implant insertion torque ≥ 40 Ncm	Passive fit with the luting technique
Angled implants in native bone	Acrylic resin occlusal surfaces
Angled conical abutments	No distal cantilevers
No bone regenerative techniques	Immediate functional load 24–48 h after surgery

Table 2.1

Insertion of a dental implant causes a localized inflammatory reaction in the narrow spaces between the implant surface and the host bone. Osteogenesis restores the bone volumes between these two surfaces. This restorative process leads to wound healing according to a biologic sequence that has evolved over time.

The biologic mechanisms of bone repair are independent from the stimulus causing the trauma, be it accidental or iatrogenic. Wound healing is dependent on the type of skeletal bone involved. The chronologic sequence of the tissue responses implies common aspects and times in wound healing, including systems of cascade compensation controlled by local and systemic factors that are biohumoral and mechanical in nature.[1]

Bone is an evolved expression of connective tissues and always forms through the substitution

of preexisting support tissues. During the repair of a bone wound, bone rebuilds directly in connective tissue, a process called *intramembranous ossification*. It is produced by osteoblasts, specialized cells that cover all surfaces showing active bone formation. Osteoblasts are characterized by their inability to migrate and reproduce. Therefore, they cannot proliferate inside a bone defect.[2]
During intramembranous bone repair, mesenchymal stem cells migrate to the abundantly vascularized wound. There they differentiate into osteoblasts, which start producing an extracellular matrix rich in collagen, called *osteoid*, that later mineralizes into new bone tissue.[3]
This type of newly formed bone can be defined in different ways: as *primitive*, *fibrous*, or *woven bone*. It represents the immature or young form of bone tissue characterized by a trabecular structure of collagen fibrils arranged in an irregular fashion. The disorganization of this tissue appears even more evident if it is observed under light microscopy with polarized light that highlights the presence of clear or dark refractory areas arranged irregularly (Fig 2.1). From the biomechanical point of view, the lack of structural organization results in lower bone quality in comparison with other bone tissues.[4,5]
In adults, this type of bone tissue serves as an emergency tissue since it can fill "gaps" in a relatively short period of time: an average of 150 μm per day in an animal model[6] (rabbit) and 30 to 50 μm per day in humans.[7] Later, the woven fibril tissue is substituted with lamellar bone. Although lamellar bone forms more slowly than osteoid, it is the most abundant type of bone in adult skeletons. The formation of lamellar bone requires a stable surface supplied by the framework of fibrous bone on which collagen fibrils can be deposited in regular lamellar layers termed *bone lamellae*.
Lamellar tissue analyzed with polarized light microscopy shows regular, dense deposits of lamellar formations (clear) alternating with less dense, sloppy deposits (dark) (Fig 2.2). The alternating opacity of the lamellae is the consequence of the regular deposition of collagen fibrils lying parallel to each other in each lamella yet perpendicular to the collagen fibrils of the contiguous lamellae.

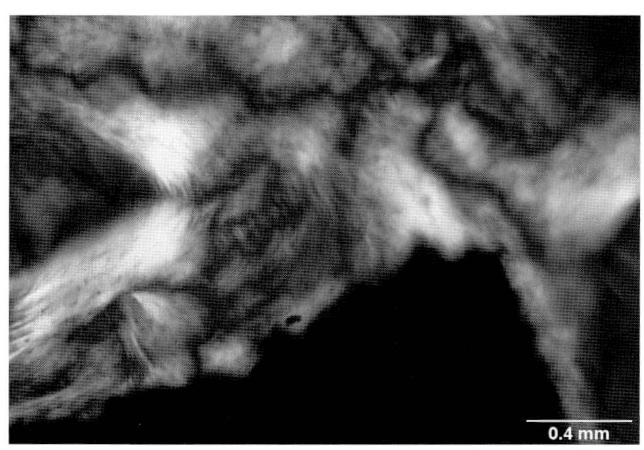

Fig 2.1 - Woven bone. Light microscopy with circular polarized light (original magnification ×400). (*Courtesy of Dr Tonino Traini and Dr Sergio Caputi, Chieti, Italy.*)

The speed of formation of lamellar bone in humans is 0.6 to 1 μm per day. The formation of parallel fibril bone tissue is mainly stimulated by the load to which the tissue is submitted. Even if bone tissue has the capacity of self-repair in its DNA, clinical observations show that some dental and orthopedic implants do not osseointegrate in the adjacent bone tissue, as the fractures refuse to heal and require reconstructive surgical intervention.

This chapter briefly describes the biologic principles of osseointegrated implants. The knowledge and the acquisition of this basic concept are even more important in treating patients when immediate loading is applied.

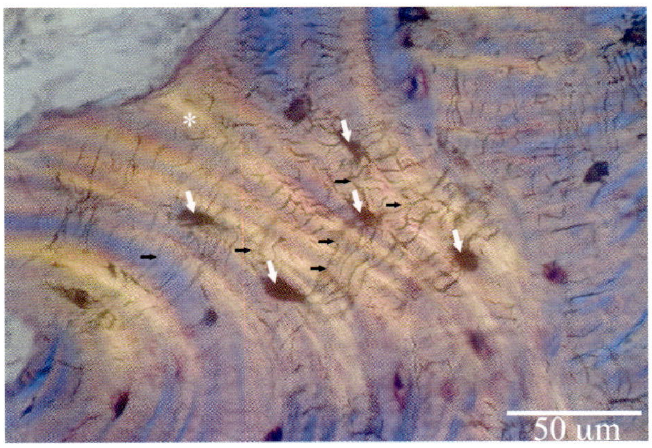

Fig 2.2 - Lamellar bone. Light microscopy with circular polarized light (original magnification ×400). Osteocyte cell bodies are visible (*white arrows*). Cytoplasmic extensions of the osteocyte network are also visible (*black arrows*). (*Courtesy of Dr Tonino Traini and Dr Sergio Caputi, Chieti, Italy.*)

HEALING OF ALVEOLAR BONE

Bone healing has been histologically studied for the last 100 years, and much attention has been given to the healing mechanisms of bone fractures.[8,9] Today, the most credited theories derive from those written by Urist in 1952.[10]

The healing of a postextraction socket (an intraoral wound) can be viewed as a prototype for osseous healing.[11] Within 30 minutes after a tooth has been extracted, the space occupied by the roots fills with blood cells, serum, and saliva. This results in a coagulum rich in fibrin.

The hemolytic processes start 24 hours later when spaces produced by inflammatory cells fill with serum in the central area of the coagulum. The formation of granulation tissue starts within 48 to 72 hours postextraction, mainly from the apical third of the extraction socket. Approximately 1 week postextraction, almost all of the new tissue consists of fibroblasts, new collagen fibrils, and blood vessels. The osteoblasts responsible for bone remodeling are present at the margins of the alveolus. At the same time, osteoblasts and osteoid appear in the bottom of the extraction socket. The granulation tissue is reorganized through the formation of osteoid trabeculae starting from the walls of the socket and growing in a coronal direction. Some trabeculae start mineralizing 3 weeks after extraction. After 6 weeks, conventional radiography can document the formation of new woven bone. The soft tissue of the wound closes with epithelium.

Complete bony fill of the extraction socket can require up to 4 months. Bone fill generally does not reach the coronal levels of the alveolar bone at the adjacent teeth.

This sequence of the events is regulated by precise chemical mediators.[12] Following surgical trauma, blood platelets are activated and release the content of their granules (platelet degranulation). This stimulates vasoconstriction of the surrounding microvasculature, and the cascade toward coagulation leads to the formation of the reticular network of fibrin and the coagulum. The coagulum releases a series of chemotactic growth factors such as platelet-derived growth factor (PDGF), transforming growth factor-β (TGF-β), and vascular endothelial growth factor (VEGF) and supplies a provisional extracellular matrix on which the inflammatory cells (neutrophil granulocytes at first, and monocytes and macrophages later) can adhere.

Formation of the hematoma starts with vasodilation at the periphery of the surgical wound that allows mature cellular elements and precursors of the cells associated with wound healing to enter the surgical wound. The fibrin-rich coagulum is then replaced with granulation tissue secondary to the proteolitic action of plasmin. Plasmin is activated by plasminogen, and this by the tissue-type plasminogen activators released by cells that have invaded the coagulum (macrophages). Granulation tissue is quite vascularized (60% of the mass) and rich in collagen, hyaluronic acid, proteoglycans, fibronectin, and mesenchymal stem cells.

Stem cells are derived from bone marrow, periosteum, adjacent soft tissues, and circulating blood. Even if rare, these cells have high proliferating capacities and are attracted to the surgical wound by bone morphogenetic proteins (BMPs) and other molecules (eg, systemic hormones, such as estradiol). Stem cells are stimulated to multiply and differentiate into osteoblasts.

New blood capillaries form by the sprouting of endothelial cells from the wall of blood vessels adjacent to the wound and proliferate continuously during removal of the coagulum. A highly vascular network is formed and, in a short time, establishes blood circulation inside the lesion or wound. Neoangiogenesis and the consequent restoration of the normal values of oxygen tension (pO_2), carbon dioxide (pCO_2), and pH are the essential premises for the regeneration processes to start. The coagulum is then replaced, secondary to the action of the fibroblasts, with loosely arranged connective tissue, properly termed *fibrocellular blastema*, which has significant regenerative possibilities. In the presence of satisfactory blood flow, which guarantees a sufficient pO_2, and intimate contact between the damaged bone surfaces and granulation tissue, bone healing occurs according to the predetermined cascade of intramembranous ossification. On the other hand, a low pO_2 results in hypoxia and favors cellular differentiation toward chondroblastic cells. Angiogenesis is essential in the bone healing mechanism since it guarantees tissue perfusion for maintenance of adequate levels of oxygen.[13–16]

The mineralized tissue, which first appears at the margins of the primitive bone tissue, is woven bone. Woven bone appears first because its rapid formation succeeds in filling the structural defects inside the wound within a short period of time, even if it lacks the biomechanical properties of mature lamellar bone. Lamellar bone is subject to continuous remodeling due to osteoclastic and osteoblastic activity that avoids the accumulation of microfractures and adapts bone to the functional demands (Fig 2.3).

Not all of the cellular and molecular mechanisms associated with bone healing are known. However, three conditions seem to be essential for bone wound healing, and consequently, the failure of bone to heal could result from the lack of one or more of these factors:

- A sufficient number of mesenchymal stem cells
- A matrix or framework onto which the stem cells can migrate and adhere
- The presence of signal molecules that attract stem cells to the bone healing site and stimulate their mitogenic activity and osteogenic differentiation

FORMATION OF NEW BONE TISSUE AROUND DENTAL IMPLANTS

Bone regeneration describes the formation of new bone tissue in a repair process.[17,18] Bone regeneration around dental implants is not different from the description in the previous paragraphs on the healing of a generic bone wound. In both cases, extravasated blood is present. The preparation of an osteotomy with rotary instruments causes not only the interruption of bone continuity but also the rupture of soft tissues and vascular structures in the implant surgical site. After hemorrhagic extravasation, the vessels, specifically capillaries, are obliterated by the formation of the hematoma. Blood flow stops at the limits of the wound.

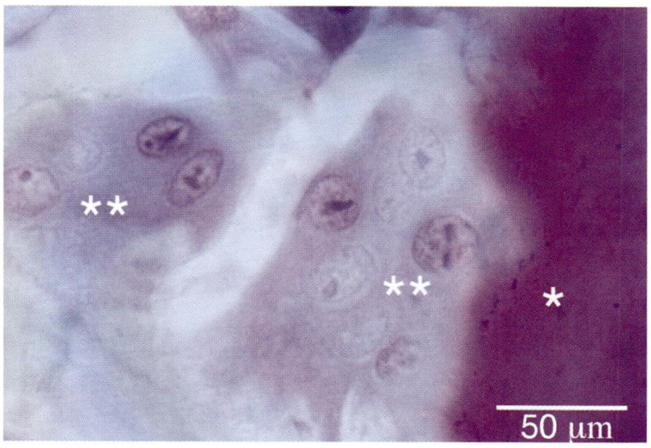

Fig 2.3 - Light microscopic image of bone tissue in the resorption phase (toluidine blue and acid fuchsin (Original magnification ×1000). Mineralized bone tissue (*) osteoclasts in active phase (**). (*Courtesy of Dr Tonino Traini and Dr Sergio Caputi, Chieti, Italy.*)

If preparation of the implant site has been performed correctly, there will be intimate bone-implant contact (BIC) between the osteotomy walls and implant surface. This contact will allow the initial healing processes–defined by Brånemark as the formation of a hematoma in a closed cavity with dimensions of 100 to 200 μm[19]–to begin.

Interruption of circulation causes a local reduction in pO_2 accompanied by an increase in pCO_2 and a corresponding reduction in pH. These changes produce anoxic damage in the adjacent tissues.[20] Therefore, the mechanical trauma associated with osteotomy preparation causes interruptions in the systems that normally maintain the vitality of the cellular elements of the skeletal segment involved. Wound repair also depends on the degree of vascularization of the involved structures and, in this specific case, the architecture of the bone (Box 2-1).[21] In compact bone, interruption of the vascular structures causes damage that spreads to some distance from the focus of the wound. In contrast, spongious (trabecular) bone has a higher ratio of vessels to bone mass, resulting in greater vascular support and less metabolic damage. It is believed that at least 0.5 to 1 mm of peri-implant bone becomes necrotic in the immediate postsurgical phases.[22]

The events involved in the first weeks of healing after implant placement have been well documented in two experimental studies by Berglundh and Abrahamsson in animal mandibles.[23,24] Osseointegration in 20 Labrador retriever dogs was followed step-by-step from the first hours after implant placement until the 12th week. A summary of the most relevant observations follows.

Two hours after implant placement, a coagulum rich in fibrin and erythrocytes, representing 50% of the volume, is present. Bone fragments produced during the surgical procedures sometimes remain trapped in the coagulum. Initially, contact between the implant and mineralized bone tissue happens only at the most protruding part

BOX 2.1 - FACTORS AFFECTING BONE HEALING

- Type of bone (cortical or cancellous)
- Position of the wound or implant
- Degree of trauma at level of the fracture or of the implant
- Degree of fixation during healing of the two bone segments or primary stability of the implant
- Animal species involved
- Age of the subject
- Drug intake

of the implant threads (major diameter). The BIC observed by the authors is approximately 6.5% of the total bone-implant interface. This situation tends to remain unchanged during the first week and is responsible for the primary stability of implants. On the fourth day, richly vascularized granulation tissue extending from the bone walls starts to form. However, numerous erythrocytes still remain in contact with the implant surface. Osteoclasts involved in the remodeling process are present on the residual bone walls and on the bone fragments trapped in the coagulum. This phenomenon partly explains the mechanism of decreasing implant stability during the first several weeks following implant placement.

After 1 week, the first processes of new bone formation are observed. The new tissue, woven bone, appeared both as an extension, if the bone tissue already existed (distance osteogenesis), and in direct contact with the implant surface (contact osteogenesis) (Figs 2.4 and 2.5).[25–27] The total volume occupied by woven bone has been reported to be 1.6% of the bone-implant interface. By the end of the first week after implant placement, BIC increases, reaching approximately 24.8%.

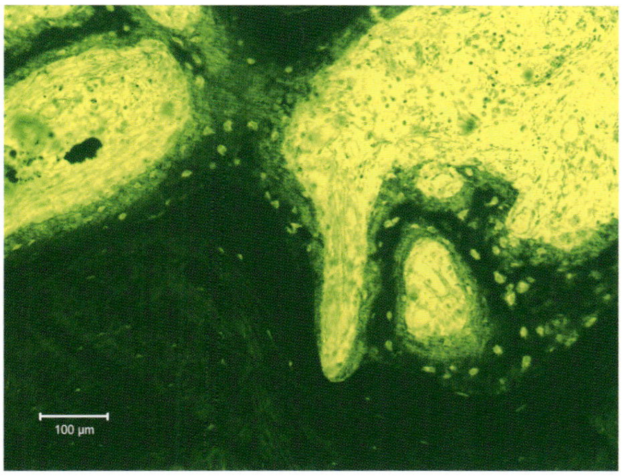

Fig 2.4 - Distance osteogenesis. Confocal scanning laser microscopy of peri-implant bone tissue (original magnification ×100). New bone formation proceeds from the bone to the implant surface. Osteoid tissue (*green*); mineralized bone tissue (*yellow*). (*Courtesy of Dr Tonino Traini and Dr Sergio Caputi, Chieti, Italy.*)

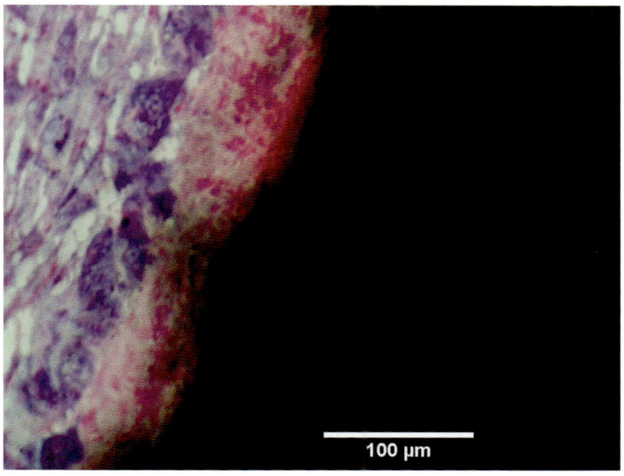

Fig 2.5 - Contact osteogenesis. Light microscopic image of peri-implant tissue (toluidine blue and acid fuchsin; original magnification ×1200). A stratum of osteoid with osteoblastic cells close to the implant surface is in the active phase of osteoid deposition. (*Courtesy of Dr Tonino Traini and Dr Sergio Caputi, Chieti, Italy.*)

Two weeks later, the quantity of bone tissue continues to increase. The total volume occupied by woven bone is now approximately 20.3%, and lamellar bone formation has begun (2%).[28] After surgery, the rate of new bone formation reaches its peak relatively quickly, at 2 to 3 weeks, and decreases rapidly thereafter.

Four weeks after implant placement, a large part of woven bone is substituted with lamellar bone (19.2%). In this phase, BIC is approximately 65% and remains almost unchanged until the 12th week.

Six weeks after implant placement, bone continues to undergo remodeling with the formation of secondary osteons (Fig 2.6); the total volume occupied by lamellar bone increases to approximately 30%. The observations reported by Berglundh and Abrahamsson[23,24] are in line with those previously described by Amler[11] as to post-extraction alveolar processes and by other authors in different clinical situations.[29–36] The events involved in implant wound healing and, particularly, in bone healing follow a biologic sequence that typically cannot be changed or influenced by the presence of modern-day dental implants. Osseointegration appears to be a dynamic phenomenon during both its attainment and its maintenance. Bone tissue, once submitted to load, modifies its original structure according to Wolff's law of bone adaptation,[9] which states that bone tissue adapts to functional mechanical conditions. In fact, dental implants could not survive functionally in trabecular bone because most of the contact surface would be touching bone marrow.[37] Histologic sections of peri-implant bone obtained by removal of implants secondary to prosthetic component fracture 3 years post-loading have demonstrated the transformation of trabecular bone into compact bone with osteons oriented according to the direction and magnitude of the functional loads.

Albrektsson et al have studied the behavior of osseointegrated implants in 17 patients. They have reported average BIC values of 84.9% following implant removal at least 1 year after occlusal loading.[38] The adaptation phase is not

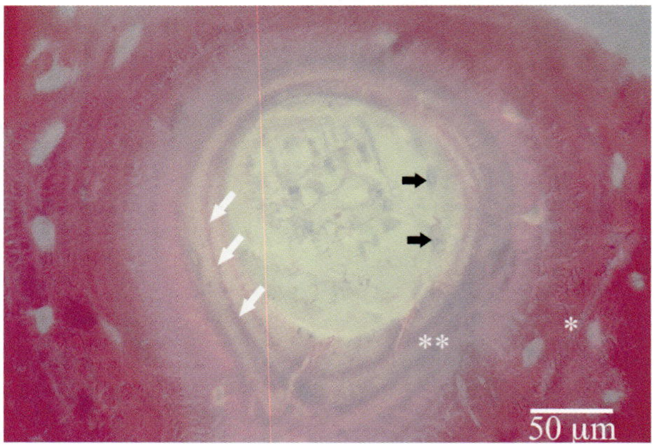

Fig 2.6 - Light microscopic image of a secondary osteon in formation phase (toluidine blue and acid fuchsin (original magnification ×400). Mineralized bone tissue (*); osteoid at different mineralization stages (**); cement line (*white arrows*); active osteoblasts (*black arrows*). (*Courtesy of Dr Tonino Traini and Dr Sergio Caputi, Chieti, Italy.*)

BOX. 2.2 - HEALING OF PERI-IMPLANT BONE TISSUE IN HUMANS (THREE PHASES)	
Phase 1	Formation of woven bone (4-6 weeks after surgery)
Phase 2	Formation of lamellar bone (6-12 weeks after surgery)
Phase 3	Bone remodeling depending on the load (3 months after surgery)

as intense as the regenerative phase, yet it lasts for a longer period (some months)—until the physiologic range for bone turnover of the segment involved has been reestablished (Fig 2.7). The most important phases of osseointegration are summarized in Box 2-2.[39]

Traditionally, it was thought that implant immobility and osseointegration could not be achieved without an adequate healing period in the absence of functional loads.[40]

BONE REGENERATION AROUND DENTAL IMPLANTS SUBJECTED TO IMMEDIATE LOADING

Historical Outline

Wound healing in bone tissue, the most specialized connective tissue, is initially conditioned by mesenchymal cells. Mesenchymal cells, secondary to their differentiation, are affected only by the conditions present in the receiving bed. At the bone-implant interface, these conditions depend on the physical and chemical characteristics of titanium and the immobility of the implant.

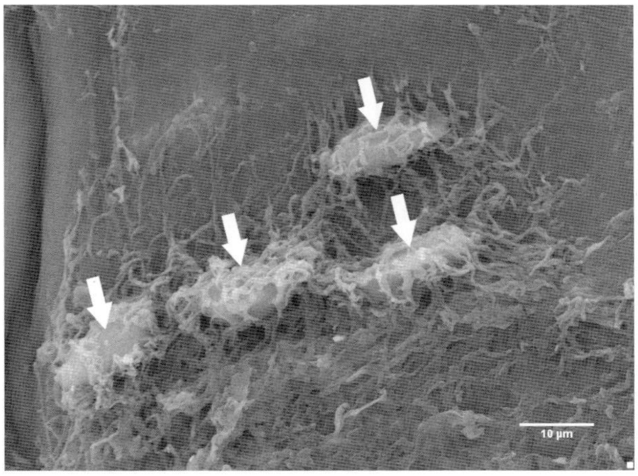

Fig 2.7 - Scanning electron microscope (SEM) image of human peri-implant bone tissue that demonstrates osteocyte cell bodies (*white arrows*) completely coated by cytoplasmic extensions of the "osteocytes network" (original magnification ×2000). (*Courtesy of Dr Tonino Traini and Dr Sergio Caputi, Chieti, Italy.*)

Early protocols called for unloaded healing periods of 3 months for edentulous mandibles and 6 months for edentulous maxillae. The period of functional load absence was established empirically by Brånemark with several clinical evaluations–but without scientific evidence proving that such a waiting period was essential.

The original protocol with unloaded healing has enabled dentists to obtain predictable and repeatable clinical results. However, implant loading protocols have continued to change over the past 40 years, and some clinicians have elected not to use unloaded healing protocols. At the end of the 1960s and during the following decades, several authors proposed immediate-loading protocols in an approach diametrically opposed to the original Brånemark protocol. Their work made use of various types of implants (blades or cylinders) immediately loaded with full functional occlusion after implant placement.[41,42] With these protocols, healing at the bone-implant interface was obtained not via direct contact with bone, but through apposition of fibrous tissues rich in collagen fibrils aligned parallel to the body of the implants. This histologic condition, where collagen fibrils were equated to Sharpey fibers, was compared to a "pseudoperiodontal" ligament. The resulting implant mobility was caused by mechanical adaptation of the adjacent bone to the occlusal loading. The biologic cost of this situation resulted in instability of the marginal seals around the implants. In fact, the scarce vascularization and reduced presence of cells also made this fibrous tissue less effective in protecting against possible infections. Localized infections could expand rapidly, resulting in bone loss and, ultimately, loss of the implants. This process, termed *fibrointegration*, proved to be deleterious to the long-term survival of dental implants. Fibrointegration yielded clinical results with high failure rates and was characterized by unpredictable prognoses.[43,44]

In light of these published results, immediate occlusal loading was regarded negatively since it produced the interposition of fibrous tissue between bone and implant surfaces. That is, micromotion within the implant sites compromised implant stability and interrupted normal bone healing because it induced stem elements to differentiate into fibroblasts instead of osteoblasts.[45]

With a careful analysis of the first studies on immediate occlusal loading, Szmukler-Moncler observed that, disregarding the material used, screw-type implants were not used.[46] The common factor in all of these cases that he did find was one often highlighted by the researchers themselves: the occurrence of micromotion of at least 150 μm at the bone-implant interface.

Many subsequent studies have proven that the healing of immediately loaded implants could occur without interposition of fibrous tissue at the bone-implant interface if certain conditions were met: *(1)* implants were shaped similar to screws; *(2)* a high degree of primary stability was achieved; and *(3)* micromotion was limited to 50 to 100 μm, or certainly not greater than 150 μm. If these conditions were satisfied, then healing would result in direct BIC.[47–55]

In a study on rabbit tibia, micromotion from 0 to 90 μm had a statistically significant effect on tissue differentiation around immediately loaded titanium screw implants. As uncontrolled micromotion increased, the probability of obtaining direct BIC decreased.[56] Furthermore, an analysis of the literature demonstrated that it was not the timing of occlusal loading that prevented osseointegration but the inability to eliminate micromotion induced by functional loads or to minimize it below a certain threshold.[57]

In the preceding paragraphs, the healing processes occurring after dental implant placement have been compared to bone wound healing. In normal bone wound healing, where micromotion is believed to be noxious, orthopedic procedures immobilize fractured segments to minimize micromotion between bony segments. However, it is not correct to affirm that optimal healing of bone fractures is obtained in the absence of micromotion. In orthopedics, the possibility of reducing and containing bone fragments is obtained by using one of two opposite therapeutic extremes: rigid or dynamic osteosynthesis. Rigid osteosynthesis is the model of bone consolidation employed in situations of rigid fixation or deformability between segments tending to zero. In contrast, dynamic osteosynthesis[58] is the model of bone consolidation employed in cases of "more elastic" implants (Figs 2.8 and 2.9).

Bone synthesis with rigid fixation devices implies that there are biomechanical problems associated with the static conditions of the materials used.[59] In fact, the mechanical stresses conveyed toward the rigid fixation devices do not propagate along the natural directions of bone load; they bypass the fracture and do not produce eutrophic stimulations.[60] This situation leads to asymmetric healing with a bone callous that is stimulated to remodel in compartments with compact and trabecular frameworks only after removal of the rigid fixation devices and the return of functional loads along the preexisting normal bone load trajectories. On the other hand, osteogenesis through dynamic devices causes an effective stabilization of the segments. It allows the transmission of axial and rhythmic mechanical stimulations to the approximated bone segments, which are able to amplify the response of the periosteal callous.

Fixation of fractured bone segments in long lower bones, in association with the application of controlled, compressive axial forces, leads to better quality ossification of the bone callous.[61,62] The orthopedic literature includes scientific evidence proving that the application of a light, precocious load to bone can accelerate the repair process of bone wounds.[63,64] Fractures submitted to cyclical movements have healed in shorter times than those not submitted to cyclical, mechanical stimuli.[65] Theoretically, the fibrocellular blastema (mass of undifferentiated cells) present in the area of the wound should be mechanically stimulated while also remaining immobile.

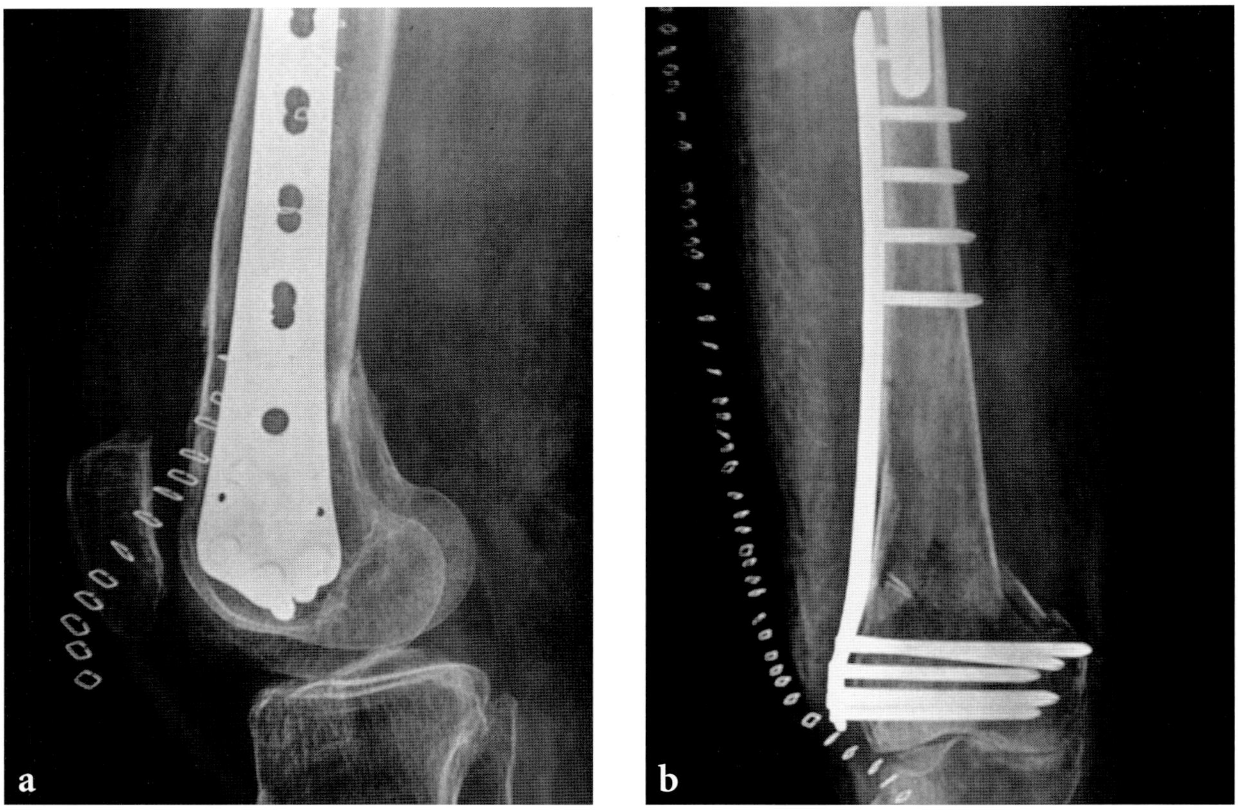

Fig 2.8 - *(a and b)* These radiographs demonstrate a condylar fracture of a femur treated with a LISS plate (Less Invasive Stabilization System plate), with internal rigid stabilization of the fracture (direct or first intention ossification). This represents a new concept in plating called "angular stability" since the screws were tightened both in the bone and in the plate *(right)*. *(Courtesy of Dr Benedetto di Santo, Italy.)*

Goodship and Kenwright[65,66] analyzed the influence of micromotion on fractures induced in the shin bones of experimental animals by applying probes on the bone and testing its deformation. The results highlighted some extremely interesting aspects associated with deforming mechanical loads, such as their direct effect on the consolidation of the fractures. The use of fixation systems that allowed for a controllable micromotion of both bone fragments proved that the proliferation of the new bone was stimulated in direct proportion to the resilience of the fixation.

This biologic behavior indicated that the ratio between tissue differentiation and the consolidation process was not only induced but also accelerated if an adequate stimulus was applied at the most suitable moment.[67,68]

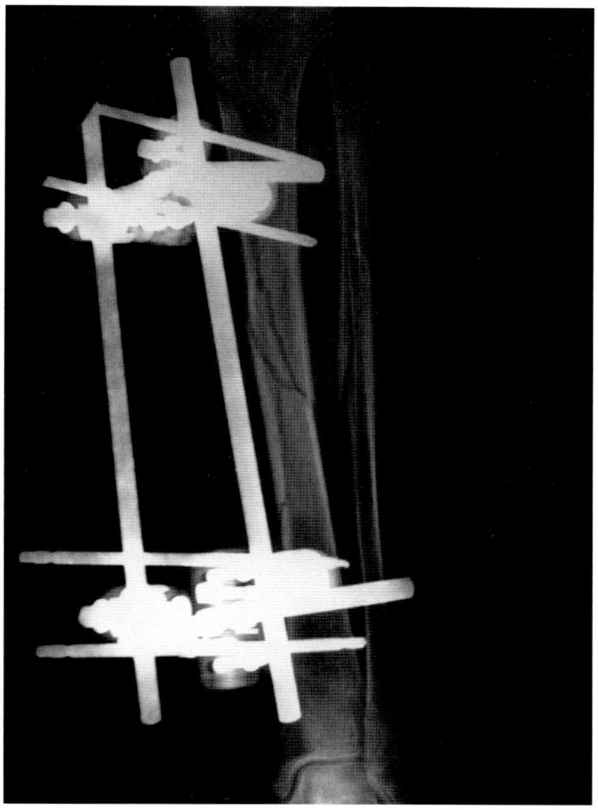

Fig 2.9 - This radiograph demonstrates a fracture in the tibia and fibula that was treated with Hoffman osteotaxis through external axial fixation. Elastic, external stabilization allowed only compression forces to be exerted onto the fractured segments. This was regarded as useful for the stimulation and formation of the bone callus–periosteal or second intention–by preventing torsion forces, scissor movements (rotation on its own axis), and varus-valgus movements. The lateral forces are considered harmful since they may break the callus and predispose healing as a "pseudoarthrosis" pathology of the bone callus (*left*). (*Courtesy of Dr Benedetto di Santo, Italy.*)

Histologic Topics

Starting with the concept that osseointegration can also be attained with immediate occlusal loading, several researchers examined the histology of early loaded, screw-type implants in animal models and humans.[69] Although the basic biology of bone tissue in animal models (dog, monkey, rabbit, rat, sheep and swine) is analogous to the human model, differences in metabolism, turnover rates of bone tissue, and hormone levels mean that results obtained in animal models cannot always be extrapolated to human clinical situations.[58] Occlusal loads applied 1 week after the insertion of dental implants in dogs does not necessarily correlate with the occlusal loading of dental implants 1 week after implant placement in humans. Theoretically, immediate loading in animal models may be equivalent to early loading in humans. Some researchers have indicated that healing processes occur 1.5 times quicker in dogs than in humans. Others have reported that the turnover rate of bone in rabbits is about three times more rapid than the rate in humans; in the rhesus macaque monkey, 15 days of healing appear to equal 7 to 8 weeks of healing in humans.[70–72]

In a 1993 study in three rhesus macaque monkeys, Piattelli et al observed that 30 days after implant placement, early loaded titanium screw implants were surrounded by thicker, cortical lamellar bone than were implants placed with an unloaded healing protocol.[73] Similar results were reported by Piattelli et al in another animal study.[74] Implants subjected to immediate occlusal loading showed a more compact peri-implant bone and statistically higher BIC than did implants placed with an unloaded healing protocol.

In two studies on *Macaca fascicularis* monkeys, Romanos and coworkers observed that osseointegration can be attained with immediate occlusal loading.[75,76] They showed evidence of higher bone density between the threads of implants submitted to immediate loading than in those placed with an unloaded healing protocol. Romanos et al affirmed that immediate loading seems to increase the ossification of alveolar bone around immediately loaded splinted implants.

Early functional stress not only induces more intense osteogenic responses than does unloaded healing but also shortens the healing time frame. Thus, early functional stress exploits the greater regenerative potential that occurs during wound healing, whereas unloaded healing makes use of the lesser possibility of structural adaptation after months of functional rest.

A study by Siar et al highlighted that, in animals, the dimensions of the peri-implant soft tissues were within the normal biologic range and were not affected by immediate occlusal loading.[77] Similar conclusions on soft tissues were drawn by Rocci et al in a study in humans.[78] Other researchers, studying minipigs, concluded that immediate occlusal loading can be used without disturbing the biologic processes of osseointegration.[79–82]

Since 1997, numerous case reports have been published concerning implant placement in the mandibles and maxillae of humans.[83–93] A number of these scientific works have reported the results of rough-surfaced implants with various surface characteristics, and they have confirmed that in certain clinical situations, immediate occlusal loading can yield results consistent with the results obtained with unloaded or early loading protocols.

In recent years, the School of Dentistry at Chieti (Italy) has distinguished itself for its histologic studies on the characteristics of peri-implant bone submitted to loads. Traini and colleagues have investigated the orientation of the collagen fibrils surrounding 20 implants inserted into the mandibles of 10 patients.[94] The content and disposition of the collagen fibrils were evaluated in alveolar bone at the moment of implant placement and around the implants (peri-implant bone) 6 months postloading. A statistically significant increase in transverse collagen fibrils was noted in the peri-implant bone, and these fibrils were more abundant on the lower side of the implant threads where the load was compressive in nature.

In contrast, in bone adjacent to the points of the implant threads, the collagen fibrils had more longitudinal orientations secondary to loads that expressed more tensile vectors (Fig 2.10). The longitudinal fibrils were present in a lower percentage compared with the presence of transverse fibrils in alveolar bone. An analysis with scanning electron microscopy established that in the bone layers immediately adjacent to the implants, there was a nonlinear orientation of the collagen fibrils (Fig 2.11).

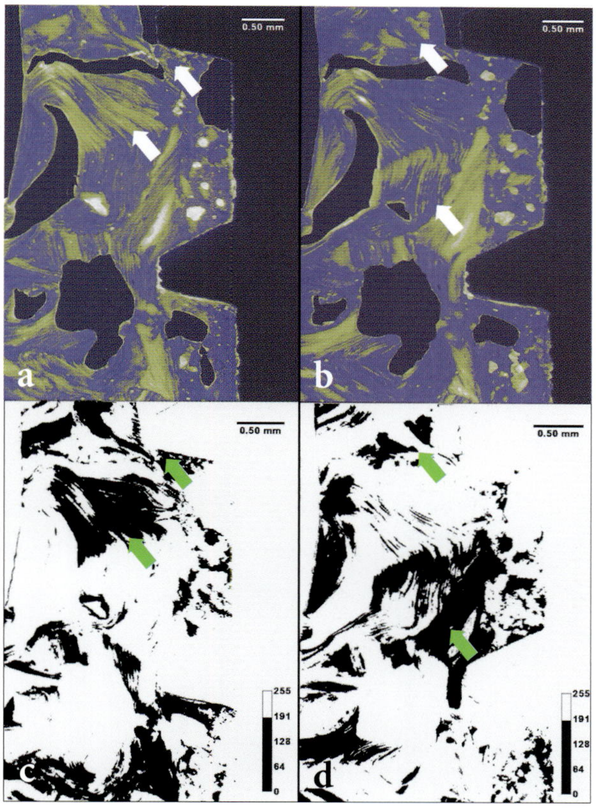

Fig 2.10 - Light microscopic image of a bone-implant interface under polarized light after 6 months of functional loading (original magnification ×100). *(a)* Transverse collagen fibers in yellow (*white arrows*). *(b)* Longitudinal collagen fibers in yellow (*white arrows*). *(c)* Re-sampling of the image with threshold values for the measurements. The *green arrows* indicate the same points as the *white arrows* in Fig 2.10a. *(d)* Re-sampling of the image with threshold values for the measurements. The *green arrows* indicate the same points as the *white arrows* in Fig 2.10b *(d)*. (*Courtesy of Dr Tonino Traini and Dr Sergio Caputi, Chieti, Italy.*)

In a case report in humans, Iezzi and coworkers confirmed the different orientations of collagen fibrils relative to implant threads.[95] In another study in humans, Traini et al evaluated the orientation of collagen fibrils on implants subject-

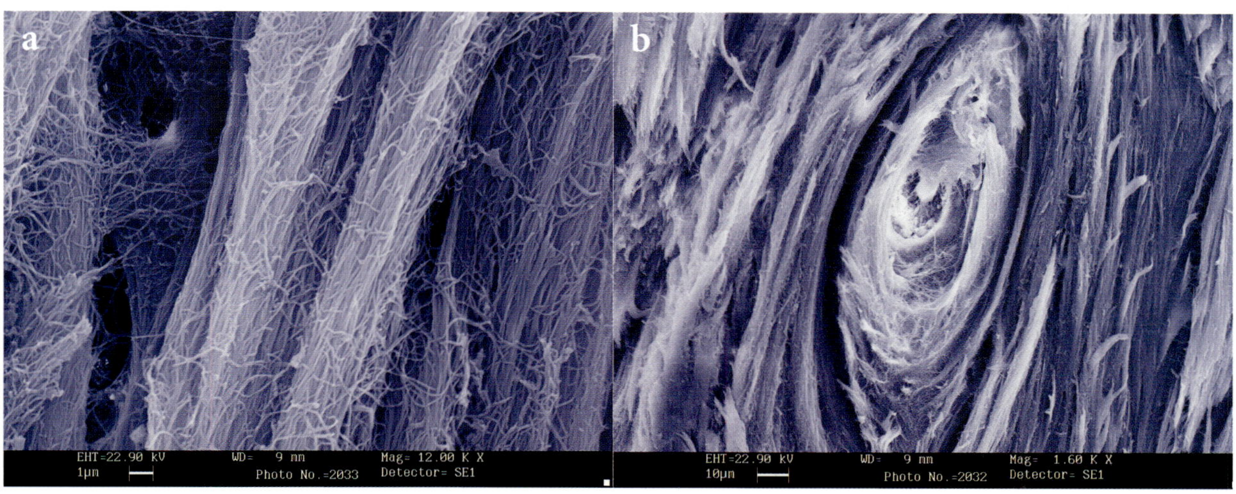

Fig 2.11 - *(a)* Woven alveolar bone (original magnification ×12,000). *(b)* Lamellar bone (osteon) (original magnification ×1,680). These SEM image shows that even if there is a nonlinear arrangement in the orientation of the collagen fibers in the first bone layers nearest the implant, fibers located farther away are organized according to the classic schemes of bone architecture. (*Courtesy of Dr Tonino Traini and Dr Sergio Caputi, Chieti, Italy.*)

ed to immediate occlusal loading and compared them with implants not subjected to immediate occlusal loading.[96] Transverse collagen fibrils were significantly more abundant around implants submitted to immediate occlusal loading than around nonloaded implants whereas longitudinal collagen fibrils were abundant around nonloaded implants. Therefore, immediate occlusal loading seems to affect the orientation of collagen fibrils through a mechanism of functional remodeling that adapts to the mechanical conditions of the load. These

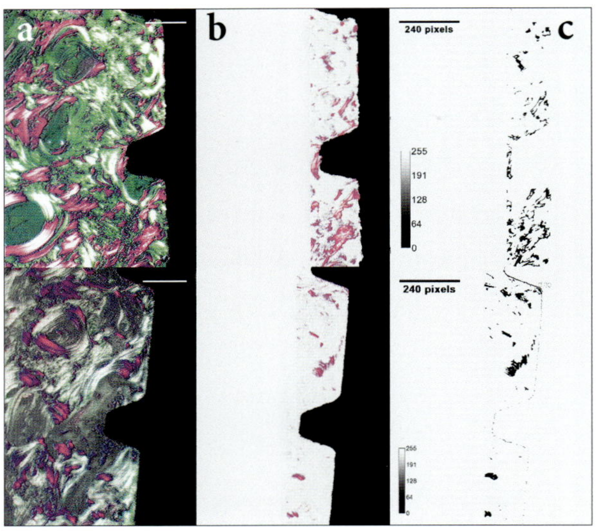

Fig 2.12 - Light microscopic image (polarized light) of an implant submitted to immediate occlusal loading in a minipig and removed 4 months after occlusal loading. Transverse collagen fibers running from the section plane of the image (*pink*). Longitudinal collagen fibers running perpendicular to the plane of the image (*gray-white*). The transverse collagen fibers in the implants submitted to load are mainly associated with compression zones (lower part of the thread). The line in *a* is 0.25 mm. The zone where transverse collagen fibers are present are mathematically separated from their context in *b*. Calculation of the pixels corresponding to the transverse collagen fibers (*original magnification ×50*). The total area covered by these collagen fibers is 112.453 ± 4.605 pixels in *c*. (*Courtesy of Dr Tonino Traini and Dr Sergio Caputi, Chieti, Italy.*)

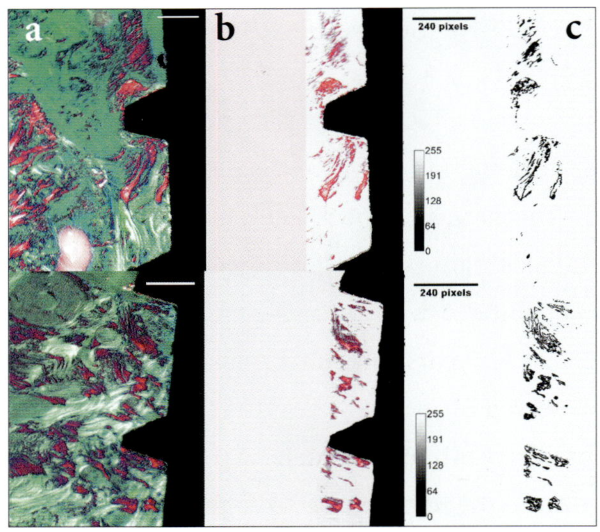

Fig 2.13 - Light microscopic image (polarized light) of a nonloaded implant in minipig and removed 4 months after placement. Transverse collagen fibers (*pink*). Longitudinal collagen fibers (*gray-white*). In implants not submitted to load, the transverse collagen fibers are distributed at random in the peri-implant bone. The line in *a* is 0.25 mm. The zones with transverse collagen fibers present are mathematically separated from their context in *b*. Calculation of the pixels corresponding to the transverse collagen fibers (*original magnification ×50*). The total area covered by these collagen fibers is 87.256 ± 2.428 pixels in *c*. This data is statistically significant when compared with that of Fig 2.12 per $P < .05$. (*Courtesy of Dr Tonino Traini and Dr Sergio Caputi, Chieti, Italy.*)

observations were later reconfirmed by Neugebauer et al in an animal study on minipigs.[97]

In a 2006 case study, Traini and colleagues evaluated the behavior of collagen fibrils around implants subjected to immediate occlusal loading (Figs 2.12 and 2.13).[98] Two implants were removed from the maxilla, at 4 months and at 12 years postloading. No statistically significant differences in the distribution of the transverse collagen fibrils were noticed in the peri-implant bone of the implants. The Traini group concluded that occlusal loading seems to determine and maintain the orientation of the collagen fibrils over time.

In another case report, Ledermann et al reported histologic data for four mandibular implants rehabilitated with a bar-supported overdenture after 12 years of functional loading.[99] The observed BIC varied from 70% to 80%, and signs of active bone remodeling were still present around the implant surfaces.

The data reported here demonstrate encouraging results on the use of immediate implant loading techniques. Nevertheless, some contrary reports have demonstrated slightly higher levels of crestal bone resorption around implants submitted to immediate occlusal loading than around those treated with traditional, unloaded healing protocols.[100,101] However, these articles present heterogenous sets of data, in terms of the material used and the surgical or prosthetic protocols followed.

The literature includes a limited number of articles with histology on maxillary implants subjected to immediate occlusal loading. Tealdo and others published a case report of a 69-year-old man who underwent complete, full-arch rehabilitation[102] (Figs 2.14 to 2.16). Ten implants were placed to support a fixed prosthesis.

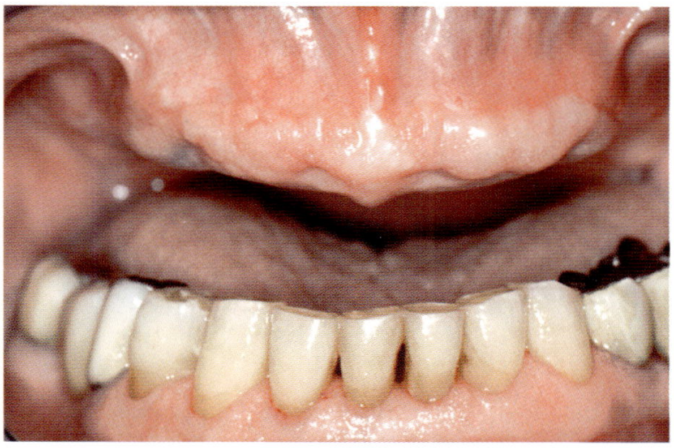

Fig 2.14 - Preoperative clinical image of edentulous maxilla prior to treatment.

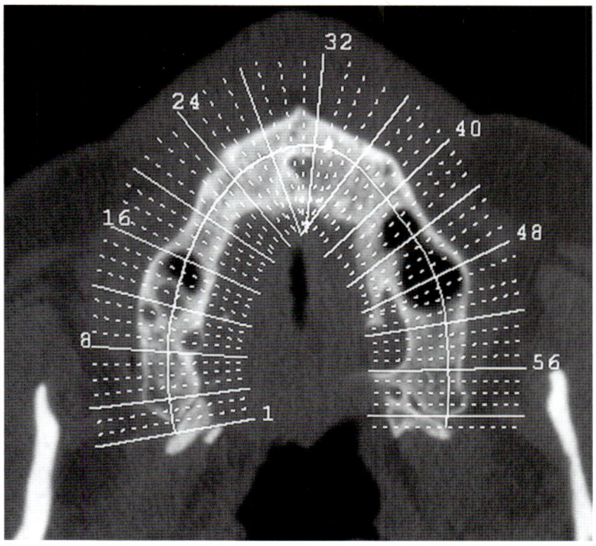

Fig 2.15 - Occlusal image of a computerized tomographic scan prior to treatment planning.

Two additional implants were positioned with the consent of the patient, which were to be removed and submitted for histologic analysis. Of these two implants, one was located in position 24 (maxillary left premolar region, test implant, 1) and was loaded immediately. The second implant was located in position 12 (maxillary right lateral incisor area, control implant, 2) and was allowed to heal unloaded according to the classic Brånemark protocol. All implants demonstrated insertion torques of 40 to 50 Ncm. Twenty-four hours after implant placement, the patient was provisionally rehabilitated with a fixed, screw-retained prosthesis. The prosthesis was made with a metal alloy framework; the rest of the prosthesis was made with acrylic resin and acrylic resin denture teeth. The prosthesis was screw retained by four implants distributed throughout the maxilla. The immediate prosthesis contained 10 masticatory units. The prosthesis did not have any cantilevered segments, and its occlusal morphology respected the long centric concept (Figs 2.17 to 2.22). All implants not loaded immediately were allowed to heal unloaded and were submerged beneath the soft tissues. Four months later, the radiographs did not show any radiolucencies on the test or control implants (Figs 2.23 and 2.24).

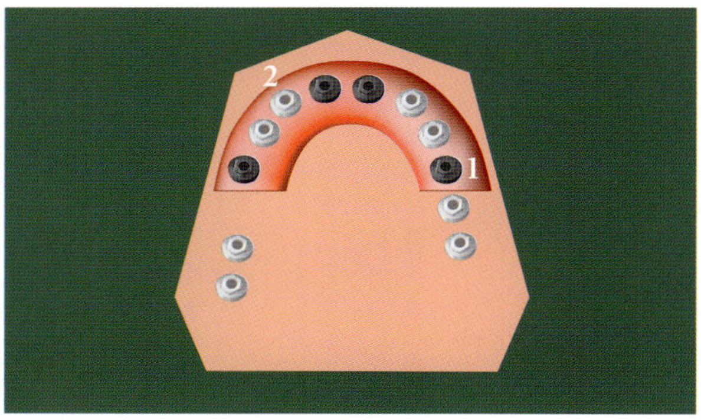

Fig 2.16 - Illustration of the scheme of the planned implant distribution. Loaded implants (*black*); nonloaded implants (*gray*); test implant (1); Control implant (2).

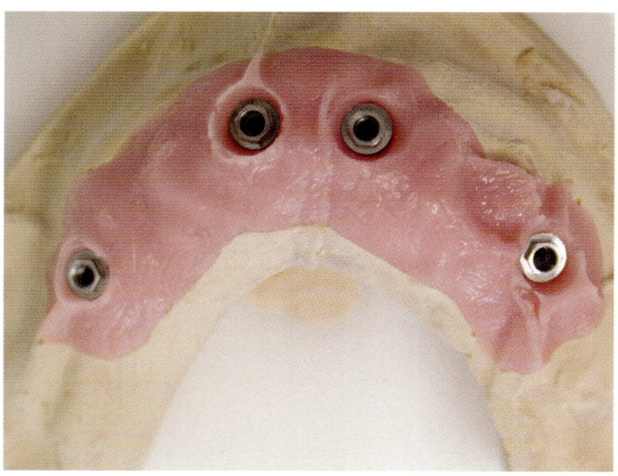

Fig 2.17 - Master cast with the four implant lab analogs that correspond to the loaded implants. This arrangement demonstrates the quadrilateral support that the implants will provide to the provisional prosthesis.

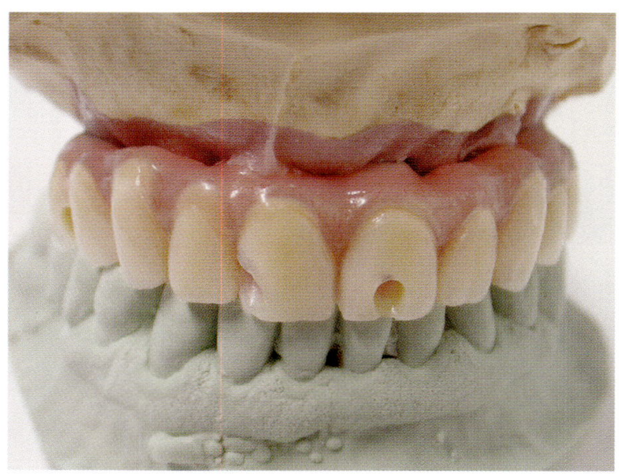

Fig 2.18 - Laboratory image of the provisional fixed prosthesis in the maxillary master cast mounted in centric occlusion in an articulator. This prosthesis was fabricated directly on the implant analogs without using conical angled abutments.

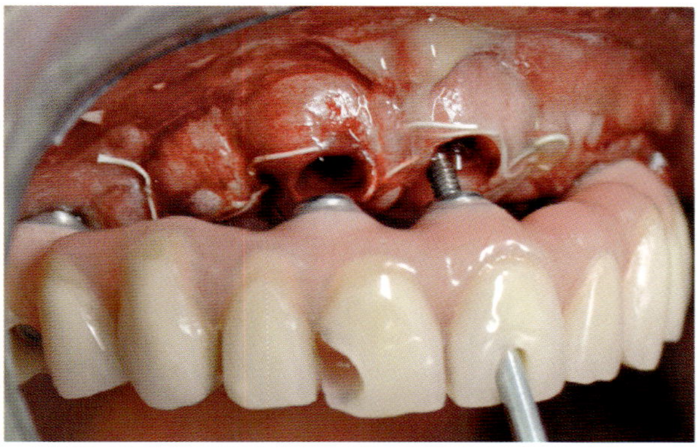

Fig 2.19 - Clinical image of the screw-retained provisional prosthesis to be placed 24 hours after surgery. The screw access openings for the anterior teeth were located within the facial surfaces of the artificial teeth.

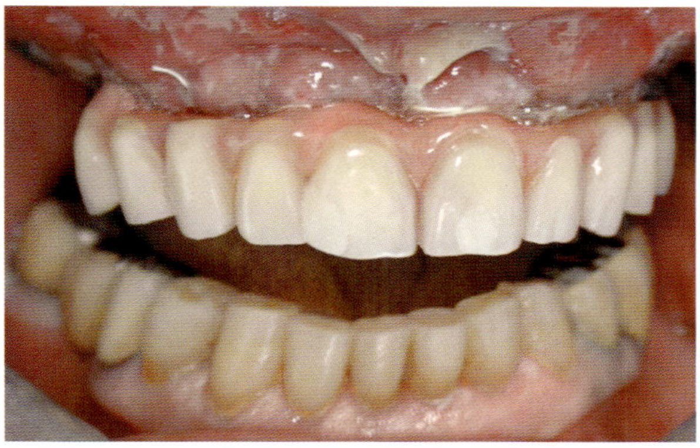

Fig 2.20 - Clinical image of the screw-retained provisional prosthesis after the screw access openings were restored with composite resin.

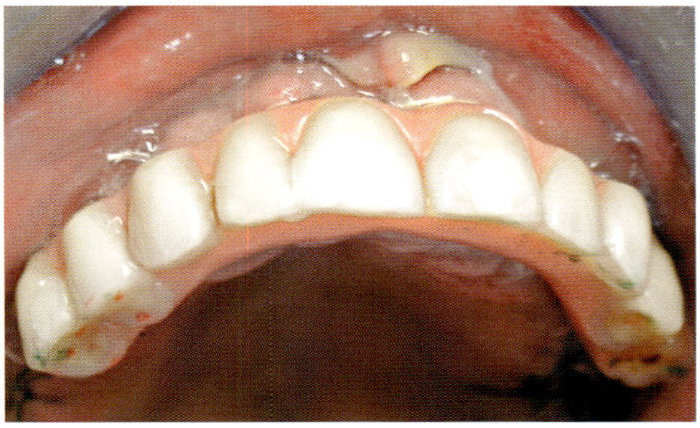

Fig 2.21 - Clinical image of the occlusal surface of the provisional prosthesis. The occlusal marks indicate that the prosthesis was inserted with full occlusal contacts and function.

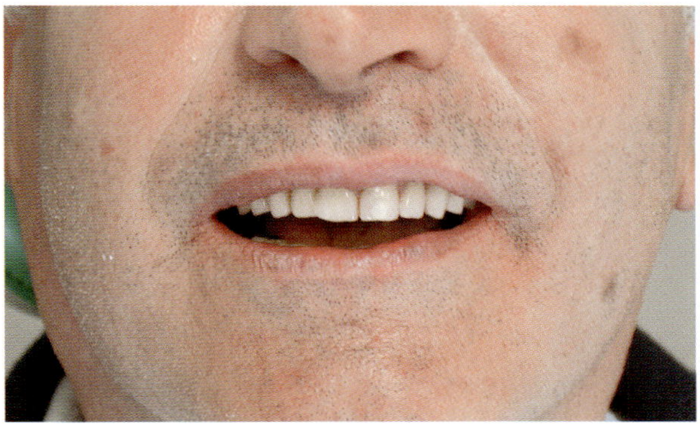

Fig 2.22 - Clinical image of the patient with the provisional prosthesis in place 24 hours after implant placement.

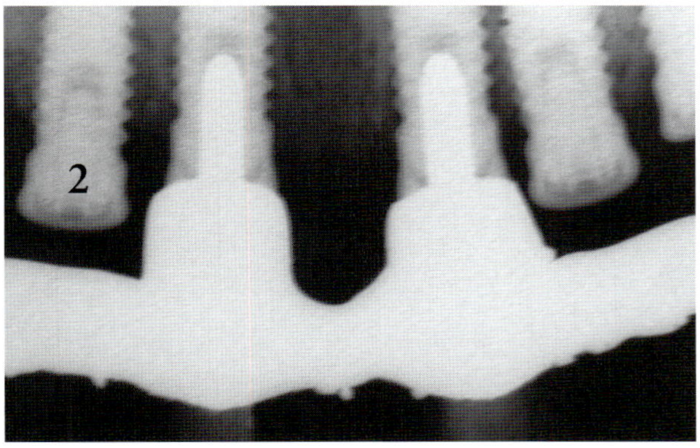

Fig 2.23 - Intraoral radiograph 4 months postsurgery. The control implant (2) was allowed to heal beneath the soft tissues and was not subject to immediate occlusal loading.

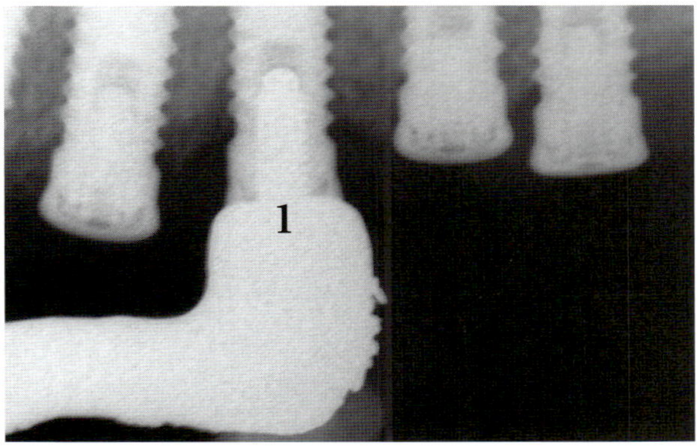

Fig 2.24 - Intraoral radiograph 4 months postsurgery. The test implant (1) was connected to the provisional prosthesis and was subjected to immediate occlusal loading.

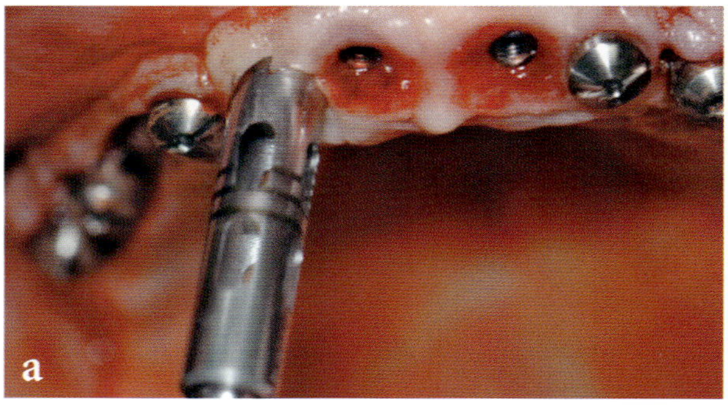

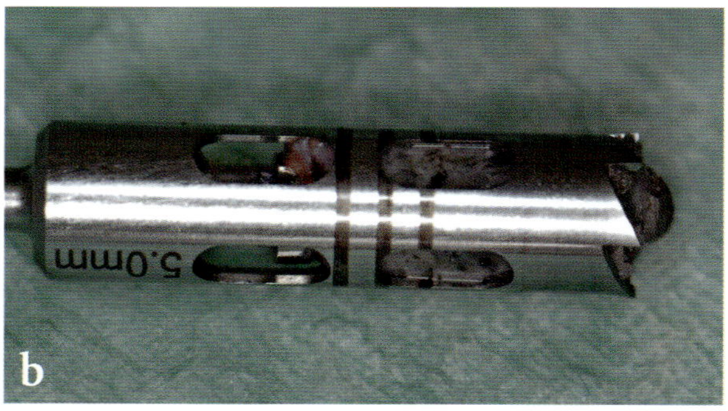

Fig 2.25 - (*a*) Clinical removal of the control implant with a trephine. (*b*) The trephine drill after remov from the surgical site. The control implant was contained within the trephine.

The two experimental implants, which clinically appeared to be osseointegrated, were removed with the aid of a trephine bur, while the other submerged implants were uncovered for the definitive prosthodontic treatment (Fig 2.25).
The two removed implants were placed into a solution of 10% buffered formalin and prepared for histologic analysis. Light microscopic examination (under normal and polarized light) showed that the implant submitted to immediate occlusal loading, which was rigidly splinted via the prosthesis to the other maxillary implants, had woven bone in strict contact with the implant threads. No connective tissue was seen along the bone-implant interface.

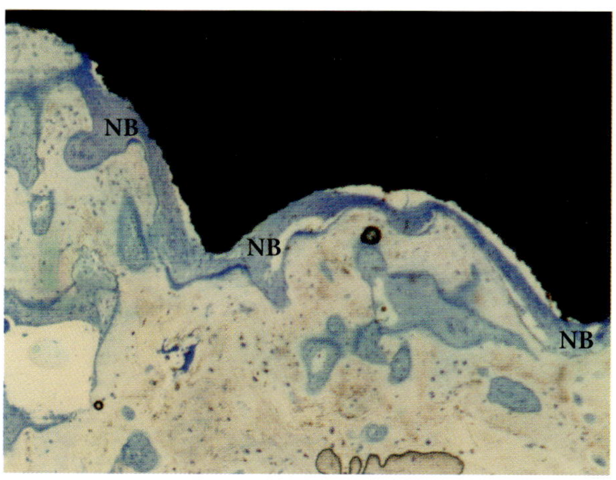

Fig 2.26 - Light microscopic image of the histologic section of the test implant that demonstrated bone-implant contact with new bone formation (NB) on the threads of the implant (toluidine blue; original magnification ×50).

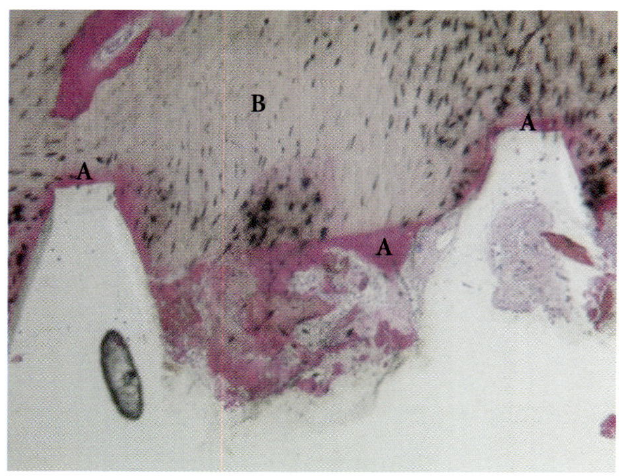

Fig 2.27 - Light microscopic image of the control implant that demonstrates a prevalent amount of compact bone (B), presumably representing preexisting bone tissue. A thin layer of tissue adjacent to the section of the slide that was previously occupied by the implant threads appears highly colored by the fuchsin acid stain. This section demonstrates the characteristics of the osteoid matrix that was not yet mineralized (A) (toluidine blue and fuchsin acid; original magnification ×50).

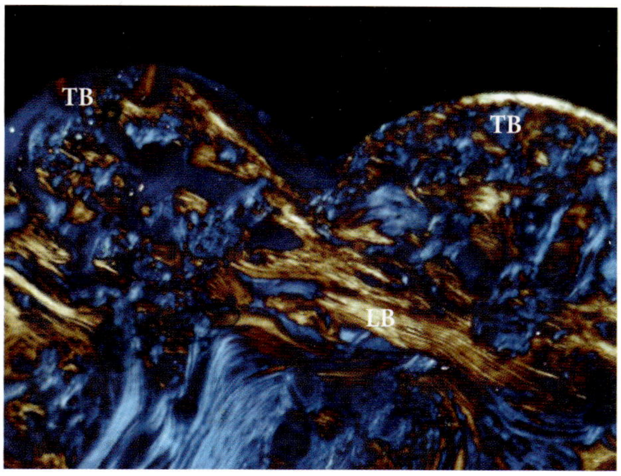

Fig 2.28 - Light microscopic image (polarized light) of the test implant. In general, the implant threads were in contact with woven bone (TB). There was a disorganized orientation of the collagen fibers. In the areas distant from the implant threads, there was lamellar bone (LB), distinguishable by a more regular arrangement of collagen (original magnification ×50).

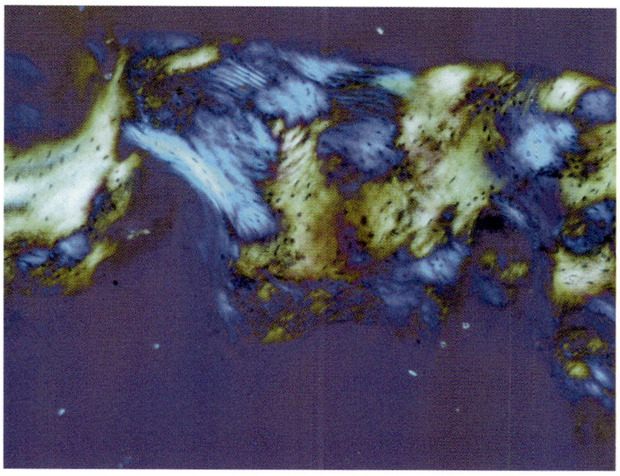

Fig 2.29 - Light microscopic image (polarized light) of the control implant. Despite difficulties in reading the image, it can be asserted that there was woven bone present in the areas previously occupied by the implant threads (original magnification ×50).

Lamellar bone was present distant from the implant and plausibly represented host bone. The marrow spaces of the trabecular bone adjacent to this implant presented numerous active osteoblasts. On the other hand, the implant that was not loaded, even in the presence of osseointegration, showed a less marked metabolism with fewer active osteoblasts (Figs 2.26 to 2.29).

Tealdo et al[102] reasserted the concept that prosthetic factors, including the timing of occlusal loading, play a key role in reaching and maintaining osseointegration in areas of poor bone quality, as typically seen in edentulous maxillae. This case report confirmed that where stabilization of implants can be obtained and maintained, immediate occlusal loading in edentulous patients should no longer be regarded as having risk factors higher or greater than the risk factors associated with implant placement and unloaded healing protocols.

REFERENCES

1. Ricciardi L (ed). Il Trattamento delle Fratture con il Fissatore Esterno di Hoffmann. Biologia, Diagnostica Strumentale, Risultati. Padova: Piccin Nuova Libraria, 1991.
2. Lang NP, Becker W, Karring T. La formazione dell'osso alveolare. In: Lindhe JL (ed). Parodontologia e Implantologia Dentale. Milano: Ermes, 1998: 906–912.
3. Friedenstein AJ. Determined and inducible osteogenic precursor cells. In: Elliott K, Fitzsimons DW (eds). Hard Tissue Growth, Repair and Remineralization. Ciba Foundation symposium 11. 1973: Amsterdam, NY: Associated Scientific, 169–181.
4. White AA, Panjabi MM, Southwick WO. The four biomechanical stages of healing. J Bone Joint Surg Am 1977;59:188–192.
5. Christel P, Cerf C, Pilla A. Time evolution of the mechanical properties of the callus of fresh fractures. Ann Biomed Eng 1981;9:383–391.
6. Albrektsson T, Bach A, Edshage S, Jonsson A. Fibrin adhesive system (FAS) influence on bone healing rate: A microradiographical evaluation using the bone growth chamber. Acta Orthop Scand 1982;53:757–763.
7. Roberts WE, Turley PK, Brezniak N, Fielder PJ. Implants: Bone physiology and metabolism. CDA J 1987;15:54–61.
8. Bruns P. Die allgemeine Lehre von den Knochenbrüchen. Deutsche Chirurgie 1982;27:1–400.
9. Wolff JL (ed). Das Gesetz der Transformation der Knochen. Berlin: Hirschwald, 1892.
10. Urist MR, McLean FC. Osteogenetic potency and new-bone formation by induction in transplants to the anterior chamber of the eye. J Bone Joint Surg Am 1952;34:443–476.
11. Amler MH. The time sequence of tissue regeneration in human extraction wounds. Oral Surg Oral Med Oral Pathol 1969;27:309–318.
12. Gruber R, Fuerst G. Experimental approaches in bone regeneration. In: Watzek G (ed). Implants in Qualitatively Compromised Bone. Surrey: Quintessence, 2004;9:95–99.
13. Winet H, Albrektsson T. Wound healing in the bone chamber: Neovascularization during transition from the repair to the regenerative phase in the rabbit tibial cortex. Int J Oral Maxillofac Implants 1988;3:99–107.
14. Albrektsson T, Eriksson AR, Jacobsson M, Kälebo P, Strid KG, Tjellström A. Bone repair in implant models: A review with emphasis on the harvest chamber for bone regeneration studies. Int J Oral Maxillofac Implants 1989;4:45–54.
15. Winet H, Bao JY, Moffat R. A control model for tibial cortex neovascularization in the bone chamber. J Bone Miner Res 1990;5:19–30.
16. Boyan BD, Hummert TW, Dean DD, Schwartz Z. Role of material surfaces in regulating bone and cartilage cell response. Biomaterials 1996;17:137–146.
17. Brighton CT. Principles of fracture healing. In: Murry JA (ed). Instructional Course Lectures. St Louis: Mosby, 1984:60–82.
18. Walter JB, Talbot IC. Wound healing. In: Walter JB, Israel MS (eds). General Pathology. New York: Churchill Livingstone, 1996;165–180.
19. Brånemark PI. Introduction to Osseointegration. In: Brånemark PI, Zarb GA, Albrektsson T (eds). Tissue-Integrated Prostheses: Osseointegration in Clinical Dentistry. Berlin: Quintessence, 1987:11–76.
20. Brighton CT. The biology of fracture repair. Instr Course Lect 1984;33:60–82.
21. Davies JE, Hosseini MM. Histodynamics of endosseous wound healing. In: Davies JE (ed). Bone Engineering. Toronto: Em Squared, 2000:1–14.
22. Rhinelander FW. Tibial blood supply in relation to fracture healing. Clin Orthop Relat Res 1974;(105):34–81.
23. Berglundh T, Abrahamsson I, Lang NP, Lindhe J. De novo alveolar bone formation adjacent to endosseous implants. A model study in the dog. Clin Oral Implants Res 2003;14:251–262.

24. Abrahamsson I, Berglundh T, Linder E, Lang N, Lindhe J. Early bone formation adjacent to rough and turned endosseous implant surfaces. Clin Oral Implants Res 2004;15:381–392.
25. Osborn JF, Newesely H. Dynamic aspects of the implant-bone interface. In: Heimke G (ed). Dental Implants, Materials and Systems. Munchen: Hanser Verlag, 1980;111–123.
26. Davies JE. Mechanisms of endosseous integration. Int J Prosthodont 1998;11:391–401.
27. Davies JE. Understanding peri-implant endosseous healing. J Dent Educ 2003;67:932–949.
28. Schenk RK. Bone regeneration: Biologic basis. In: Buser D, Dahlin C, Schenk RK (eds). Guided Bone Regeneration in Implant Dentistry. Chicago: Quintessence, 1994:49–100.
29. Cardaropoli G, Araùjo MG, Lindhe J. Dynamics of bone tissue formation in tooth extraction sites. An experimental study in dogs. J Clin Periodontol 2003;30:809–818.
30. Araùjo MG, Berglundh T, Lindhe J. On the dynamics of periodontal tissue formation in degree III furcation defects. J Clin Periodontol 1997;24: 738–746.
31. Araùjo MG, Berglundh T, Lindhe J. GTR treatment of degree III furcation defects with two different resorbable barriers. An experimental study in dogs. J Clin Periodontol 1998;25:253–259.
32. Kostopoulos L, Karring T. Augmentation of the rat mandible using the principles of guided tissue regeneration. Clin Oral Implants Res 1994;5:75–82.
33. Kostopoulos L, Karring T, Uraguchi R. Formation of jawbone tuberosities by guided tissue regeneration. An experimental study in the rat. Clin Oral Implants Res 1994;5:245–253.
34. Hämmerle CHF, Schmid J, Olah AJ, Lang NP. A novel model system for the study of experimental guided bone formation in humans. Clin Oral Implants Res 1996;7:38–47.
35. Botticelli D, Berglundh T, Buser D, Lindhe J. The jumping distance revisited. An experimental study in dog. Clin Oral Implants Res 2003;14:35–42.
36. Botticelli D, Berglundh T, Lindhe J. Appositional bone growth in marginal defects at implants. An experimental study in dog. Clin Oral Implants Res 2003;14:1–9.
37. Di Silvestro S, Poli O, Confalone L. Aspetti di fisiologia osteoimplantare. Quintessenz Int 1997;3:73–80.
38. Albrektsson T, Eriksson AR, Friberg B, et al. Histologic investigations on 33 retrieved Nobelpharma implants. Clin Mater 1993;12:1–9.
39. Shenk RK, Buser D. Osseointegration: A reality. Periodontol 2000 1998;17:22–35.
40. Brånemark PI. Osseointegration and its experimental background. J Prosthet Dent 1983;50:399–410.
41. Linkow LI, Glassman PE, Asnis ST. Macroscopic and microscopic studies of endosteal bladevent implants (six month dog study). Oral Implantol 1973;3:281–309.
42. Babbush CA. Endosteal blade-vent implants. Dent Clin North Am 1980;24:421–440.
43. Kapur KK. Veterans administration cooperative dental implant study. Comparisons between fixed partial dentures supported by blade-vent implants and removable partial dentures. Part II. Comparisons of success rates and periodontal health between two treatment modalities. J Prosthet Dent 1989;62:685–703.
44. Spiekermann H. Clinical and animal experiences with endosseous metal implants. In: Heimke G (ed). Dental Implants: Materials and Systems. Munchen: Hanser Verlag, 1980;49–54.
45. Uhthoff HK, Germain JP. The reversal of tissue differentiation around screws. Clin Orthop 1975;123:248–252.
46. Szmukler-Moncler S, Salama H, Reingewirtz Y, Dubruille JH. Timing of loading and effect of micromotion on bone-dental implant interface: Review of experimental literature. J Biomed Mater Res 1998;43:192–203.
47. Fradsen PA, Christoffersen H, Madsen T. Holding power of different screws in the femoral head. A study in human cadaver hips. Acta Orthop Scand 1984;55:349–351.

48. Cameron H, Macnab I, Pilliar R. Porous surfaced Vitallium staples. S Afr J Surg 1972;10:63–70.
49. Cameron HU, Pilliar RM, MacNab I. The effect of movement on the bonding of porous metal to bone. J Biomed Mater Res 1973;7:301–311.
50. Brunski JB. Influence of biomechanical factors at the bone-biomaterial interface. In: Davies JE (ed). The Bone-Biomaterial Interface. Toronto: University of Toronto, 1991:391–404.
51. Brunski JB. Biomechanical factors affecting the bone-dental implant interface. Clin Mater 1992;10:153–201.
52. Brunski JB. Avoid pitfalls of overloading and micromotion of intraosseous implants. Dent Implantol Update 1993;4:77–81.
53. Pilliar RM, Lee JM, Maniatopoulos C. Observation on the effect of movement on bone in-growth into porous-surfaced implants. Clin Orthop 1986; 208:108–113.
54. Szmukler-Moncler S, Salama H, Reingewirtz Y, Dubruille JH. Time of loading and effect of micromotion on bone-dental implant interface: Review of experimental literature. J Biomed Mater Res 1998;43:192–203.
55. Szmukler-Moncler S, Piattelli A, Favero GA, Dubruille JH. Considerations preliminary to the application of early and immediate loading protocols in dental implantology. Clin Oral Implants Res 2000;11:12–25.
56. Duyck J, Vandamme K, Geris L, et al. The influence of micro-motion on the tissue differentiation around immediately loaded cylindrical turned titanium implants. Arch Oral Biol 2006;51:1–9.
57. Testori T, Del Fabbro M. Carico precoce, carico occlusale immediato, carico non occlusale immediato degli impianti endossei orali. Basi scientifiche ed esperienze cliniche. In: Malchiodi L (ed). Chirurgia Implantare. Bologna: Martina, 2003:369–89.
58. Bianchi A (ed). Implantologia e Implantoprotesi. Basi Biologiche, Biomeccanica, Applicazioni Cliniche. Torino: UTET, 2004:116–120.
59. Uhthoff HK, Dubuc FL. Bone structural changes in the dog under rigid internal fixation. Clin Orthop 1971;81:165–170.
60. Tonino AJ, Davidson CL, Klopper PJ, Lincalan LA. Protection from stresses in bone and its effect. J Bone Joint Surg Br 1976;58:107–112.
61. De Bastiani G, Aldegheri R, Renzi-Brivio L. Dynamic axial fixation. A rational alternative for the external fixation of fractures. Int Orthop 1986;10:95–99.
62. De Bastiani G, Aldegheri R, Renzi-Brivio L, Trivella G. Limb lengthening by callus distraction (callotasis). J Pediatr Orthop 1987;7:129–134.
63. Sarmiento A, Schaeffer JF, Beckermann L, Latta LL, Enis JE. Fracture healing in rat femora is affected by functional weight bearing. J Bone Joint Surg Am 1977;59:369–375.
64. Goodman S, Aspenberg P. Effects of mechanical stimulation on the differentiation of hard tissues. Biomaterials 1993;14:563–569.
65. Kenwright J, Richardson JB, Cunningham JL, et al. Axial movement and tibial fractures. A controlled randomised trial of treatment. J Bone Joint Surg Br 1991;73:654–659.
66. Goodship AE, Kenwright J. The influence of induced micromovement upon the healing of experimental tibia fractures. J Bone Joint Surg Br 1985;67:650–655.
67. Vandamme K, Naert I, Geris L, Vander Sloten J, Puers R, Duyck J. The effect of micro-motion on the tissue response around immediately loaded roughened titanium implants in the rabbit. Eur J Oral Sci 2007;115:21–29.
68. Vandamme K, Naert I, Geris L, Sloten JV, Puers R, Duyck J. Histodynamics of bone tissue formation around immediately loaded cylindrical implants in the rabbit. Clin Oral Implants Res 2007;18:471–480.
69. Romanos G. Immediate Loading of Endosseous Implants in the Posterior Area of the Mandible: Animal and Clinical Studies. Berlin: Quintessence, 2005.
70. Roberts WE. Bone tissue interface. J Dent Educ 1988;52:804–809.
71. Vrespa G. Il sistema implantare PHI una filosofia nuova per l'osteointegrazione. Quintessenza Int 1993;9:117–119.

72. Piattelli A, Corigliano M, Scarano A, Quaranta M. Bone reactions to early occlusal loading of two-stage titanium plasma-sprayed implants: A pilot study in monkeys. Int J Periodontics Restorative Dent 1997;17:162–169.
73. Piattelli A, Ruggeri A, Franchi M, Romasco N, Trisi P. An histologic and histomorphometric study of bone reactions to unloaded and loaded non-submerged single implants in monkeys: A pilot study. J Oral Implantol 1993;19:314–320.
74. Piattelli A, Corigliano M, Scarano A, Costigliola G, Paolantonio M. Immediate loading of titanium plasma-sprayed implants: An histologic analysis in monkeys. J Periodontol 1998;69:321–327.
75. Romanos G, Toh CG, Siar CH, et al. Peri-implant bone reactions to immediately loaded implants. An experimental study in monkeys. J Periodontol 2001;72:506–511.
76. Romanos GE, Toh CG, Siar CH, Swaminathan D. Histologic and histomorphometric evaluation of peri-implant bone subjected to immediate loading: An experimental study with Macaca fascicularis. Int J Oral Maxillofac Implants 2002;17:44–51.
77. Siar CH, Toh CG, Romanos G, et al. Peri-implant soft tissue integration of immediately loaded implants in the posterior macaque mandible: A histomorphometric study. J Periodontol 2003; 74:571–578.
78. Rocci A, Martignoni M, Burgos PM, Gottlow J, Sennerby L. Histology of retrieved immediately and early loaded oxidized implants: Light microscopic observations after 5 to 9 months of loading in the posterior mandible. Clin Implant Dent Relat Res 2003;5(suppl 1):88–98.
79. Meyer U, Wiesmann HP, Fillies T, Joos U. Early tissue reaction at the interface of immediately loaded dental implants. Int J Oral Maxillofac Implants 2003;18:489–499.
80. Meyer U, Joos U, Mythili J, et al. Ultrastructural characterization of the implant/bone interface of immediately loaded dental implants. Biomaterials 2004;25:1959–1967.
81. Nkenke E, Fenner M, Vairaktaris EG, Neukam FW, Radespiel-Troger M. Immediate versus delayed loading of dental implants in the maxillae of minipigs. Part II: Histomorphometric analysis. Int J Oral Maxillofac Implants 2005;20:540–546.
82. Joos U, Buchter A, Wiesmann HP, Meyer U. Strain driven fast osseointegration of implants. Head Face Med 2005;1:1–6.
83. Testori T, Szmukler-Moncler S, Francetti L, et al. Immediate loading of Osseotite implants: A case report and histologic analysis after 4 months of occlusal loading. Int J Periodontics Restorative Dent 2001;21:451–459.
84. Testori T, Szmukler-Moncler S, Francetti L, Del Fabbro M, Trisi P, Weinstein RL. Healing of Osseotite implants under submerged and immediate loading conditions in a single patient: A case report and interface analysis after 2 months. Int J Periodontics Restorative Dent 2002;22:345–353.
85. Degidi M, Petrone G, Iezzi G, Piattelli A. Histologic evaluation of a human immediately loaded titanium implant with a porous anodized surface. Clin Implant Dent Relat Res 2002;4:110–114.
86. Degidi M, Scarano A, Petrone G, Piattelli A. Histologic analysis of clinically retrieved immediately loaded titanium implants: A report of 11 cases. Clin Implant Dent Relat Res 2003;5:89–93.
87. Degidi M, Petrone G, Iezzi G, Piattelli A. Histologic evaluation of 2 human immediately loaded and 1 titanium implants inserted in the posterior mandible and submerged retrieved after 6 months. J Oral Implantol 2003;29:223–229.
88. Degidi M, Scarano A, Iezzi G, Piattelli A. Periimplant bone in immediately loaded titanium implants: Histologic and histomorphometric evaluation in human. A report of two cases. Clin Implant Dent Relat Res 2003;5:170–175.
89. Degidi M, Scarano A, Piattelli M, Piattelli A. Histologic evaluation of an immediately loaded titanium implant retrieved from a human after 6 months in function. Oral Implantol 2004;30:289–296.

90. Degidi M, Scarano A, Piattelli M, Perrotti V, Piattelli A. Bone remodeling in immediately loaded and unloaded titanium dental implants: A histologic and histomorphometric study in humans. J Oral Implantol 2005;31:18–24.
91. Degidi M, Scarano A, Iezzi G, Piattelli A. Histologic and histomorphometric analysis of an immediately loaded implant retrieved from man after 14 months of loading. J Long Term Eff Med Implants 2005;15:489–498.
92. Degidi M, Scarano A, Iezzi G, Piattelli A. Histologic analysis of an immediately loaded implant retrieved after 2 months. J Oral Implantol 2005;31:247–254.
93. Piattelli A, Paolantonio M, Corigliano M, Scarano A. Immediate loading of titanium plasma-sprayed screw-shaped implants in man: A clinical and histological report of two cases. J Periodontol 1997;68:591–597.
94. Traini T, Degidi M, Strocchi R, Caputi S, Piattelli A. Collagen fiber orientation near dental implants in human bone: Do their organization reflect differences in loading? J Biomed Mater Res B Appl Biomater 2005;74:538–546.
95. Iezzi G, Pecora G, Scarano A, Perrotti V, Piattelli A. Histologic evaluation of 3 retrieved immediately loaded implants after a 4-month period. Implant Dent 2006;15:305–312.
96. Traini T, Degidi M, Caputi S, Strocchi R, Di Iorio D, Piattelli A. Collagen fiber orientation in human peri-implant bone around immediately loaded and unloaded titanium dental implants. J Periodontol 2005;76:83–89.
97. Neugebauer J, Traini T, Thams U, Piattelli A, Zöller JE. Peri-implant bone organization under immediate loading state. Circularly polarized light analyses: A minipig study. J Periodontol 2006;77:152–160.
98. Traini T, Pecora G, Iezzi G, Piattelli A. Preferred collagen fiber orientation human peri-implant bone after a short- and long-term loading period: A case report. J Oral Implantol 2006;32:177–181.
99. Ledermann PD, Schenk RK, Buser D. Long-lasting osseointegration of immediately loaded, bar-connected TPS screws after 12 years of function: A histologic case report of a 95-year-old patient. Int J Periodontics Restorative Dent 1998;18:552–563.
100. Akagawa Y, Ichikawa Y, Nikai H, Tsuru H. Interface histology of unloaded and early loaded partially stabilized zirconia endosseous implant in initial bone healing. J Prosthet Dent 1993;69:599–604.
101. Romanos GE, Testori T, Degidi M, Piattelli A. Histologic and histomorphometric findings from retrieved, immediately occlusally loaded implants in humans. J Periodontol 2005;76:1823–1832.
102. Tealdo T, Bevilacqua M, Orsini G, Caputi S, Pera P. Histological evaluation of bone healing around rough surface implants in different loading conditions in edentulous maxilla: Report of a case. Doctor Os 2007;18(suppl 2):42–46.

CHAPTER 3
PRESURGICAL DIAGNOSTIC PROCEDURES

COLUMBUS BRIDGE PROTOCOL	
SURGICAL PROTOCOL	**PROSTHETIC PROTOCOL**
External hex rough-surface implants	Screw-retained fixed prosthesis
Implant length ≥ 13 mm, Ø 4 mm	Plaster impression with pickup technique
Underprepared osteotomy	Rigid splinting with metal framework
Implant insertion torque ≥ 40 Ncm	Passive fit with the luting technique
Angled implants in native bone	Acrylic resin occlusal surfaces
Angled conical abutments	No distal cantilevers
No bone regenerative techniques	Immediate functional load 24–48 h after surgery

Table 3.1

Rehabilitative prosthetic treatment in patients with an edentulous maxilla is determined by an evaluation of the anatomy and function. The main objectives of rehabilitation include the restoration of *(1)* optimal esthetics and phonetics; *(2)* masticatory function; *(3)* a physiologic ratio among tongue, lips, and cheeks; and *(4)* an optimal skeletal maxillomandibular relationship (Fig 3.1).

In many societies, loss of the maxillary anterior teeth is regarded as a major disability that negatively affects a person's interpersonal relationships, social life, and working capacity. In such situations, patients tend to be extremely concerned about phonetics and esthetics.

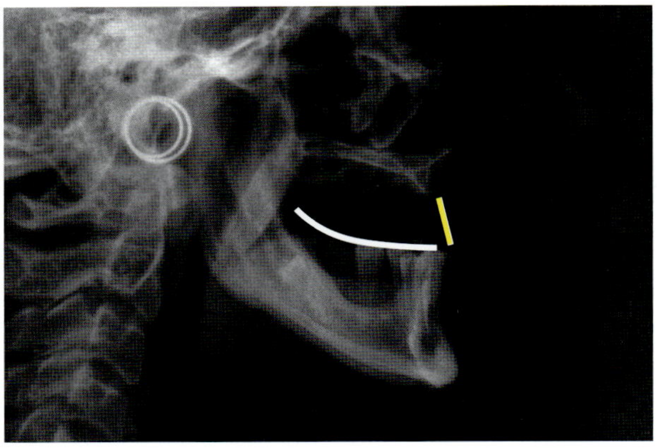

Fig 3.1 - Assessment of the skeletal jaw relationship between maxilla and mandible on the horizontal and vertical planes is essential for optimal treatment in the edentulous patient. Occlusal plane (*white line*), anteroposterior position in the sagittal plane of the labial surfaces of the maxillary anterior teeth (*yellow line*).

The maxillary anterior teeth affect the tongue-to-teeth ratio and, therefore, phonetics. Furthermore, these teeth not only are the most prominent portion of the smile but also support the cheeks and lips. Without the natural support of the teeth and alveolar bone, the cheeks and lips become hollow, negatively affecting the appearance of the entire face. Therefore, the first goal of treatment is to reestablish optimal esthetics and function by replacing the maxillary anterior teeth.

Loss of the maxillary teeth also compromises masticatory function. Mastication and the ability to taste food are important contributors to quality of life. Studies on edentulous patients rehabilitated with removable dental prostheses have demonstrated that gastric function is not improved by mastication of a food bolus with the dentures in place.[1] In contrast, a study by Pera et al[2] suggests that poor digestion could result from inadequate mastication. They demonstrated that sound dentition resulted in more efficient mastication and significantly improved digestive processes, thus contributing to the overall health of patients.

In the prediagnostic work-ups of patients with edentulous maxillae, all elements that may affect treatment, including design and durability of the prostheses, are evaluated. Independent of the type of prosthesis, the work-up must start with a review of the patient's medical history. It is essential that any diseases that could affect treatment planning and surgery be recognized during this initial step. Next, the morphostructural and functional status of the stomatognathic system is evaluated. The health of the stomatognathic apparatus is defined as the *(1)* absence of pain, abnormal sensations, and noise during mandibular movements; *(2)* presence of free-flowing, symmetric mandibular movements; and *(3)* functional harmony between positions guided by the muscles of mastication and maximum intercuspation. The main symptomatology of the stomatognathic apparatus, therefore, is characterized by pain in the muscles of mastication, pain and noise in the temporomandibular joint(s), and limitation in mandibular movements.

Primary dysfunction is the expression of an overload of muscular and/or skeletal structures generated by prolonged muscle hyperactivity, the genesis of which is considered multifactorial. Before prosthodontic treatment begins, it is advisable to perform a careful investigation of craniomandibular conditions that could affect treatment planning. In particular, special attention must be given to the evaluation of masticatory function in patients with craniomandibular conditions. The presence of craniomandibular pathology can require the use of long-term, provisional prostheses designed for solving functional problems before proceeding to treatment with definitive prostheses.

Definitive prosthetic treatment may warrant supportive therapies such as occlusal guards and physical therapy after placement of the definitive prostheses. Protocols defined by the European Academy of Craniomandibular Disorders (EACD) may be helpful for general dentists who find themselves treating patients with craniomandibular disorders.[3] These tools will enable the dentists to evaluate and treat patients by identifying the necessary measures of prophylaxis and therapy that have proven useful in the diagnosis of functional disorders.[4]

In review, the authors want to stress the necessity of devoting the utmost attention to the diagnostic phases of treatment and treatment planning, well before commencing the surgical-prosthetic treatment phases. This principle is important in *(1)* cases of traditional rehabilitative treatment of edentulous maxillae with removable prostheses and *(2)* cases of fixed rehabilitation on implants when immediate occlusal loading has been selected as the optimal treatment.

TEMPLATES

The primary purposes of prosthetic rehabilitation are restoration of masticatory function, long-term occlusal stability, and optimal esthetics. Correct positioning of the artificial teeth is a key component of implant-prosthetic therapy.[5] Templates for implant positioning can be divided into four groups: *(1)* surgical, *(2)* radiographic-surgical, *(3)* stereolithographic, and *(4)* surgical-prosthetic.

Modica et al have asserted that optimal implant positioning is more likely to be achieved if surgical templates are used.[6] An ideal implant template should allow for:

- The correct insertion of implants
- A certain freedom in decision making for the implant surgeon
- Satisfactory irrigation of the implant site during osteotomy preparation

In addition, an ideal template also should be:

- Retentive and stable
- Noninvasive
- Sterilizable
- Comfortable for patients
- Usable during radiographic studies
- Manufacturable by every dental laboratories
- Inexpensive

Surgical Templates

Surgical templates are used for positioning implants during surgery. The Brånemark System Novum protocol (Nobel Biocare) and the All-on-

4 technique (Nobel Biocare) make use of these kind of templates. Surgical templates are most widely known for their use in the rehabilitation of edentulous patients. In the Novum protocol, four prefabricated templates are used for the insertion of three implants into the interforaminal regions of mandible.[7] They are the *(1)* guide template, *(2)* evaluation template, *(3)* positioning template, and *(4)* V-template (Fig 3.2). The templates dictate the positions of the implants in a preestablished tripod configuration. This protocol requires accurate, optimal patient selection and can be considered advanced level surgey. The surgical template used for the All-on-4 technique is less invasive compared to Novum protocol ones. The template is retained on the median line of edentulous jaws by an articulated pin, 2 mm in diameter (Fig 3.3).[8,9] The titanium device may be bent to adapt to the profile of the crest of the edentulous jaw. The vertical indicator lines allow the gradient of the distal implants to be visualized according to the technique proposed by Maló.[8] This protocol is described in detail in Chapter 6. A characteristic unique to surgical templates is that they are prefabricated by the implant manufacturer. Therefore, the location of the implant prosthesis within the residual edentulous structures is guided by the prefabricated surgical template, without any prosthetic reference to the location of the teeth in the implant rehabilitation.

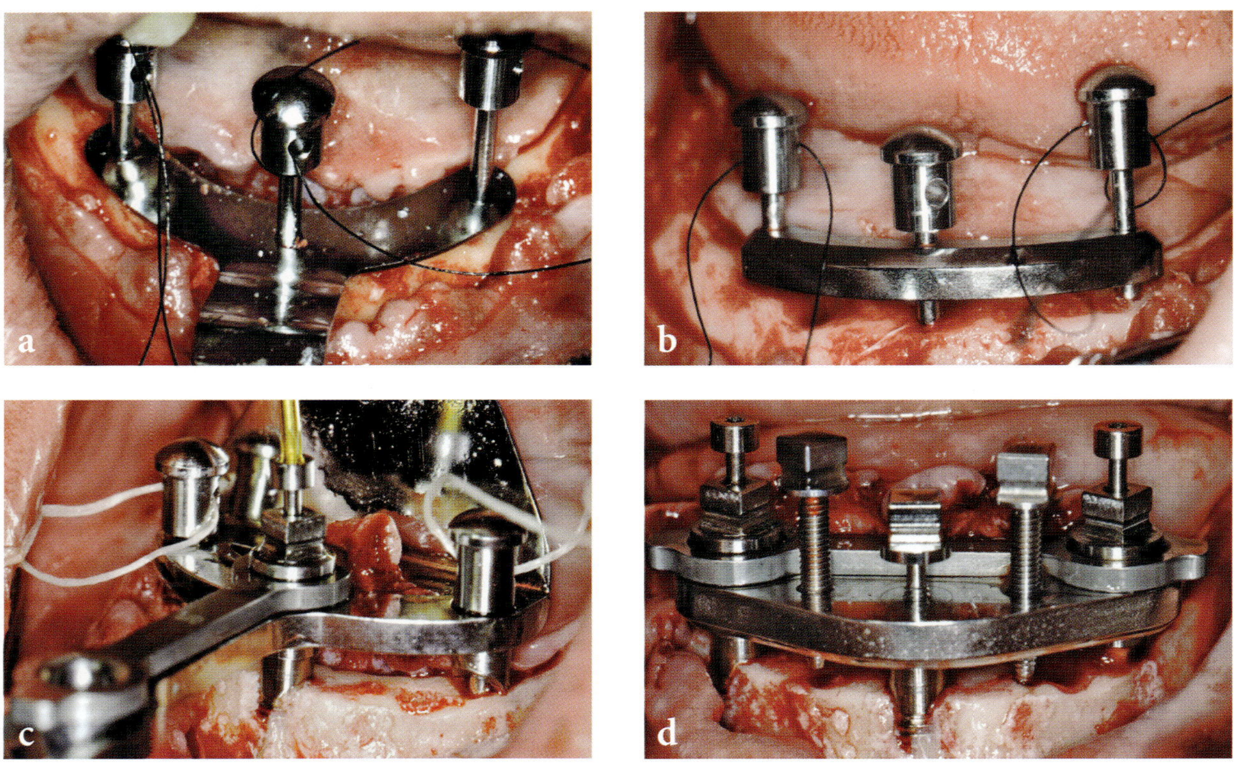

Fig 3.2 - Clinical photographs of a surgical templates in the Brånemark System Novum. This patient was scheduled for placement of three implants into the anterior mandible: guide template *(a)*, evaluation template *(b)*, positioning template *(c)*, and V-template *(d)*.

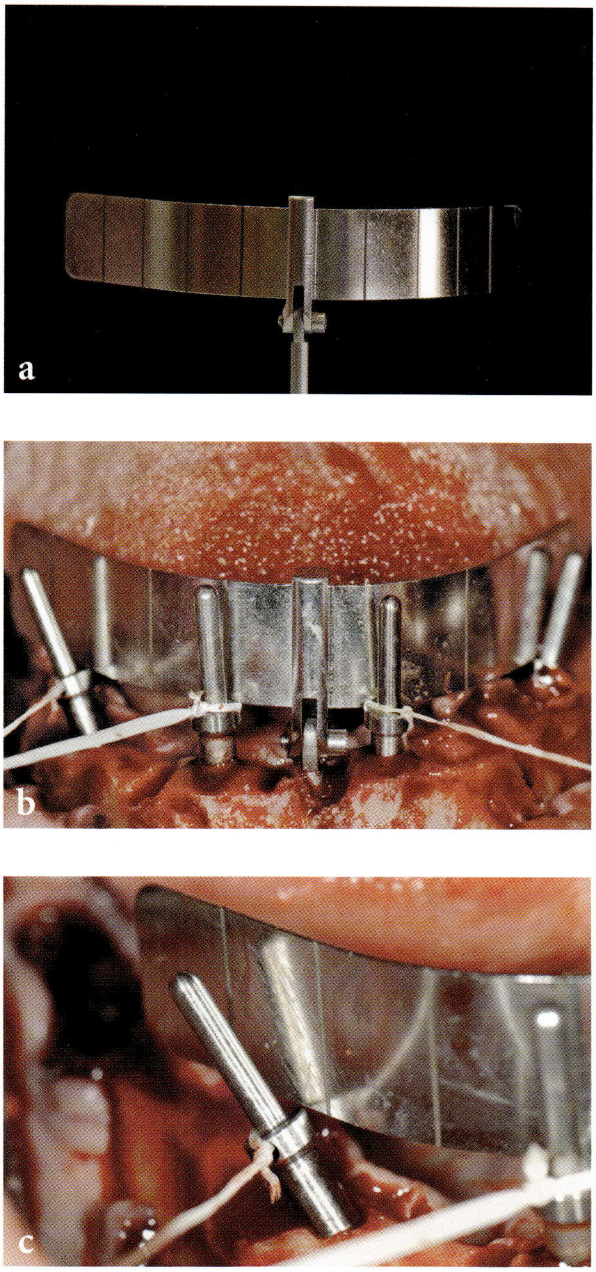

Fig 3.3 - *(a)* Surgical guide used with the All-on-4 technique. *(b)* The All-on-4 surgical guide was anchored into the mandibular midline by means of an articulated pin. *(c)* This image clearly shows the vertical lines in the surgical guide; the implant was placed with a distal inclination of 45 degrees (± 10 degrees).

Radiographic-Surgical Templates

In general, radiographic-surgical templates are made in acrylic resin. They are duplicated from satisfactory preexisting dentures or from wax trial dentures (Fig 3.4). The templates are radiopaque, so they can be worn during radiographic surveys (Fig 3.5). A radiopaque image of an artificial tooth in computerized axial tomography is called a computer profile image (CPI) (Fig 3.6).[10,11] The CPI serves as a reference. It gives clinicians a starting point from which to analyze the position of the tooth relative to the crest of the residual ridge or edentulous site. The position of the CPI in relation to the alveolar bone supplies important diagnostic data that enables the clinician to determine the most suitable implant

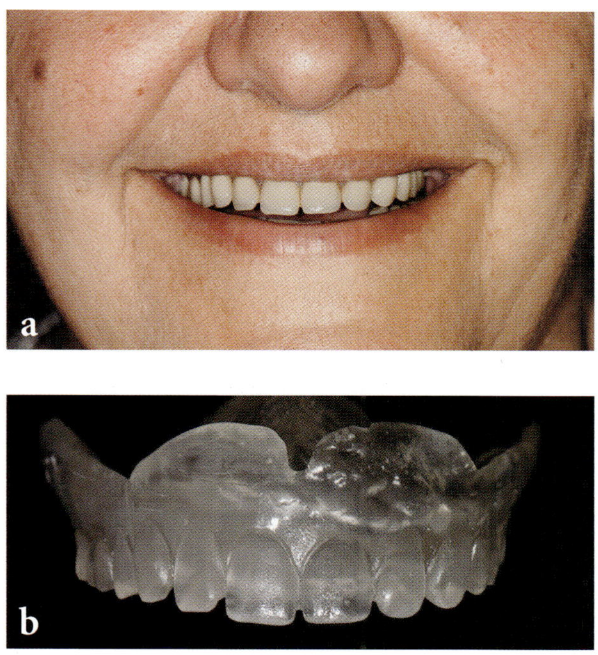

Fig 3.4 - *(a)* Preoperative photograph of a patient with a maxillary complete denture in place. The patient liked the esthetics of the existing denture. *(b)* The maxillary complete denture was duplicated in clear acrylic resin.

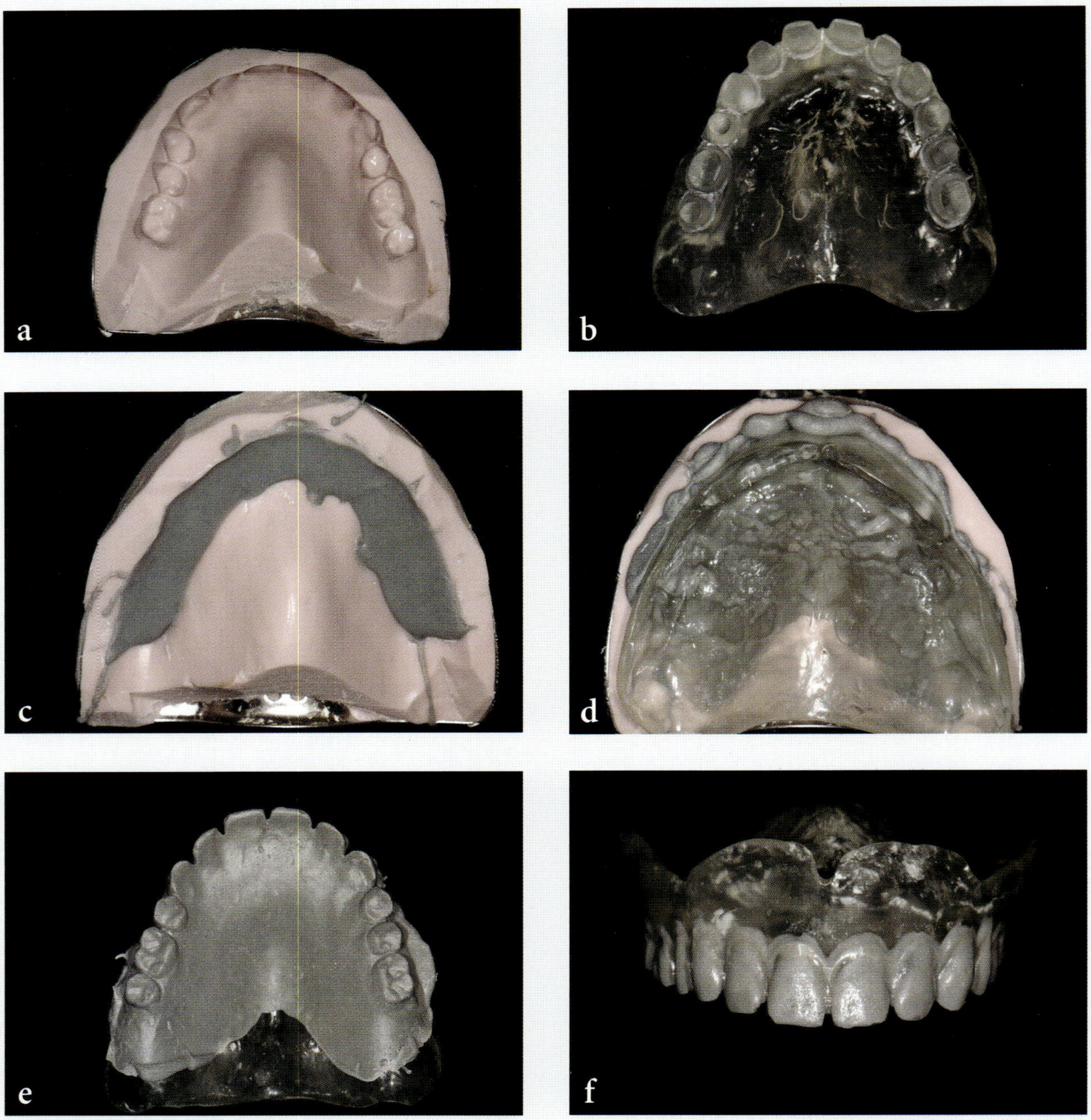

Fig 3.5 - *(a)* Fabrication of the scanning appliance begins with a silicone impression of the occlusal surface of the duplicate of the preexisting maxillary complete denture. *(b)* The occlusal, labial, and palatal surfaces of the teeth in the surgical guide are reduced by approximately 2 mm. *(c)* Autopolymerizing acrylic resin is mixed in the usual proportions. Approximately 20% amalgam powder (volume) is added to the mix. The resin is poured into the occlusal portion of the silicone impression. *(d)* The clear duplicate denture that was modified is repositioned in the mold. *(e and f)* After the resin polymerized, the scanning appliance is removed from the silicone impression, and the appliance is finished and polished. *(g)* Prior to sending the patient for scanning, the scanning appliance is tried into the patient's mouth and adjusted as needed. The scanning appliance must fit comfortably, be stable and retentive, and reproduce the occlusal relationship of the preexisting denture.

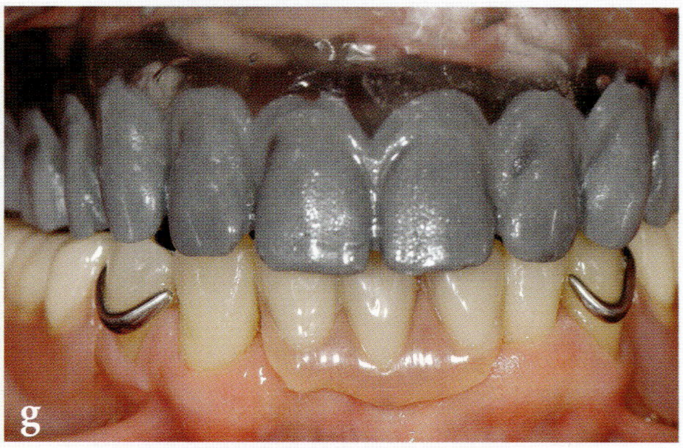

site for an optimal restoration. Later, this same template may be modified for clinical use during the surgical treatment phase (Fig 3.7).[12] Note, however, that a CPI should not be used with implants placed immediately after tooth extraction.

Stereolithographic Templates

Stereolithography is a computer-guided process that creates three-dimensional models using a laser beam that polymerizes liquid resin per digitized data from a computed tomography (CT) scan.[13] These surgical templates were conceived for a type of implant placement surgery called *flapless surgery*.[14-19] Flapless surgeries eliminate incisions and reflecting surgical flaps, which significantly reduces operating times and the postoperative swelling, pain, and edema that are secondary to the soft tissue trauma caused by full-thickness flaps.[20] Because this laser-guided process depends on digitized data, a preoperative CT scan is necessary. Consequently, stereolithographic templates cannot be made in conventional dental laboratories. Rather, they are produced in specialized centers that have purchased the expensive, sophisticated equipment needed to carry out the procedure (Figs 3.8 and 3.9). Stereolithographic templates can be used for edentulous and partially edentulous patients and may be tooth, mucosa, or bone supported.[21-23] They generally do not prove satisfactory in treating

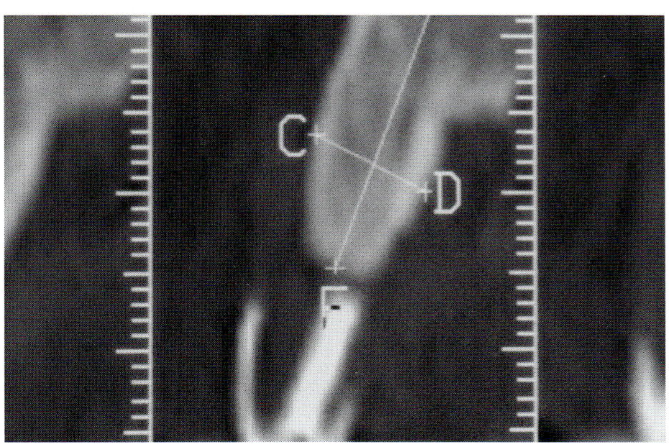

Fig 3.6 - The scanning appliance is radiopaque and identifies the location of the teeth in the scan. Clinicians now can visualize the planned location of the teeth relative to the amount of bone in a given location. This facilitates the selection of optimal implant lengths and diameters.

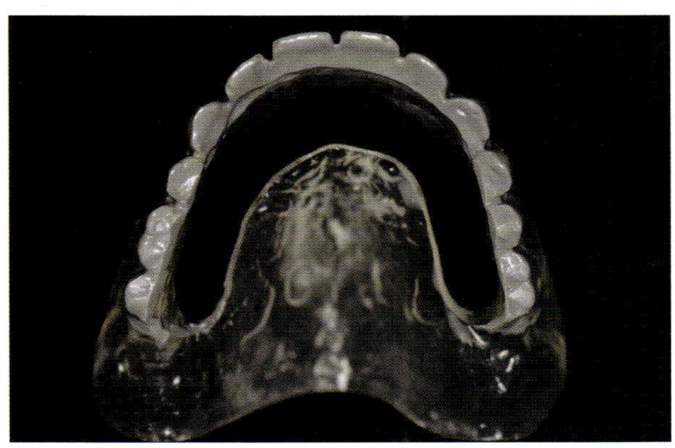

Fig 3.7 - The scanning appliance is further modified for clinical use during the implant surgery by removing the occlusal and palatal aspects of the artificial teeth. The flanges should be approximately 2 mm thick.

multiple dental extractions and alveoloplasties, however, since the postextraction contours of the alveolus cannot be estimated accurately. Difficulties in three-dimensional reconstruction sometimes arise in the rehabilitations of maxillary segments, as modern volumetric tomography has a precision of 70% to 80% in the maxilla. Furthermore, conventional CT scanning does not guarantee 100% accuracy. Some of the commercially available CT protocols use digitized data from the original CT scan to guide construction of the definitive prosthesis and its metal framework. Currently, these procedures do not possess the required accuracy for constructing definitive metal frameworks that will fit passively and accurately onto implants for immediate occlusal loading. One manufacturer has tried to overcome this deficiency by manufacturing special components that eliminate misfit that may exist between the

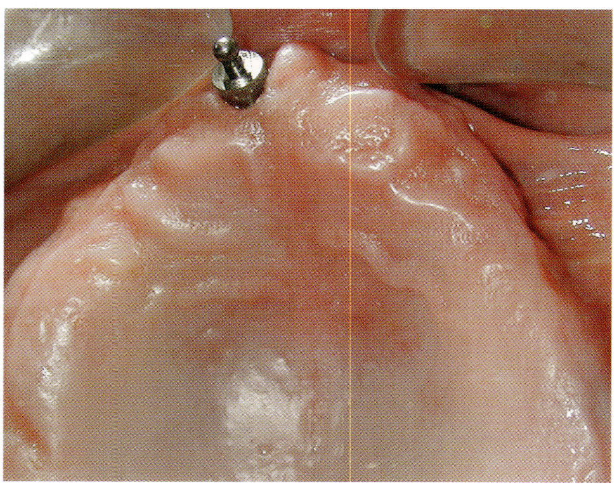

Fig 3.8 - Clinical occlusal image of a patient with an edentulous maxilla. This patient will be treatment planned using the NobelGuide system for CT treatment planning, including a stereolithographic surgical guide.

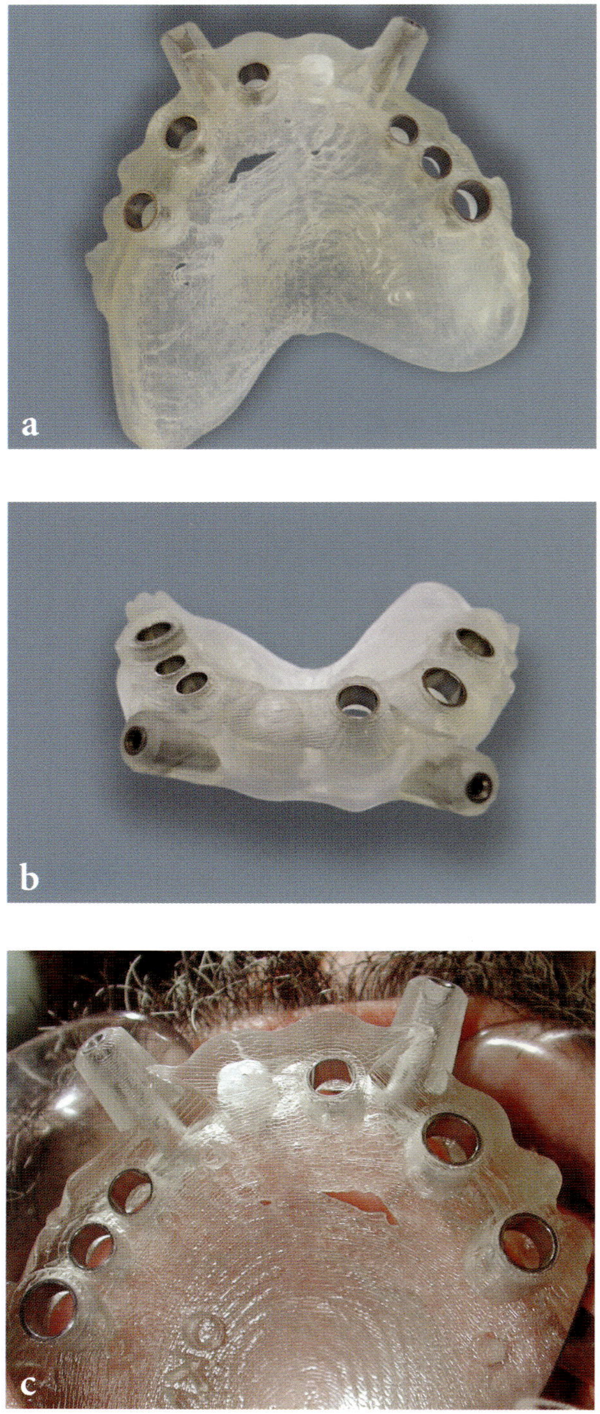

Fig 3.9 - (*a to c*) Images of a NobelGuide stereolithographic template designed for the insertion of six implants with a flapless surgical protocol. Two horizontal fixation screws were treatment planned to anchor the guide into the maxilla. (*Courtesy of Dr Ilario Peano and Dr Roberto Simondi, Italy.*)

implants and frameworks.[24] Particularly, Teeth-in-an-Hour (Nobel Biocare) was a concept developed for immediate loading where the implant process started with the partial denture construction away from the patient, thus saving chair time. However, problems could occur with the partial denture delivery. Adjustable abutments (interlocked, two-piece sleeves) were constructed to eliminate misfit between the implants and the framework. Theoretically, this technique was extremely convenient, but in reality, the definitive partial denture precision was debatable. So, Teeth-in-an-Hour was relegated early on, and no scientific follow-up was carried out except for a 12-month study.[25] The specific indications and high costs associated with stereolithography limit its wide-scale use. At present, stereolithographic templates are suitable for use in only a select group of patients.[17]

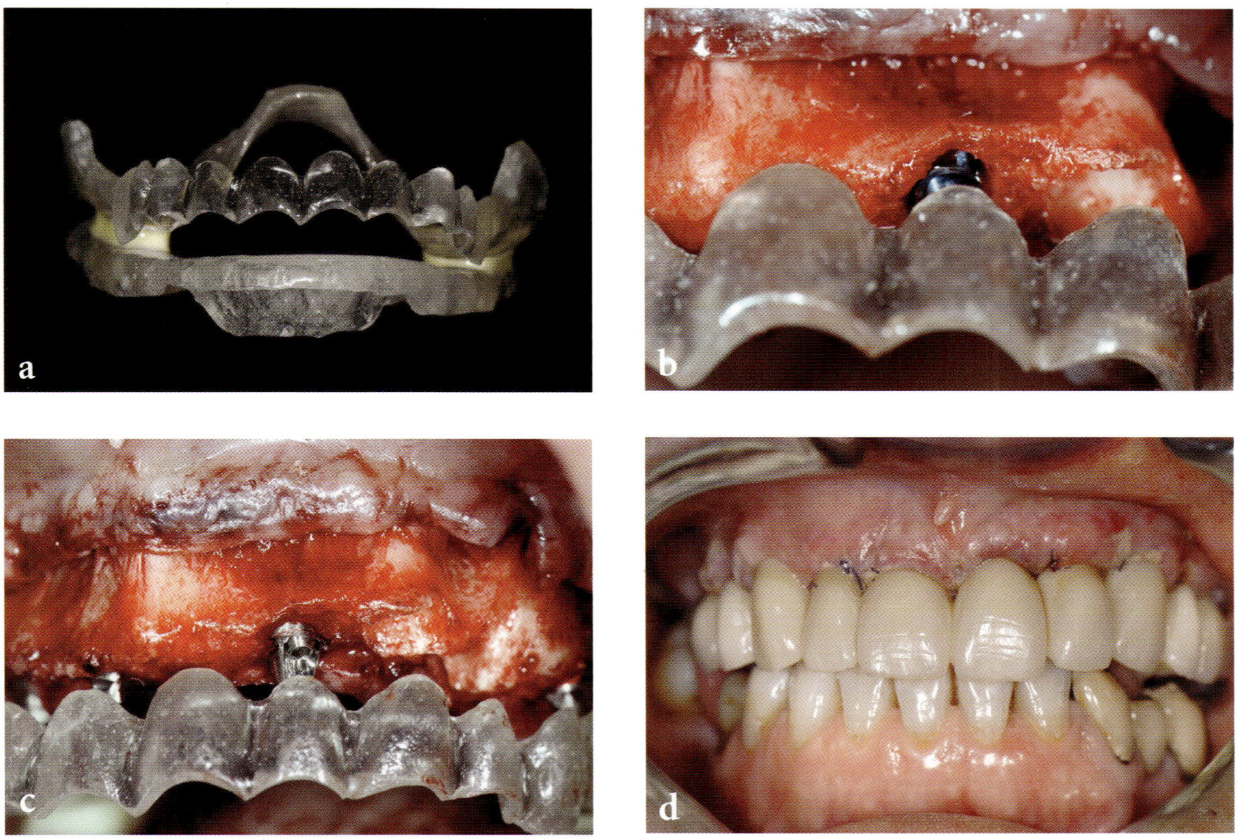

Fig 3.10 - Columbus Bridge Protocol. *(a)* Facial image of an acrylic resin surgical-prosthetic template for use with immediate-loading procedures. *(b)* Clinical image of a surgical-prosthetic template in place. An implant has been placed consistent with the location of the maxillary left lateral incisor. *(c)* Clinical image of a surgical-prosthetic template in place. The preangled abutments have been placed consistent with the location of the teeth in the surgical template. *(d)* Clinical image of a patient immediately after insertion of a maxillary provisional implant prosthesis that demonstrates the correlation between the anticipated position of the implants during the treatment planning process and the actual location of the implants. The emergence profiles of the implants and abutments and the location of the screw access openings were anatomically correct.

Surgical-Prosthetic Templates

Surgical-prosthetic templates were created specifically for an immediate occlusal loading protocol where clinicians need a surgical guide for the correct positioning of the implants and for the correct choice and orientation of the abutments within the implant fixed prosthesis. These templates are made with conventional prosthodontic materials and according to conventional prosthetic treatment planning (Fig 3.10). The diagnostics and construction of these surgical templates are described in the rest of the chapter.

DIAGNOSTIC PROCEDURES

Diagnostic procedures include a series of evaluations that enable clinicians to choose the type of fixed prosthesis most suitable for patients who may be candidates for the Columbus Bridge Protocol. Candidate patients may already be edentulous, with healed extraction sites, or they may be made edentulous at the time of implant placement. Fixed prosthetic options include a full-arch fixed prosthesis either *(1)* with (Toronto bridge; Fig 3.11) or *(2)* without reconstruction of the soft tissues (natural fixed bridge; Fig 3.12).

Edentulous Patients

When treating edentulous patients, clinicians must evaluate the esthetic and functional characteristics of the existing complete dentures. If a prosthesis is satisfactory for the patient and the clinician, it can be used as the starting point in implant-prosthetic

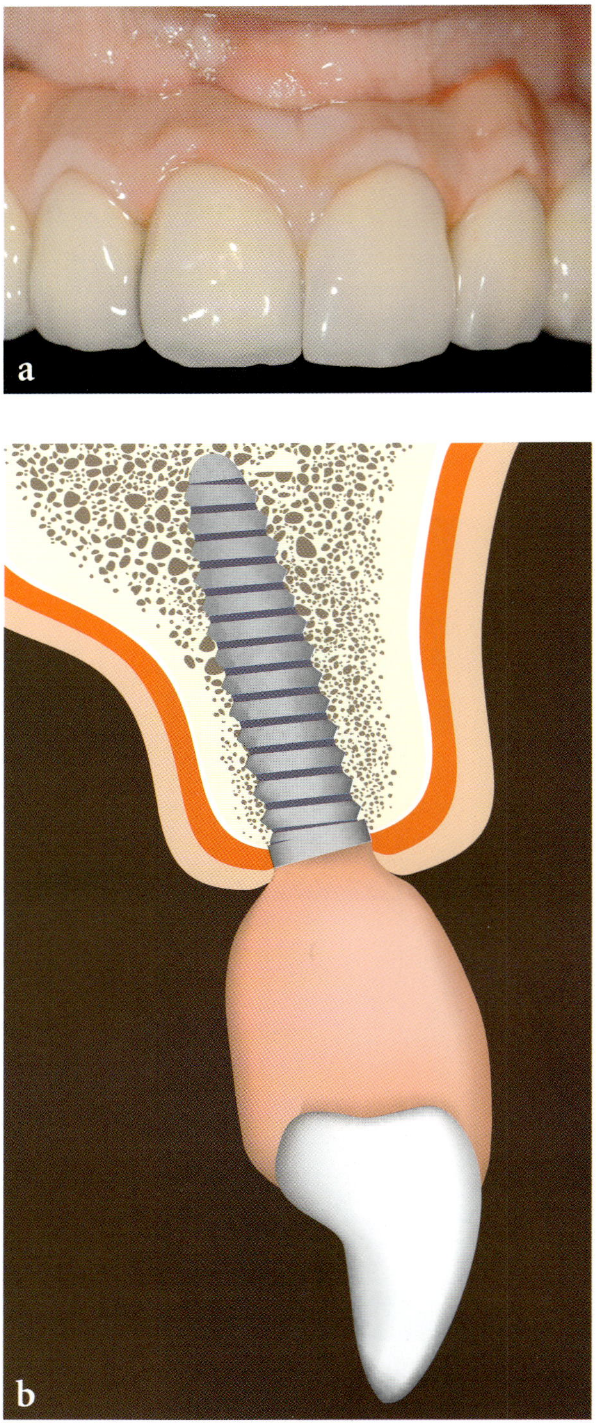

Fig 3.11 - *(a)* Clinical anterior image of a patient who was treated with a Toronto bridge. The missing soft tissues were replaced with gingiva-colored composite resin on the prosthesis. *(b)* Cross-sectional schematic illustration of the anterior portion of a Toronto bridge.

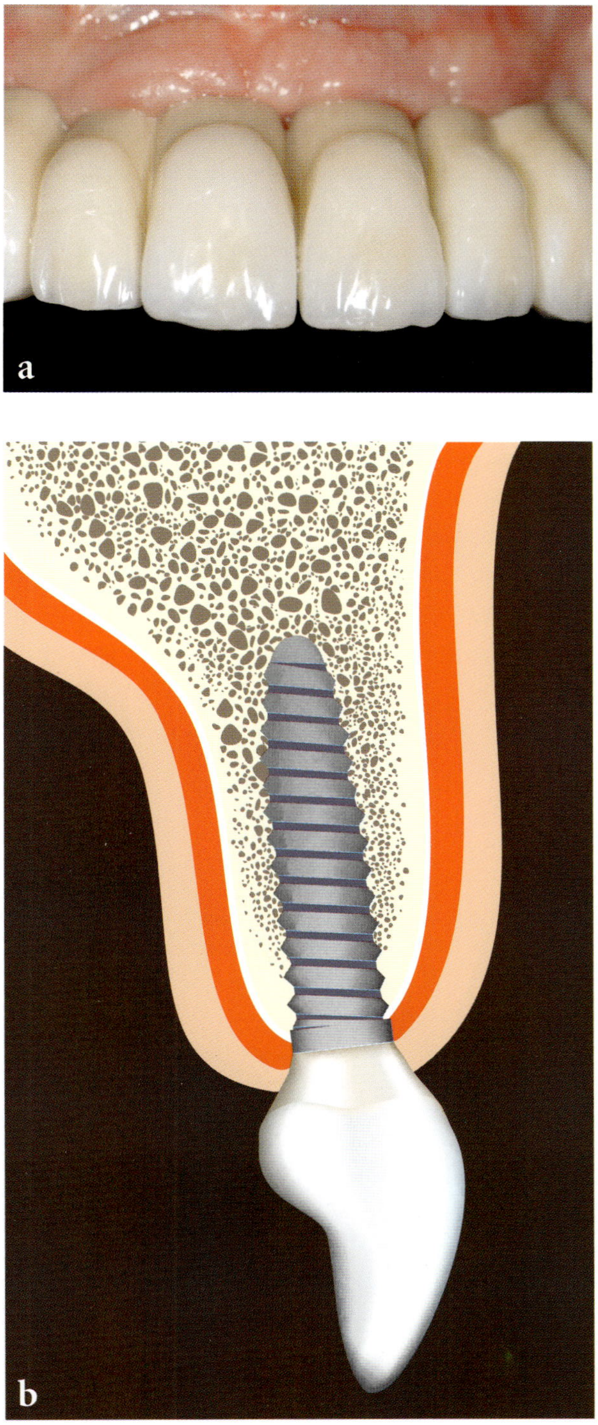

Fig 3.12 - *(a)* Clinical anterior image of a patient who was treated with a fixed prosthesis who did not need replacement of the soft tissues. This type of prosthesis is called a *natural fixed bridge. (b)* Cross-sectional schematic illustration of the anterior portion of a natural fixed bridge.

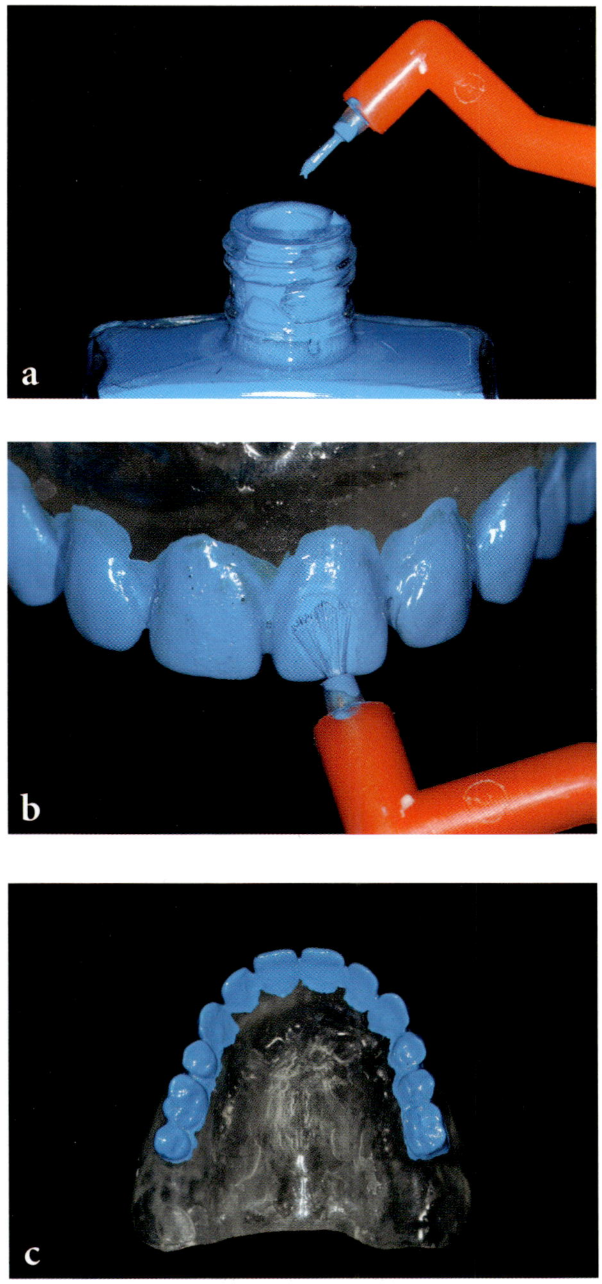

Fig 3.13 - (*a to c*) Laboratory images of another technique used to fabricate a radiopaque scanning appliance. This technique calls for placing multiple layers of a radiopaque liquid onto the labial and palatal surfaces of an acrylic resin template. This method is practical, quickly accomplished, and inexpensive.

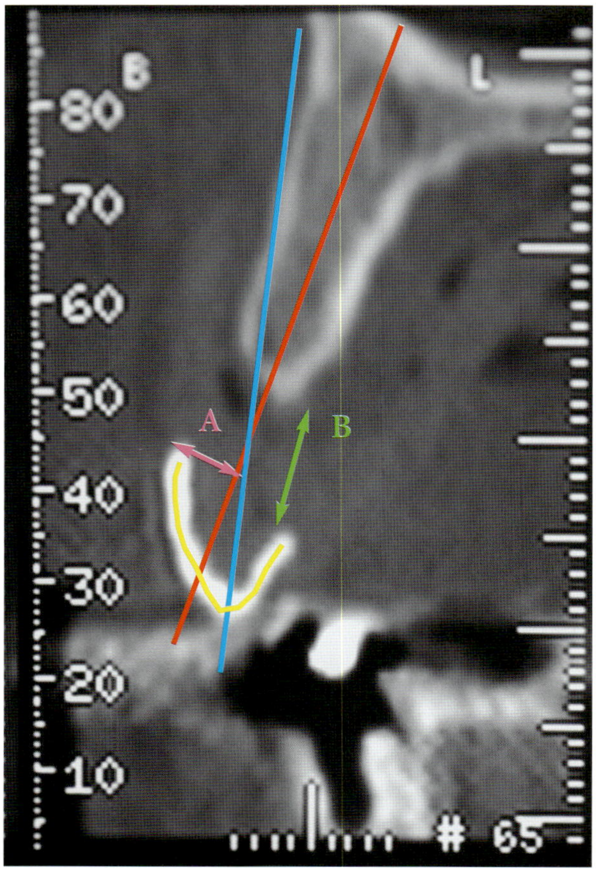

Fig 3.14 - Cross-sectional image of a CT scan with a scanning appliance in place. Labial profile of the artificial tooth (*yellow*); long axis of the tooth (*blue*); long axis of the implant (*red*); distance between the labial surface of the artificial tooth and the long axis of the implant (*arrow A*); distance between the cervical portion of the artificial tooth and the crest of the edentulous ridge (*arrow B*).

Fig 3.15 - *(a)* Clinical profile image of a patient with a maxillary complete denture in place. *(b)* Clinical profile of the same patient without the maxillary complete denture. This image demonstrates the amount of support the maxillary labial flange provides to the patient's upper lip. A fixed prosthesis is contraindicated in this case because of the anterior cantilever and the difficulties associated with oral hygiene. *(c)* Cross-sectional schematic illustration of an anterior maxillary overdenture designed with a labial flange that would support the upper lip.

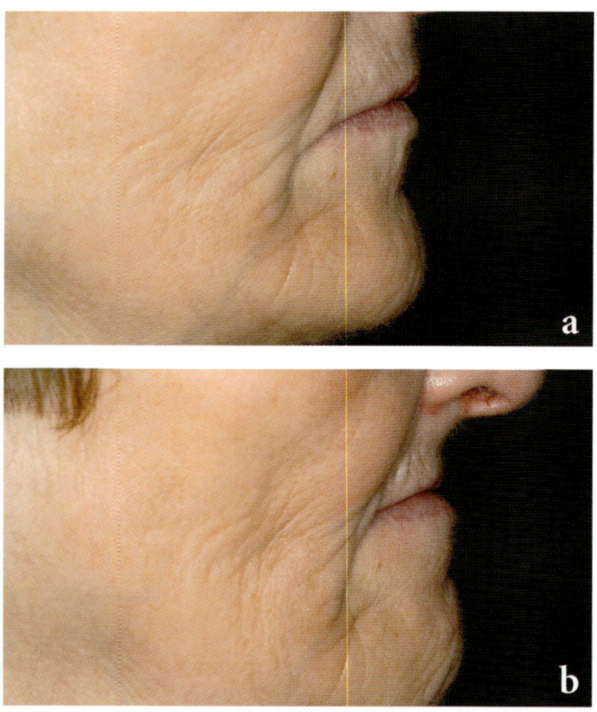

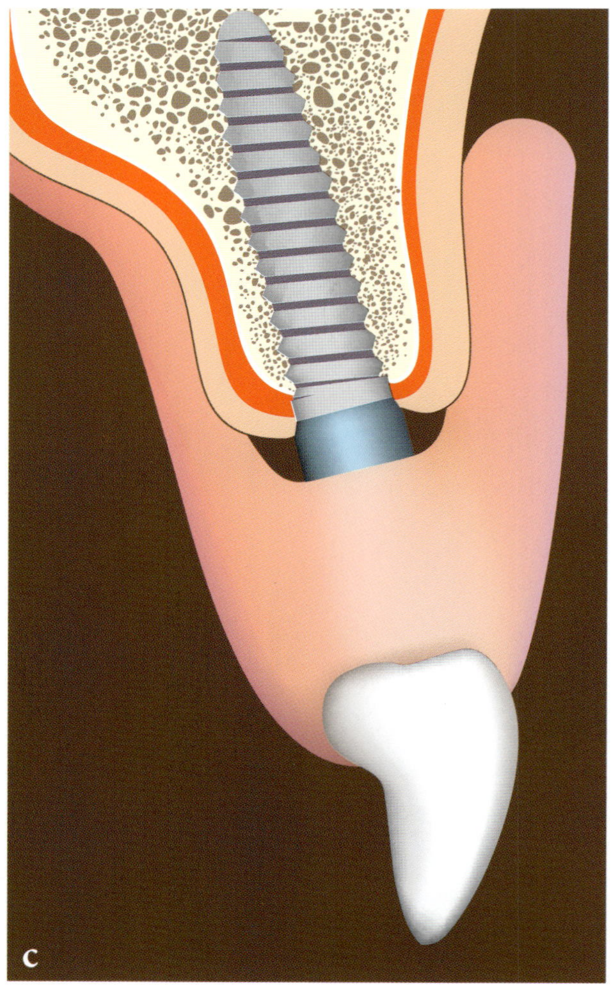

treatment. If the prosthesis is unsatisfactory to the patient or clinician, new prostheses will have to be fabricated so the surgeon can identify the implant locations relative to the planned positions of the artificial teeth. In either case, the prostheses are duplicated with autopolymerizing acrylic resin for use as radiographic templates per Mecall and Rosenfeld.[10,11] These templates can be made radiopaque quickly and inexpensively by painting them with four to five layers of spacer, to which has been added amalgam powder (20% in volume) for each artificial tooth (Fig 3.13). The radiographic template is placed into the patient's mouth, and a CT scan is made, after which the CPI is evaluated, and the definitive treatment planning process begins (Fig 3.14). Clinical situations with marked residual ridge or bone resorption and significant prosthetic overjet (see Fig 3.14; A > 5 mm) require maxillary implant-retained overdentures with labial flanges (Fig 3.15), a design that is easily and predictably accomplished. Overdentures are also required in the treatment of other clinical situations as well–for patients who have high smile lines or unacceptable phonetics with fixed prostheses or certain biomechanical situations–but these cases are not discussed in this textbook. When the distance between the cervical portion of the artificial teeth and the implant restorative platform is greater than 25% of the length of the artificial tooth (Fig 3.16; B > 25%), the recommended treatment protocol should include soft tissue reconstruction, ie, a Toronto bridge prosthesis. When the distance between the cervical portion of the artificial teeth and the implant restorative platform is less than 25% of the length of the

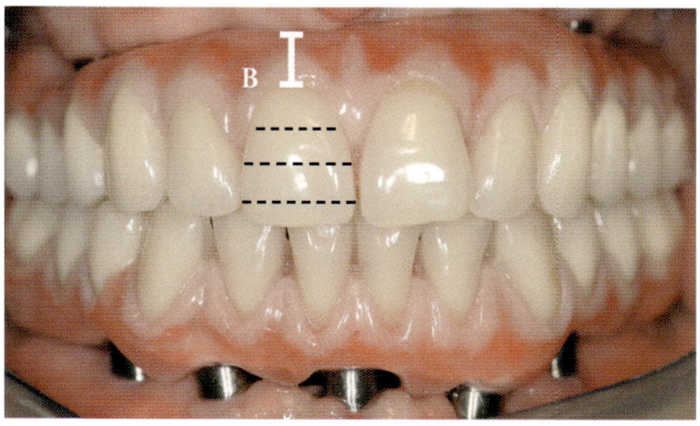

Fig 3.16 - Clinical anterior image of a patient treated with maxillary and mandibular fixed prostheses. If distance B is greater than 25% of the clinical length of the central incisor (artificial tooth), it is advisable to fabricate a prosthesis that replaces the missing soft tissues.

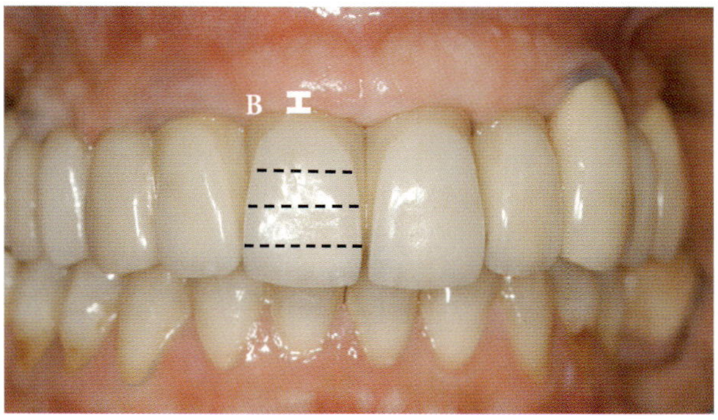

Fig 3.17 - Clinical anterior image of a patient treated with a maxillary fixed prosthesis. If distance B is less than 25% of the clinical length of the central incisor (artificial tooth), it is possible to fabricate the prosthesis without replacing the soft tissues since minimal resorption has occurred and soft tissue replacement is not required.

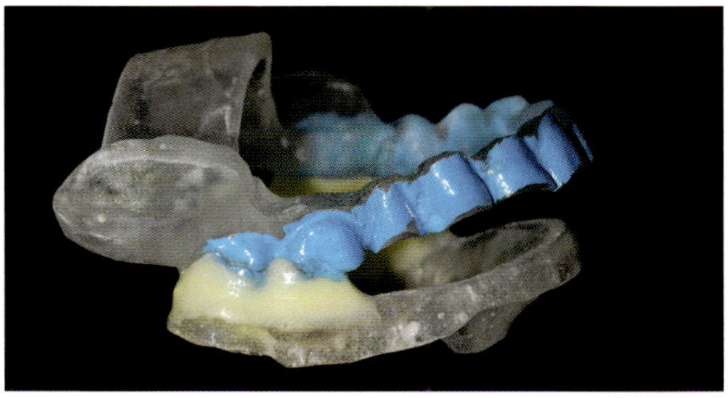

Fig 3.18 - Laboratory image of a finished surgical-prosthetic template. This maxillary portion was also used as the scanning appliance. Note the blue radiopaque material that was placed onto the labial surfaces of the maxillary teeth.

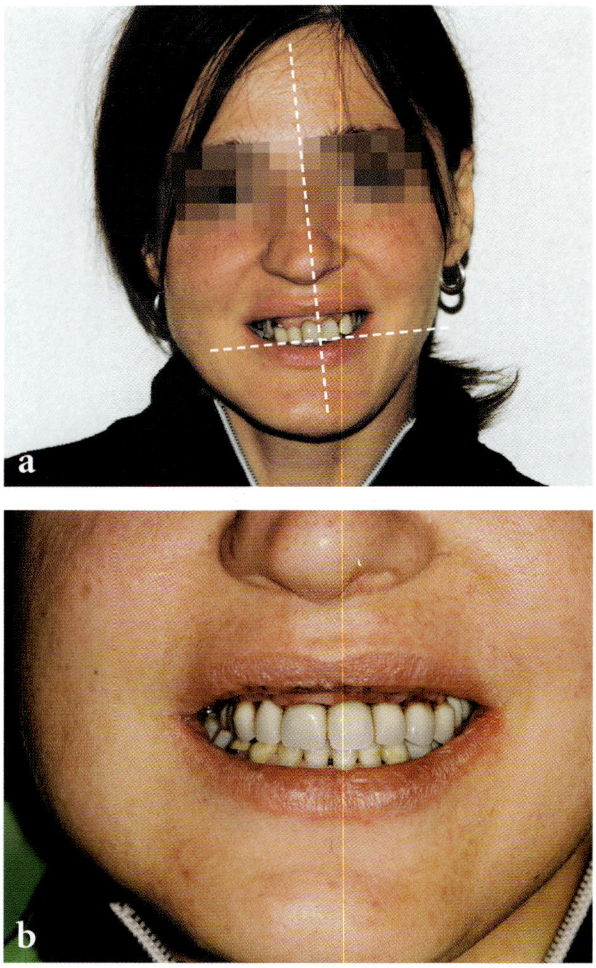

Fig 3.19 - *(a)* Facial, preoperative anterior image of a patient with marked asymmetries of the gingival architecture and occlusal plane. *(b)* Facial, postoperative anterior image of the patient 24 hours after extractions, implant placement, and insertion of an immediate fixed provisional prosthesis. The asymmetries were corrected with the maxillary prosthesis.

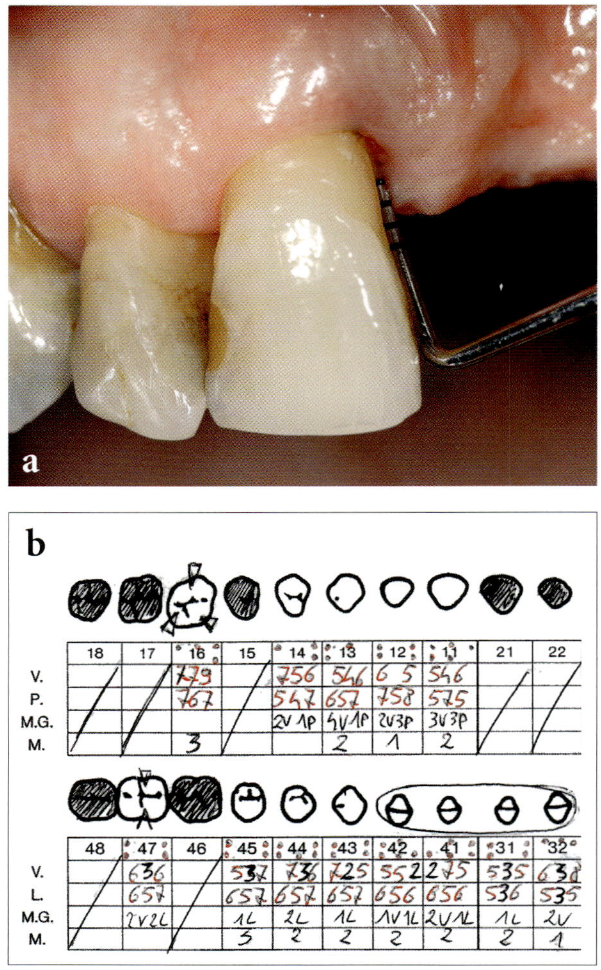

Fig 3.20 - *(a)* Clinical image of a periodontal probe in place in the mesiobuccal gingival sulcus of a maxillary right central incisor. Probing is one of the most important factors in determining the prognosis of a given tooth and developing treatment plan options. *(b)*Preoperative periodontal chart.

artificial tooth (Fig 3.17; B < 25%), the recommended treatment protocol should be similar to the natural dentition, ie, a natural fixed bridge. Before proceeding with the surgical treatment, the template must be modified so that it is retained and stabilized on the occlusal and incisal edges of the mandibular dentition per the technique in the following paragraphs (Fig 3.18).

Patients Made Edentulous at the Time of Implant Placement

The initial esthetic evaluation must include the analysis of the symmetries of the occlusal plane in the frontal plane, the positioning of the interincisal line (Fig 3.19), and the type and location of the smile line (high, medium, low). Periodon-

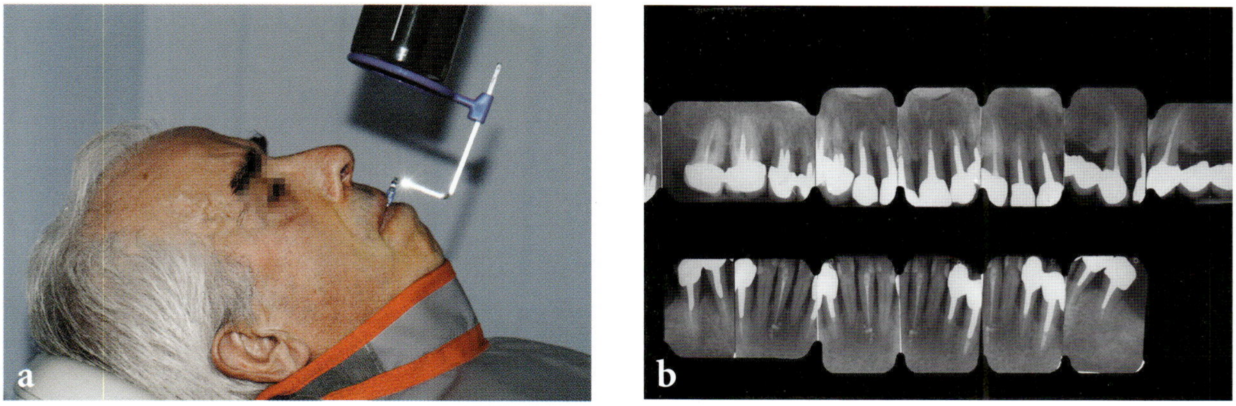

Fig 3.21 - *(a)* Clinical image of a patient in position for maxillary periapical radiographs. The parallel technique should be used for intraoral radiographs. *(b)* Example of an intraoral periapical radiographic series.

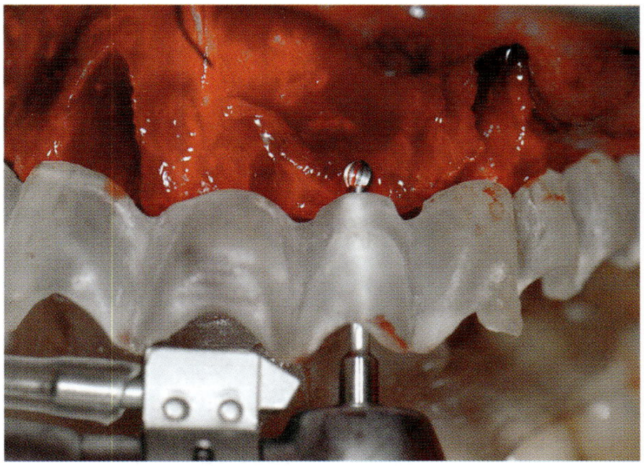

Fig 3.22 - This patient's maxillary dentition is going to be restored with a natural fixed bridge. This is a clinical image with the surgical-prosthetic template in place. A round bur was used to identify the planned location of the implant consistent with the locations of the teeth in the template. With this type of prosthesis, the location of the osteotomy must be consistent with the location of the artificial tooth.

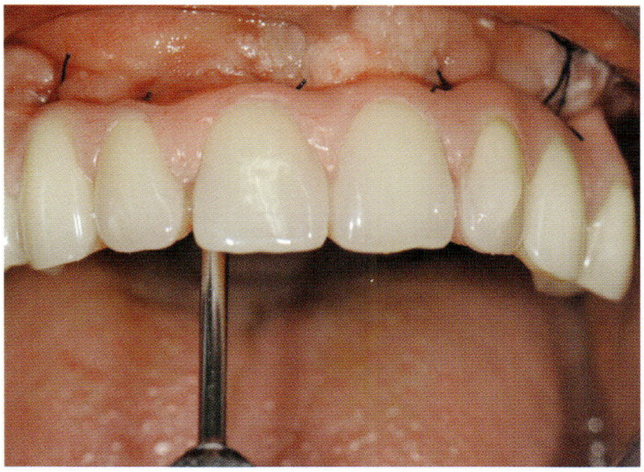

Fig 3.23 - Clinical anterior image of a patient treated with a fixed Toronto bridge. The orientation of the screwdriver indicates that this implant was inserted only consistent with the buccal and palatal profiles of the planned future prosthesis.

tal probing of the natural teeth completes the examination (Fig 3.20).

Thorough evaluation of the residual dentition (Fig 3.21) requires a systematic intraoral radiographic examination. In the case of large edentulous areas, a CT scan is also required for treatment planning. Severe horizontal bone loss with periodontal pocket measurements of approximately 5 mm is an indication for a prosthesis that replaces the hard and soft tissues associated with attachment loss (ie, Toronto bridge). For patients presenting with periodontal pockets less than 5 mm deep and with natural teeth compromised secondary to dental caries and/or endodontic failures, the indicated implant-prosthetic treatment would likely consist of a prosthesis that does not replace soft tissues (ie, natural fixed bridge). The accurate determination of the most appropriate prosthetic design is essential to optimal treatment because of its impact on implant placement. In the full-arch fixed prosthesis without reconstruction of the soft tissues, implant position is critical to developing optimal emergence profiles of the future artificial teeth (Fig 3.22). In the full-arch fixed prosthesis with replacement of the soft tissues, the implants must be positioned inside the volume of the planned future prosthesis–although the authors believe it is not necessary to place the implants within the mesiodistal emergence profiles of the planned future teeth (Fig 3.23). In both of these cases, the screw access openings of the abutments should be positioned so that the prosthetic retaining screws are contained within the occlusal and palatal surfaces of the artificial teeth (Fig 3.24).

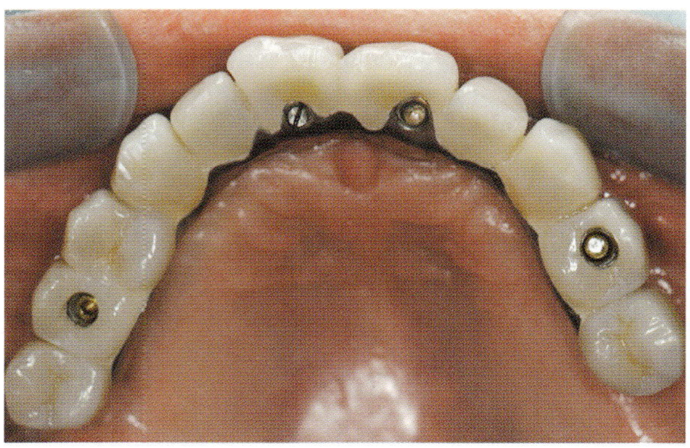

Fig 3.24 - Occlusal view of a screw-retained fixed prosthesis. In this prosthesis, all of the access openings were located within the boundaries of the occlusal table.

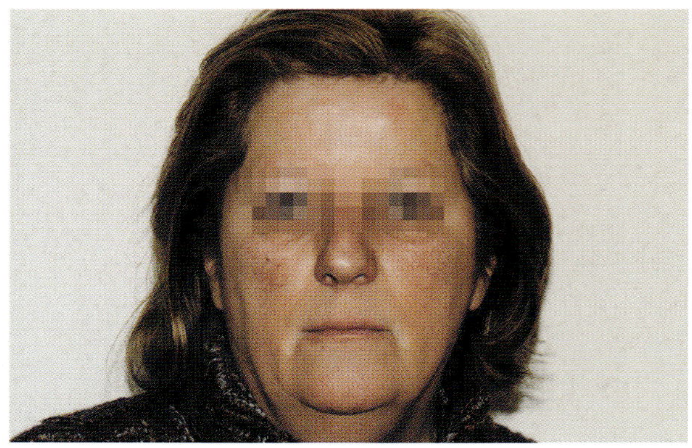

Fig 3.25 - Clinical frontal image of the patient at rest with the prosthesis in place and her lips closed.

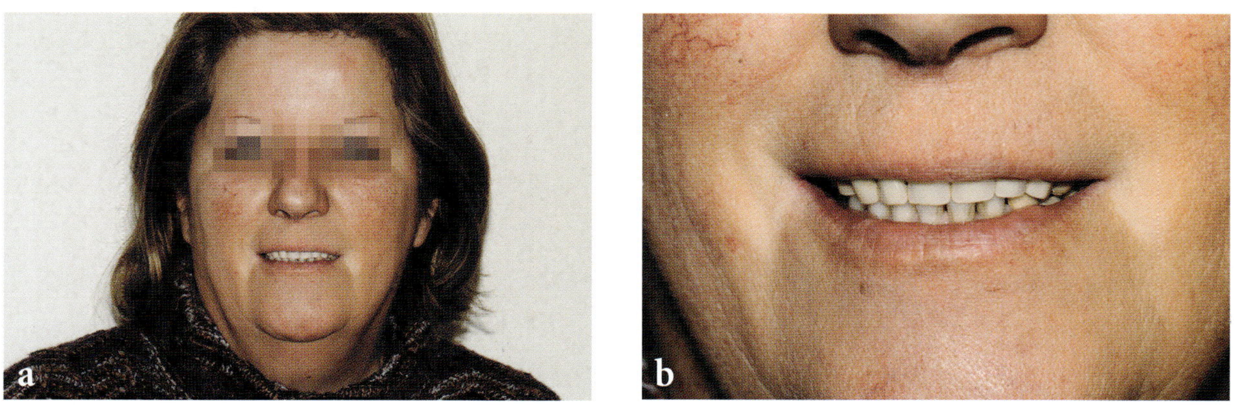

Figs 3.26 - *(a)* Clinical frontal image of the patient smiling with the prosthesis in place. *(b)* Clinical anterior close-up image of the patient with the prosthesis in place and smiling.

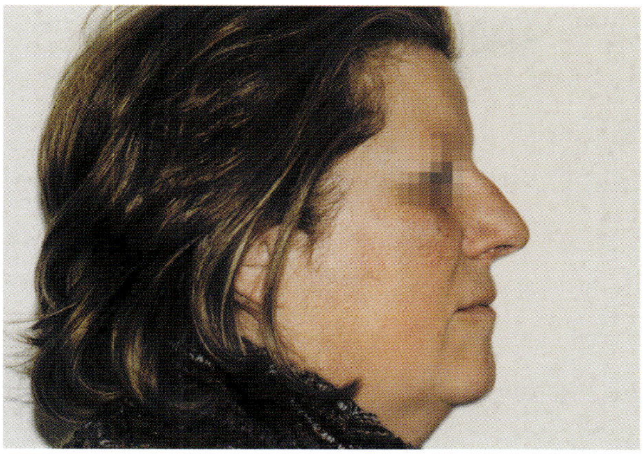

Fig 3.27 - Clinical profile image of the patient at rest with her lips closed.

FABRICATION OF A SURGICAL-PROSTHETIC TEMPLATE ACCORDING TO THE COLUMBUS BRIDGE PROTOCOL

Initially, the clinician takes a series of photographs of the patient that will convey important clinical characteristics of the preoperative condition to the dental laboratory technicians. It is important that the clinician position herself or himself directly in front of the patient to avoid making geometric distortions of the images.

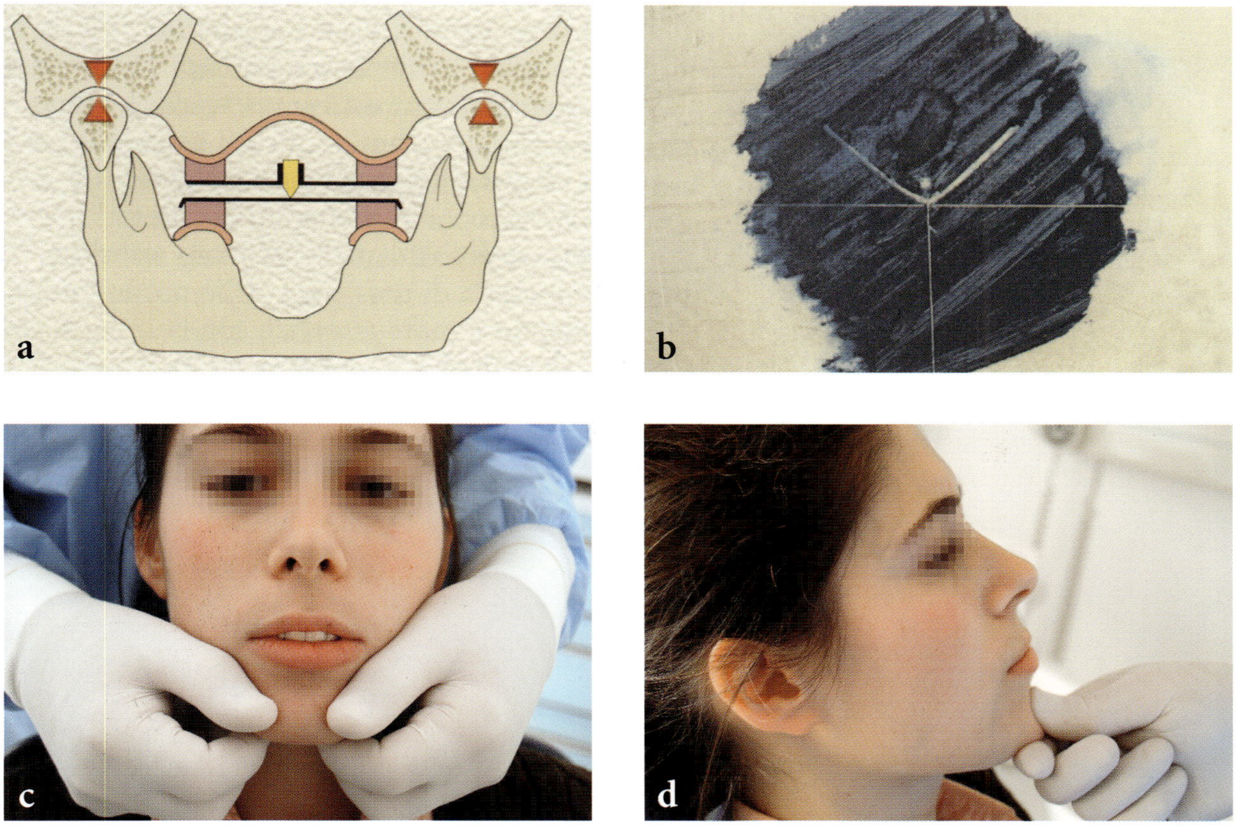

Fig 3.28 - *(a and b)* Schematic illustration of a centric relation record with a Gothic arch tracing and a central bearing point. (Reprinted from Preti and Gassino[4] with permission). *(c)* Clinical image of recording centric relation with bimanual mandibular manipulation according to Dawson. *(d)* Clinical image of recording centric relation according to the chin-point technique by McCollum.

Frontal photographs should include closed mouth (Fig 3.25), frontal smiling (Fig 3.26), and lateral profile, not smiling (Fig 3.27).

Centric relation is then measured and recorded. The recording of the centric relation position depends mainly on manipulation of the mandible, consistent with the patient's neuromuscular relaxation. In patients who cannot be manipulated, the best method to obtain centralization of the condyles in the glenoid fossae is to use the central bearing point technique of McGrane, with the subsequent recording of a Gothic arch tracing.[26] In patients who can be manipulated, two interocclusal wax records are made by guiding the mandible into centric relation through bimanual manipulation of the mandible, according to Dawson,[27] or through guiding the gnathion (chin point), according to McCollum (Fig 3.28).[28]

Thanks to the interocclusal wax records, the maxillary and mandibular casts are mounted into an articulator. The centric relation is a useful reference because it is a limit position, independent of tooth contact, reproducible even when the patient is made edentulous.[29] After 4 months, at the time of constructing the definitive prosthesis, the centric relation position is checked and reevaluated.[30] In the Columbus Bridge Protocol, the interocclusal records are made with Hard Beauty Pink Wax (Miltex) softened in a bowl with hot water. The first wax record preserves the intermaxillary position at the correct vertical dimension of occlusion. This wax record is called the *thin wax record* and is made from one or two sheets of material (Figs 3.29a and 3.29b).

The second wax interocclusal record is called the *thick wax record* (Fig 3.29c) and is made from three to five sheets of Hard Beauty Pink Wax.

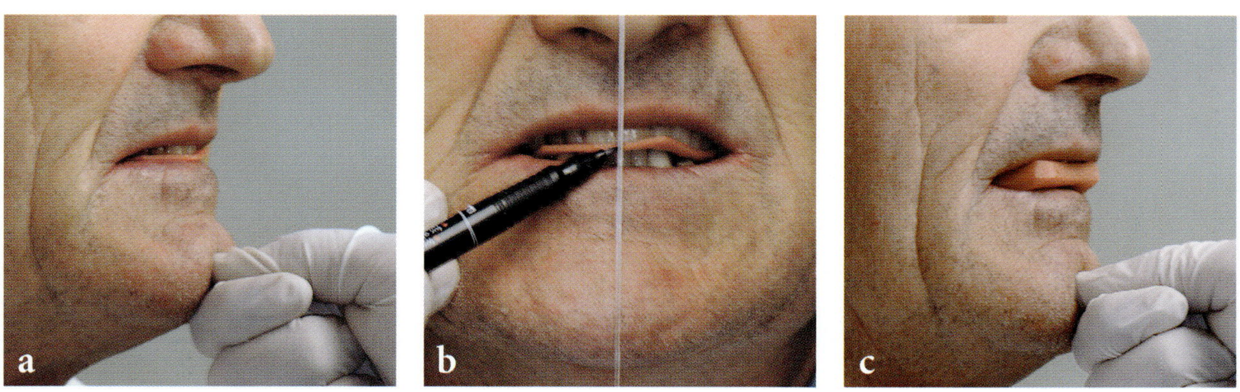

Fig 3.29 - *(a)* Thin wax record made with a thin wax wafer at the correct vertical dimension of occlusion. *(b)* The facial midline is marked onto the thin wax interocclusal record. *(c)* Thick wax record made with a thick wax wafer that should contain the movement of the mandible to rotation, avoiding translation.

The increase in the vertical dimension of occlusion induced by the thick wax record is insignificant provided that the increase is moderate since it is made in the context of the terminal hinge axis. This results in pure rotation of the condyles without translation. Clinically, the increased vertical dimension caused by the thickness of the interocclusal records allows the clinician the requisite visual access to the surgical field. The symmetric center of the face is marked on the thin wax record with an indelible felt-tip pen, and the interocclusal wax records are carefully cooled with a spray of air and water before being removed from the oral cavity. An alginate impression is made of the treatment arch for construction of a diagnostic cast, and two alginate impressions are made of the opposing dentition. At the end of this appointment, three impressions and three casts will have been made (Box 3.1). The working casts are made with type IV plaster. The thin wax record is used to help fit the casts into an articulator at medium values. The original opposing cast is removed from the articulator, and the second opposing cast is mounted into the articulator with the thick wax record. The incisal guide pin is not changed. The second opposing cast articulation, with the increased interocclusal distance, will be used in the last preoperative phase in constructing the surgical template.

The clinician evaluates the articulator mounting with the thin wax record, the photographs, and the findings associated with the esthetics of the existing dentition and patient perceptions to make decisions regarding the overall treatment. These decisions may be consistent with the preoperative condition, or they may warrant a new esthetic setup. In the latter case, the dental technician will reduce the bone crest (on the diagnos-

BOX 3.1 - PREOPERATIVE CLINICAL RECORDS

- Clinical frontal image of the patient at rest with closed lips
- Clinical frontal image of the patient smiling
- Clinical profile image of the patient with closed lips
- Thin wax record
- Thick wax record
- Alginate impression of the treatment arch
- Two alginate impressions of the opposite dentition
- Preoperative periodontal chart

tic cast) based on the depths of the periodontal pockets and attachment loss supplied by the dentist (Figs 3.30 to 3.33). The esthetic setup is carried out with artificial denture teeth.

A silicone index is then made in the laboratory. It records the contours and arrangement of the artificial teeth that are considered optimal for the patient. The first surgical-prosthetic template for the maxilla is manufactured in acrylic resin (ProBase, Ivoclar Vivadent). The autopolymerizing acrylic resin is poured into the silicone mold to create a duplicate of the maxillary teeth. The inner portion of the template is removed, leaving a buccal boundary 2 mm thick and a palatal portion that supports the maxillary surgical guide in

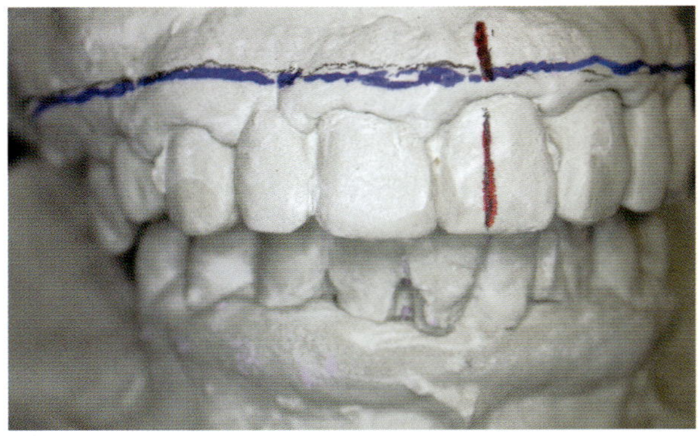

Fig 3.30 - Laboratory image of mounted diagnostic casts for construction of the surgical-prosthetic template according to the Columbus Bridge Protocol. The casts were mounted into the articulator, set with medium values, with the thin wax record. The facial midline marked on the thin wax record is reported as a red line on the casts. Average sulcular depths obtained from the clinical pocket measurements were also marked directly on the cast (*blue line*).

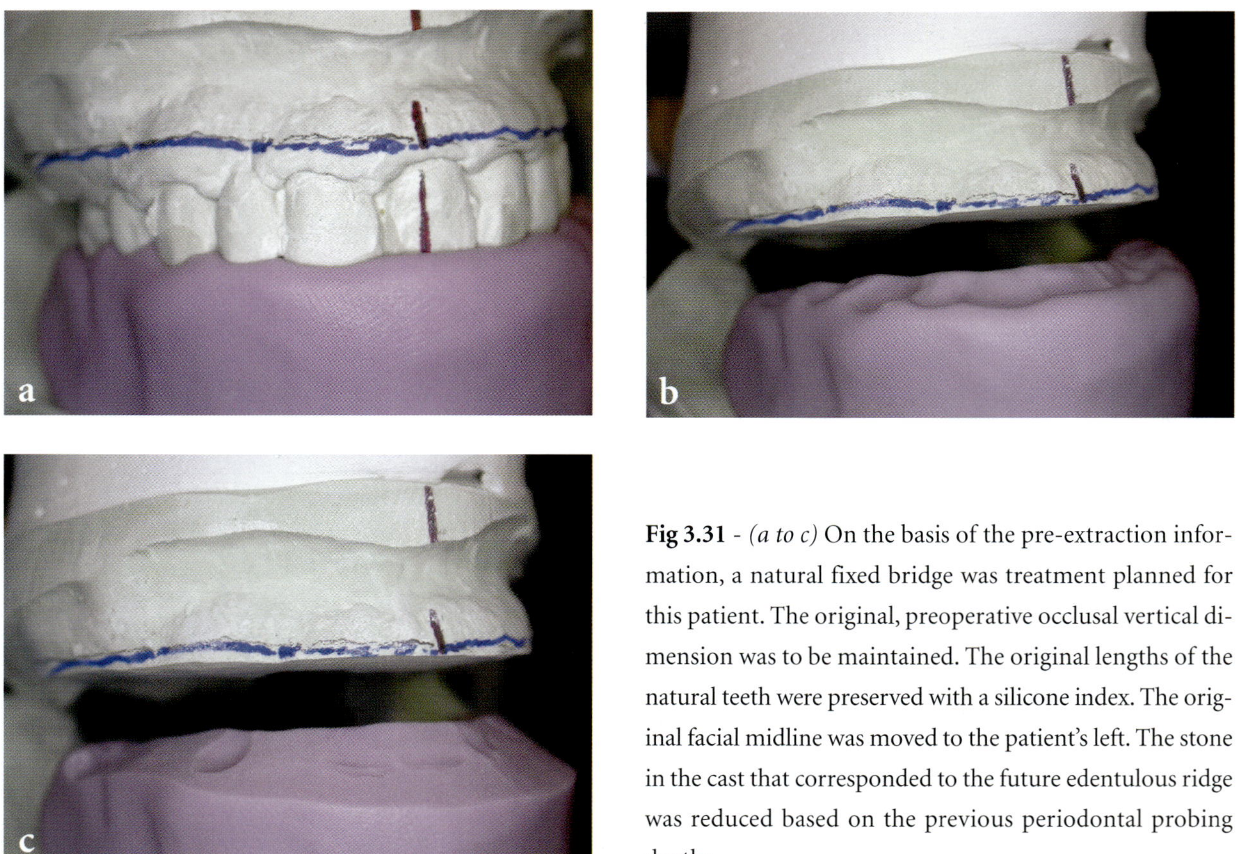

Fig 3.31 - *(a to c)* On the basis of the pre-extraction information, a natural fixed bridge was treatment planned for this patient. The original, preoperative occlusal vertical dimension was to be maintained. The original lengths of the natural teeth were preserved with a silicone index. The original facial midline was moved to the patient's left. The stone in the cast that corresponded to the future edentulous ridge was reduced based on the previous periodontal probing depths.

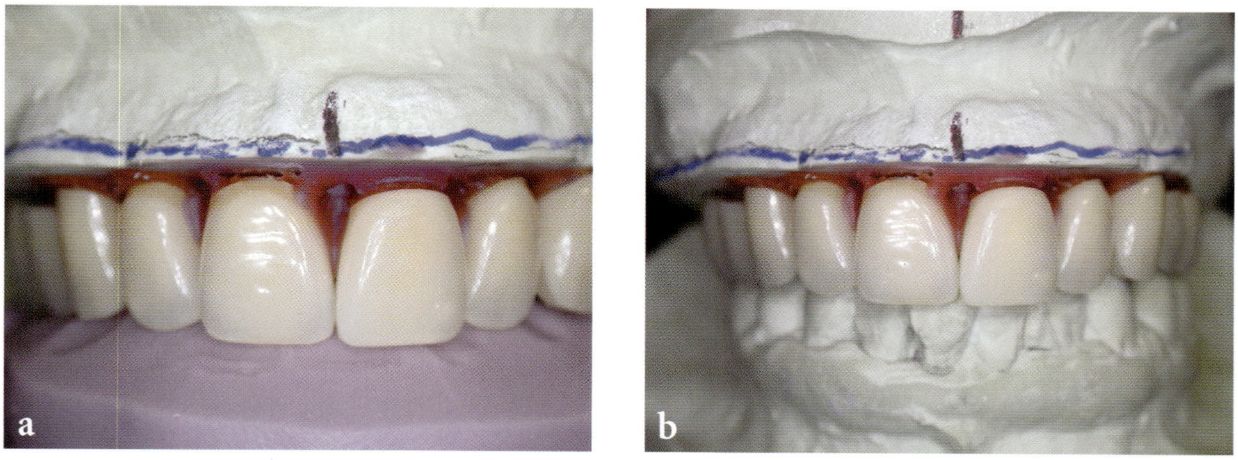

Fig 3.32 - *(a and b)* Artificial denture teeth were placed into their correct positions using the laboratory silicone index.

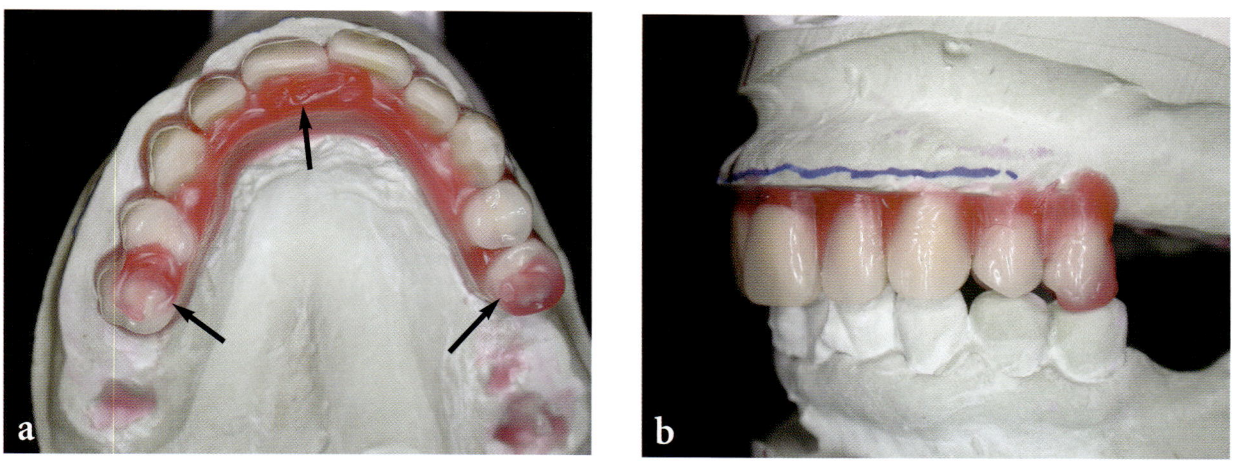

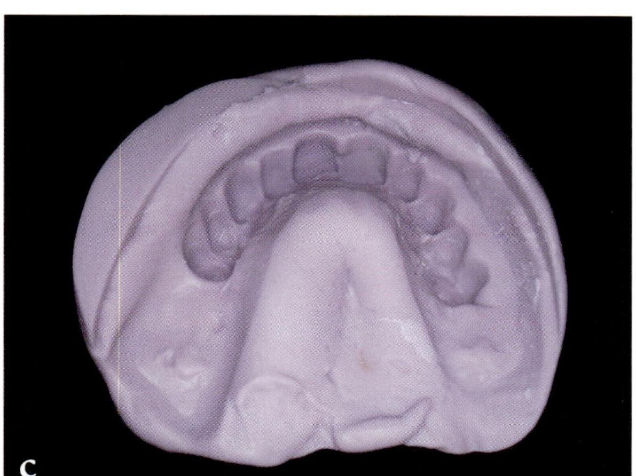

Fig 3.33 - *(a and b)* Prior to processing the surgical-prosthetic template, three occlusal stops are waxed onto the palatal and occlusal surfaces of the wax prosthesis (*black arrows*). *(c)* A silicone index was made of the wax prosthesis. Autopolymerizing acrylic resin was poured into the silicone impression, replicating the contours of the wax prosthesis. The device will occlude against the opposing cast as well as the original wax prosthesis did. This appliance will be used after surgery to fabricate the fixed provisional prosthesis (see Fig 9.29).

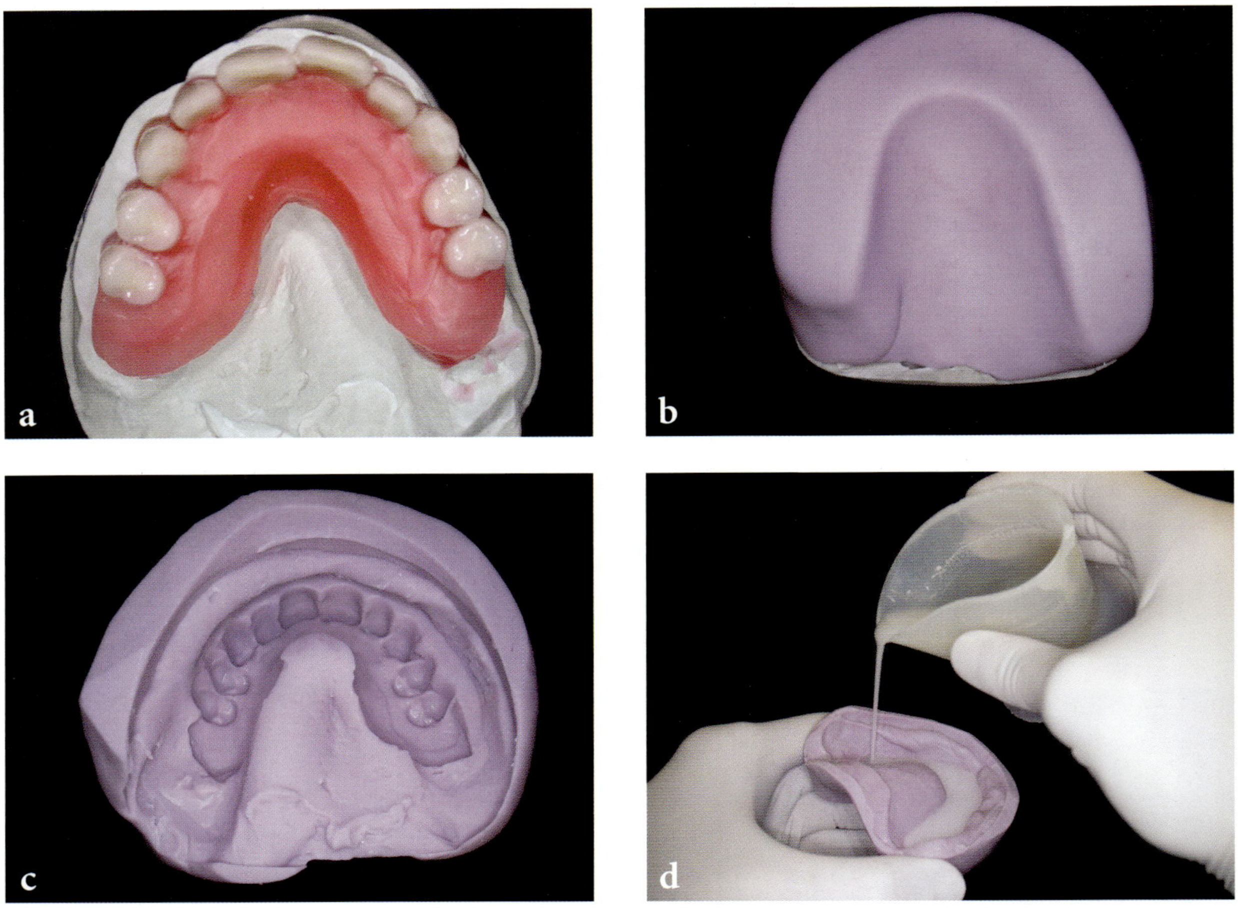

Fig 3.34 - *(a)* The occlusal stops were removed; the palatal surface of the denture setup was thickened with additional layers of baseplate wax for increased strength of the template. *(b and c)* An update silicone index was created with laboratory silicone putty. *(d)* The first part of the surgical template was created by pouring acrylic resin into the mold of the laboratory silicone impression.

its correct position during the surgery. The material is allowed to polymerize fully. Additional acrylic resin is mixed, placed onto the occlusal and incisal edges of the teeth in the mandibular cast, and allowed to polymerize (Figs 3.34 and 3.35). On the casts mounted with the thick wax record, the two resin surgical prosthetic template are luted together. This stabilizes the surgical-prosthetic template intraorally because the mandibular dentition remains unchanged during the maxillary treatment (Figs 3.36 and 3.37). In maxillary treatment, the inferior part of the template is retained by the mandibular teeth and/or mucosa while the superior part is supported partly by the maxillary tuberosities and partly by the palatal vault; it is important that the surgeon leave some soft tissue uninvolved with the surgical site (elevation of the flap) to support the surgical template. In mandibular rehabilitations, the superior part of the template is retained and supported by the maxillary teeth and/or mucosa; the inferior portion is supported by the retromolar pads.

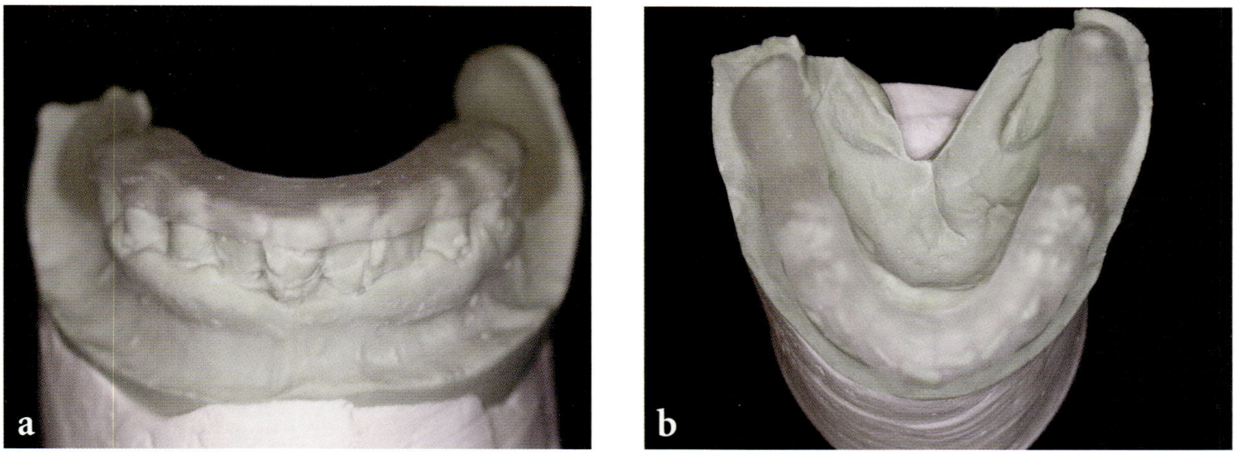

Fig 3.35 - A flat occlusal splint was fabricated in acrylic resin on the opposing mandibular cast. *(a)* Facial view. *(b)* Occlusal view.

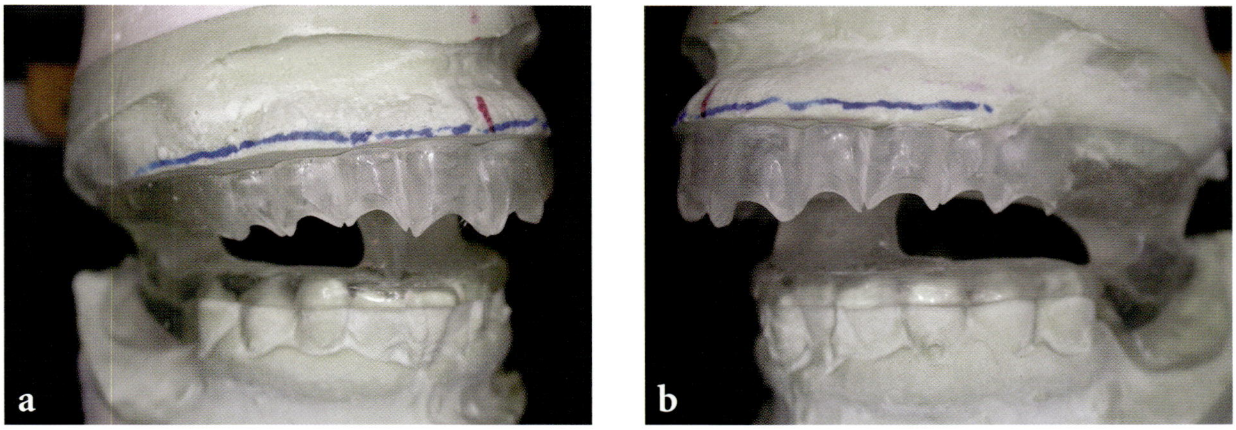

Fig 3.36 - At this point, the maxillary portion of the template was connected to the mandibular portion of the splint with acrylic resin struts. This procedure is carried out on the working casts mounted according to the thick wax record. *(a)* Right lateral view. *(b)* Left lateral view.

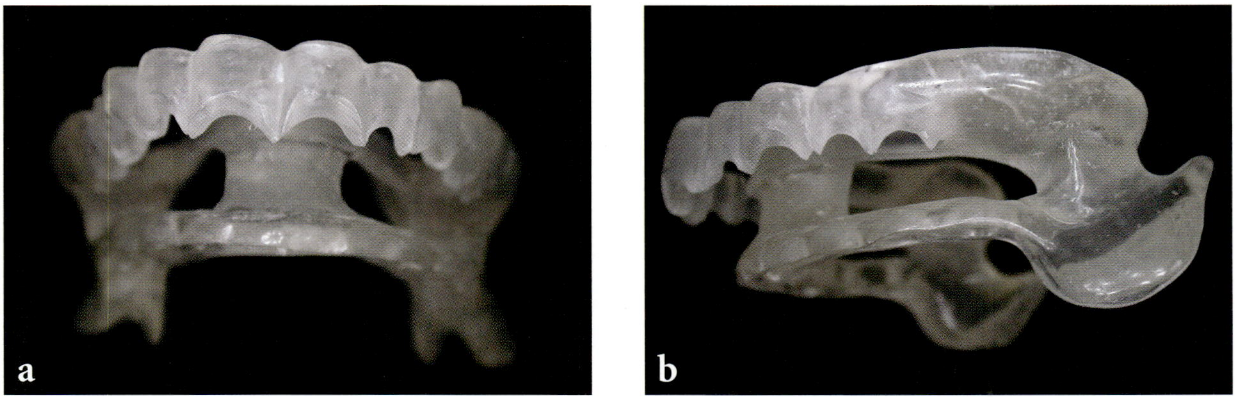

Fig 3.37 - After the acrylic resin set, the surgical-prosthetic template was removed from the casts. It was finished and polished. *(a)* Anterior view. *(b)* Left lateral view.

The surgical template must be finished and polished in such a way that the surgeon can easily insert and remove the template from the oral cavity. Before surgery, the surgical template must be submerged for at least 15 minutes in a bath of disinfectant and then rinsed with physiologic saline solution. The possibility of easily inserting and removing the template according to the operator's necessity provide adequate room for optimal irrigation during osteotomy preparation, a factor more difficult to control when templates for implant positioning are mucosa or bone supported.[31] The removability advantage is exploited twice: first, when the clinician chooses the positions of the implants; second, in the choice and correct positioning of the abutments. In the Columbus Bridge Protocol, the abutment setup is performed prior to closing the surgical flaps (Figs 3.38 to 3.41).

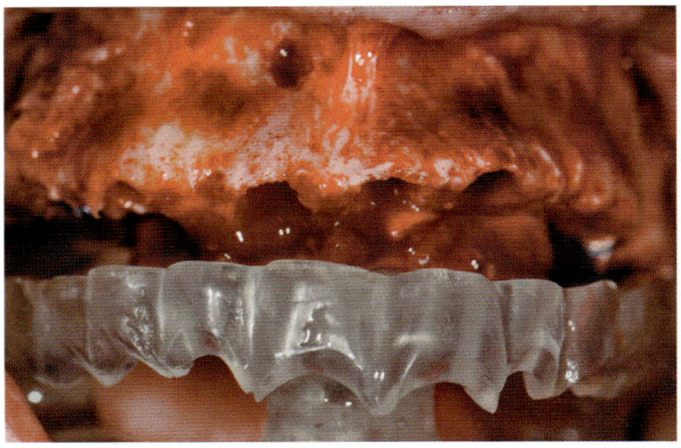

Fig 3.38 - Clinical image of the surgical-prosthetic template in place after removal of the maxillary teeth. The surgical-prosthetic template was retained by the mandibular teeth.

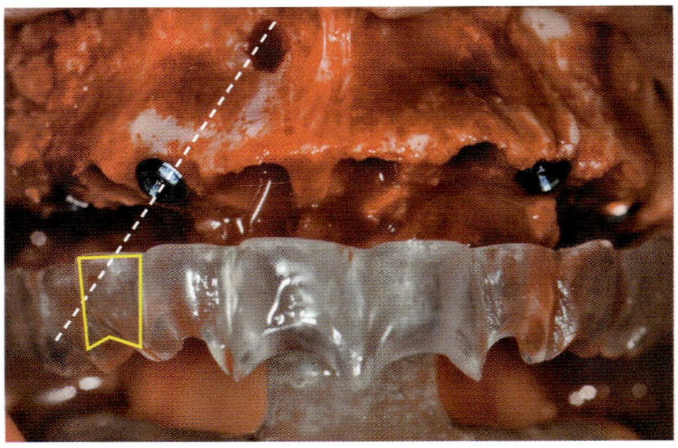

Fig 3.39 - Clinical image with the implants in place. Note that the implant emergence (*dotted line*) respects the mesiodistal emergence profile of the future artificial teeth (*yellow line*).

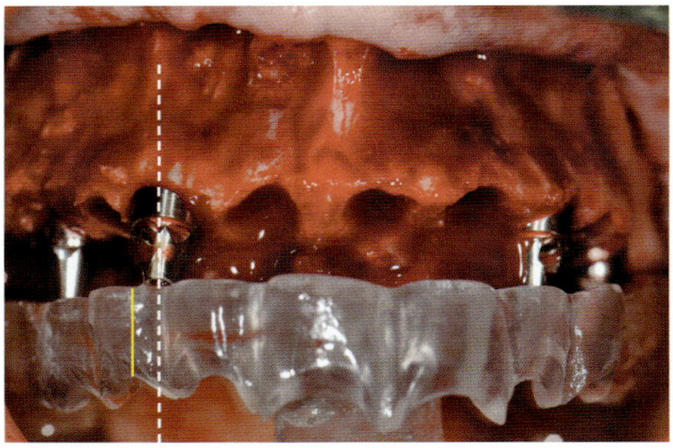

Fig 3.40 - The implant angulations were corrected with the use of preangled conical abutments that placed the screw access openings (*dotted line*) palatal to the facial surfaces of the template (*yellow line*). This orientation was necessary to fabricate a screw-retained prosthesis with optimal esthetics.

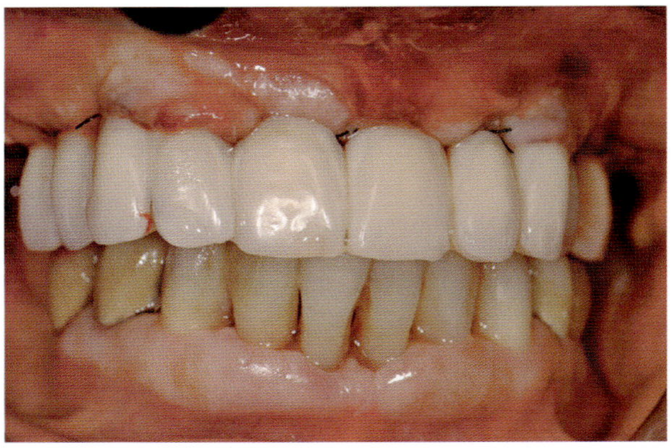

Fig 3.41 - Clinical image immediately after insertion of the maxillary fixed provisional prosthesis. The prosthesis was inserted less than 24 hours after the surgical phase was completed.

REFERENCES

1. Poitras P, Boivin M, Morais J, Picard M, Mercier P. Gastric emptying of solid food in edentulous patients. Digestion 1995;56:483–487.
2. Pera P, Bucca C, Borro P, Bernocco C, De Lillo A, Carossa S. Influence of mastication on gastric emptying. J Dent Res 2002;81:179–181.
3. De Boever JA, Nilner M, Orthlieb JD, Steenks MH. Recommendations by the EACD for examination, diagnosis, and management of patients with temporomandibular disorders and orofacial pain by the general dental practitioner. J Orofac Pain 2008; 22:268–278.
4. Preti G, Gassino G (eds). Management of the Edentulous Patient: A Biological Approach. Berlin: Quintessence, 2008.
5. Assémat-Tessandier X, Sansemat JJ. Surgical guide for prosthetic technic for Brånemark osseointegrated implants [in French]. Cah Prothese 1990;(69):76–87.
6. Modica F, Fava C, Benech A, Preti G. Radiologic prosthetic planning of the surgical phase of the treatment of edentulism by osseointegrated implants: An in vitro study. J Prosthet Dent 1991;65:541–546.
7. Brånemark PI, Engstrand P, Ohrnell LO, et al. Brånemark Novum: A new treatment concept for rehabilitation of the edentulous mandible. Preliminary results from a prospective clinical follow-up study. Clin Implant Dent Relat Res 1999;1:2–16.
8. Maló P, Rangert B, Nobre M. "All-on-Four" immediate-function concept with Brånemark System implants for completely edentulous mandibles: A retrospective clinical study. Clin Implant Dent Relat Res 2003;5(suppl 1):2–9.
9. Maló P, Rangert B, Nobre M. All-on-4 immediate-function concept with Brånemark System implants for completely edentulous maxillae: A 1-year retrospective clinical study. Clin Implant Dent Relat Res 2005;7(suppl 1):88S–94S.
10. Mecall RA, Rosenfeld AL. The influence of residual ridge resorption patterns on implant fixture placement and tooth position. Part I. Int J Periodontics Restorative Dent 1991;11:9–24.
11. Mecall RA, Rosenfeld AL. The influence of residual ridge resorption patterns on implant fixture placement and tooth position. Part II. Presurgical determination of prosthesis type and design. Int J Periodontics Restorative Dent 1992;12:32–51.
12. Ganz CH. Radiopaque surgical stents: A practical office technique. Dent Econ 1995;85:100–101.
13. van Steenberghe D, Naert I, Andersson M, Brajnovic I, Van Cleynenbreugel J, Suetens P. A custom template and definitive prosthesis allowing immediate implant loading in the maxilla: A clinical report. Int J Oral Maxillofac Implants 2002;17:663–670.
14. Hahn J. Single-stage, immediate loading, and flapless surgery. J Oral Implantol 2000;26:193-198.
15. Kan JY, Rungcharassaeng K, Ojano M, Goodacre CJ. Flapless anterior implant surgery: A surgical and prosthodontic rationale. Pract Periodontics Aesthet Dent 2000;12:467–474.
16. Rocci A, Martignoni M, Gottlow J. Immediate loading in the maxilla using flapless surgery, implants placed in predetermined positions, and prefabricated provisional restorations: A retrospective 3-year clinical study. Clin Implant Dent Relat Res 2003;5(suppl 1):29–36.
17. Becker W, Goldstein M, Becker BE, Sennerby L. Minimally invasive flapless implant surgery: A prospective multicenter study. Clin Implant Dent Relat Res 2005;7(suppl):21S–27S.
18. Calandriello R, Tomatis M. Simplified treatment of the atrophic posterior maxilla via immediate/early-function and tilted implants: A prospective 1-year clinical study. Clin Implant Dent Relat Res 2005;7(suppl):1S–12S.
19. Rao W, Benzi R. Single mandibular first molar implants with flapless guided surgery and immediate function: Preliminary clinical and radiographic study. J Prosthet Dent 2007;98(suppl):3–14.

20. Esposito M, Grusovin MG, Maghaireh H, Coulthard P, Worthington HV. Interventions for replacing missing teeth: Management of soft tissues for dental implants. Cochrane Database Syst Rev 2007;18:CD006697.
21. Sarment DP, Sukovic P, Clinthorne N. Accuracy of implant placement with a stereolithographic surgical guide. Int J Oral Maxillofac Implants 2003; 18:571–577.
22. Marchack CB, Moy PK. The use of a custom template for immediate loading with the definitive prosthesis: A clinical report. J Calif Dent Assoc 2003;31:925–929.
23. Parel SM, Triplett RG. Interactive imaging for implant planning, placement, and prosthesis construction. J Oral Maxillofac Surg 2004;62:41–47.
24. Marchack CB, Moy PK. The use of a custom template for immediate loading with the definitive prosthesis: A clinical report. J Calif Dent Assoc 2003;31:925–929.
25. van Steenberghe D, Glauser R, Blombäck U, et al. A computed tomographic scan-derived customized surgical template and fixed prosthesis for flapless surgery and immediate loading of implants in fully edentulous maxillae: A prospective multicenter study. Clin Implant Dent Relat Res 2005;7 (suppl):111S–120S.
26. Gerber A. Registrirtechnik fur prothetik okklusiondiagnostik, okklusionterapie [manual]. Zurich: Condylator Service, 1974.
27. Dawson PE. Centric relation. Its effect on occlusomuscle harmony. Dent Clin North Am 1979;23: 169–180.
28. Castellani D (ed). Elementi di Occlusione. Bologna: Martina, 1998.
29. Palla S. Myoarthropathien des Kausystems und Orofaziale Schmerzen [thesis]. Zurich: University of Zurich, 1998.
30. Bassi F, Carossa S, Gassino G, et al (eds). Advances in Clinical Prosthodontics. Padova: Piccin, 1999.
31. Eriksson A, Albrektsson T, Grane B, McQueen D. Thermal injury to bone. A vital-microscopic description of heat effects. Int J Oral Surg 1982;11:115–121.

CHAPTER 4
CHOICE OF IMPLANT TYPE

COLUMBUS BRIDGE PROTOCOL	
SURGICAL PROTOCOL	**PROSTHETIC PROTOCOL**
External hex rough-surface implants	Screw-retained fixed prosthesis
Implant length ≥ 13 mm, Ø 4 mm	Plaster impression with pickup technique
Underprepared osteotomy	Rigid splinting with metal framework
Implant insertion torque ≥ 40 Ncm	Passive fit with the luting technique
Angled implants in native bone	Acrylic resin occlusal surfaces
Angled conical abutments	No distal cantilevers
No bone regenerative techniques	Immediate functional load 24–48 h after surgery

Table 4.1

The materials of choice for manufacturing endosseous implants are commercially pure (cp) titanium and titanium alloyed with other elements such as aluminium, iron, molybdenum, niobium, and zirconium. Titanium is well suited for endosseous implants. It has excellent physical properties, and it may offer even better mechanical properties as an alloy than its cp form.[1] Because of titanium's high level of corrosion resistance, it has proven extremely biocompatible. This characteristic can also be attributed to the spontaneous passivation of titanium–that is, in the presence of oxygen, titanium reacts to form a thin surface layer of titanium oxide[2,3] (mainly TiO_2 but also Ti_2O_3 and TiO depending on the depth to which the implant is inserted into the tissue*).

This inert layer protects and insulates the metal from the organism, thus preventing the release of metal ions into the external environment.[5] These ions are thought to be at least partly responsible for activating the phagocytic and immune responses that can lead to implant failure.[6,7]

The cp titanium used for implants is classified into four grades (I to IV) that are differentiated by the percentage of minor elements contained in them and, as a result, by different mechanical properties (Table 4.2). Grades II and

TABLE 4.2 - CHEMICAL COMPOSITION (MAXIMUM %) OF CP TITANIUM AND ITS ALLOYS[8]

TITANIUM	N	C	H	Fe	O	Al	V	Ti
cp grade I	0.03	0.010	0.015	0.02	0.18	-	-	Balance
cp grade II	0.03	0.010	0.015	0.03	0.25	-	-	Balance
cp grade III	0.03	0.010	0.015	0.03	0.35	-	-	Balance
cp grade IV	0.03	0.010	0.015	0.05	0.40	-	-	Balance
grade V (Ti6Al4V)	0.05	0.08	0.015	0.30	0.20	5.5–6.8	3.5–4.5	Balance

TABLE 4.3 - MECHANICAL PROPERTIES OF CP TITANIUM AND ITS ALLOYS**

TITANIUM	Young modulus (GPa)	Resistance to traction (MPa)	Yield strenght (MPa)	Elongation (%)	Density (g/cm^3)
cp grade I	102	240	170	24	4.5
cp grade II	102	345	275	20	4.5
cp grade III	102	450	380	18	4.5
cp grade IV	104	550	483	15	4.5
grade V (Ti6Al4V)	113	860	795	10	4.4

* In fact the Ti/O stoichiometric relationship varies with the distance from the external environment, which is richer in oxygen.[4]

** Data are from the American Society for Testing and Materials, Standard specification for unalloyed titanium for surgical implant applications. Philadelphia: Annual Book of ASTM Standards, 1995:67-95.

IV are the most widely used types of cp titanium. Grade V titanium is an alloy containing 6% aluminium and 4% vanadium (Ti6Al4V). Its elastic modulus (113 GPa) is slightly higher than that measured for grade IV cp titanium (104 GPa) (Table 4.3). The yield strength* of grade V titanium is also dramatically higher: 795 MPa for grade V titanium versus 483 MPa for grade IV cp titanium. This increased resistance to load is favorable for endosseous implants since they will better resist fracture and/or deformations associated with occlusal loading. Because the elastic modulus is relatively low, this property also permits better distribution of loads at the bone-implant interface. For these reasons, grade V titanium alloy is recommended in the treatment of patients with parafunctional habits or in cases where previous implants have fractured.[5]

The various types of cp titanium have different physical properties due to structural differences at the atomic level. At temperatures below 884°C, titanium crystallizes into a compact hexagonal system (phase α); at higher temperatures, it crystallizes into a cubical system (phase β).[2] In the Ti6Al4V alloy, vanadium stabilizes the phase β, allowing a combination of both phase α and phase β to be maintained. The combination of these two systems results in increased fracture resistance with Ti alloy.[5] It is essential for clinicians to understand the general properties of titanium dental implants. The first atomic layers of the titanium implant are exposed to the external world and direct the interaction between implant surfaces and bone. Thus it has a dramatic impact on the bone healing process.[9]

Current dental literature is replete with studies reporting on the physical properties of implants and the molecular dynamics occuring at the bone-implant interface after implant placement, and these properties help to determine the survival or failure of dental implant treatment. This chapter provides information that clinicians may use to select a well-suited implant for a particular patient. Clinicians must consider several different factors prior to choosing an implant for use. Some of the more controversial and important factors are the surface characteristics of the implant.

IMPLANT DESIGN CHARACTERISTICS

In today's market, clinicians may choose from quite a number of dental implant companies and dental implant designs. Clinicians are advised to focus on the following characteristics.[1,9,10]

* The *yield strenght* or *yield point* of a material is defined as the stress at which a material begins to plastically deform. Prior to the yield point, the material will deform elastically and will return to its original shape when the applied stress is removed. Once the yield point is passed, some fractions of the deformation will be permanent and nonreversible.

Macrostructure, or macroarchitecture, is the overall macroscopic shape of an implant. Implants are available in the following shapes: cylindric, conical (tapered or root-form), blade, disc, pin, and others (including different morphologies used at various times in history).

Microstructure, or implant profile, is determined by the geometry of the threads, including factors such as quantity, height, thickness, and pitch. The macroscopic morphology being equal, the profile may be linear, with threads or tiered. Such elements also may have different geometries and dimensions. These characteristics affect the direction that vector loading forces exert on adjacent bone.

Microtopography is determined by implant surface treatment. Implants may show machining striations from the turning (machining) process. Such implants are called *machined surface implants* and may show various degrees of roughness (different types and variable entities) according to specific manufacturing processes.

Chemical structure is determined by the chemical composition of the surface secondary to the production process. An implant's chemical structure is essential in establishing a healthy, viable bone-implant interface because it determines the implant biocompatibility. It regulates the ionic exchanges occurring between implant and osteotomy walls, is the basis for cytotoxic and inflammatory reactions, and affects the deposition and adsorption of proteins from blood.

Both implant macrostructure and microstructure affect the biomechanical behavior of implants. The macrostructure and microstructure of an implant relate directly to implant primary stability[11] and affect the distribution of forces at the bone-implant interface after occlusal loading. In contrast, to evaluate the biologic behavior of the bone-implant interface, the microtopography and superficial chemical structure of the dental implants must be investigated.[11,12]

Implant Macrostructure

Cylindric implants vs conical (tapered) implants

Currently, cylindric implants are the most widely used implant, and their use is supported by the greatest number of publications. Cylindric implants have parallel walls and flat apices. They were introduced by Brånemark with the first studies on osseointegration.[13] More recently, conical (also *tapered* or *root-form*) implants that reproduce the shape of tooth roots[14,15] have been manufactured for clinical use.

At present, the literature reports no clear indications on which implant shape should be used in different circumstances.[15] Conical implants may prove easier to place into osteotomies due to their smaller apical diameters when underpreparation of the implant site is required for increased primary stability (as in trabecular bone or in a postextraction site). In these clinical situations, conical, self-tapping implants with tapered apices may facilitate implant placement (see also chapter 5).

Internal hexagon vs external hexagon implant-abutment connections

Another feature clinicians need to consider in selecting a dental implant for clinical use is the type of implant-abutment connection. Currently, the two most often used connections are the external hexagon connection and the internal hexagon connection. Neither implant-abutment connection seems to influence the distribution of stress to peri-implant bone.[14,15]

The internal hexagon implant-abutment connection used for single-tooth replacement has a low reported incidence of complications secondary to screw loosening. However, in splinted full-arch implant treatment, internal connection implants may be more difficult to record in full-arch impressions. In contrast, impressions are easily recorded with external hex implants. According to the authors, the clinician could encounter great difficulties while using a rigid impression material such as impression plaster in making full-arch impressions of tilted, internal connection implants. In addition, they believe that the conical abutments are easier to align with external hex implants (see also chapter 5). Therefore, internal connection implants are contraindicated for use in the Columbus Bridge Protocol.

Microstructure

The development of new thread geometries have helped to increase the level of primary implant stability and removal torque values. With respect to nonthreaded implant designs, threaded implants evenly distribute the stresses from masticatory loads throughout the implant and avoid dangerous concentrations of forces at the apex of cylindric, nonthreaded implants. The width, profile (pitch), and spacing of the thread design may help determine the success or failure of osseointegration and implant survival.

In fact bone is a dynamic tissue characterized by high metabolic activity that produces a continuous exchange of its organic and inorganic components. The balance of the metabolic changes is influenced by endocrine and metabolic factors. Moreover, bone, as defined in Wolff's law,[16] remodels and adapts in response to the functional loads applied to it.

Microtopography

Superficial morphology

Implants are made with a variety of surface textures. Over the past 10 years, implant manufacturers have changed from producing implants with machined surfaces to implants with roughened surfaces. Roughened surfaces provide greater surface area for increased bone-implant contact and facilitate micromechanical retention between implants and bone.[17]

More recent studies have concentrated on the ability of implants with roughened surfaces to increase the amount of cellular activity and differentiation after implant placement.[9] Biochemical modifications of implant surfaces are another topic of current interest because it is well known

that bioengineered surfaces are able to direct bone healing and bone-implant interaction through the local activation of site-specific genes.[18–20]
In vitro and in vivo studies[21–24] have demonstrated that the microscopic topography of implant surfaces could guide osteoblastic activity and differentiation. Cells of mesenchymal origin interact with proteins adsorbed onto the titanium surfaces through focal adhesions in their cytoskeletons. This adhesion process is made possible by integrins, adhesive glycoproteins that enable cells to adhere to the substratum, and the number and distribution of these contact points can influence cells' genetic expression. Therefore, the importance of implant surface microtopography in the determination of cell shape, migration, and differentiation[25–33] is evident.

Modification processes of superficial morphology

The most extensively used implant surface treatments are:[34–36]

- Machining (turned or machined implants)
- Sandblasting (Al_2O_3, ZrO_2, TiO_2, SiC)
- Anodization (through galvanic baths)
- Acid etching (H_2SO_4, HCl, HF)
- Apposition (plasma-spray, hydroxyapatite, nanometric apposition)

Machining

Machining (Fig 4.1) is the production of implants by industrial milling units,[37] and this process results in a "turned" surface. Turned implants are not submitted to any other treatment after production; that is, their surface morphology is not

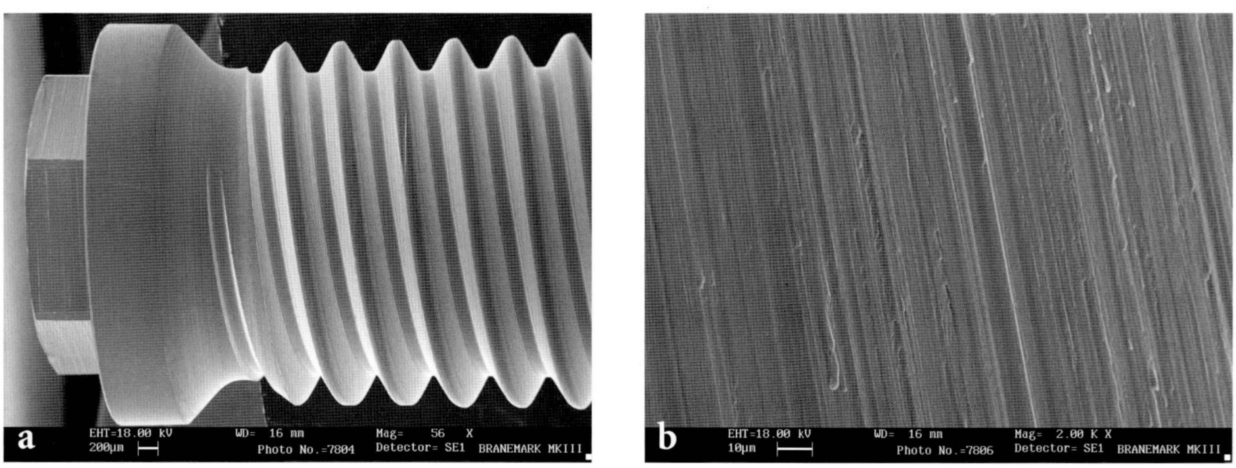

Fig 4.1 - *(a)* Scanning electron microscopy (SEM) of the machined surface of a Brånemark (Nobel Biocare) implant (original magnification ×56). *(b)* Higher magnification SEM of the same implant surface (original magnification ×2,000).

altered. Machining was the first process used in manufacturing dental endosseous implants. At the microscopic level, the surface shows minor, circumferential, horizontal striping produced by the milling cutters during machining.

The striping varies according to the protocol of the manufacturer, the hardness or grade of titanium used, and the sharpness of the rotating instruments. The striping is generally less than 1 μm in width. Turned surfaces have been tested extensively in a large number of clinical and experimental studies. Long-term reports have proven the predictability of this type of surface.[38,39]

Machined surface implants also may be modified with various modification treatments, as described in the following sections.

Sandblasting

Sandblasting (Fig 4.2) was one of the first processes used to create roughened implant surfaces. Sandblasting physically modifies implant surfaces by subtraction. Implants are subjected to an air stream, under high pressure, of hard particles approximately 10 μm in diameter. The particles may consist of aluminium trioxide (Al_2O_3), hydroxyapatite, zirconium dioxide (ZrO_2), titanium oxide (TiO_2), or silicone carbide (SiC). The plastic deformation produced by the particles hitting the implant surfaces creates a series of microscopic craters with dimensions that depend on the original dimensions of the particles and the force of the impacts. In general, protocols for sandblasted implants also call for removal of the particles with acid treatments.

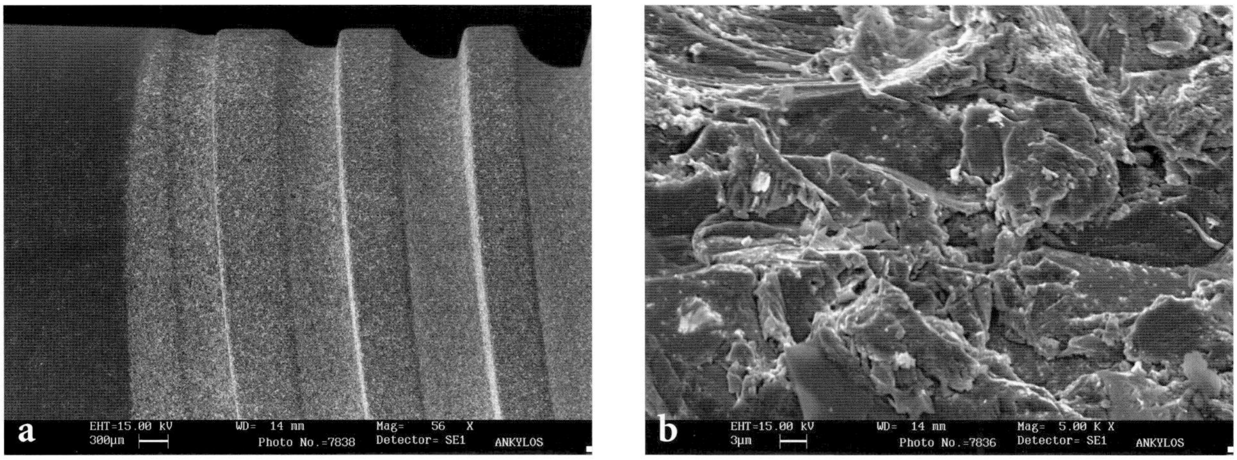

Fig 4.2 - *(a)* SEM of the sandblasted surface of an Ankylos (Dentsply) implant (original magnification ×56). *(b)* Higher magnification SEM of the same implant (original magnification ×5,000).

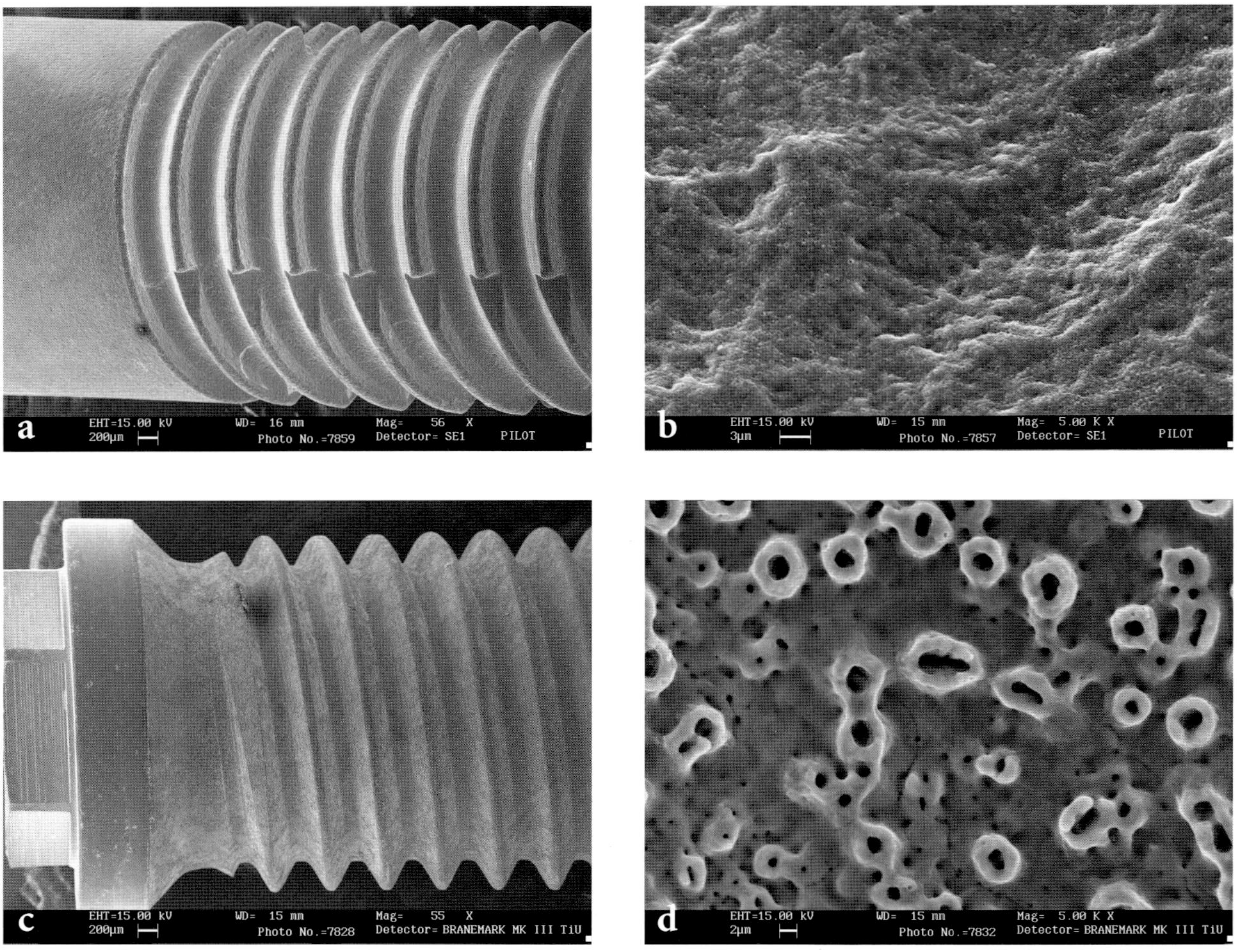

Fig 4.3 - *(a)* SEM of the oxidized surface of a Pilot (Sweden & Martina) implant (original magnification ×56). *(b)* Higher magnification SEM of the same implant surface shown in *a* (original magnification ×5,000). *(c)* SEM of the oxidized surface of a Brånemark Mk III TiUnite (Nobel Biocare) implant (original magnification ×55). *(d)* Higher magnification SEM of the same implant surface shown in *c* (original magnification ×5,000).

Anodization with galvanic baths

Anodization with galvanic baths is an electrochemical method of surface modification (Fig 4.3). In this technique, implants are immersed in electrolyte baths to which a certain voltage has been applied.[40] The passage of the electric current between the anode and cathode in the galvanic bath results in the development of a thickened, irregular layer of titanium oxide on the implant surface.

Acid etching

Acid etching (Fig 4.4) is a chemical procedure that uses acid to partially dissolve the titanium surface. It results in a roughened implant surface by subtraction. Acid etching of titanium was originally studied in the military aerospace industry. The most commonly used agents to roughen implants are sulphuric acid (H_2SO_4), hydrochloric acid (HCl), and hydrofluoric acid (HF).

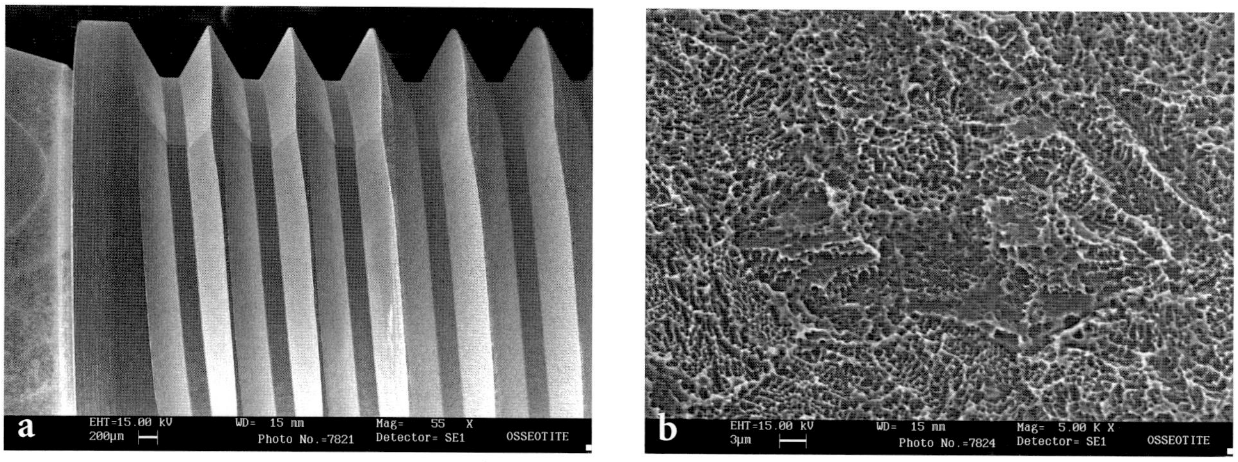

Fig 4.4 - *(a)* SEM of the etched surface of an Osseotite (Biomet 3i) implant manufactured with double etching in HCl and H_2SO_4 (original magnification ×56). *(b)* Higher magnification SEM of the same implant (original magnification ×5,000).

Titanium is soluble in HF by the action of the fluoride ions in the acid.

A combination of hydrochloric acid and sulphuric acid (HCl-H_2SO_4) is used to modify the surface morphology of two popular dental implants: Straumann implants, with sandblasted, large grit acid-etched (SLA) surfaces, and Osseotite implants (Biomet 3i), with dual acid-etched (DAE) surfaces. For both products, the surface modification process starts with sand-blasting. This step both increases the microscopic surface area of the implants and makes the implants more sensitive to acid etching with HCl-H_2SO_4. Before treatment with HCl-H_2SO_4, the Osseotite implant is also treated with HF, the extra step suggested by the name *dual acid-etched*. The implants then undergo additional processing to remove the residual acid and other contaminants.

Apposition

The plasma-spray technique (Fig 4.5) is one of the most commonly used procedures for altering implant surface morphology. Like sand-blasting, it too is a physical method for surface roughening. Apposition alters dental implants by adding particles to the surface, ie, by depositing hydroxyapatite or titanium particles after the implants have been machined. The semifinished implants are sprayed with melted titanium drops (titanium plasma spray) in suitable reactors at controlled pressures. The droplets solidify on the surfaces of the implants, creating a surface that is generally rougher than the surfaces created with sand-blasting.

A *plasma* is a partially ionized gas (eg, flames, lightening, boreal dawns). Technologic development allowed for the laboratory generation of high-pressure plasma (thermal plasma), which enabled achievement of sufficiently high temperatures. With these high temperatures, deposition of layers of inorganic materials (plasma spray) onto the implant surfaces was obtained. During this process, the noble gas argon is "cracked" into ions and electrons (plasma). The gas is compressed through a light beam at high temperature (15,000°C to 20,000°C) and at high speed (3,000 m/s), along with particles of titanium powder in the form of titanium hydrogenate. In the gas beam, the titanium hydrogenate decomposes, and the melted particles hit the implants at a distance of 15 to 20 cm and melt into the implant surfaces.

Recently, Biomet 3i has patented a new technique of calcium phosphate (CaP) nanocrystalline deposition onto metal implant surfaces. With this process, CaP particles are suspended in solution and then induced to assemble onto the titanium oxide present on the implant surfaces. This new implant is called *NanoTite* (Fig 4.6). The new surface is derived from the preexisting Osseotite surface technology (DAE) that is currently being used and has been clinically tested for more than a decade.[41-46] All NanoTite implants are manufactured from Osseotite implants. This process of depositing nanometer-sized crystals of CaP onto the DAE Osseotite implant surface is called *discrete crystalline deposition (DCD)*; it has been patented by Biomet 3i. The DCD process was developed to provide quicker rates of osseointegration with more predictable results. It was also developed for use in advanced implant treatments that involved greater risks, such as immediate or early loading protocols, immediate implant placement into postextraction sites, implant positioning concurrent with regenerative bone surgery, and positioning of implants into poor quality bone or into esthetic areas where bone preservation is essential. Quicker osseointegration during initial wound healing after implant placement should reduce implant vulnerability to micromovements and early failure. Prospective clinical studies are necessary to test these expectations.

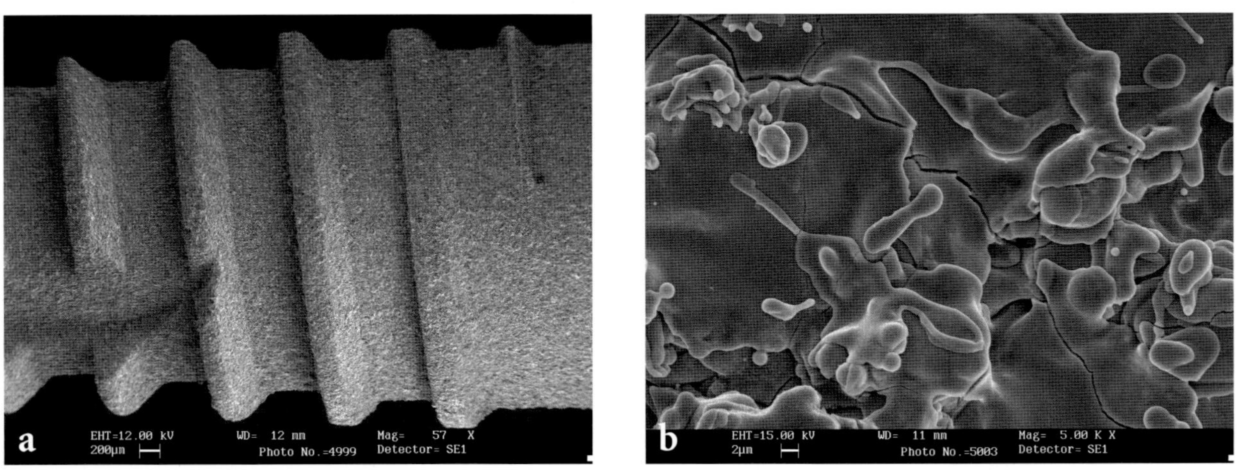

Fig 4.5 - *(a)* SEM of an implant at the conclusion of the surface-roughening process through plasma-spray treatment (original magnification ×57). *(b)* Higher magnification SEM of the surface-treated implant in *a* (original magnification ×5,000). *(Courtesy of Dr Clara Cassinelli and Dr Marco Morra, Nobil Bio Ricerche, Villafranca d'Asti, Italy.)*

Roughness and osteogenesis

Modification of implant surfaces was designed to improve the rates of osseointegration. Initially, the trend toward modified implant surfaces, and away from smooth implant surfaces, was justified because rough surfaces have greater surface areas and increased bone-implant contact, which further increases micromechanical retention at the bone-implant interface as well. Since that time, correlations between surface modifications and cellular behavior have also been established. Conserva et al[47] performed an in vitro study of the effect of dental implants on adhesion, diffusion, migration, and proliferation in osteoblastic cells SaOS-2 (an immortalized cell line with an osteoblastic phenotype deriving from a human sarcoma) and, through modifications of cytoskeletons, cellular metabolism.

The group examined 10 types of dental implants:

- Brånemark System: machined surface
- Ankylos: sandblasted surface
- Silhouette Screw (Biolok): sandblasted surface
- Galant System: experimental implant with sandblasted surface
- Osseotite: dual acid-etched surface
- Straumann Standard RN: acid-etched surface
- MK IV (Nobel Biocare): etched surface experimental implant
- Calcitek MP-1 (Sulzer Calcitek): hydroxyapatite surface
- Pilot: anodized surface
- TiUnite: oxidized surface conditioned in a specific way

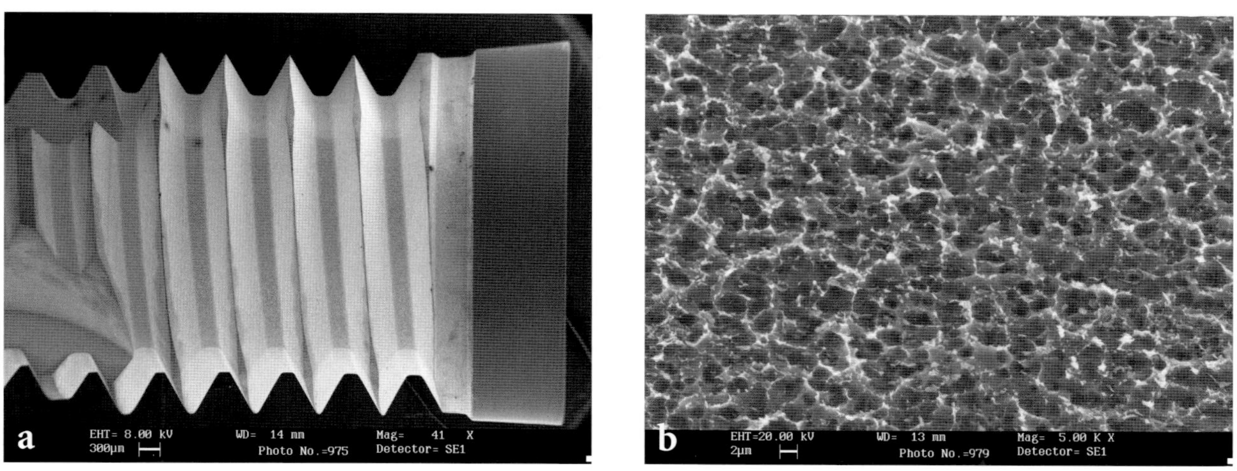

Fig 4.6 - *(a)* SEM of the appositional surface of a NanoTite implant (original magnification ×41). *(b)* Higher magnification SEM of the same surface (original magnification ×5,000).

A key element of the study was that the researchers used dental implants as received from the manufacturers instead of using modified implant forms such as discs that only simulate implant surfaces. Sometimes, these models may have different macro- and microsurface geometries when compared with clinical implants, so results obtained with these simulations may not apply to clinical implant dentistry in humans. In fact, industrial modifications to implant surface microtopography change the implants so that they do not have the same effects on flat surfaces, such as a disc, as they do on three-dimensional complex surfaces, such as implants with variable geometries and threads. Conserva's team established that at 72 hours, implants with roughened surfaces exhibited higher levels of cellular proliferation than did those with smooth surfaces.

The effect of implant surface roughness on cell behavior and the production of specific biochemical molecules by bone was examined in a series of studies in the late 1990s.[48-50] Investigators observed that cells could not become completely flattened when implant surface roughness was less than cellular dimension.

This stimulated osteoblastic activity and led to the concept of modulating osteogenesis through modified implant surfaces.[51] A smooth implant surface (Ra < 2 µm*) (machined) allowed osteoblastic cells to assume a flat shape, similar to fibroblasts; the cells were undifferentiated and did not behave as osteoblasts (Fig 4.7a). In contrast, implants with rough, acid-etched surfaces (ie, with distances between the peaks that were smaller than cell dimensions (Ra > 2 µm; RSm < 10 µm) did not permit cell flattening.

As a result, the cells maintained an osteoblastic phenotype that favored the development of osseointegration (Fig 4.7b). If the peaks were vertically higher than those noted above, yet spaced with horizontal gaps that were larger than the cells (Ra > 2 µm, RSm > 10 µm), then the

* A roughness value can either be calculated on a profile or on a surface. The profile roughness parameters (Eg, Ra, RSm) are more common. Each of the roughness parameters is calculated using a formula for describing the surface. There are many different roughness parameters in use, but Ra is by far the most common.

- Ra: The mean height of the roughnes, ie the arithmetic average of the absolute values of surface height deviations
- RSm: The mean distance between the peaks

osteoblasts perceived the surfaces as "smooth".[9] A second important factor, the role of blood coagulation in bone healing, has also been described.[52–54] Initially, the implant site is occupied by blood coagulum that forms around the implant as soon as it is placed into the osteotomy. Connective tissue cells migrate through the coagulum, and when pluripotential mesenchymal cells reach the implant surface, they operate in the environment generated by the blood-titanium interaction. Platelet activation is critical in releasing growth factors and cytokines. These molecules accelerate formation of a three-dimensional reticulum of fibrin that facilitates the migration of osteogenic cells to implant surfaces (osseoconduction). If the roughened (osseoconductive) surface of a dental implant retains this fibrin coagulum, then the osteogenic cells will produce bone directly on the implant surface (called *contact osteogenesis*). But a smooth implant surface (non-osseoconductive) does not inhibit retraction of the fibrin coagulum; therefore, new bone is deposited onto the surface of the preexisting bone and not directly onto the implant (called *distance osteogenesis*),[22] which may compromise osseointegration. Since implant surface morphology influences the quality and quantity of platelet activation,[53] it is possible that implant roughness contributes to healing through its specific effect on platelet interaction.

The concepts described above introduced a biochemical dimension into a context previously dominated by physical and mechanical considerations. It is worth remembering that in both the correlation between surface roughness and osteoblasts and the correlation between surface

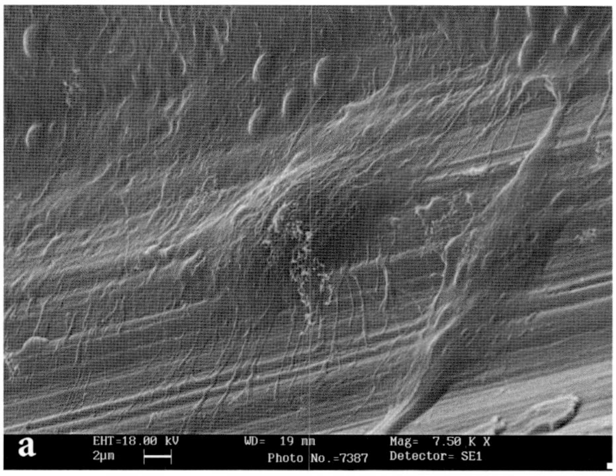

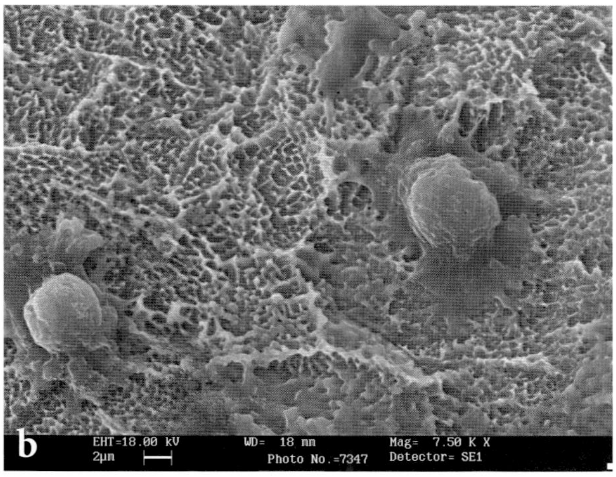

Fig 4.7 - Difference in osteoblastic adhesion after 24 hours between a machined surface (Brånemark, Nobel Biocare) *(a)* and an Osseotite surface *(b)*.

roughness and platelet activation, the surface roughness that influences cellular behavior has dimensions comparable to or smaller than cell dimensions. Numerous studies have estimated that dimension–the average distance between peaks–to be less than 10 μm.[48–50,52–54]

In conclusion, an implant surface will only influence cellular behavior if its surface roughness is much finer than the surface roughness of the implants commonly used in the past. These levels may be difficult to obtain with traditional sandblasting processes or deposition via plasma spray. It is appropriate to note that in the references cited above, the investigators included acid etching to obtain the requisite roughness.

Chemical composition of implant surfaces

Superficial properties of titanium

For all medical materials, cell-material contact does not occur directly. It occurs through microproteins that, in the first moments of exposure to biologic fluids, bind to surfaces in a process called *adsorption*.[55,56] Because proteins are smaller than cells, they have higher diffusion coefficients and transfer speeds, so after implant placement, they reach the implant surfaces in advance of the cells. The proteins of blood and the plasma of adjacent tissues attach to the implant surfaces, forming a medium for cells to colonize the implants.[57] Some of these proteins have receptors that can bind to cells and promote cellular adhesion. The composition of the protein bed depends on the composition of the implant surface; therefore, cellular adhesion depends on the implant surface.[58] It is important to understand that even though dental implants may be made from cp titanium, with titanium concentrations equal to or greater than 99%, their surface composition is not completely predictable. Analyses of the chemical composition of implant surface topography have demonstrated great variability.[9] Modifications to implant surface topography may alter their chemical composition, energy, and charge.

Techniques of surface analysis

The investigation techniques revealing the surface chemical composition of a material must be able to process data from as thin an external layer as possible and to distinguish it from the prevailing signals of subjacent materials. Among these techniques, x-ray photoelectron spectroscopy (XPS), also called electron spectroscopy for chemical analysis (ESCA), is one of the most widely used.[59] In XPS analysis, the sample, positioned in a high vacuum chamber, is irradiated by x-rays and, consequently, emits electrons. The electrons are collected by an analyzer that measures the energy reflected from the object. The energy of the electrons emitted by every element has a typical value that identifies the elements present, while their numbers may quantify the mass of the object. It is important to note that only the electrons emitted by a thin superficial layer (4 to 5 nm) succeed in reaching the analyzer. This explains the high sensitivity of the technique.

Auger electron spectroscopy (AES) is another widely used technique to study surface chemical composition. This technique, discovered by the French physician who gave his name to it, studies the effects of electron emission. In this process, the sampled depth is also several nanometers thick. This process differs from XPS analysis in that the surface of the sample is hit with a beam of electrons. Since focusing electrons is relatively easy while focusing x-rays is difficult, AES offers the possibility of analyzing very small zones (high lateral resolution) with respect to XPS. In the case of XPS, the analyzed material is several hundred microns in depth. This aspect must be considered when the data obtained with the two research methods are compared. One of the disadvantages associated with these techniques is the great expense associated with the studies.

A commonly used investigative technique that is often erroneously applied to define surface "cleanness" is energy dispersive x-ray analysis (EDX). EDX is not a surface analysis technique. It uses a microprobe, together with a scanning electronic microscope. The sample is exposed to electrons that are diffused by the material and generate an image. One of the effects associated with exposure to a stream of electrons is that the samples will emit x-rays. The energy of the x-rays emitted is specific for the elements present in the sample. In comparison to the previously described techniques, EDX analyzes a depth that is approximately a thousand times thicker than the previous methods. EDX therefore offers limited information about surface chemistry. However, it can provide information about the chemical nature of inclusions and impurities at the micron level, such as alumina grains present on the surface of sand-blasted implants.

Scanning electron microscopy (SEM) supplies only qualitative observations relative to surface morphology; it does not supply quantitative topographic data or information regarding chemical type. SEM does provide visualization of particles within the limits of its resolution.

If the electron acceleration potential (EHT) is reduced, electrons reaching the surface to be analyzed will have less energy and will remain more confined to the surface. In this way, a high level of contrast can be created between the metallic (titanium implant) and organic (contaminants) parts. If compared with the topographic images of conventional SEM, the acquisition of SEM images with low-acceleration voltage (low-voltage SEM) improves the superficial sensitivity of the technique and adds "chemical" information limited to organic contaminants.[60] That is, low-voltage SEM can identify contaminants that conventional SEM cannot.

SEM morphologic analysis and XPS chemical analysis on different implant surfaces

Many studies have reported that superficial topography of dental implants plays an essential role in the regulation of the biologic functions of osteoblasts during osseointegration. It must be remembered that surface modifications to dental implants may lead to changes in the chemical composition of implant surfaces.[61] Since the chemical composition of implant surfaces affects cellular behavior,[21] the University of Genoa developed a comparative analysis regarding the microtopography and surface chemical compositions of machined implants versus "third generation" implants treated with processes that altered the microtopography of the surfaces in order to fasten osteoblastic adhesion and to decrease prosthetic loading times.

Four types of implants were studied:

- ICE (Biomet 3i): machined surface
- Osseotite: DAE surface with machined coronal portion
- Full Osseotite: fully DAE surface
- NanoTite: apposition-modified surface

The implants were tested as they were supplied by the manufacturer, as if for clinical use; they were not specially designed for laboratory research since design modifications could affect the macro- and microstructures of implants and therefore influence the results.

Implant microtopography was analyzed using an SEM LEO 420 (Leo Electron Microscopy) with a magnifying range from ×50 to ×7,000. The salient parameters of the analysis (EHT = electron high tension, WD = working distance, MAG = magnification) were reported on black strips under each photograph. The chemical composition of the surfaces were analyzed with the XPS technique performed with a Perkin Elmer PHI 5400 ESCA System instrument (Perkin Elmer).[60] This instrument is equipped with an x-ray source (magnesium anode) maintained at 10 kV with 200 W of power. The pressure inside the analytic chamber was maintained at 10^{-8} Pa. XPS studies are designed to obtain qualitative and quantitative analyses of the most external layers of the materials under examination. In the case of dental implants, the depths were approximately 5 nm. XPS studies provided the chemical composition of the layers of the material directly in contact with the bone.

Considering the data specific to an XPS investigation surface analysis of the various implants, three elements were expected to be found: titanium; oxygen, because titanium oxide is present on the surface; and carbon (CO_2 or composite of hydrocarbons), which is inevitably present in Earth's atmosphere.[61]

The surface of the metals combined with carbon (phenomenon of adsorption). Carbon was found through a specific surface analysis with XPS; it would not be visible with more conventional methods of analysis. Carbon may also be present secondary to contamination by contact with oils or grease during implant machining. To distinguish between "natural" carbon and external contaminated carbon, it was necessary to consider quantitative analysis. Carbon residue in the range of 30% to 40% is considered normal; higher percentages indicate contamination.

As for dental implants, the maximum percentage of titanium theoretically observable through surface analysis is approximately 33%; the remaining 67% would be represented by oxygen because of the presence of TiO_2 on the surface. The inevitable presence of carbon, as described above, further lowers the theoretical limit. Therefore, the maximum concentration of titanium observed with XPS analysis would be about 14% to 19%. The data obtained in this study are reported in Table 4.4.

The results demonstrated that titanium, oxygen, and carbon, as well as various other elements, were present on all of the implant surfaces. Elements with the lower concentrations (≤ 2%) were commonly observed on the surfaces of implants that are currently commercially available and should not be considered an anomaly. Both Osseotite and Full Osseotite demonstrated low quantities of sulphur on the surface. This was attributed to the surface treatment associated with sulphuric and hydrochloric acid baths. Other identified elements included calcium, phosphorus, and chlorine. They were probably derived from washing processes and were not considered to be anomalies at these low concentrations.

ICE implants (machined) appeared to be "dirtier" (in terms of carbon) when compared with the other implants. There have been reports[35,61] that machined surfaces often present with higher carbon to titanium ratios than those observed on acid-etched implant surfaces. This is thought to occur because the acid-etching process includes total immersion of the implants into acid baths, thereby dissolving the most external

TABLE 4.4 - SURFACE COMPOSITION (ATOMIC %) OBTAINED THROUGH XPS ANALYSIS

Sample	C	O	Ti	N	S	Si	P	Ca	Al	Cl
ICE	66.1	22.3	8.6	0.6		1.8				0.6
Osseotite	42.2	33.5	18.1	0.8	0.5	2.1	0.4	0.4		
Full Osseotite	42.2	36.6	18.8	0.9	0.1	1.1		0.3		
NanoTite	35.1	34.9	6.4	0.5		0.7	7.5	14.3	0.6	

surface of the implants. The acid bath removes most of the residuals of the machining process, which are not always completely removed in the washing processes. Therefore, from a chemical point of view, etching has the effect of "cleaning" implant surfaces.

However, to distinguish between natural carbon and carbon secondary to contamination, it was necessary to perform an XPS investigation with a time-of-flight secondary ion mass spectrometry analysis (ToF-SIMS analysis). This test also accounted for qualitative differences. In fact, this technique identified the precise amount of energy for each atom bonded with carbon that was dissipated at the moment of the detachment:

- C-C, C-H, C-Si, (approximately 284 to 285 eV)
- C-O (286 eV)
- C-O-O (288 to 289 eV)[62]

In comparison with the other samples, NanoTite implants demonstrated reduced amounts of carbon. The surfaces of these implants appeared to be cleaner than the surfaces of the other implants. It is important to note that significant levels of calcium and phosphorus were present, with a ratio close to 2 (Fig 4.8).

These data corresponded to information provided by the manufacturer, which stated that the surfaces of NanoTite implants were enriched with nanocrystals of calcium phosphate. This implant also demonstrated the presence of aluminium, an observation consistent with the fact that the implants were manufactured with grade V titanium alloy (Ti6Al4V).

The results of the SEM morphologic observations and the relevant XPS graphics are reported in Figs 4.9 to 4.16 for each implant type.

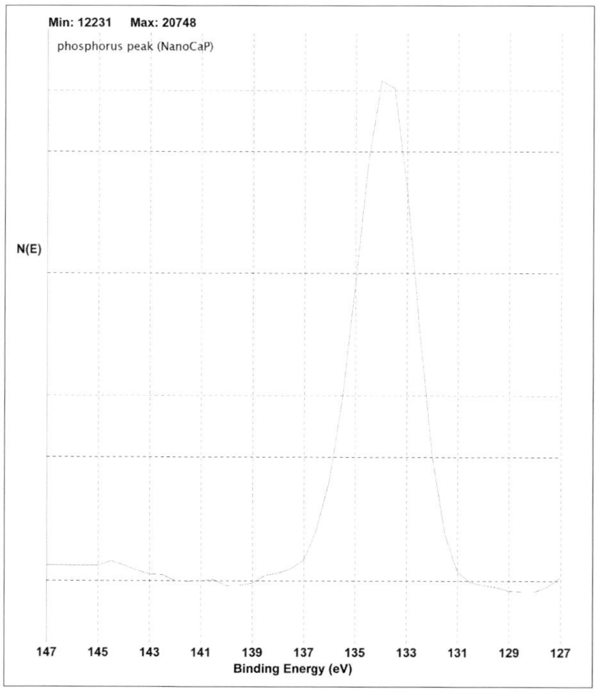

Fig 4.8 - XPS analysis of a NanoTite implant. The phosphorus peak is at 134 eV and is consistent with the presence of phosphate.

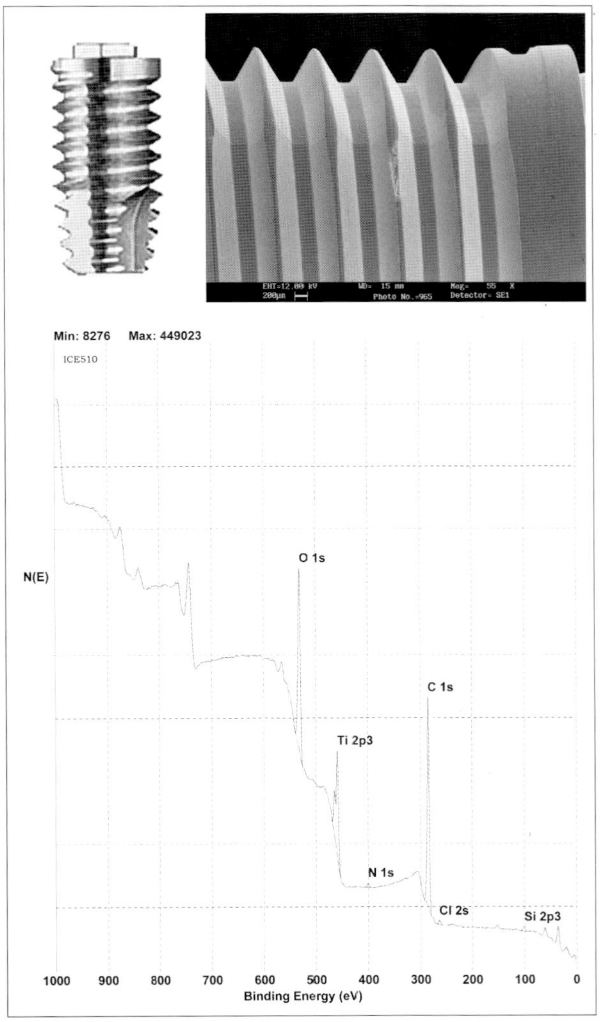

Fig 4.9 - ICE (Biomet 3i) implant (*top left*). SEM (original magnification ×55) (*top right*). Chart of the XPS surface analysis (*bottom*). Notice that the carbon peak (C1s) is high because of unavoidable contamination of hydrocarbons in the air.

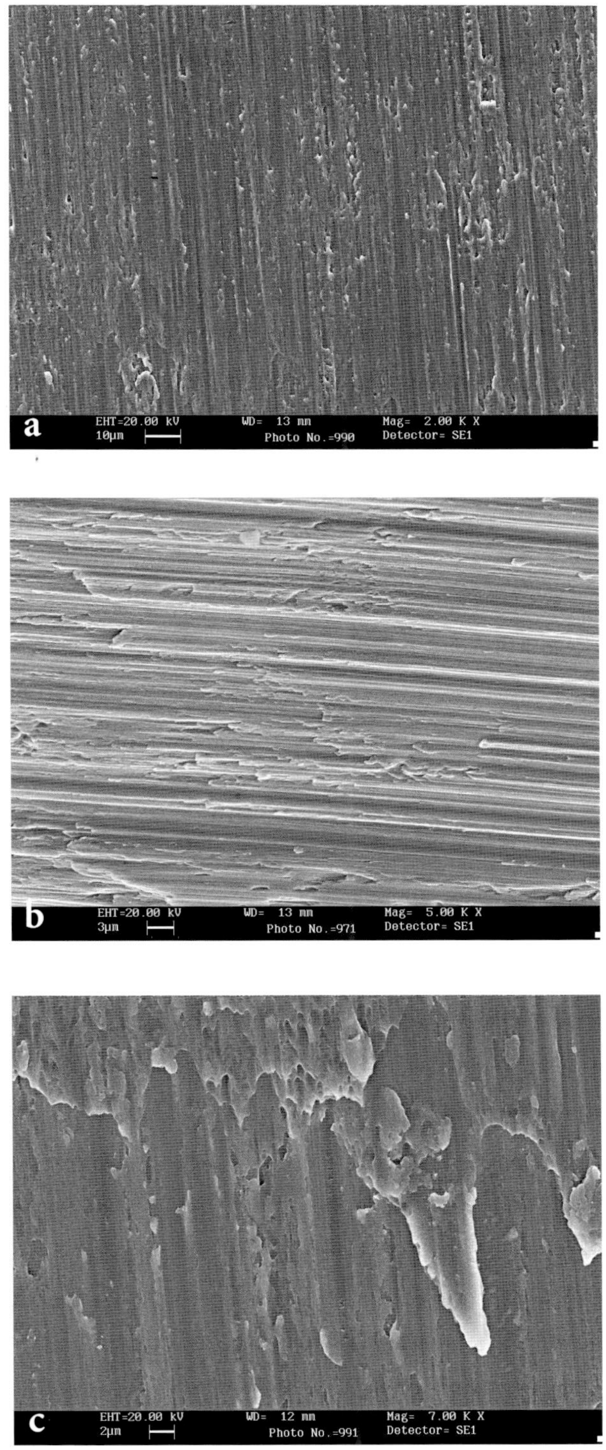

Fig 4.10 - SEMs of ICE surface (original magnification ×2,000, *[a]*; ×*5,000 [b]*, ×*7,000 [c]*).

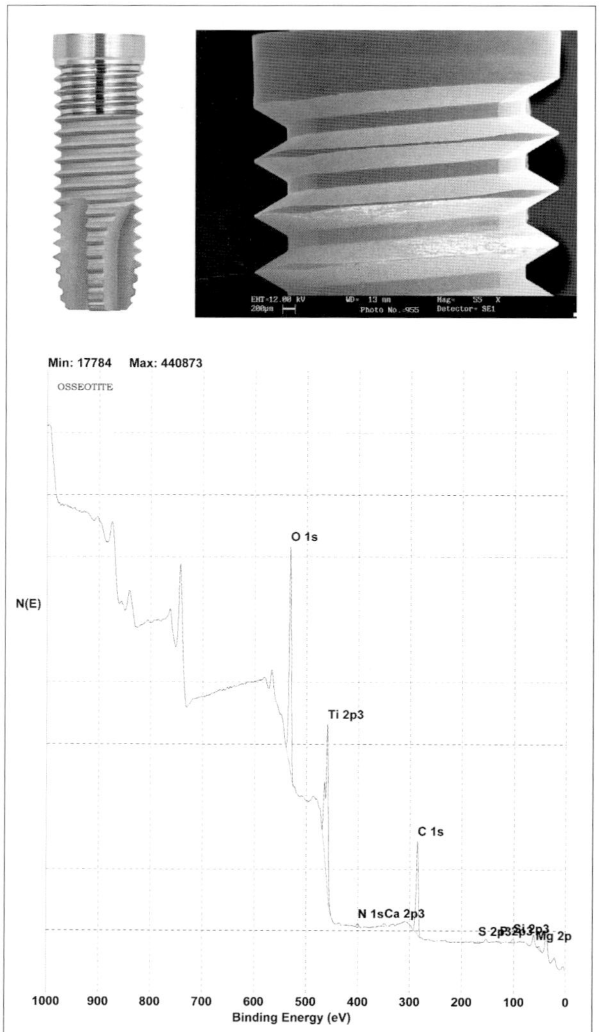

Fig 4.11 - Osseotite implant (*top left*). SEM of the cervical threads not submitted to dual acid etching (original magnification ×55) (*top right*). XPS analysis of the surface of an Osseotite implant (*bottom*).

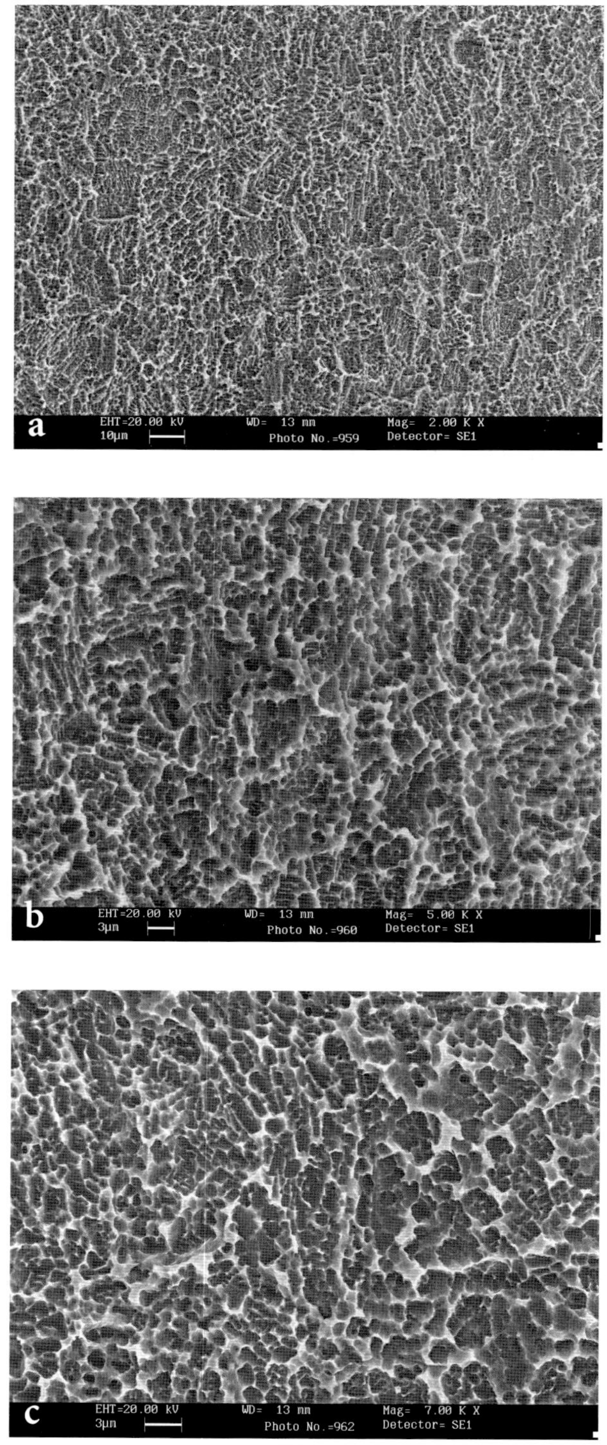

Figs 4.12 - SEMs of an Osseotite surface (original magnification ×2,000 *[a]*; ×*5,000 [b]*; ×*7,000 [c]*).

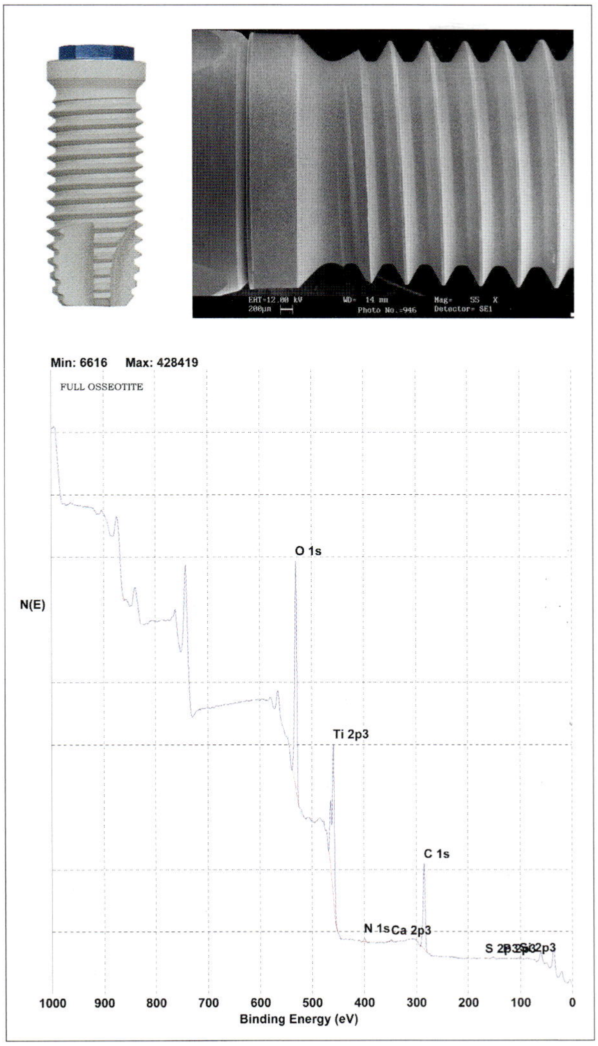

Fig 4.13 - Full Osseotite implant (*top left*). SEM demonstrates the homogeneity of the etching treatment extended to the margin of the implant platform (original magnification ×55) (*top right*). XPS analysis of the surface of a Full Osseotite implant (*bottom*).

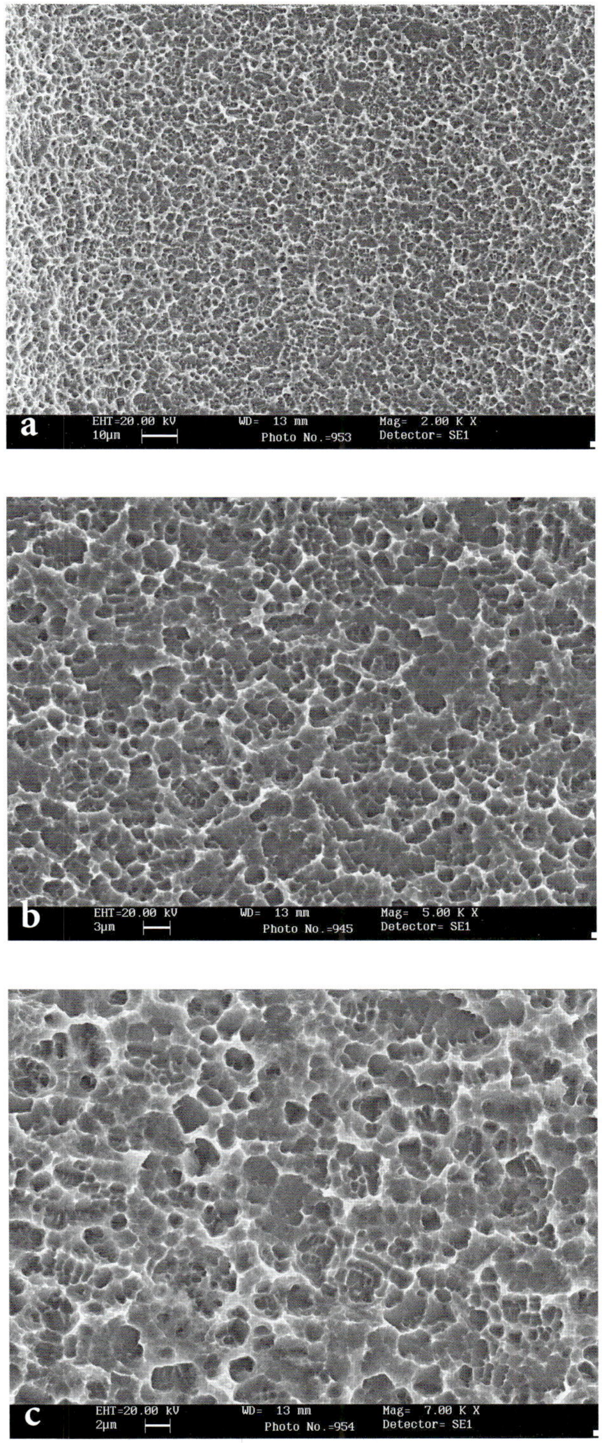

Figs 4.14 - SEMs of a Full Osseotite surface (original magnification ×2,000 *[a]*; *×5,000 [b]*; *×7,000 [c]*).

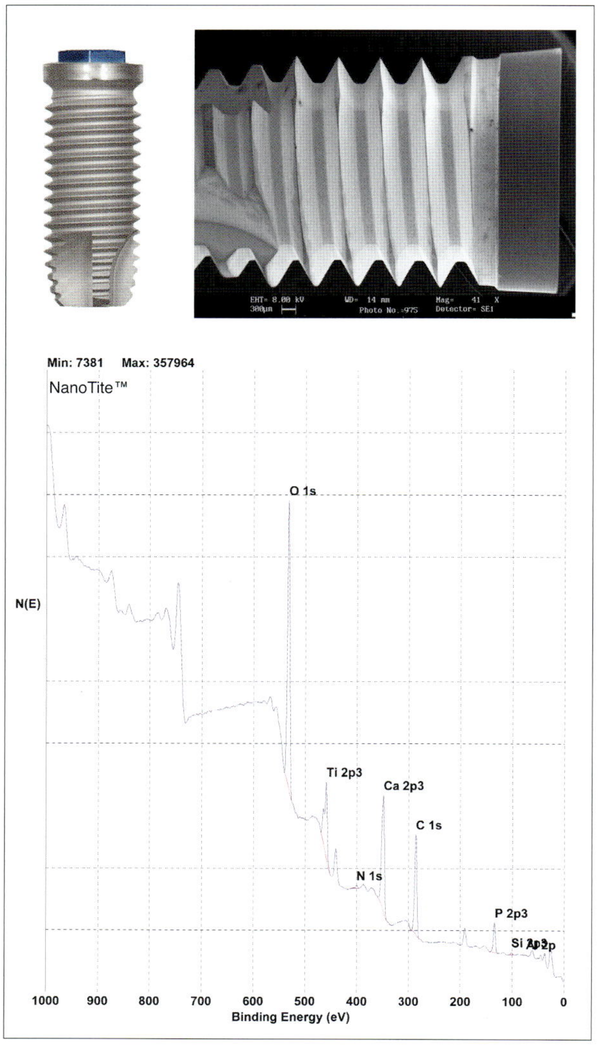

Fig 4.15 - NanoTite implant (*top left*). SEM (original magnification ×41) (*top right*). XPS analysis of the surface (*bottom*). Note the presence of calcium and phosphorus due to the surface deposition of calcium phosphate.

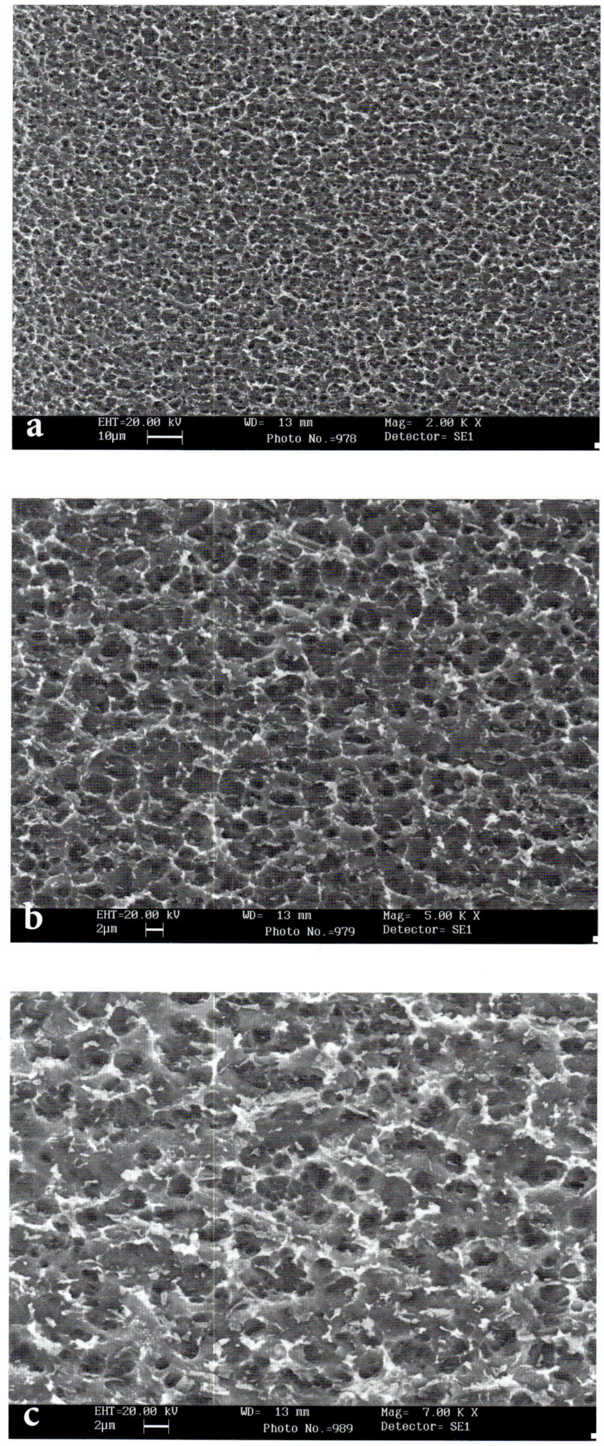

Figs 4.16 - SEMs of a NanoTite surface (original magnification ×2,000 *[a]*; *×5,000 [b]*; *×7,000 [c]*).

In review, the XPS chemical analysis demonstrated:

- Acid etching treatments "clean" implant surfaces by removing much of the residual debris from the machining process. This has been confirmed by the high atomic percentage of carbon remaining on the machined surface of the ICE implant (66.1%). When these data were compared with acid-etched implant surfaces (Osseotite and Full Osseotite), the acid-etched surfaces demonstrated a lower atomic percentage of surface carbon (42.2%).
- The NanoTite implant demonstrated a further reduction in the quantity of superficial carbon (35.1%). NanoTite implants had significant levels of aluminium (0.6%) and high percentages of calcium (14.3%) and phosphorus (7.5%). These data are consistent with the manufacturing process that includes deposition of nanocrystals of calcium phosphate, which is a specific characteristic of this implant.

Nanomodified implants: Stability and osseoconduction

The use of dental and orthopedic implants enriched with CaP* was originally developed in the mid-1980s as a way to accelerate peri-implant bone healing and to make implant surfaces favorable to bonding with bone.[63–66] CaP particles were originally applied to implant surfaces with the plasma-spray technique and created a layer that was 50 to 100 μm thick.

The layers deposited at high temperature with the plasma-spray technique resulted in an inhomogeneous distribution of crystals, causing macroscopic and microscopic defects in the coatings. This led to the presence of amorphous and crystalline phases of CaP with different degrees of solubility and high susceptibility to events such as delamination or dissolution of the amorphous content of the coating,[5,34,67] and ultimately, to a subsequent increase in the risk for peri-implantitis. In fact, the large hydroxyapatite crystals generated with this process could not be absorbed by macrophages via phagocytosis; this generated significant inflammatory reactions within the peri-implant soft tissues. In the process, inflammation and bacterial contamination reduced the tissue pH, increased the dissolution of the amorphous phase, and further increased the release of crystalline bodies from the surfaces of the implants.

The prosthodontic department of the University of Genoa conducted two studies and confirmed what was previously reported in the literature.[48,68] In vitro tests with SaOS-2 osteoblasts demonstrated that Calcitek MP-1 implants, with hydroxyapatite surface coatings, initially demonstrated optimal biocompatibility, high cellular affinity, and higher cellular proliferation with respect to the other implants tested.

* Calcium phosphate, in the form of hydroxyapatite [$Ca_{10}(PO_4)_6(OH)_2$] is the mineral component of bone matrix.

After 72 hours, Calcitek MP-1 implants also revealed delamination of the hydroxyapatite coatings from the implants. In fact, after 72 hours, the Calcitek MP-1 sample demonstrated hydroxyapatite precipitates detached from the implant surfaces.

With the new technique of hydroxyapatite crystalline deposition on metal surfaces (DCD), the advantages associated with hydroxyapatite (biocompatibility and affinity for osteogenic cells) have been potentiated while their limitations (delamination of the coating) have been minimized or eliminated. With the DCD method, nano-size particles of calcium phosphate (nano-CaP) are not applied with the plasma-spray process. The crystals are suspended in solution and are induced to self-assemble on the titanium oxide on the implant surfaces. This technique is used to modify the DAE surfaces of Osseotite implants that already have proven clinical success.[41–45]

The DCD technique results in the deposition of 20- to 100-nm discrete crystalline CaP that occupies approximately 50% of the Osseotite implant surface. The total quantity of CaP is small (≤ 20 µg; 1,000 times less than CaP crystals placed onto implant surfaces with the plasma-spray technique). The surface (NanoTite) is characterized by nanostructural morphology where the crystals are less than 1 µm in diameter, and the average diameter is in the order of 100 nm. Therefore, NanoTite surfaces demonstrate morphologic elements with dimensions less than cellular bodies. These dimensions are consistent with the findings described previously.[48,50–54]

Evaluation of the stability of the NanoTite surface

Research was developed at the University of Genoa to evaluate variations in the chemical composition of NanoTite implant surfaces during time with the XPS technique. To perform this study, Nano Tite implants were immersed in phosphate-buffered saline solution for variable periods.

A NanoTite implant, as supplied by the manufacturer for clinical use, was submitted to the first XPS analysis at time zero. Then the implant was placed into a sterile plastic test tube containing 4 mL of Dulbecco's phosphate-buffered saline solution (Sigma Aldrich) with a pH of 7.4. The test tube, with the implant inside it, was closed and placed into an incubator at 5% CO_2, 99% humidity, and a constant temperature of 37°C, for 3 months. After the 1-month immersion, the implant was removed from the test tube with sterile titanium forceps and washed with ultrapure filtered water (Milli-Q, Millipore). The implant dried under a laminar air flow cover. After the XPS analysis was performed, the implant was placed again into 4 mL of fresh Dulbecco's phosphate-buffered saline solution inside a new sterile test tube, which was placed into an incubator under the same conditions described above, and finally a second and a third XPS analysis were made after 2 and 3 months of immersion. The results of this experiment are reported in Table 4.5 and described in Fig 4.17. The alterations in the chemical composition of the surfaces were similar to the ion exchange reactions that occur when a metal is immersed in solution. Ion release (eg, Ca^{2+}, P^{3-}, Si^{4+}) from the implant surface is an inevitable physiologic process, provided that ion release remains in the range of the reference values codified by Iyengar in 1989.[69]

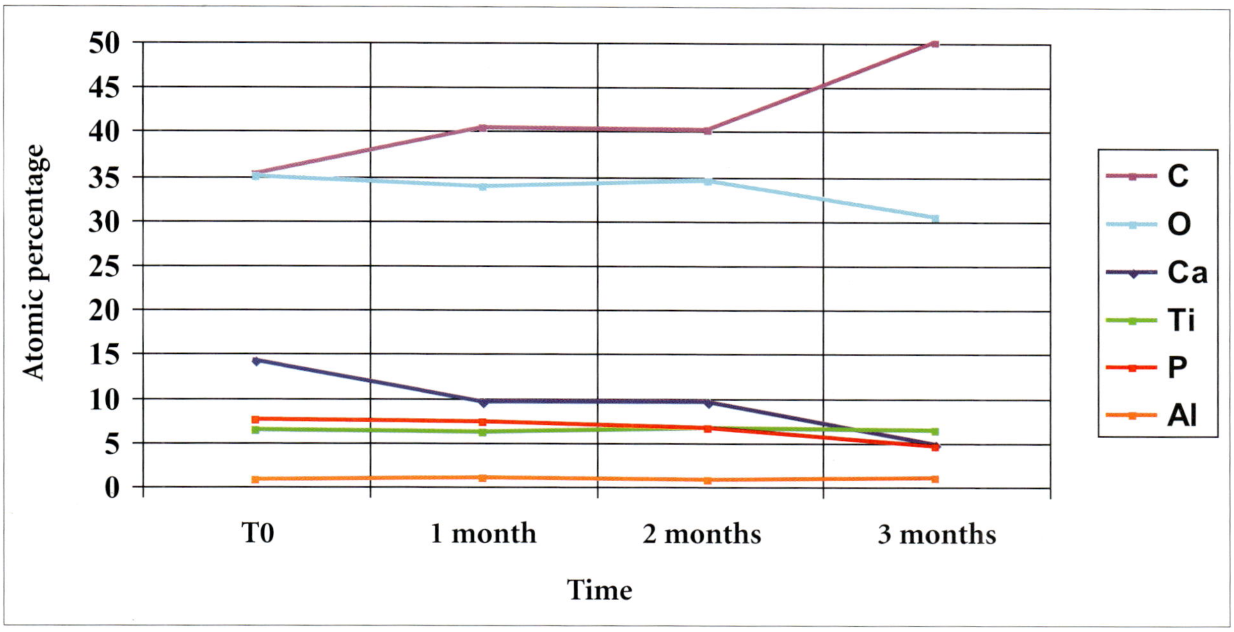

Fig 4.17 - Variation of the atomic percentage of the chemical composition of the NanoTite sample submitted to four evaluations (from time 0 to 3 months).

TABLE 4.5 - SURFACE COMPOSITION OF NANOTITE IMPLANTS (ATOMIC %) OVER TIME, OBTAINED THROUGH XPS ANALYSIS

Sample	C	O	Ti	N	Si	P	Ca	Al
Time 0	35.1	34.9	6.4	0.5	0.7	7.5	14.3	0.6
1 month	40.3	33.8	6.0	1.7	0.7	7.3	9.4	0.8
2 months	40.0	34.4	6.5	1.8	0.5	6.6	9.4	0.7
3 months	50.1	30.4	6.2	2.0	1.3	4.4	4.7	0.9

Several studies have demonstrated that excessive metal ion release can affect cellular metabolism and impair bone mineralization of the peri-implant bone in contact with the implant interface.

It must be noted that the phosphorus-to-titanium ratio remained unchanged until the second month of the study, and then it was lowered at the end of the third month (Table 4.6). Also the calcium-to-phosphorus ratio decreased from 1.9 to 1.4 at the end of the second month of immersion to 1.1 at the end of the third month of immersion.

In this specific instance, Ca^{2+} cations released into solution were hydrated and formed calcium hydroxide ($Ca(OH)_2$). Calcium hydroxide is a strong base and contributed to an increase in the pH of the solution, although this effect was hidden by the buffered solution. The most plausible hypothesis to explain these findings is that the most superficial layer of the CaP layer must be completely hydrated before it can detach from the implant surface. A confirmation of this phenomenon was noted by the increase in the atomic percentage of exposed carbon.

This variation in calcium levels was evident from the comparison of the peaks in the graphics of the XPS analysis performed at different times (Fig 4.18). The red curve shows that calcium dissolution occurred mainly during the first month of immersion and then stabilized with constant atomic percentages of 9.4%. Later, during the third month of immersion, the calcium loss was almost 50%.

The variation in the results is even more evident when observing the histogram of the dissolution of calcium phosphate in toto (Fig 4.19). From the histogram, it can be inferred that the reduction in the percentages of calcium and phosphorus is not homogeneous: calcium loss was larger than the phosphorus loss. This occurred because the two elements possess different chemical properties and underwent different chemical reactions. The calcium loss was probably the consequence of ion exchange reac-

TABLE 4.6 - PERCENTAGES OF SOME CHEMICAL ELEMENTS IN NANOTITE IMPLANTS OVER TIME

Sample	Ca/Ti	P/Ti	Ca/P
Time 0	2.2	1.2	1.9
1 month	1.6	1.2	1.3
2 months	1.7	1.2	1.4
3 months	0.8	0.7	1.1

tions with H_3O^+ ions coming from water. This reaction occurred rapidly. The phosphorus loss probably occurred through dissolution only when ceramic crystal hydration (through calcium substitution) reached the point at which ceramic becomes water soluble.

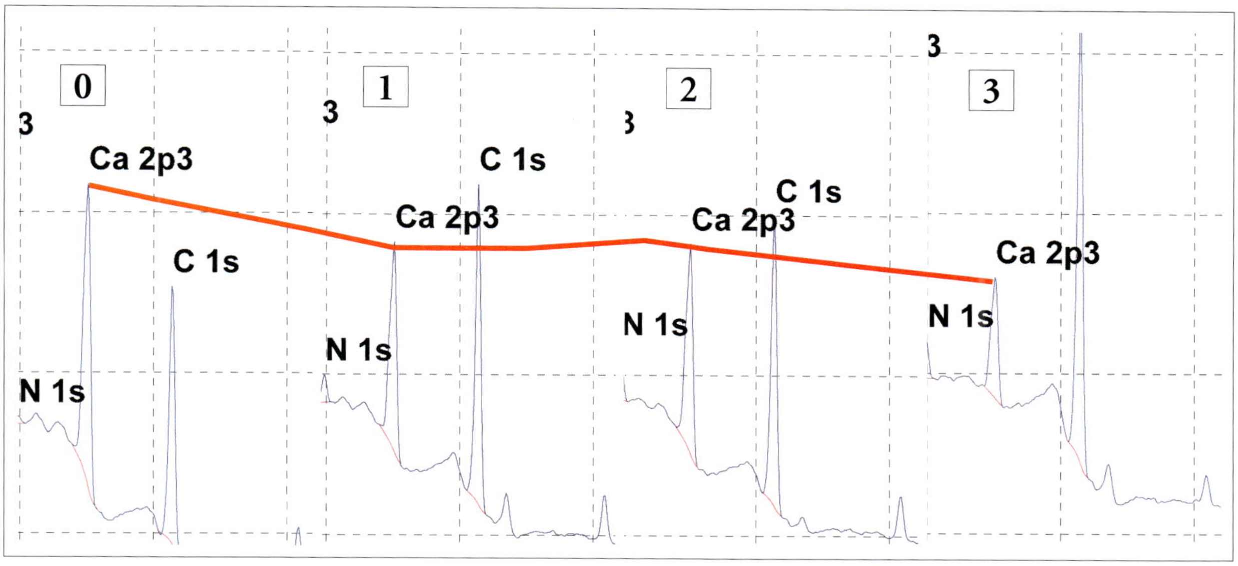

Fig 4.18 - Comparison of calcium (Ca) peaks in the XPS charts. Chart of the XPS analysis at time zero (0); chart of the XPS analysis 1 month post-immersion in Dulbecco's phosphate-buffered saline solution (1); chart of the XPS analysis 2 months postimmersion (2); chart of the XPS analysis 3 months postimmersion (3).

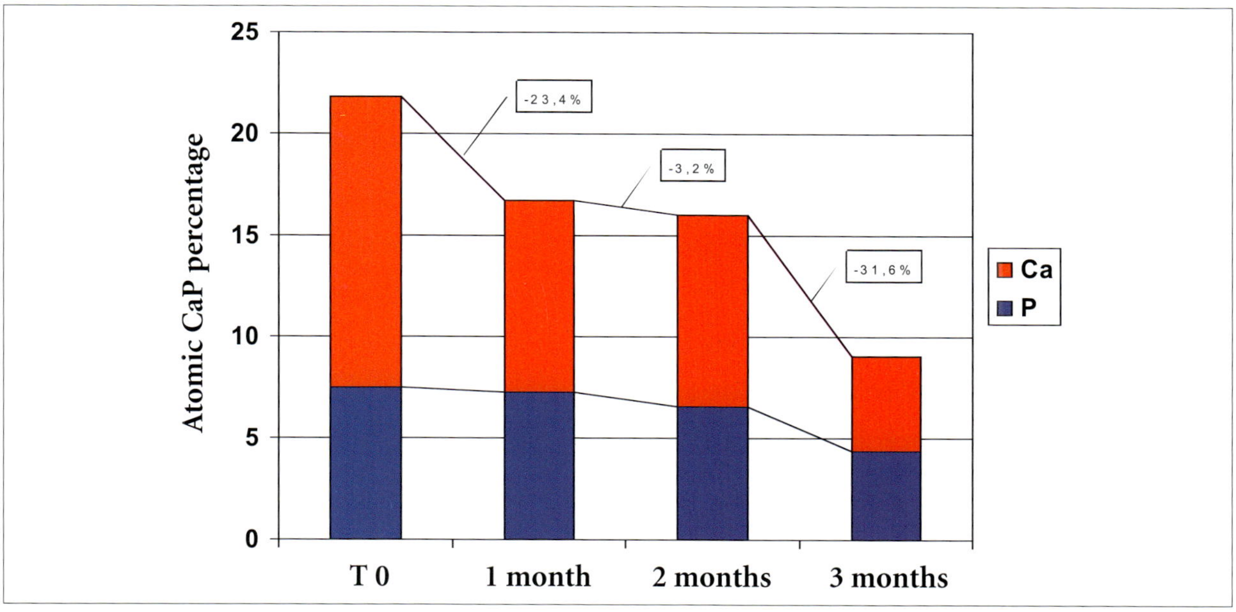

Fig 4.19 - Variation of the atomic percentage of calcium phosphate ($Ca_3(PO_4)_2$) in the NanoTite sample submitted to four evaluations.

This study followed the interaction between ceramic crystals and the adjacent aqueous environment that initially led to the expected variation in the calcium to phosphorus ratio and then to an actual reduction of phosphorus, as shown by the phosphorus to titanium ratio. Because the total quantity of calcium on the implant surface is about 20 µg and the variation of atomic composition is greater than 50%, the quantity of calcium dispersed into solution should be approximately 13 µg. Since the sampling depth of XPS is only several nanometers, the results of this experiment demonstrated a loss of crystalline coating consistent with a depth of several nanometers. The authors, drawing on the fact that the XPS analysis did not report the presence of elemental titanium after 3 months, postulated that about 1 hundredth of 1 µm was lost, which they judged to be minimal. It is also important to remember that after 3 months, peri-implant bone tissue is undergoing active remodeling, and gaps of several nanometers are not a cause for concern. To put this into proper perspective, remember that one osteoblast is approximately 1,000 times larger than this gap.

The results of this study demonstrated that the surface dissolution of CaP is not complete and that it was limited to several nanometers in depth. Dissolution of the CaP crystals occurred only when the implant surface was in direct contact with the adjacent, newly formed bone. At this point, the behavior of CaP nanocrystals is no longer determined only by the interaction with the adjacent aqueous environment but also as a result of the complex interaction of deposition and remodeling normally associated with dynamic bone physiology.

In review, the following should be remembered when using implant surfaces treated with CaP apposition:

- Implants treated with apposition of hydroxyapatite crystals have optimal biocompatibility and favor osseointegration when compared with machined implants. But a major limitation is the potential for the hydroxyapatite coating to undergo delamination and dissolution.
- The NanoTite surface, manufactured with the DCD method, maintains the advantages of surfaces coated with hydroxyapatite (biocompatibility and high level of cellular affinity) while dramatically reducing the problem of delamination. Reductions of surface calcium (possibly because of hydration reactions) by 67.13% and of surface phosphorus by 41.33% after 3 months were recorded. This corresponded to a loss of a minimal number of nanocrystals and occurred approximately 2 to 3 months after implant placement, when the implant was in contact with newly formed bone tissue that, by then, was not affected by coating gaps of these dimensions.

Peri-implant tissues and surface modification of dental implants

Peri-implant hard tissues

The connection between hard peri-implant tissue (bone) and the various types of implants with surface modifications has already been described.
In review:

- Modified implant surfaces favor osteogenesis. This is especially true in the first stages of wound healing, immediately after implant placement. These surfaces are preferred to classic machined implant surfaces, especially when for use with immediate-loading protocols.
- Ideal surface roughness should be in the order of magnitude of the cell dimensions (average distance between peaks < 10 μm).
- The nanomodified implant surface seems to favor osseoconduction and exhibits in vitro biocompatibility.

Peri-Implant Soft Tissues

The dental literature about osseointegration has devoted significant attention to the bone-implant interface and the phenomena leading to direct contact between bone and alloplastic implants.[70–73]

Direct contact between living bone and the surfaces of load-carrying implants is necessary for implant success. A significantly smaller number of studies evaluated the behavior of soft tissues adjacent to different implant surfaces, which also are important in maintaining the health and integrity of implant sites[74] by forming barriers against external factors.[75]
Peri-implant soft tissues also contribute to the esthetic and functional success of prosthetic treatment.[74] This is particularly important today when, to improve the bone-implant interface, there has been a trend toward modified implant surfaces as opposed to machined titanium implant surfaces.[76] Moreover, many manufacturers now modify implant surfaces along the entire length of the implants.
The specific type of treatment that implant surfaces receive becomes particularly important when, in the case of complications such as peri-implantitis or inappropriate positioning of an implant, the modified surface may be in contact not only with bone but also with peri-implant mucosal soft tissues. A particularly problematic case could arise when two or more implant threads have been exposed into the oral cavity since the exposure of a rough surface to the oral cavity may favor plaque accumulation,[77,78] lead to peri-implant inflammatory processes,[79] and even result in the loss of the implant.[80–81]

Evaluation of the behavior of soft tissues in contact with different implant surfaces

A randomized prospective study was designed and carried out at the University of Genoa to evaluate the response of peri-implant tissues to plaque accumulation after insertion of Osseotite implants and Full Osseotite implants.[83] The Osseotite implants are cp titanium implants with DAE-treated surfaces. However, the occlusal three threads of these implants are not acid-etched; rather, the coronal portion of the Osseotite implants has machined surfaces.

The Full Osseotite implants are titanium implants, similar to the Osseotite implants, except that the implant bodies are DAE treated up to and including most of the implant collars (Fig 4.20). In the study described above, eight patients were selected according to a rigid protocol that included placement of standard Osseotite implants as controls and Full Osseotite implants as experimental variables. Ten sets of implants were placed.

Machined healing abutments were placed onto the Osseotite implants; DAE healing abutments were placed onto the Full Osseotite implants (see Fig 4.20). The implant sites were submitted to histologic, microbiologic, and radiographic analysis with customized intraoral devices; plaque accumulation analysis and bleeding indices were recorded. The patients' progress was followed for 12 months.

Plaque indices were recorded before and after professional oral hygiene sessions. The results demonstrated that the healing abutments with the modified surfaces (DAE) accumulated higher quantities of plaque ($P < .0006$) when compared with plaque accumulations on the machined healing abutments, and the plaque accumulated on DAE surfaces was more difficult to remove during oral hygiene sessions compared with machined surfaces ($P < .0143$) (Figs 4.21 and 4.22).

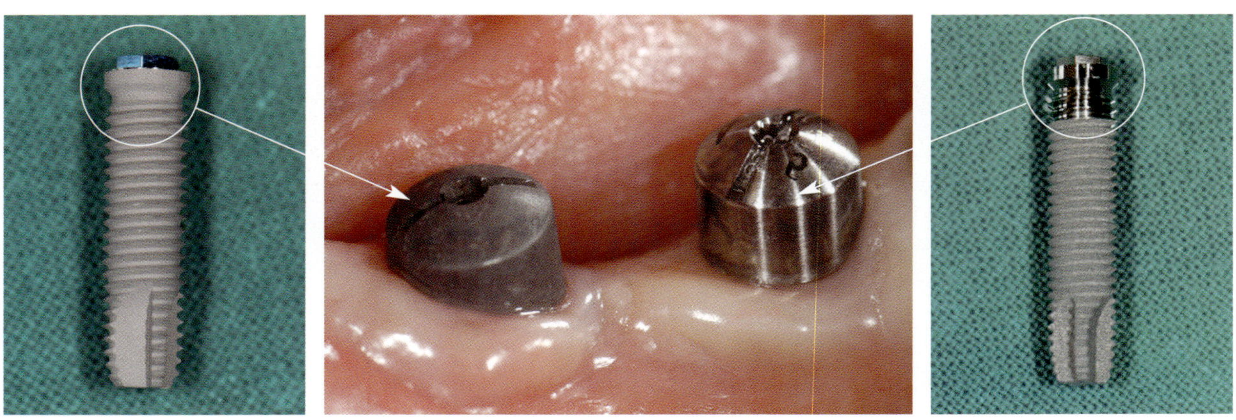

Fig 4.20 - Healing abutments in place *(middle)*. The healing abutment on the left side has a dual acid-etched surface and was screwed on a full Osseotite implant (*left*). The healing abutment on the right side has a machined surface and was connected on an Osseotite implant with a machined coronal surface (*right*).

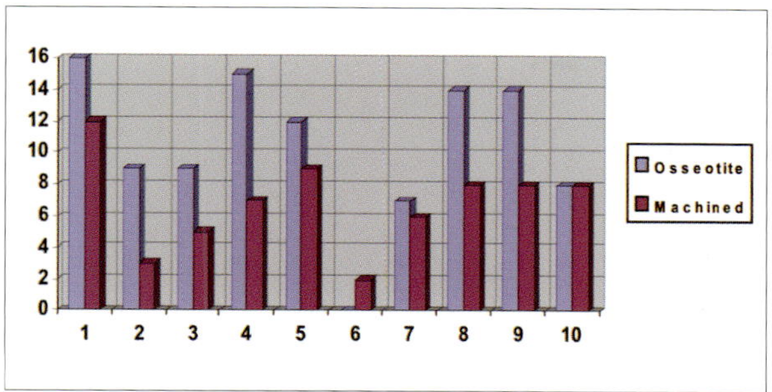

Fig 4.21 - Plaque accumulation before oral hygiene procedures. The numbers on the x-axis correspond to the number of implants examined. The numbers on the y-axis report the cumulative number of healing abutment surfaces that have plaque at the recording visits.

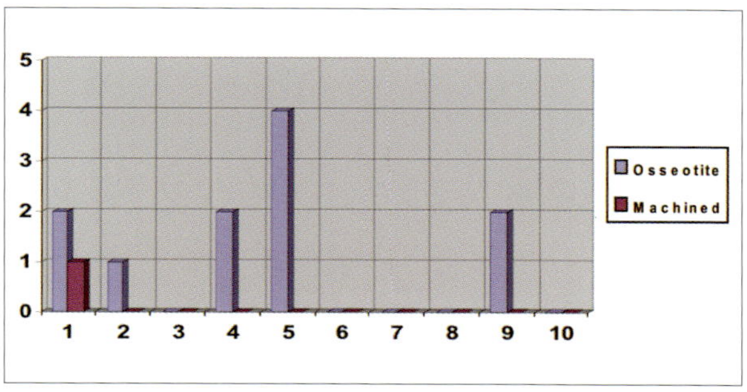

Fig 4.22 - Plaque accumulation after oral hygiene procedures. The numbers on the x-axis correspond to the number of implants examined. The numbers on the y-axis report the cumulative number of healing abutment surfaces that have plaque.

Bleeding indices did not show significant differences between the two sites (Figs 4.23 and 4.24). In most cases, this indicated the absence of inflammation. These data were confirmed by SEM analysis of the healing abutments: plaque was present in larger quantities on the acid-etched healing abutments but did not result in pathology in the peri-implant soft tissues (Figs 4.25 to 4.28).

The histologic (Fig 4.29) and microbiologic (Table 4.7) analyses of the peri-implant soft tissues did not show any differences between the two types of implants. Both sites demonstrated normal healing without significant differences as to inflammatory infiltrate, and the microbiotic populations were consistent with normal oral flora. These findings corresponded to results reported by other authors[77,84,85]: roughened surfaces accumulated larger quantities of plaque when compared with machined surfaces, but the plaque composition was similar in both groups.

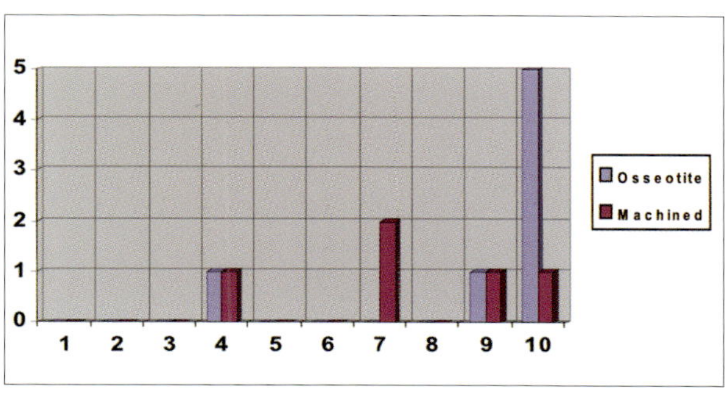

Fig 4.23 - Bleeding index before oral hygiene procedures in the 4 months after implant placement. The numbers on the x-axis correspond to the number of implants examined. The numbers on the y-axis report the cumulative number of healing abutment surfaces that demonstrated bleeding during the follow-up visits.

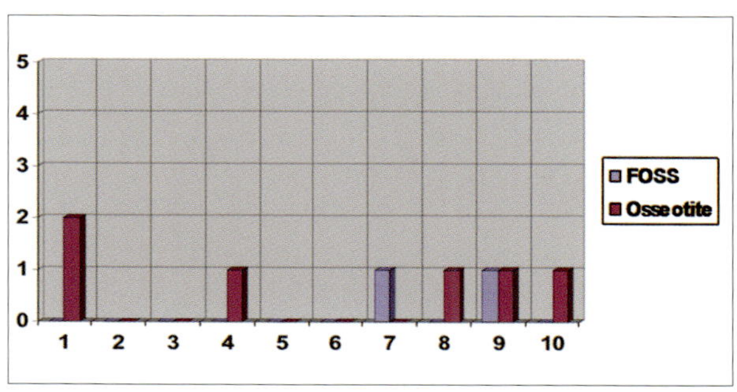

Figs 4.24 - Bleeding index at 12 months of healing. The numbers on the x-axis correspond to the number of implants examined. The numbers on the y-axis report the number of the healing abutment surfaces that demonstrated bleeding during the follow-up visits.

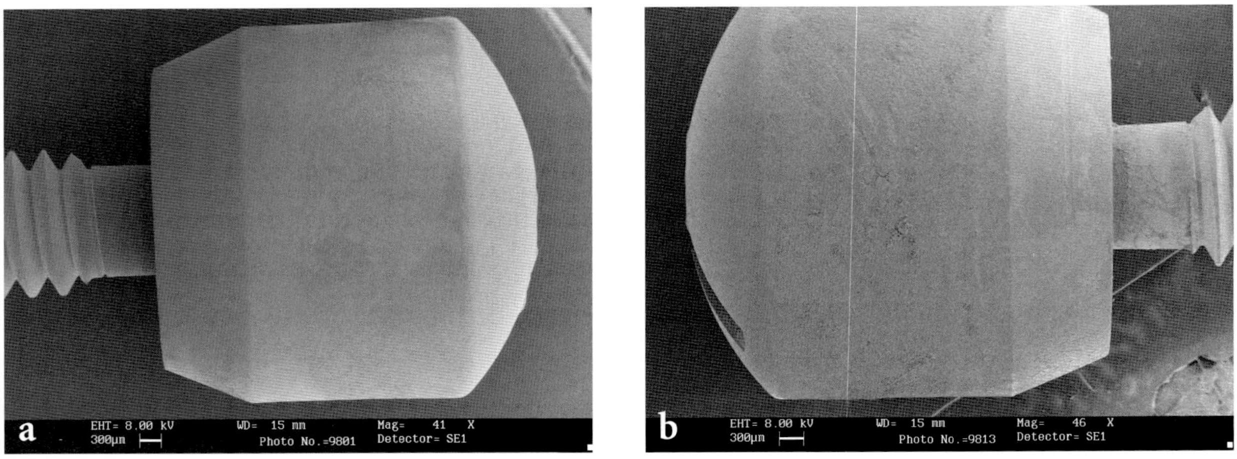

Fig 4.25 - *(a)* SEM of a machined healing abutment (Biomet 3i) (original magnification ×41). *(b)* SEM of an Osseotite abutment (original magnification ×46). Both healing abutments were removed from the same patient at 5 months after placement.

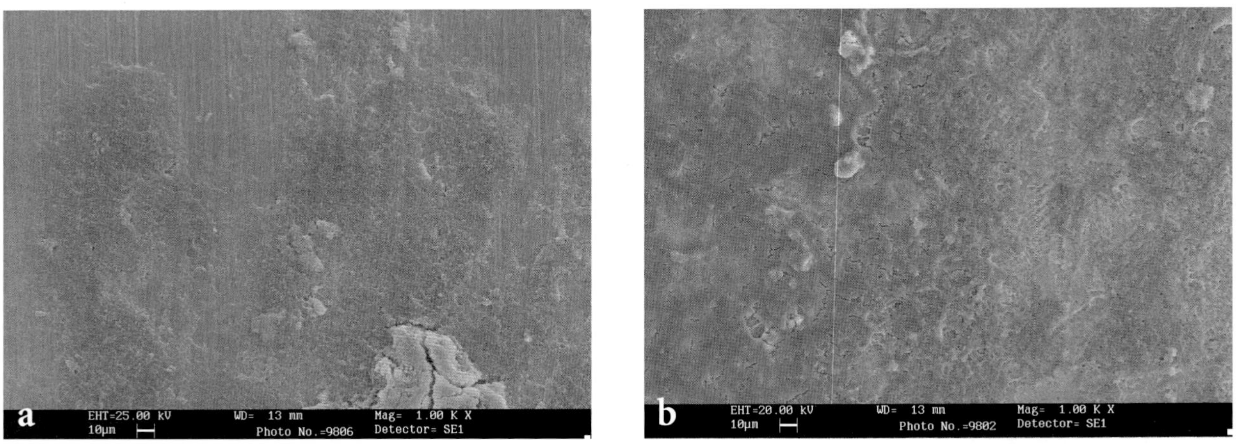

Fig 4.26 - *(a)* SEM of a machined abutment (Biomet 3i) (original magnification ×1,000). *(b)* SEM of an Osseotite abutment (original magnification ×1,000). Both healing abutments were removed from the same patient 5 months after placement.

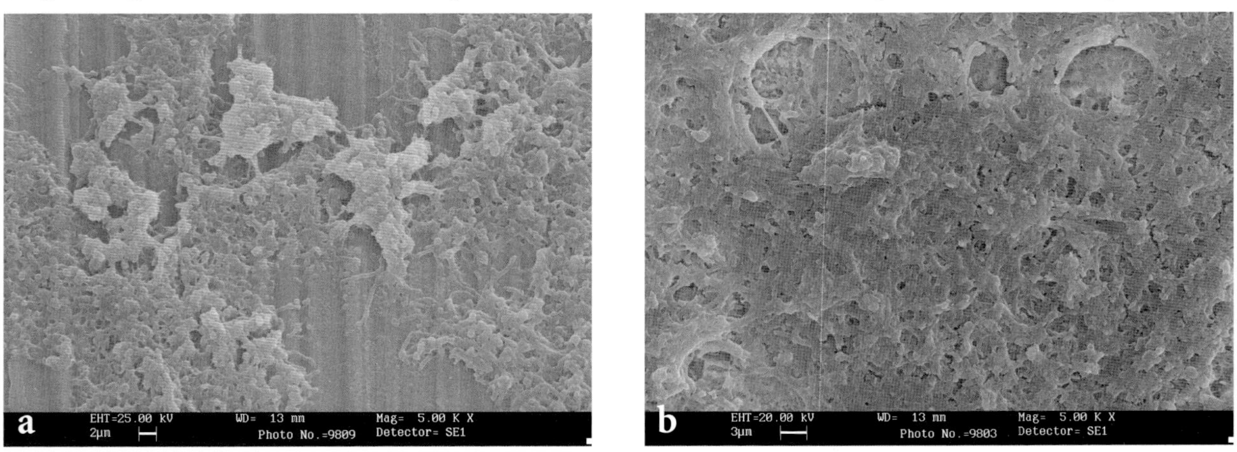

Fig 4.27 - *(a)* SEM of a machined abutment (Biomet 3i) (original magnification ×5,000). *(b)* SEM of an Osseotite abutment (original magnification ×5,000). Both healing abutments were removed from the same patient 5 months after placement.

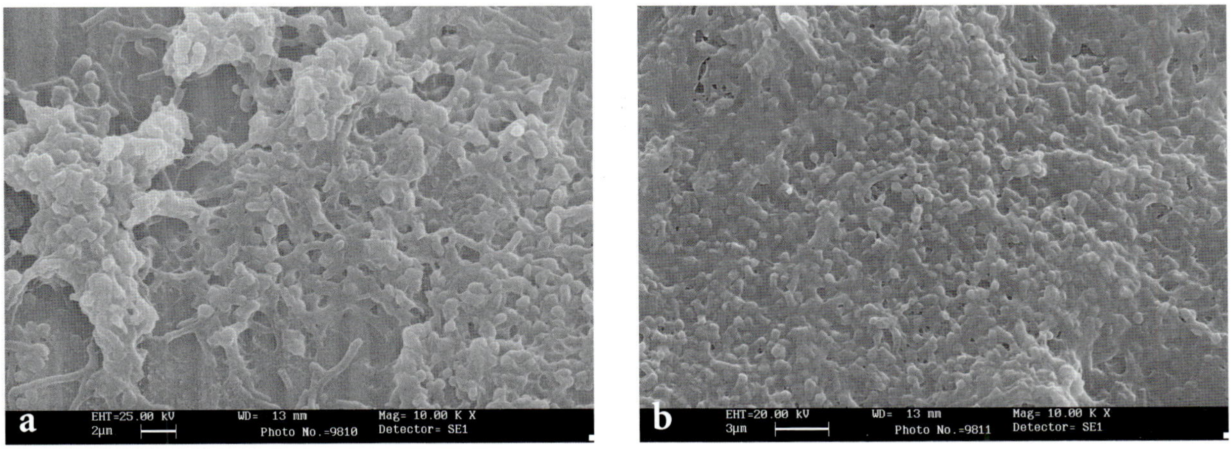

Fig 4.28 - *(a)* SEM of a machined abutment (Biomet 3i) (original magnification ×10,000). *(b)* SEM of an Osseotite abutment (original magnification ×10,000). Both healing abutments were removed from the same patient 5 months after placement. The surface of the machined abutment was still visible in some areas. The surface of the dual acid-etched abutment was completely covered with plaque.

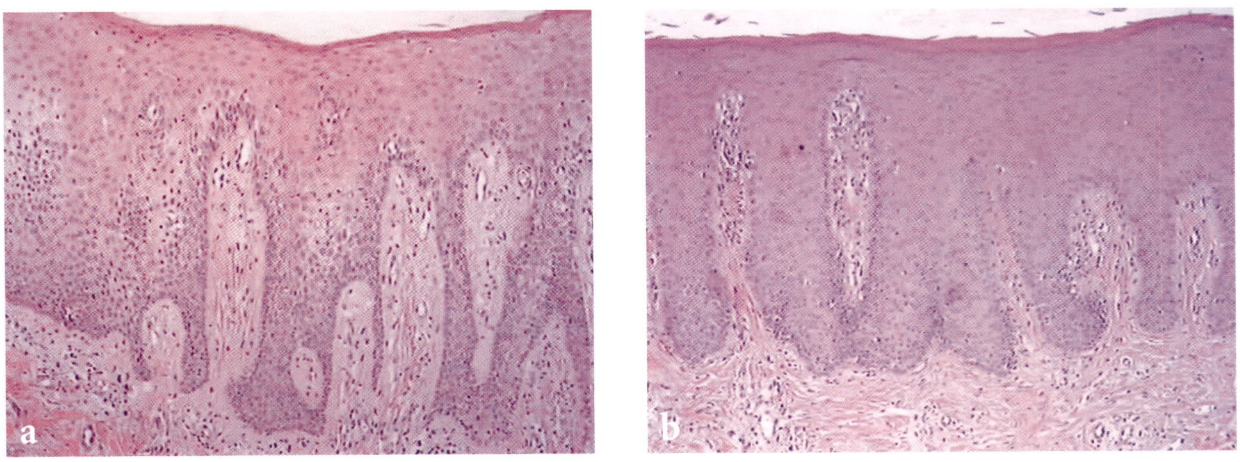

Fig 4.29 - *(a)* Light microscopic image of peri-implant mucosa taken in a zone adjacent to an Osseotite standard implant with a machined abutment. *(b)* Light microscopic image of peri-implant mucosa taken in a zone adjacent to a Full Osseotite implant with an Osseotite abutment after 3 months of healing. No significant differences were noted.

The presence of pathologic bacteria and their quantities appeared to be linked more to the conditions of the oral cavity than to the type of implant surface.

Measurement of peri-implant bone resorption, through intraoral radiographs, showed more coronal peri-implant bone resorption at the level of the standard Osseotite implants (average bone resorption was 1.45 mm after 6 months; 1.47 mm after 1 year) when compared with peri-implant bone resorption of Full Osseotite implants (average bone resorption was 0.45 mm after 6 months; 0.61 mm after 1 year) (Fig 4.30) ($P < .0174$). All patients' progress was followed according to a rigid protocol. They had excellent levels of oral hygiene and demonstrated high

TABLE 4.7 - BACTERIA FOUND AT THE LEVEL OF THE TWO IMPLANT SITES		
Clinical case	**OSSEOTITE**	**FULL OSSEOTITE**
01	–	*Veillonella* spp
02	–	*Peptococcus prevotii*
03	**Staphylococci**, Streptococci, *Prevotella intermedia*	**Staphylococci**, Streptococci, *Prevotella intermedia*
04	***Staphylococcus warneri***, *Streptococcus constellatus, Lactococcus lactis cremoris*	*Lactococcus lactis cremoris*, ***Staphylococcus capitis***, *Streptococcus mitis*
05	*Lactococcus garviae, Gemella morbillorum*	*Leuconostoc, Gemella morbillorum, Neisseria* spp, *Peptostreptococcus asaccharolyticus, Propionibacterium granulosum, Capnocytophaga*
06	***Pseudomonas aeruginosa***, *Neisseria* spp, *Pastorella multocida, Lactococcus lactis cremoris, Gemella haemolysans, Staphylococcus saccharolyticus*	*Neisseria* spp, ***Micrococcus* spp**, *Gemella haemolysans, Peptostreptococcus anaerobius*
07	*Prevotella intermedia*	***Pseudomonas aeruginosa***
08	–	***Prevotella oralis***
09	–	–
10	–	–

Table 4.7 - The bacteria not found in the normal oral flora are in bold print.

motivation. Therefore, it was not possible to evaluate the consequences of poor oral hygiene on implant thread exposure in the oral cavity, nor the effects of longer follow-up periods.

Many studies reported in the literature confirmed the results of this research: Surfaces modified with DAE favor the osseointegration process,[41–44,86, 87] and peri-implant soft tissues are not affected by the type of titanium surface adjacent to them (machined or modified).[88–92] Other studies have affirmed that implant surface roughness can favor the formation of a wider connective tissue seal and inhibit apical downgrowth of epithelium.[76,93–96]

Lin et al[97] reported more plaque accumulations and greater inflammation on modified implant surfaces when compared with smooth surfaces. However, the team's implant surfaces were modified via apposition of hydroxyapatite with a plasma-spray technique, not with the DAE treatment received by the implants in the research reported above. A significant number of studies reported in the literature concerning implant-soft tissue responses are based on animal research.[88–92,94,96,97] These studies do not represent clinical situations with osseointegrated implants in humans, nor do they represent the complex (physical and chemical) phenomena to which dental implants are subjected in the human oral cavity. The authors believe that it is extremely important to perform and report the results of in vivo clinical research in humans.

On the basis of the data from the University of Genoa research reported above, it is possible to affirm that, in patients with satisfactory oral hygiene, Full Osseotite implants yield preferential results when compared with standard Osseotite implants. In fact, modified surfaces favor bone healing and osseointegration. On the basis of this study, there were no negative side effects noted with the use of DAE surfaces in contact with peri-implant soft tissues.

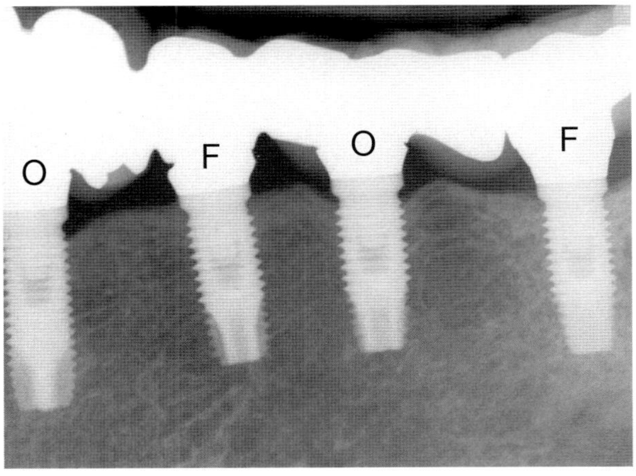

Fig 4.30 - Intraoral periapical radiograph of a clinical case of two standard Osseotite implants (O) and two Full Osseotite implants (F), 1 year after placement. The Osseotite implants demonstrated greater crestal bone loss than either of the Full Osseotite implants.

In review, the in vivo comparison between Osseotite and Full Osseotite implants and healing abutments, where the peri-implant soft tissue response was evaluated, yielded the following results:

- Healing abutments with the Osseotite surface treatment (DAE) resulted in larger accumulations of plaque than did healing abutments with machined surfaces ($P < .0006$).
- Plaque removal from the DAE healing abutments was more difficult ($P < .0143$) than plaque removal from machined healing abutments.
- Plaque accumulations from the DAE healing abutments did not reveal microbiologic or qualitative histologic differences in adjacent tissues when compared with machined surfaces.
- Bleeding indices did not differ significantly between the two groups in the first year after implant placement.
- Full Osseotite implants demonstrated minor peri-implant bone resorption (averages of 0.45 mm after 6 months; 0.61 after 1 year) when compared with Osseotite implants (averages of 1.45 mm after 6 months; 1.47 mm after 1 year). This difference between the two implants was statistically significant ($P < .0174$).

Use of cDNA microarray in dental research on different implant surfaces

The use of cDNA microarray allows for the simultaneous evaluation of the expression of tens of thousands of genes and, as described in a review of 2002,[98] represents a new promising method for use in dental research.[99] A DNA microarray is done on a surface to which sequences of DNA (called "probes") are attached. These sequences are then exposed to a target represented by mRNA extracted from the cells under examination. Microarrays allow for quantitative evaluation of genetic expression by measuring the mRNA hybridization levels with the probes immobilized on the surface. So far, microarrays have been used in dental research mainly for the study of tumors of the oral cavity. More recently, some researchers have used this technology to analyze the behavior of osteoblastic cells in contact with different implant surfaces. This type of research performed on osteoblast-like cell lines (MG-63 or SaOS-2) or on cells derived from human bone (HBDC) has shown that the expression of genes coding for key proteins in osteogenesis is dependent on the implant surface studied.[100–107]

The genes most frequently involved were associated with various cellular activities, in particular with vesicular transport, signal transduction, regulation of the cell cycle, apoptosis, and structural and metabolic functions. Therefore they affected cellular adhesion, growth, and differentiation. The items analyzed showed that modified implant surfaces were able to increase the expression of osteogenic genes when compared with surfaces of machined titanium implants. The authors believe that these data must be taken into consideration, especially relative to implant surgery in areas of high risk, as well as in immediate-loading protocols, where it is important to adopt procedures that promote osseointegration and make results more predictable.

REFERENCES

1. Schierano G, Pera P, Macaluso MM, Galli C, Conserva E. Impianti dentari. In: Preti G (ed). Riabilitazione Protesica. Torino: UTET, 2005;341–367.
2. Pappalardo G. Materiali per implantologia. In: Pappalardo G (ed). Manuale di Materiali Dentari. Padova: Piccin, 1997:251–260.
3. Ellingsen JE, Thomsen P, Lyngstadaas P. Advances in dental implant materials and tissue regeneration. Periodontol 2000 2006;41:136–156.
4. Steinemann S. Metal implants and surface reactions. Injury 1996;27(3, suppl):16SC–22SC.
5. Lacefield WR. Materials characteristics of uncoated/ceramic-coated implant materials. Adv Dent Res 1999;13:21–26.
6. Sawase T, Hai K, Yoshida K, Baba K, Hatada R, Atsuda M. Spectroscopic studies of three osseointegrated implants. J Dent 1998;26:119–124.
7. Thompson GJ, Puleo DA. Effects of sublethal metal ion concentrations on osteogenic cells derived from bone marrow stromal cells. J Applied Biomater 1995;6:249–258.
8. McCracken M. Dental implant materials: Commercially pure titanium and titanium alloys. J Prosthodont 1999;8:40–43.
9. Morra M, Cassinelli C, Di Carlo F. Le superfici implantari. In: Malchiodi M (ed). Chirurgia Implantare. Bologna: Martina, 2003.
10. Pera P, Conserva E, Pin D, et al. Analisi "in vitro" della citotossicità di differenti sistemi implantari in relazione al tipo di microtopografia di superficie. Implantologia 2004;3:207–217.
11. Arcelli D, Palmieri A, Pezzetti F, Brunelli G, Zollino I, Carinci F. Genetic effects of a titanium surface on osteoblasts: A meta-analysis. J Oral Sci 2007;4:299–309.
12. Li LH, Kong YM, Kim HW, et al. Improved biological performance of Ti implants due to surface modification by micro-arc oxidation. Biomaterials 2004;25:2867–2875.
13. Brånemark PI, Zarb GA, Albrektsson T (eds). Osseointegrazione tissutale. Osseointegrazione in Odontoiatria. Berlin: Quintessenz, 1987.
14. Cehreli M, Duyck J, De Cooman M, Puers R, Naert I. Implant design and interface force transfer. A photoelastic and strain-gauge analysis. Clin Oral Implants Res 2004;15:249–257.
15. Jokstad A, Braegger U, Brunski JB, Carr AB, Naert I, Wennerberg A. Quality of dental implants. Int Dent J 2003;53:409–443.
16. Wolff J. Das Gesetz der Transformation der Knochen. Berlin: Hirschwald, 1982.
17. Cochran DL. A comparison of endosseous dental implant surfaces. J Periodontol 1999;70:1523–1539.
18. Morra M. Biochemical modification of titanium surfaces: Peptides and ECM proteins. Eur Cell Mater 2006;12:1–15.
19. Yamamichi N, Pugdee K, Chang WJ, et al. Gene expression monitoring in osteoblasts on titanium coated with fibronectin-derived peptide. Dent Mater J 2008;27:744–750.
20. Stanford CM. Surface modifications of dental implants. Aust Dent J 2008;53:S26–S33.
21. Cassinelli C, Morra M, Bruzzone G, et al. Surface chemistry effects of topographic modification of titanium dental implant surfaces: In vitro experiments. J Oral Maxillofac Implants 2003;18:46–52.
22. Davies JE. Mechanisms of endosseous integration. Int J Prosthodont 1998;11:391–401.
23. Albrektsson T, Brånemark PI, Hansson HA, et al. The interface zone of inorganic implants in vivo: Titanium implants in bone. Ann Biomed Eng 1983;11:1–27.
24. Soskolne WA, Cohen S, Sennerby L, Wennerberg A, Shapira L. The effect of titanium surface roughness on the adhesion of monocytes and their secretion of TNF and PGE2. Clin Oral Implants Res 2002;13:86–93.
25. Viornery C, Guenther HL, Aronsson BO, Pechy P, Descouts P, Gratzel M. Osteoblast culture on polished titanium disks modified with phosphoric acids. J Biomed Mater Res 2002;62:149–155.

26. Sul YT, Johansson CB, Kang Y, Jeon DG, Albrektsson T. Bone reactions to oxidized titanium implants with electrochemical anion sulphuric acid and phosphoric acid incorporation. Clin Implant Dent Relat Res 2002;4:78–87.
27. Sul YT. The significance of the surface properties of oxidized titanium to the bone response: Special emphasis on potential biochemical bonding of oxidized titanium implant. Biomaterials 2003;24: 3893–3907.
28. Cordioli G, Majzoub Z, Piattelli A, Scarano A. Removal torque and histomorphometric investigation of 4 different titanium surfaces: An experimental study in the rabbit tibia. Int J Oral Maxillofac Implants 2000;15:668–674.
29. Sul YT, Johansson CB, Jeong Y, Wennerberg A, Albrektsson T. Resonance frequency and removal torque analysis of implants with turned and anodized surface oxides. Clin Oral Implants Res 2002;13:252–259.
30. Sul YT, Johansson CB, Roser K, Albrektsson T. Qualitative and quantitative observations of bone tissue reactions to anodized implants. Biomaterials 2002;23:1809–1817.
31. Lincks J, Boyan BD, Blanchard CR, et al. Response of MG63 osteoblast-like cells to titanium and titanium alloy is dependent on surface roughness and composition. Biomaterials 1998;19:2219–2232.
32. Mustafa K, Wroblewski J, Hultenby K, Lopez BS, Arvidson K. Effects of titanium surfaces blasted with TiO2 particles on the initial attachment of cells derived from human mandibular bone. A scanning electron microscope and histomorphometric analysis. Clin Oral Implants Res 2000;11:116–128.
33. Anselme K, Bigerelle M, Noël B, Iost A, Hardouin P. Effect of grooved titanium substratum on human osteoblastic cell growth. J Biomed Mater Res 2002;60:529–540.
34. Le Guèhennec L, Soueidan A, Layrolle P, Amouriq Y. Surface treatments of titanium dental implants for rapid osseointegration. Dent Mater 2007; 23:844–854.
35. Massaro C, Rotolo P, De Riccardis F, et al. Comparative investigation of the surface properties of commercial titanium dental implants. Part I: Chemical composition. J Mater Sci Mater Med 2002; 13:535–548.
36. Rodriguez-Rius D, Garcia-Saban FJ. Physico-chemical characterization of the surface of 9 dental implants with 3 different surface treatments. Med Oral Patol Oral Cir Bucal 2005;10:58–65.
37. Lorenzetti M, Menicucci G, Mozzati M, Polizzi G. Implantologia: Nuove acquisizioni e aspetti clinici. In: Preti G (ed). Riabilitazione Protesica. Torino: UTET, 2003:185–261.
38. Adell R, Lekholm U, Rockler B, Brånemark PI. A 15-year study of osseointegrated implants in the treatment of the edentulous jaw. Int J Oral Surg 1981;10:387–416.
39. Adell R, Eriksson B, Lekholm U, Brånemark PI, Jemt T. Long-term follow-up study of osseointegrated implants in the treatment of totally edentulous jaws. Int J Oral Maxillofac Implants 1990;5:347–359.
40. Park KH, Heo SJ, Koak JY, et al. Osseointegration of anodized implants under different current voltages: A rabbit study. J Oral Rehabil 2007; 34:517–527.
41. Mayer TM, Hawley CE, Gunsolley JC, Feldman S. The single-tooth implant: A viable alternative for single tooth replacement. J Periodontol 2001;3: 687–693.
42. Testori T, Woolfe S, Porter SS, Wiseman L. A prospective multicenter clinical study of the Osseotite implant: A four-year interim report. Int J Oral Maxillofac Implants 2001;16:193–200.
43. Grunder U, Gaberthuel T, Boitel N, et al. Evaluating the clinical performance of the Osseotite implant: Defining prosthetic predictability. Compend Contin Educ Dent 1999;20:628–640.
44. Sullivan DY, Sherwood RL, Porter SS. Long-term performance of Osseotite implants: A 6-year clinical follow-up. Compend Contin Educ Dent 2001;22:326–328,330,332–334.

45. Sullivan DY, Sherwood RL, Mai TN. Preliminary results of a multicenter study evaluating a chemically enhanced surface for machined commercially pure titanium implants. J Prosthet Dent 1997; 78:379–386.
46. Stach RM, Kohles SS. A meta-analysis examining the clinical survivability of machined-surfaced and Osseotite implants in poor-quality bone. Implant Dent 2003;12:87–96.
47. Conserva E, Tealdo T, Acquaviva A, Bevilacqua M, Volpara G, Pera P. Analisi morfologica e valutazione della proliferazione cellulare in relazione a differenti trattamenti di superficie impiantare: Studio in vitro. Implantologia 2005;4:1–15.
48. Cochran DL, Boyan BD. Effect of titanium surface roughness on proliferation, differentiation and protein synthesis of human osteoblast-like cells (MG63). J Biomed Mater Res 1995;29:389–401.
49. Kieswatter K, Schwartz Z, Hummert TW, et al. Surface roughness modulates the local production of growth factors and cytokines by osteoblast-like MG-63 cells. J Biomed Mater Res 1996;32:55–63.
50. Boyan BD, Batzer R, Kieswetter K, et al. Titanium surface roughness alters responsiveness of MG63 osteoblast-like cells to 1 alpha, 25-(OH)2D3. J Biomed Mater Res 1998;39:77–85.
51. Boyan BD, Schwartz Z. Modulation of osteogenesis via implant surface design. In: Davies JE (ed). Bone Engineering. Toronto: Em Squared, 2000:232–239.
52. Davies JE, Housseini MM. Histodynamics of endosseous wound healing. In: Davies JE (ed). Bone Engineering. Toronto: Em Squared, 2000;1–14.
53. Park JY, Gemmel CH, Davies JE. Platelet interactions with titanium: Modulation of platelet activity by surface topography. Biomaterials 2000; 22:2671–2682.
54. Park JY, Davies JE. Red blood cell and platelet interactions with titanium implant surfaces. Clin Oral Implants Res 2000;11:530–539.
55. Wojciechowski PW. Transport and adsorption of protein and cells at interfaces. In: Brash PL, Wojciechowski PW (eds). Interfacial Phenomena and Bioproducts. New York: Marcel Dekker, 1996:109–230.
56. Kasemo B, Gold J. Implant surfaces and interface processes. Adv Dent Res 1999;13:8–20.
57. Ellingsen JE. A study on the mechanism of protein adsorption to TiO2. Biomaterials 1991;12:593–596.
58. Deligianni DD, Katsala N, Ladas S, Sotiropoulou D, Amedee J, Missirlis YF. Effect of surface roughness of the titanium alloy Ti-6Al-4V on human bone marrow cell response and on protein adsorption. Biomaterials 2001;22:1241–1251.
59. Vörös J, Wieland M, Ruiz-Taylor L, Textor M, Brunette DM. Characterization of titanium surfaces. In: Brunette DM, Tengvall P, Textor M, Thomsen P (eds). Titanium in Medicine. Berlin: Springer, 2001:87–144.
60. Morra M, Cassinelli C. Evaluation of surface contamination of titanium dental implants by LV-SEM: Comparison with XPS measurements. Surf Interface Anal 1997;25:983–988.
61. Morra M, Cassinelli C, Bruzzone G, et al. Surface chemistry effects of topographic modification of titanium dental implant surfaces. 1: Surface analysis. Int J Oral Maxillofac Implants 2003;18:40–45.
62. Wieland M, Sitting C, Brunette DM, Textor M, Spencer ND. Measurement and evaluation of the chemical composition and topography of titanium implant surfaces in bone engineering. In: Davies JE (ed). Bone Engineering. Toronto: Em Squared, 2000:163–182.
63. Block MS, Kent JN, Kay JF. Evaluation of hydroxylapatite-coated titanium dental implants in dogs. J Oral Maxillofac Surg 1987;45:601–607.
64. Block MS, Finger IM, Fontenot MG, Kent JN. Loaded hydroxylapatite-coated and grit-blasted titanium implants in dogs. Int J Oral Maxillofac Implants 1989;4:219–225.
65. Sun L, Berndt CC, Gross KA, Kucuk A. Material fundamentals and clinical performance of plasma-sprayed hydroxyapatite coatings: A review. J Biomed Mater Res 2001;58:570–592.
66. Steflik DE, Corpe RS, Young TR, Sisk AL, Parr GR. The biologic tissue responses to uncoated and coated implanted biomaterials. Adv Dent Res 1999;13:27–33.

67. Ellingsen JE, Thomsen P, Lyngstadaas SP. Advances in dental implant materials and tissue regeneration. Periodontol 2006;41:136–156.
68. Pera P, Conserva E, Tealdo T. Analisi in vitro della citotossicità di differenti sistemi implantari in relazione al tipo di microtopografia di superficie. Implantologia 2004;3:215–217.
69. Iyengar GV. Elemental Analysis of Biological Systems. Biological, Medical, Environmental, Compositional, and Methodological Aspects, vol 1. Boca Raton: CRC, 1989.
70. Brunski JB. In vivo bone response to biomechanical loading at the bone/dental-implant interface. Adv Dent Res 1999;13:99–119.
71. Davies JE. Understanding peri-implant endosseous healing. J Dent Educ 2003;67:932–949.
72. Cehreli MC, Akca K. Mechanobiology of bone and mechanocoupling of endosseous titanium oral implants. J Long Term Eff Med Implants 2005; 15:139–152.
73. Joos U, Wiesmann HP, Szuwart T, Meyer U. Mineralization at the interface of implants. Int J Oral Maxillofac Surg 2006;35:783–790.
74. Myshin HL, Wiens JP. Factors affecting soft tissue around dental implants: A review of the literature. J Prosthet Dent 2005;94:440–444.
75. Rompen E, Domken O, Degidi M, Pontes AEF, Piattelli A. The effect of material characteristics, of surface topography and of implant components and connections on soft tissue integration: A literature review. Clin Oral Implants Res 2006;17:55–67.
76. Schwartz Z, Nasazky E, Boyan BD. Surface microtopography regulates osteointegration: The role of implant surface microtopography in osteointegration. Alpha Omegan 2005;98:9–19.
77. Quirynen M, van der Mei HC, Boleen CML, et al. An in vivo study on the influence of the surface roughness of implants on the microbiology of supra- and subgingival plaque. J Dent Res 1993;72:1304–1309.
78. Rimondini L, Fare S, Brambilla E, et al. The effect of surface roughness on early in vivo plaque colonization on titanium. J Periodontol 1997;68:556–562.
79. O'Mahony A, MacNeill SR, Cobb CM. Design features that may influence bacterial plaque retention: A retrospective analysis of failed implants. Quintessence Int 2000;31:249–256.
80. Ericsson I, Berglundh T, Marinello CP, Liljenberg B, Lindhe J. Long-standing plaque and gingivitis at implants and teeth in the dog. Clin Oral Implants Res 1992;3:99–103.
81. Abrahamsson I, Berglundh T, Glantz PO, Lindhe J. The mucosal attachment at different abutments. A comparison study in dog. J Clin Periodontol 1998;25:721–727.
82. Abrahamsson I, Berglundh T, Lindhe J. Soft tissue response to plaque formation at different implant systems. A comparative study in the dog. Clin Oral Implants Res 1998;9:73–79.
83. Baldi D, Menini M, Pera F, Ravera G, Pera P. Plaque accumulation on exposed titanium surfaces and peri-implant tissue behavior. A preliminary 1-year clinical study. Int J Prosthodont 2009;22:447–455.
84. Quirynen M. The clinical meaning of the surface roughness and the surface free energy of intra-oral hard substrata on the microbiology of the supra- and subgingival plaque: Results of in vitro and in vivo experiments. J Dent 1994;22(1, suppl):13S–16S.
85. Li X, Guo T, Zhou Z. Influence of surface roughness of pure titanium on accumulation of bacterium. Zhonghua Kou Qiang Yi Xue Za Zhi 2001; 36:289–291.
86. Khang W, Feldman S, Hawley CE, Gunsolley J. A multi-center study comparing dual acid-etched and machined-surfaced implants in various bone qualities. J Periodontol 2001;72:1384–1390.
87. Trisi P, Lazzara R, Rebaudi A, Rao W, Testori T, Porter SS. Bone-implant contact after 2 months of healing in the human maxilla. J Periodontol 2003;74:945–956.
88. Abrahamsson I, Berglundh T, Wennström J, Lindhe J. The peri-implant hard and soft tissues at different implant systems. A comparative study in the dog. Clin Oral Implants Res 1996;7:212–219.

89. Çomut AA, Weber HP, Shortkroff S, Cui FZ, Spector M. Connective tissue orientation around dental implants in a canine model. Clin Oral Implants Res 2001;12:433–440.
90. Abrahamsson I, Zitzmann NU, Berglundh T, Linder E, Wennerberg A, Lindhe J. The mucosal attachment to titanium implants with different surface characteristics: An experimental study in dogs. J Clin Periodontol 2002;29:448–455.
91. Zitzmann NU, Abrahamsson I, Berghlund T, Lindhe J. Soft tissue reactions to plaque formation at implant abutments with different surface topography. An experimental study in dogs. J Clin Periodontol 2002;29:456–461.
92. Watzak G, Zechner W, Tangl S, Vasak C, Donath K, Watzek G. Soft tissue around three different implant types after 1.5 years of functional loading without oral hygiene. A preliminary study in baboons. Clin Oral Implants Res 2006;17:229–236.
93. Glauser R, Schüpbach P, Gottlow J, Hämmerle CH. Periimplant soft tissue barrier at experimental one-piece mini-implants with different surface topography in humans: A light-microscopic overview and histometric analysis. Clin Implant Dent Relat Res 2005;7(1, suppl):44S–51S.
94. Kim H, Murakami H, Cherhoudi B, Textor M, Brunette DM. Effects of surface topography on the connective tissue attachment to subcutaneous implants. Int J Oral Maxillofac Implants 2006; 21:354–365.
95. Zhao BH, Lee SI, Bai W, Cui FZ, Feng HL. Improvement of fibroblast adherence to titanium surface by calcium phosphate coating formed with IBAD. Surf Coat Technol 2005;193:366–371.
96. Zhao BH, Han I, Feng HL, Bai W, Cui FZ, Lee SI. Histological and histomorphometrical study of connective tissue around calcium phosphate coated titanium dental implants in a canine model. Surf Coat Technol 2006;201:5696–5700.
97. Lin H, Van't Veen SJ, Klein CP. Permucosal implantation pilot study with HA-coated dental implant in dogs. Biomaterials 1992;13:825–831.
98. Kuo PW, Whipple ME, Sonis ST, Ohno-Machado L, Jenssen TK. Gene expression profiling by DNA microarrays and its application to dental research. Oral Oncol 2002;38:650–656.
99. Mittermayer C, Eblenkamp M, Richter HA, Zwadlo-Klarwasser G, Bhardwaj RS, Klosterhalfen B. Pathology of implants. Kongressbd Dtsch Ges Chir Kongr 2002;119:491–497.
100. Carinci F, Volinia S, Pezzetti F, Francioso F, Tosi L, Piattelli A. Titanium-cell interaction: Analysis of gene expression profiling. J Biomed Mater Res B Appl Biomater 2003;66:341–346.
101. Carinci F, Pezzetti F, Volinia S, et al. Analysis of osteoblast-like MG63 cells' response to a rough implant surface by means of DNA microarray. J Oral Implantol 2003;29:215–220.
102. Kim Y, Jang JH, Ku Y, et al. Microarray-based expression analysis of human osteoblast-like cell response to anodized titanium surface. Biotechnol Lett 2004;26:399–402.
103. Knabe C, Berger G, Gildenhaar R, Klar F, Zreiqat H. The modulation of osteogenesis in vitro by calcium titanium phosphate coatings. Biomaterials 2004; 25:4911–4919.
104. Carinci F, Pezzetti F, Volinia S, et al. Analysis of MG63 osteoblastic-cell response to a new nanoporous implant surface by means of a microarray technology. Clin Oral Implants Res 2004; 15:180–186.
105. Kim CS, Sohn SH, Jeon SK, Kim KN, Ryu JJ, Kim MK. Effect of various implant coatings on biological responses in MG63 using cDNA microarray. J Oral Rehabil 2006;33:368–379.
106. Sohn SH, Jun HK, Kim CS, et al. Biological responses in osteoblast-like cell line according to thin layer hydroxyapatite coatings on anodized titanium. J Oral Rehabil 2006;33:898–911.
107. Baldi D, Longobardi MG, Cartiglia C, et al. Dental implants osteogenic properties evaluated by cDNA microarrays. Clin Implant Dent; 2011;20:299–305.

CHAPTER 5
PRIMARY STABILITY

COLUMBUS BRIDGE PROTOCOL	
SURGICAL PROTOCOL	**PROSTHETIC PROTOCOL**
External hex rough-surface implants	Screw-retained fixed prosthesis
Implant length ≥ 13 mm, Ø 4 mm	Plaster impression with pickup technique
Underprepared osteotomy	Rigid splinting with metal framework
Implant insertion torque ≥ 40 Ncm	Passive fit with the luting technique
Angled implants in native bone	Acrylic resin occlusal surfaces
Angled conical abutments	No distal cantilevers
No bone regenerative techniques	Immediate functional load 24–48 h after surgery

Table 5.1

As described in chapter 2, bone healing relies upon the presence of undifferentiated mesenchymal cells that are affected by conditions in the receptor bed. At the bone-implant interface, these conditions consist of the chemical and physical characteristics of titanium and the immobility of the implant. Many authors believe that the primary stability of dental implants is an essential prerequisite for osseointegration.[1–9] Primary stability can be assessed by the absence of mobility between implants and osteotomies immediately following implant placement. Based on clinical findings, implant mobility is classified as follows:[10]

- *Absence of mobility:* The implant is mechanically stable, and no movement can be detected.
- *Partial mobility:* The implant cannot move horizontally, but rotation is possible.
- *Lateral and/or vertical mobility:* The implant is not secure within the osteotomy.

A mobile implant should be removed immediately and, if possible, substituted with another implant with a larger diameter or length.[11] Friberg and colleagues reported a failure rate of 32% in implants that did not demonstrate primary stability.[12]

ASSESSING PRIMARY STABILITY

Implant stability may be assessed with invasive or noninvasive techniques. Removal torque, an invasive technique, is used almost exclusively for scientific research in animals.[13–17] Noninvasive techniques are suitable for use in humans as well as in animal research. They include:

- Percussion
- Insertion torque
- Periotest (Medizintechnik Gulden)
- Resonance frequency analysis (Ostell AB)
- Radiographs

Invasive technique: removal torque

Removal torque is an invasive technique that applies force counterclockwise to an implant to test its degree of osseointegration. Force is placed on the implant until the biologic bone-implant connection is broken. Johansson and Albrektsson[18] reported that a torque value of 11 Ncm is necessary to remove an implant 3 weeks after implant placement; after 3 and 12 months, that value increases to 68 and 88 Ncm, respectively. Reverse torque testing implies that the implant will be removed; therefore, this test is not clinically relevant in human patients.

Noninvasive techniques

Percussion is the simplest of the methods that use vibration to interpret implant stability. It is based on the difference in the sound made by percussing an osseointegrated implant versus a fibrointegrated or nonintegrated implant. When percussed with a metallic instrument, integrated implants emit a sharp sound. In comparison, fibrointegrated or nonintegrated implants produce dull, flat sounds. Note that percussion supplies only qualitative, not quantitative, data.[19]

One of the most easily applicable and reliable quantitative methods to assess bone-implant contact during surgery is the *insertion torque value*, first proposed in 1994 by Johansson and Strid[20] (Fig 5.1).

Higher insertion torque values are correlated with more stable implants (primary stability).[21] Insertion torque represents the moment, expressed in Ncm, required to screw implants into bone. The major disadvantage of this measurement is that it is not repeatable in real time. It can be obtained only at the time of implant placement. Its primary advantage is that it can be easily checked. The insertion torque value is normally visualized on the display of the drill unit motor in a range from 10 to 50 Ncm.

Once the motor stops at the maximum value, it still is possible to improve the seating of the implant with the use of a dynamometric wrench that can reach insertion values of up to 70 Ncm (Fig 5.2). Insertion torque values greater than 40 to 50 Ncm have been associated with problems in the local microcirculation and, consequently, with necrosis (pressure necrosis) of osteocytes and bone resorption.[22,23] It should be noted that in the original articles by Niimi et al[22] and O'Sullivan et al,[23] pressure necrosis is not mentioned. More recently, Trisi et al[24] concluded that exceeding a certain insertion torque value, rather than causing bone necrosis, stimulates bone remodeling.

By conducting removal torque tests in dog femurs, Okazaki et al[25] observed that primary stability decreased within 1 week after implant placement, a characteristic already observed by other authors.[26]

During the first weeks after implant placement, high insertion torque values result in high levels of implant primary stability and improved mechanical retention in bone.

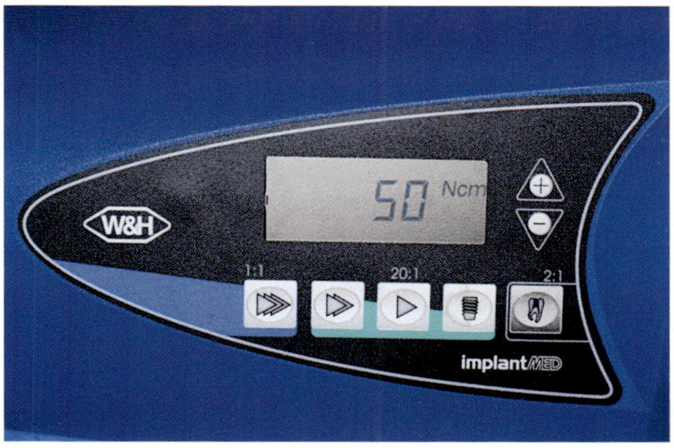

Figs 5.1 - Digital display of an implant drilling unit that identifies the amount of torque generated through the handpiece and applied to an implant. In this case, the torque value was 50 Ncm.

Presumably, this decrease is caused by osteoclastic remodeling of the necrotic bone that results from damage inflicted during the surgical preparation of the implant sites.[27,28]

The *Periotest* is an instrument designed to assess dental mobility by measuring the resiliency of the periodontal ligament.[29] Some authors promote its use in assessing the degree of osseointegration of dental implants.[30,31] Others discount its use because of the Periotest's limited sensitivity (values range from −8 to +50).[32] A new noninvasive technique based on *resonance frequency analysis* (Osstell) was introduced in 1996.[33] The Osstell system generates a number called the *implant stability quotient* (ISQ) that ranges in value from 1 to 100. The ISQ appears to provide data regarding the macroscopic behavior of the bone-implant system, and the Osstell system was rapidly accepted and proved helpful in both research and clinical practice, especially with the advent of immediate and early loading protocols (Fig 5.3). What the Osstell system actually measures, however, is unknown.[34,35] Some authors have reported a correlation between ISQ values and the amount of bone-implant contact (BIC).[36,37] However, this value does not correlate with the degree of osseointegration because *(1)* implants with different BIC values may show similar ISQ values[38]; *(2)* implants with similar BIC values may show different ISQ values; and *(3)* implants with similar bone fixation may record different ISQ values.[39] Therefore, the Osstell device cannot diagnose the implants that have lost stability and become mobile. It can reasonably be assumed that resonance frequency analysis does not give only information regarding bone-implant interfaces, but it primarily measures the bone tissue–implant behaviors according to the bone volume in a specific area.

Intraoral radiography, though unable to provide quantitative values of the primary stability of implants, may prove useful in the presurgical

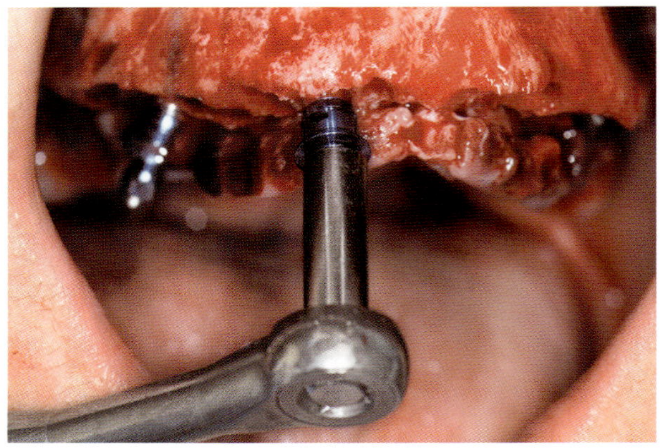

Fig 5.2 - Hand wrench driver that may be used for final positioning of an implant. Generally, this instrument is used when the drill unit reaches its maximum torque value of 50 Ncm and the implant is not yet in its correct vertical position.

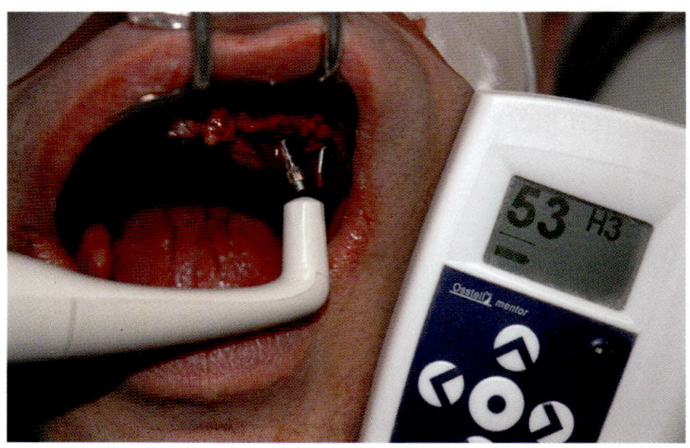

Fig 5.3 - Clinical image demonstrating the use of the Osstell system. This device measures the resonance frequency of an implant, which is then used to assess its relative stability.

diagnostic phase by assessing the amount of bone mineralization present in potential implant sites, where bone quality is highly correlated with primary stability. However, bone quality may be difficult to assess from intraoral radiographs.[40] Intraoral radiography is better suited to assessing secondary stability, despite incongruous reports in the literature concerning the two-dimensional measurement, the technique involved in the execution of the radiographs,[41,42] and the subjective interpretation of the data.[43] The study of maxillary bones with computed tomography (CT) is the best method to obtain qualitative and quantitative information about the amount of bone mineralization present in edentulous sites. In CT studies, bone density is measured in Hounsfield units (HUs), so named in honor of the English physician Sir Godfrey Hounsfield, winner of the 1979 Nobel prize in medicine for his studies on the development of computer-aided tomography. HUs are numbers that range from –1,000 (density of air) to +1,000 (density of cortical bone). The units are further divided into reference intervals that result in practical and predictable measurements regarding bone density. Cone beam CT makes use of spiral or hypocycloidal slices and reference scales called *gray scales*. In this case, variations in the relative amount of white and black (gray) indicate the density of the structure being examined (eg, air, bone, metal, soft tissue, water). The numbers of the gray scale are lower than HUs. Figure 5.4 illustrates similar panoramic images of maxillae, each having a different bone quality.

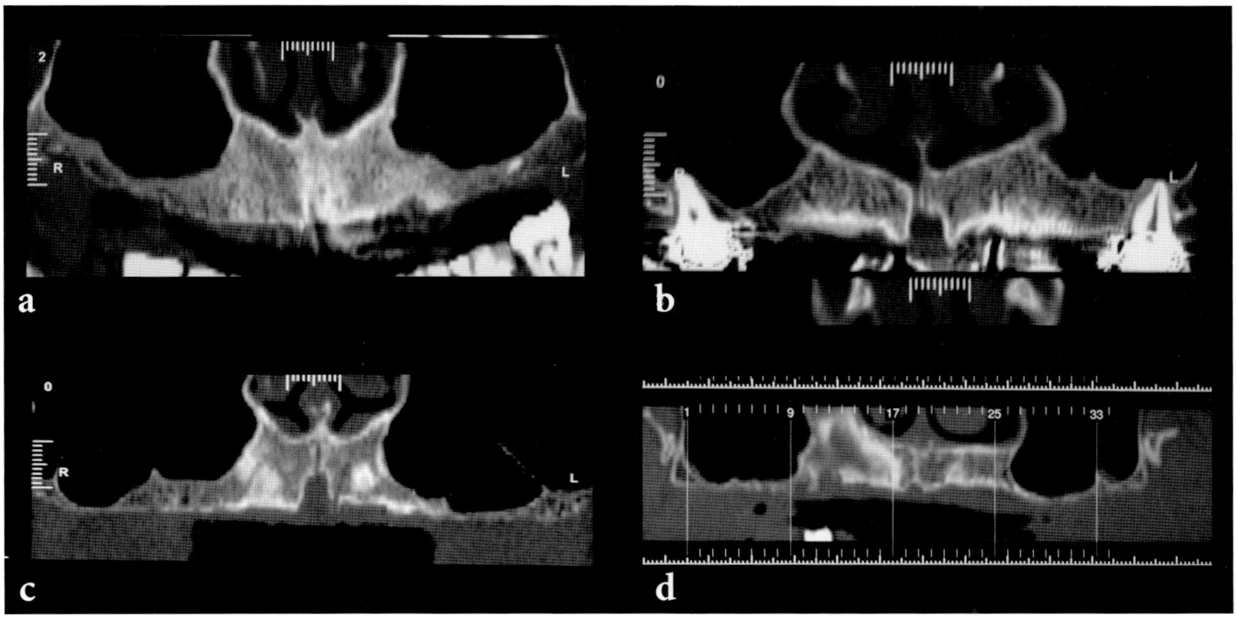

Fig 5.4 - Panoramic reformations of CT images of various maxillary dentitions. Bone classifications per Lekholm and Zarb: type 1 *(a)*, type 2 *(b)*, type 3 *(c)*, and type 4 *(d)*.

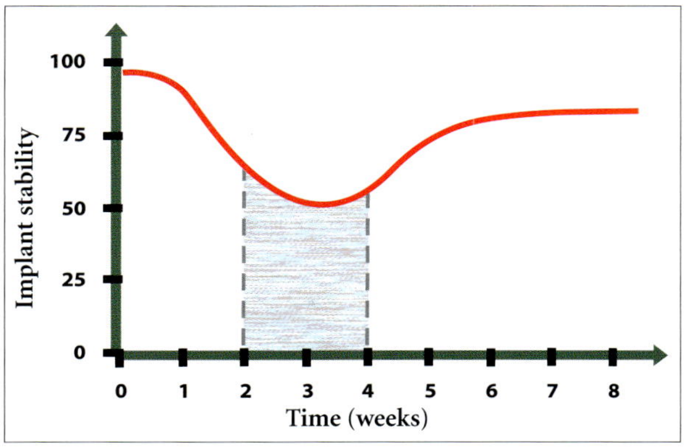

Fig 5.5 - Implant primary stability, based on mechanical concepts, is a direct function of bone quality and the type of osteotomy prepared for a given implant. Primary stability decreases from week 1 through week 4 as bone resorption begins. Implant stability increases from week 4 through week 8 as bone regeneration begins. The x-axis shows time in weeks from implant surgery (time 0) to osseointegration (week 9); the y-axis reflects implant stability.

PRIMARY STABILITY IN IMMEDIATE-LOADING PROTOCOLS

Primary stability is an essential prerequisite for immediate-loading protocols where implants are submitted to functional loads when they are mechanically stable within the osteotomies but are not yet osseointegrated. Nedir et al[44] stated that implants submitted to immediate loading receive more stress than do implants submitted to delayed loading and, as a result, they need higher levels of primary stability. When this initial stability is maintained for a considerable length of time, the implant can be considered to be osseointegrated.[45]

The term *secondary stability* indicates that a stable biologic connection has been achieved between implants and the adjacent bone through osseointegration. Its degree is mainly given by the amount of BIC. While primary stability is determined by the characteristics of the residual bone and the implant design, secondary stability is linked to the formation of new bone tissue at the bone-implant interface. Since the formation of new bone tissue does not become significant before the fourth week after implant placement, implants subjected to immediate loading may be subjected to pathologic movement secondary to occlusal loading between the second and fourth weeks[46] (Fig 5.5). Modification of the implant surface could reduce this weakness at the bone-implant interface; nevertheless, high insertion torque values and high levels of implant primary stability remain crucial factors in immediate loading protocols.

Primary stability is predominately affected by three factors:

1. Biomechanical properties of bone (quality and quantity of the host bone)
2. Osteotomy preparation (diameter and morphology of the drills; tapped or nontapped receiving sites)
3. Implant macrostructure (diameter, length, and shape)

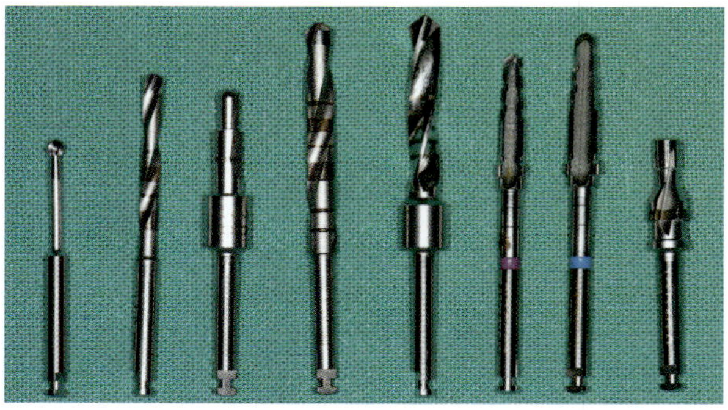

Fig 5.6 - Drills used (diameter, length and shape) for preparation of implant osteotomies should be chosen based on bone quality, implant design, and planned loading protocols.

TABLE 5.2 - DRILLING SEQUENCE FOR THE INSERTION OF 4-MM Ø IMPLANT FOLLOWING THE PRINCIPLES OF UNDERSITE PREPARATION ACCORDING TO THE COLUMBUS BRIDGE PROTOCOL			
	DENSE BONE	**INTERMEDIATE BONE**	**SOFT BONE**
Tapered implants	• Round drill • 2-mm Ø twist drill • 3.25-mm Ø tapered drill • 4-mm Ø twist drill for 2/3 of osteotomy length	• Round drill • 2-mm Ø twist drill • 3.25-mm Ø tapered drill	• Round drill • 2-mm Ø twist drill
Cylindrical implants	• Round drill • 2-mm Ø twist drill • Pilot drill • 3-mm Ø twist drill • 3.6-mm Ø twist drill	• Round drill • 2-mm Ø twist drill • Pilot drill • 3-mm Ø twist drill	Not suitable

Biomechanical properties of bone

Optimal biomechanical characteristics of bone are essential for the survival of dental implants.[47] In edentulous patients, the rate of early implant failure has been reported to be three times higher in the maxilla than in the mandible.[48] Reduced implant primary stability in soft bone (type 4 according to Lekholm and Zarb[49]) results in a reduction in implant survival, with percentages ranging from 50% to 94%.[50–54] In a meta-analysis on 2,812 implants, Esposito et al concluded that bone quality was responsible for 7.7% of all failures.[55,56] In a study of 905 implants inserted consecutively, Ostman and coworkers observed a positive correlation between bone density and primary stability.[57] Turkyilmaz et al reached similar conclusions in their own study of dental implant placement.[58]

Osteotomy preparation

While bone quality cannot be modified, clinicians can modify osteotomy preparation[59,60] and implant macrostructure[61,62] to optimize primary stability. The surgical protocol chosen may affect implant stability.[63] The surgeon can perceive bone quality manually during the first phase of osteotomy preparation,[64] and clinically, it can be divided into three categories: dense, intermediate, and soft.[65] It is imperative that surgeons make use of this qualitative assessment of bone hardness to change the use and sequence of the drills in the surgical preparation of the osteotomies (Fig 5.6) (Table 5.2).

Beer et al[66] have demonstrated a correlation between osteotomy diameter and implant stability. The group began a standard preparation in animal vertebra with a 3-mm diameter drill for the insertion of a Brånemark System Mk II implant (Nobel Biocare), 3.75 mm in diameter, but then varied the amount of insertion torque by changing the final diameter of the osteotomy. They found that a 5% reduction (to 2.85 mm) in the diameter of the osteotomy increased insertion torque by 17%. Conversely, increasing the diameter of the osteotomy by 5% (to 3.15 mm) decreased insertion torque by 21%, and increasing the osteotomy diameter by 12% (to 3.35 mm) resulted in a 50% reduction of insertion torque. The bicortical implant placement technique is generally pursued in maxillary implant sites by stabilizing the apex of implants in the cortical bone of the maxillary sinus floor and nasal cavities.[67,68] The authors believe that the use of countersink drills in trabecular bone (typically maxillary bone) should be abolished, thereby anchoring the coronal aspects of maxillary dental implants in cortical bone.[69]

Implant macrostructure

Screw-shaped implants are best suited for achieving maximum retention and reduced micromotion at the bone-implant interface.[70] Implant design has been modified to facilitate implant insertion, reduce surgical operating times, reduce trauma to bone tissue, and improve primary stability.[71–74]

In 2003, Jokstad and coworkers[75] studied more than 220 implant systems produced by approximately 80 manufacturers. Because implants can be manufactured with different dimensions, materials, and shapes, dentists must choose from among more than 2,000 types of implants. Many of the statements made by dental implant manufacturers about the superiority of a particular implant system specific to certain design characteristics are not based on long-term scientific research. As has been demonstrated by Cehreli et al on photoelastic models and with strain gauges,[76] the distribution of occlusal loads on adjacent peri-implant bone does not seem to be significantly affected by the shape of the implant connection nor by the use of internal versus external implant connections. In full-arch treatment, however, the external hexagonal connection does offer some practical advantages such as the possibility of executing pickup impressions, even in the presence of nonparallel implants,[77] and the ability to more easily orient conical abutments for screw-retained prostheses (Fig 5.7). The external connection is the implant-abutment connection most supported by long-term scientific studies.

Clinically, one determining factor of implant shape is the configuration of the apical third. Implants are produced with either parallel walls

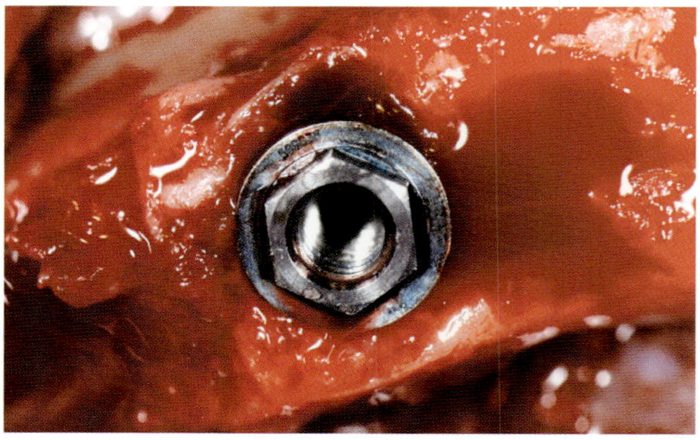

Fig 5.7 - Close-up clinical image of an implant with an external hex implant-abutment connection photographed immediately after implant placement.

(cylindric shape) (Fig 5.8) or tapered walls (conical implant) (Fig 5.9). A cylindric implant offers greater biomechanical resistance to displacing horizontal forces. A conical implant, on the other hand, can be inserted more easily into implant sites that require that osteotomies be prepared with a reduced diameter (postextraction sites[78]; type 3 or type 4 bone[79]) (Fig 5.10).

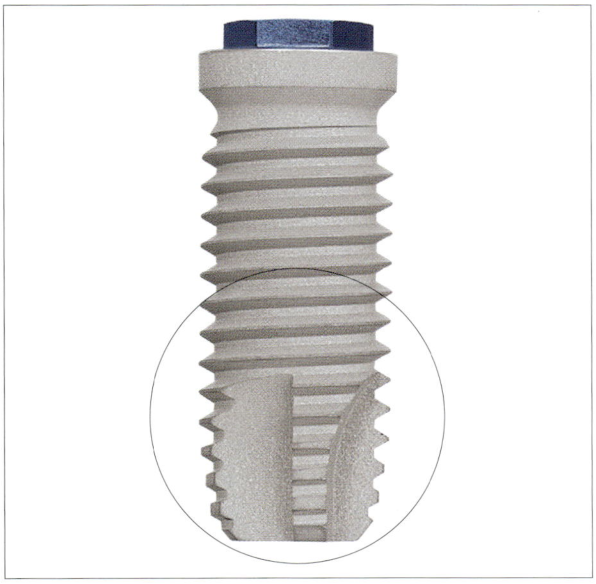

Fig 5.8 - Image of cylindric implant with an external hex implant-abutment connection. Note that the walls of this implant are parallel throughout the implant body.

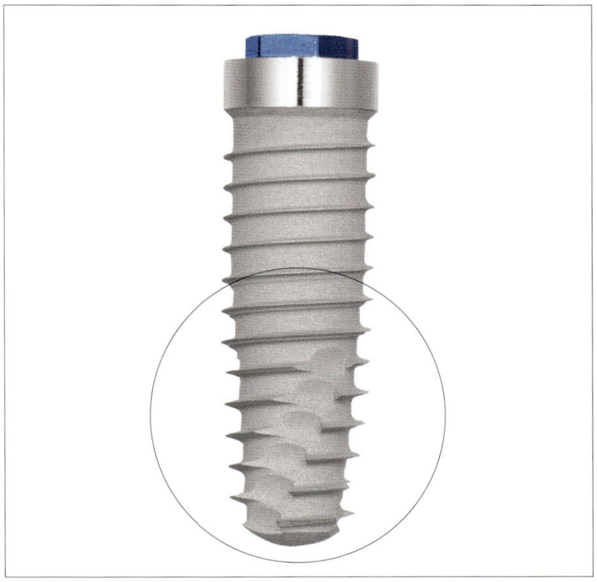

Fig 5.9 - Image of a tapered implant with an external hex implant-abutment connection. Note that the walls in the apical third of this implant are tapered and narrower than the coronal parallel walls of the implant.

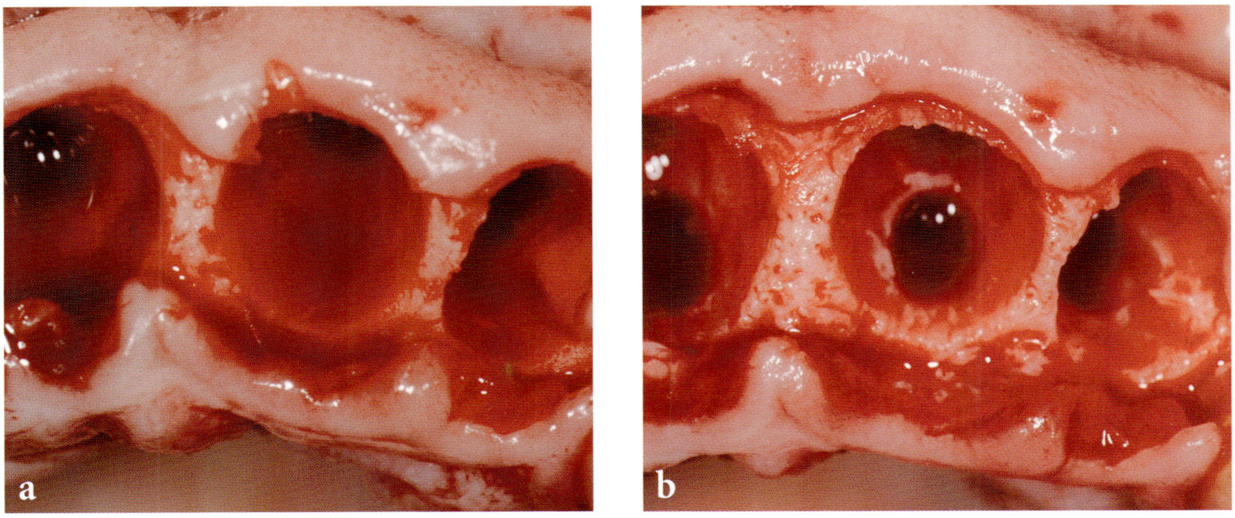

Fig 5.10 - *(a)* Close-up clinical image of an osteotomy prepared in a postextraction socket. *(b)* The direction of the osteotomy was distinctly palatal to the long axis of the socket and did not follow the direction of the root of the extracted tooth.

In these cases, implant geometry may be directly correlated with controlling loads.[80] While opinions on this matter vary,[81,82] it is clear that implant length affects primary stability, and longer lengths may result in increased survival rates in poor quality bone.[83,84]

In maxillary immediate-loading protocols, implant lengths vary, but implants that are from 13 to 18 mm in length are recommended. In the authors' opinion, implants that are 4 mm in diameter seem to be most advantageous. Ivanoff and colleagues,[85] in a retrospective study, correlated implant failure with implant diameter. They reported that implants 3.75 mm in diameter had a 5% failure rate, implants 4 mm in diameter had a 3% failure rate, and implants 5 mm in diameter had an 18% failure rate.

Threshold values for achieving primary stability

Over the last several years, many authors have attempted to identify a threshold value correlating primary stability with implant success, but their answers have differed widely. In 1999, Friberg et al stated that it was not possible to determine a threshold insertion torque value that would determine implant survival or failure.[86] Noguerol and colleagues defined a Periotest value decreasing down to –2 as the threshold in predicting early implant failures.[87] Using resonance frequency analysis, Nedir et al[44] proposed an ISQ value of 54 as the lower threshold for implants subjected to immediate loading and an ISQ value of 49 for implants subjected to delayed loading. In an in vivo study, Ottoni and coworkers recommended insertion torque values over 20 Ncm for single implants submitted to immediate load.[88] Drago and Lazzara, in a prospective study of mandibular edentulous patients treated with immediate occlusal loading, proposed an insertion torque value of at least 30 Ncm[89] as the clinical criterion. Calandriello et al, in a study published in 2003, considered 40 Ncm (with values up to 72 Ncm) to be the threshold for implant primary stability.[90] In the opinion of the authors, immediate occlusal loading has the greatest chance for success when implants are placed with insertion torque values of at least 40 Ncm. Typically, this is the endpoint of insertion torque in most drill units.

In conclusion, two different strategies can be used in planning implant-prosthetic treatment.[91] As clinical evaluation of implant micromotion is not possible, clinicians must choose the most suitable implant sites for obtaining high implant primary stability in edentulous patients. Surgical site selection also must be done with respect to the prosthetic quadrilateral support concept, which is essential in fixed prostheses made according to the Columbus Bridge Protocol.

In contrast, in patients who are missing teeth in the esthetic zone, implant positions should be determined by the position of the missing tooth as developed in the diagnostic wax pattern(s). In these cases, it is advisable to make clinical decisions that do not necessarily reflect reduced implant loading times.

REFERENCES

1. Brånemark PI, Hansson BO, Adell R, Breine U, Lindström J, Hallén O, Ohman A. Osseointegrated implants in the treatment of the edentulous jaw. Experience from a 10-year period. Scand J Plast Reconstr Surg Suppl 1977;16:1–132.
2. Adell R, Lekholm U, Rockler B, Brånemark PI. A 15-year study of osseointegrated implants in the treatment of the edentulous jaw. Int J Oral Surg 1981;10:387–416.
3. Albrektsson T, Brånemark PI, Hansson HA, Lindstrom J. Osseointegrated titanium implants. Requirements for ensuring a long-lasting, direct bone-to-implant anchorage in man. Acta Orthop Scand 1981;52:155–170.
4. Jovanovic SA, Spiekermann H, Richter EJ. Bone regeneration around titanium dental implants in dehisced defect sites: A clinical study. Int J Oral Maxillofac Implants 1992;7:233–245.
5. Meredith N. Assessment of implant stability as a prognostic determinant. Int J Prosthodont 1998;11:491–501.
6. Glauser R, Rée A, Lundgren A, Gottlow J, Hämmerle CH, Schärer P. Immediate occlusal loading of Brånemark implants applied in various jawbone regions: A prospective, 1-year clinical study. Clin Implant Dent Relat Res 2001; 3:204–213.
7. da Cunha HA, Francischone CE, Filho HN, de Oliveira RC. A comparison between cutting torque and resonance frequency in the assessment of primary stability and final torque capacity of standard and TiUnite single-tooth implants under immediate loading. Int J Oral Maxillofac Implants 2004;19:578–585.
8. Wang HL, Boyapati L. "PASS" principles for predictable bone regeneration. Implant Dent 2006;15:8–17.
9. Lioubavina-Hack N, Lang NP, Karring T. Significance of primary stability for osseointegration of dental implants. Clin Oral Implants Res 2006;17:244–250.
10. Orenstein IH, Tarnow DP, Morris HF, Ochi S. Factors affecting implant mobility at placement and integration of mobile implants at uncovering. J Periodontol 1998;69:1404–1412.
11. Langer B, Langer L, Herrmann I, Jorneus L. The wide fixture: A solution for special bone situations and a rescue for the compromised implant. Part 1. Int J Oral Maxillofac Implants 1993;8:400–408.
12. Friberg B, Jemt T, Lekholm U. Early failures in 4,641 consecutively placed Brånemark dental implants: A study from stage 1 surgery to the connection of completed prostheses. Int J Oral Maxillofac Implants 1991;6:142–146.
13. Carlsson LV, Alberktsson T, Berman C. Bone response to plasma-cleaned titanium implants. Int J Oral Maxillofac Implants 1989;4:199–204.
14. Johansson CB, Albrektsson T. A removal torque and histomorphometric study of commercially pure niobium and titanium implants in rabbit bone. Clin Oral Implants Res 1991;2:24–29.
15. Morberg P, Albrektsson T. Removal torque for bone-cement and titanium screws implanted in rabbits. Acta Orthop Scand 1991;62:554–556.
16. Johansson CB, Sennerby L, Albrektsson T. A removal torque and histomorphometric study of bone tissue reactions to commercially pure titanium and Vitallium implants. Int J Oral Maxillofac Implants 1991;6:437–441.
17. Henry PJ, Tan AES, Allan BP, Hall J, Johansson C. Removal torque comparison of TiUnite and turned implants in the greyhound dog mandible. Appl Osseointegration Res 2000;1:15–17.
18. Johansson C, Albrektsson T. Integration of screw implants in the rabbit: A 1-year follow-up of removal torque of titanium implants. Int J Oral Maxillofac Implants 1987;2:69–75.

19. Meredith N, Shagaldi F, Alleyne D, Sennerby L, Cawley P. The application of resonance frequency measurements to study the stability of titanium implants during healing in the rabbit tibia. Clin Oral Implants Res 1997;8:234–243.
20. Johansson P, Strid KG. Assessment of bone quality from cutting resistance during implant surgery. Int J Oral Maxillofac Implants 1994;9:279–288.
21. Turkyilmaz I. A comparison between insertion torque and resonance frequency in the assessment of torque capacity and primary stability of Brånemark system implants. J Oral Rehabil 2006;33:754–759.
22. Niimi A, Ozeki K, Ueda M, Nakayama B. A comparative study of removal torque of endosseous implants in the fibula, iliac crest and scapula of cadavers: Preliminary report. Clin Oral Implants Res 1997;8:286–289.
23. O'Sullivan D, Sennerby L, Meredith N. Measurements comparing the initial stability of five designs of dental implants: A human cadaver study. Clin Implant Dent Relat Res 2000;2:85–92.
24. Trisi P, De Benedittis S, Perfetti G, Berardi D. Primary stability, insertion torque and bone density of cylindric implant ad modum Branemark: Is there a relationship? An in vitro study. Clin Oral Implants Res 2011;22:567–570.
25. Okazaki J, Komasa Y, Sakai D, et al. A torque removal study on the primary stability of orthodontic titanium screw mini-implants in the cortical bone of dog femurs. Int J Oral Maxillofac Surg 2008;37:647–650.
26. Hutzschenreuter P, Claes L, Pohler O. Loosening capacity of corticalis tension screws with varying surfaces and their histological correlations (in German). Helv Chir Acta 1976;43:765–768.
27. Brånemark PI, Zarb GA, Albrektsson T (eds). Tissue-Integrated Prostheses: Osseointegration in Clinical Dentistry. Chicago: Quintessence, 1985.
28. Roberts WE, Garetto LP, DeCastro RA. Remodeling of devitalized bone threatens periosteal margin integrity of endosseous titanium implants with threaded or smooth surfaces: Indications for provisional loading and axially directed occlusion. J Indiana Dent Assoc 1989;68:19–24.
29. d'Hoedt B, Lukas D, Mühlbradt L, et al. Periotest methods: Development and clinical trial. Dtsch Zahnarztl Z 1985;40:113–125.
30. Lachmann S, Jager B, Axmann D, Gomez-Roman G, Groten M, Weber H. Resonance frequency analysis and damping capacity assessment. Part I: An in vitro study on measurement reliability and a method of comparison in the determination of primary dental implant stability. Clin Oral Implants Res 2006;17:75–79.
31. Lachmann S, Laval JY, Jäger B, et al. Resonance frequency analysis and damping capacity assessment. Part 2: Peri-implant bone loss follow-up. An in vitro study with the Periotest and Osstell instruments. Clin Oral Implants Res 2006;17:80–84.
32. Meredith N, Friberg B, Sennerby L, Aparicio C. Relationship between contact time measurements and PTV values when using the Periotest to measure implant stability. Int J Prosthodont 1998;11:269–275.
33. Meredith N, Alleyne D, Cawley P. Quantitative determination of the stability of the implant-tissue interface using resonance frequency analysis. Clin Oral Implants Res 1996;7:261–267.
34. Bischof M, Nedir R, Szmukler-Moncler S, Bernard JP, Samson J. Implant stability measurement of delayed and immediately loaded implants during healing. Clin Oral Implants Res 2004;15:529–539.
35. Zix J, Kessler-Liechti G, Mericske-Stern R. Stability measurements of 1-stage implants in the maxilla by means of resonance frequency analysis: A pilot study. Int J Oral Maxillofac Implants 2005;20:747–752.

36. Nkenke E, Hahn M, Weinzierl K, Radespiel-Tröger M, Neukam FW, Engelke K. Implant stability and histomorphometry: A correlation study in human cadavers using stepped cylinder implants. Clin Oral Implants Res 2003;14:601–609.
37. Scarano A, Degidi M, Iezzi G, Petrone G, Piattelli A. Correlation between implant stability quotient and bone-implant contact: A retrospective histological and histomorphometrical study of seven titanium implants retrieved from humans. Clin Implant Dent Relat Res 2006;8:218–222.
38. Rasmusson L, Kahnberg KE, Tan A. Effects of implant design and surface on bone regeneration and implant stability: An experimental study in the dog mandible. Clin Implant Dent Relat Res 2001;3:2–8.
39. Rasmusson L, Meredith N, Cho IH, Sennerby L. The influence of simultaneous versus delayed placement on the stability of titanium implants in onlay bone grafts. A histologic and biomechanic study in the rabbit. Int J Oral Maxillofac Surg 1999;28:224–231.
40. Mezzanotte P (ed). Le indagini radiologiche pre e post-implantari. Metodiche di esecuzione, errori, lettura. Milano: Masson, 2005:129–133.
41. Sewerin IP. Errors in radiographic assessment of marginal bone height around osseointegrated implants. Scand J Dent Res 1990;98:428–433.
42. Bauman GR, Mills M, Rapley JW, Hallmon WH. Clinical parameters of evaluation during implant maintenance. Int J Oral Maxillofac Implants 1992;7:220–227.
43. Sundén S, Gröndahl K, Gröndahl HG. Accuracy and precision in the radiographic diagnosis of clinical instability in Brånemark dental implants. Clin Oral Implants Res 1995;6:220–226.
44. Nedir R, Bischof M, Szmukler-Moncler S, Bernard JP, Samson J. Predicting osseointegration by means of implant primary stability. Clin Oral Implants Res 2004;15:520–528.
45. Corso M, Sirota C, Fiorellini J, Rasool F, Szmukler-Moncler S, Weber HP. Clinical and radiographic evaluation of early loaded free-standing dental implants with various coatings in beagle dogs. J Prosthet Dent 1999;82:428–435.
46. Raghavendra S, Wood MC, Taylor TD. Early wound healing around endosseous implants: A review of the literature. Int J Oral Maxillofac Implants 2005;20:425–431.
47. Ekfeldt A, Christiansson U, Eriksson T, et al. A retrospective analysis of factors associated with multiple implant failures in maxillae. Clin Oral Implants Res 2001;12:462–467.
48. Mailath-Pokorny G. Surgical perspectives for compromised bone. In: Watzek G (ed). Implants in Qualitatively Compromised Bone. Surrey: Quintessence, 2004:95–99.
49. Lekholm U, Zarb G. Patient selection and preparation. In: Brånemark PI, Zarb G, Albrektsson T (eds). Tissue-Integrated Prostheses. Osseointegration in Clinical Dentistry. Chicago: Quintessence, 1985:199–209.
50. Engquist B, Bergendal T, Kallus T, Linden U. A retrospective multicenter evaluation of osseointegrated implants supporting overdentures. Int J Oral Maxillofac Implants 1988;3:129–134.
51. Jaffin RA, Berman CL. The excessive loss of Brånemark fixtures in type IV bone: A 5-year analysis. J Periodontol 1991;62:2–4.
52. Johns RB, Jemt T, Heath MR, et al. A multicenter study of overdentures supported by Brånemark implants. Int J Oral Maxillofac Implants 1992;7:513–522.
53. Hutton JE, Heath MR, Chai JY, et al. Factors related to success and failure rates at 3-year follow-up in a multicenter study of overdentures supported by Brånemark implants. Int J Oral Maxillofac Implants 1995;10:33–42.

54. Jemt T, Chai J, Harnett J, et al. A 5-year prospective multicenter follow-up report on overdentures supported by osseointegrated implants. Int J Oral Maxillofac Implants 1996;11:291–298.
55. Esposito M, Hirsch JM, Lekholm U, Thomsen P. Biological factors contributing to failures of osseointegrated oral implants. (I). Success criteria and epidemiology. Eur J Oral Sci 1998;106: 527–551.
56. Esposito M, Hirsch JM, Lekholm U, Thomsen P. Biological factors contributing to failures of osseointegrated oral implants. (II). Etiopathogenesis. Eur J Oral Sci 1998;106:721–764.
57. Ostman PO, Hellman M, Wendelhag I, Sennerby L. Resonance frequency analysis measurements of implants at placement surgery. Int J Prosthodont 2006;19:77–83.
58. Turkyilmaz I, Tözüm TF, Tumer C, Ozbek EN. Assessment of correlation between computerized tomography values of the bone, and maximum torque and resonance frequency values at dental implant placement. J Oral Rehabil 2006;33: 881–888.
59. Summers RB. A new concept in maxillary implant surgery: The osteotome technique. Compendium 1994;15:154–156.
60. Adriaenssens P, Hermans M. Immediate implant function in the anterior maxilla: A surgical technique to enhance primary stability for Brånemark Mk II and Mk IV implants. A randomised, prospective clinical study at the 1-year follow-up. Appl Osseointegration Res 2001;2:17–21.
61. Glauser R, Portmann M, Ruhstaller P, Gottlow J, Schärer P. Initial implant stability using different implant designs and surgical techniques. A comparative clinical study using insertion torque and resonance frequency analysis. Appl Osseointegration Res 2001;2:6–8.
62. O'Sullivan D, Sennerby L, Meredith N. Influence of implant taper on the primary and secondary stability of osseointegrated titanium implants. Clin Oral Implants Res 2004;15:474–480.
63. Buchter A, Kleinheinz J, Joos U, Meyer U. Primary implant stability with different bone surgery techniques. An in vitro study of the mandible of the minipig [in German]. Mund Kiefer Gesichtschir 2003;7:351–355.
64. Friberg B, Sennerby L, Roos J, Johansson P, Strid CG, Lekholm U. Evaluation of bone density using cutting resistance measurements and microradiography: An in vitro study in pig ribs. Clin Oral Implants Res 1995;6:164–171.
65. Martinez H, Davarpanah M, Missika P, Celletti R, Lazzara R. Optimal implant stabilization in low density bone. Clin Oral Implants Res 2001;12: 423–432.
66. Beer A, Gahleitner A, Holm A, Birkfellner W, Homolka P. Adapted preparation technique for screw-type implants: Explorative in vitro pilot study in a porcine bone model. Clin Oral Implants Res 2007;18:103–107.
67. Brånemark PI, Adell R, Albrektsson T, Lekholm U, Lindstrom J, Rockler B. An experimental and clinical study of osseointegrated implants penetrating the nasal cavity and maxillary sinus. J Oral Maxillofac Surg 1984;42:497–505.
68. Sennerby L, Thomsen P, Ericson LE. A morphometric and biomechanic comparison of titanium implants inserted in rabbit cortical and cancellous bone. Int J Oral Maxillofac Implants 1992;7:62–71.
69. Davarpanah M, Martinez H, Tecucianu JF. Apical-coronal implant position: Recent surgical proposals. Technical note. Int J Oral Maxillofac Implants 2000;15:865–872.
70. Brunski JB. Biomechanical factors affecting the bone-dental implant interface. Clin Mater 1992;10:153–201.

71. O'Sullivan D, Sennerby L, Meredith N. Measurements comparing the initial stability of five designs of dental implants: A human cadaver study. Clin Implant Dent Relat Res 2000;2:85–92.
72. da Cunha HA, Francischone CE, Filho HN, de Oliveira RC. A comparison between cutting torque and resonance frequency in the assessment of primary stability and final torque capacity of standard and TiUnite single-tooth implants under immediate loading. Int J Oral Maxillofac Implants 2004;19:578–585.
73. O'Sullivan D, Sennerby L, Jagger D, Meredith N. A comparison of two methods of enhancing implant primary stability. Clin Implant Dent Relat Res 2004;6:48–57.
74. Sakoh J, Wahlmann U, Stender E, Nat R, Al-Nawas B, Wagner W. Primary stability of a conical implant and a hybrid, cylindric screw-type implant in vitro. Int J Oral Maxillofac Implants 2006;21:560–566.
75. Jokstad A, Braegger U, Brunski JB, Carr AB, Naert I, Wennerberg A. Quality of dental implants. Int Dent J 2003;53(6 suppl 2):409–443.
76. Cehreli M, Duyck J, De Cooman M, Puers R, Naert I. Implant design and interface force transfer. A photoelastic and strain-gauge analysis. Clin Oral Implants Res 2004;15:249–257.
77. Choi JH, Lim YJ, Yim SH, Kim CW. Evaluation of the accuracy of implant-level impression techniques for internal-connection implant prostheses in parallel and divergent models. Int J Oral Maxillofac Implants 2007;22:761–768.
78. Davarpanah M, Caraman M, Szmukler-Moncler S, Jakubowicz-Kohen B, Alcolforado G. Preliminary data of a prospective clinical study on the Osseotite NT implant: 18-month follow-up. Int J Oral Maxillofac Implants 2005;20:448–454.
79. Rompen E, DaSilva D, Hockers T, Lundgren A-K, Gottlow J, Glauser R, Sennerby L. Influence of implant design on primary fit and stability. A RFA and histological comparison of Mk III and Mk IV Brånemark implants in the dog mandible. Appl Osseointegration Res 2001;2:9–11.
80. Vandamme K, Naert I, Geris L, Vander Sloten J, Puers R, Duyck J. Influence of controlled immediate loading and implant design on peri-implant bone formation. J Clin Periodontol 2007;34:172–181.
81. Bischof M, Nedir R, Szmukler-Moncler S, Bernard JP, Samson J. Implant stability measurement of delayed and immediately loaded implants during healing. Clin Oral Implants Res 2004;15:529–539.
82. Bernard JP, Szmukler-Moncler S, Pessotto S, Vazquez L, Belser UC. The anchorage of Brånemark and ITI implants of different lengths. I. An experimental study in the canine mandible. Clin Oral Implants Res 2003;14:593–600.
83. van Steenberghe D, Lekholm U, Bolender C, et al. Applicability of osseointegrated oral implants in the rehabilitation of partial edentulism: A prospective multicenter study on 558 fixtures. Int J Oral Maxillofac Implants 1990;5:272–281.
84. Wyatt CC, Zarb GA. Treatment outcomes of patients with implant-supported fixed partial prostheses. Int J Oral Maxillofac Implants 1998;13:204–211.
85. Ivanoff CJ, Grondahl K, Sennerby L, Bergstrom C, Lekholm U. Influence of variations in implant diameters: A 3- to 5-year retrospective clinical report. Int J Oral Maxillofac Implants 1999;14:173–180.
86. Friberg B, Sennerby L, Grondahl K, Bergstrom C, Back T, Lekholm U. On cutting torque measurements during implant placement: A 3-year clinical prospective study. Clin Implant Dent Relat Res 1999;1:75–83.

87. Noguerol B, Muñoz R, Mesa F, de Dios Luna J, O'Valle F. Early implant failure. Prognostic capacity of Periotest: Retrospective study of a large sample. Clin Oral Implants Res 2006;17:459–464.
88. Ottoni JM, Oliveira ZF, Mansini R, Cabral AM. Correlation between placement torque and survival of single-tooth implants. Int J Oral Maxillofac Implants 2005;20:769–776.
89. Drago CJ, Lazzara RJ. Immediate occlusal loading of Osseotite implants in mandibular edentulous patients: A prospective observational report with 18-month data. J Prosthodont 2006;15:187–194.
90. Calandriello R, Tomatis M, Rangert B. Immediate functional loading of Brånemark System implants with enhanced initial stability: A prospective 1- to 2-year clinical and radiographic study. Clin Implant Dent Relat Res 2003;5(suppl 1):10–20.
91. Homolka P, Beer A, Birkfellner W, et al. Bone mineral density measurement with dental quantitative CT prior to dental implant placement in cadaver mandibles: Pilot study. Radiology 2002;224:247–252.

CHAPTER 6
ANGLED IMPLANTS

COLUMBUS BRIDGE PROTOCOL	
SURGICAL PROTOCOL	**PROSTHETIC PROTOCOL**
External hex rough-surface implants	Screw-retained fixed prosthesis
Implant length ≥ 13 mm, Ø 4 mm	Plaster impression with pickup technique
Underprepared osteotomy	Rigid splinting with metal framework
Implant insertion torque ≥ 40 Ncm	Passive fit with the luting technique
Angled implants in native bone	Acrylic resin occlusal surfaces
Angled conical abutments	No distal cantilevers
No bone regenerative techniques	Immediate functional load 24–48 h after surgery

Table 6.1

LITERATURE REVIEW

Mattsson and coworkers,[1] in a study published in 1999, were the first to propose the use of angled implants supporting a fixed, full-arch implant-retained prosthesis in patients with severe maxillary atrophy. The protocol consisted of creating a window in the maxillary sinus prior to inserting tilted implants that were considerably longer than those used in more conventional protocols. The longer implants were placed anterior and parallel to the anterior wall of the maxillary sinus. Mattsson's team followed the patients' progress for 45 months and reported that only one implant was lost. All 15 patients in the study were pleased with their treatments, which were provided at reasonable cost. None of the patients required bone grafting procedures during the course of the treatments. In 2000, Krekmanov and colleagues[2] proposed using angled implants to reduce the extension of distal cantilevers in clinical situations that had previously required transposing the inferior alveolar neurovascular bundle in the mandible and/or bone grafting in the maxilla. Forty-seven patients were treated per the tilted implant protocol by inserting 36 mandibular implants and 30 maxillary implants. The mandibular implants were inserted with inclinations of 25 to 35 degrees to avoid the inferior alveolar neurovascular bundle and canal; the maxillary implants were inserted parallel to the anterior wall of the maxillary sinus, with inclinations of 30 to 35 degrees. Researchers followed the progress of patients with mandibular implants for an average of 40 months, patients with maxillary implants for an average of 53 months. The mandibular angled implants allowed for a reduction of 6.5 mm in the distal prosthetic cantilevers; the maxillary implants reduced the distal cantilevers 9.3 mm. The cumulative survival rate (CSR) at 5 years was 100% for the mandibular implants and 98% for the maxillary implants. No statistically significant differences were found between the CSRs of angled and vertically placed implants.

In a later study, Krekmanov[3] described a technique for the fixed prosthetic treatment of patients with severe bone resorption in maxillary and mandibular posterior quadrants. This study reported on the survival rates for angled implants: mesial to avoid the maxillary sinus and distal to impact the pterygoid processes. Krekmanov believed that this methodology provided for better use of the maxillary residual bone volume and spared the patients the trauma associated with bone grafting. Seventy-five implants were inserted in the maxilla, and the patients' progress was followed for 1 to 10 years after delivery of the prostheses. Three maxillary implants were lost at the abutment connection appointment. One of the failed implants was inserted into a pterygoid process; the second was positioned near the rear wall of the maxillary sinus; and the third showed a remarkable inclination toward the palate. An additional implant demonstrated mobility 1 year after occlusal loading, possibly due to an ill-fitting prosthesis. The implant CSR was 94.7%.

In 2001, Aparicio et al[4] conducted research that evaluated an alternative treatment to elevation of the sinus floor in the treatment of atrophic maxillae. At the time of the report, this technique had not been universally accepted. The authors combined angled and vertical implants for treatment with fixed implant prostheses in the treatment of severely resorbed, edentulous maxillary posterior quadrants. Twenty-five patients were treated with a total of 101 implants, of which 59 were vertical and 42 were angled. The CSR at the 5-year follow-up visits was 96.5% for the vertical implants and 100% for the angled implants. Marginal bone loss averaged 0.92 mm for the vertical implants and 1.21 mm for the angled implants. During the follow-up period, all but two of the prostheses remained stable. Eighteen abutment screws and five retaining screws were reported to loosen, and two abutment screws and two occlusal surfaces fractured. In conclusion, Aparicio et al indicated that the use of angled implants provided an effective and safe alternative to the elevation of the floor of the maxillary sinus in the treatment of severely atrophic maxillae.

The following year, Fortin et al[5] published an alternative surgical-prosthetic protocol for the treatment of severely resorbed edentulous maxillae, in lieu of complete maxillary dentures without interventions for the elevation of the maxillary sinus floor. The removable prostheses were called *Marius bridges* in honor of the first patient who elected to use this treatment. Prostheses made according to this protocol are overdentures retained and supported on four to six implants. The two distal implants are inserted with the apical portions of the implants mesial to the coronal portions (mesial tilt) and parallel to the anterior sinus wall to avoid the presence of maxillary sinuses. In this study, 45 patients were treated with 245 implants. After 5 years of follow-up, five implant failures were recorded. This yielded an implant CSR of 97%. The success rate for the prostheses was 100%. The reported complications in this study were mainly prosthetic in nature. Considering the satisfactory midterm results, the authors concluded that the Marius bridge should be considered a valid alternative for maxillary implant-prosthetic treatments that reduce the need for bone grafting. This protocol uses long, angled implants to provide adequate bone-implant anchorage and prosthetic support.

In 2003, Maló and colleagues[6] described an immediate-loading approach for the fixed mandibular treatment of edentulous patients. They proposed a simplified technique for immediate occlusal loading with only four implants supporting fixed full-arch prostheses. The technique was called *All-on-4*. This paper reported the results of a retrospective study conducted on 44 patients with a total of 176 implants inserted into the interforaminal region of edentulous mandibles. Five implants were lost during the first 6 months of follow-up; the CSR was 97.1%. The prosthetic success rate was 100%. To facilitate implant positioning, a surgical guide was used. The distal implants were tilted such that the occlusal surfaces of the implants were distal to the apical portions of the implants. This orientation provided satisfactory bone anchoring (implant primary stability) secondary to increased lengths of the fixtures. This orientation also provided satisfactory anteroposterior spread and distances between implants that were suitable to obtain ideal prosthetic support. Maló et al concluded that the All-on-4 concept should be considered for immediate occlusal loading of patients with edentulous mandibles.

In another retrospective clinical study, published in 2005, Maló et al[7] evaluated the All-on-4 technique in edentulous maxillae. This study included 32 patients treated with 128 immediately loaded implants that supported fixed, full-arch acrylic resin prostheses. At the 1-year follow-up, three implants had failed. The CSR was 97.6%. Marginal bone loss measured from the abutment-implant connection was 0.9 mm. The authors concluded that the high CSR and the small amount of crestal bone loss validated the All-on-4 concept in edentulous maxillae as well as in edentulous mandibles.

That same year, Calandriello and Tomatis[8] proposed a protocol for the treatment of atrophic maxillary posterior quadrants with immediate occlusal loading on angled implants. The paper reported the results of 18 patients treated with 60 implants that supported fixed partial or full-arch prostheses. The follow-up period was at least 1 year after the delivery of the prostheses. Two implants, one vertical and one angled, were lost. The implant CSR was 96.7%. The prosthetic success rate was 100%. The reported bone resorption values were 0.82 mm for straight implants and 0.34 mm for tilted implants. The article concluded by listing some advantages of using this protocol for immediate occlusal loading, including simplified treatment, minimally invasive surgical procedures, shorter treatment times, and reduced costs.

In 2006, Maló et al[9] published another pilot work aimed at evaluating a new implant design for the treatment of edentulous jaws with immediate occlusal loading. The performance of the new proposed implant design was studied in combination with the All-on-4 immediate-loading technique described previously. A key point of the All-on-4 concept is the mesial inclination of the two distal implants. The progress of 56 patients treated with 189 fixtures was followed for at least 1 year. During that period, two implants were lost; the CSR was 98.1%. One year after immediate occlusal loading, the marginal crestal bone loss (measured from the implant-abutment junction) was 1.2 ± 0.7 mm. Maló's team reported satisfactory results for the overall health and esthetics of the soft tissues.

A 2007 retrospective study conducted by Rosen and Gynther[10] evaluated the surgical results associated with the use of angled implants in severely resorbed edentulous maxillae as an alternative to bone grafts. The investigators also reported on the prosthetic results associated with distal cantilevered extensions on angled implants. This study consisted of 19 patients who demonstrated insufficient bone volumes relative to conventional implant placement protocols for supporting fixed prostheses. These treatments were proposed as an alternative to bone grafting and were consistent with the surgical technique proposed by Mattsson,[1] which included windows into the maxillary sinus for direct observation of the residual bone volume, followed by the insertion of angled implants parallel to the anterior wall of the maxillary sinus. Rosen treated 19 patients with a two-stage surgical protocol by placing four to six implants with adequate lengths. A total of 103 implants were placed, all according to an unloaded healing protocol. Rosen and Gynther reported that three implants were lost at the abutment connection appointment prior to occlusal loading. The implant CSR was 97%. Radiographic examination showed an average crestal bone loss of 1.2 mm. This study demonstrates how a simplified surgical protocol, combined with the use of angled implants, can be regarded as a valid alternative to more complex surgical techniques such as sinus floor elevation or block bone grafting in treating patients with severely resorbed maxillae. In recent years, there has been an increase in the use of angled implants to support full-arch prostheses.[11–15] The published studies have not found statistically significant differences in crestal bone loss between straight and angled fixtures. Similarly, no significant differences exist between implant CSRs for angled implants and implants inserted orthogonally. In review, angled implants inserted with the apical portions mesial to the coronal ones can be used in both jaws. Their inclinations allow clinicians to avoid anatomical structures such as the maxillary sinus and inferior alveolar neurovascular bundle and canal. For clinicians to bypass critical anatomical structures with conventional techniques, it would require more complicated surgical treatments and would likely result in increased postoperative morbidities. Another possibility would be that clinicians would have to use shorter implants with, potentially, decreased implant primary stability and less bone-implant contact. Distal dental implant positioning generally increases cross-arch stabilization for the implant prostheses while reducing the lengths of distal cantilevered extensions by up to 1 cm (Figs 6.1 to 6.4). Longer angled implants in native host bone are a better choice in immediate occlusal loading protocols, where attaining high primary stability is critical for long-term clinical success.

Table 6.2 describes the results of the articles published on the use of angled implants.

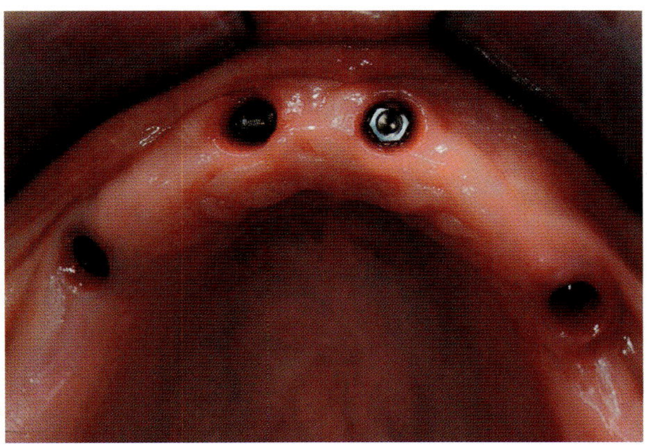

Fig 6.1 - Clinical occlusal image of edentulous maxilla treated with four implants placed according to the conventional Brånemark surgical protocol. Note that the implants are almost in a straight line, with little anteroposterior spread. This arrangement is based on the positions of the anterior walls of the maxillary sinuses.

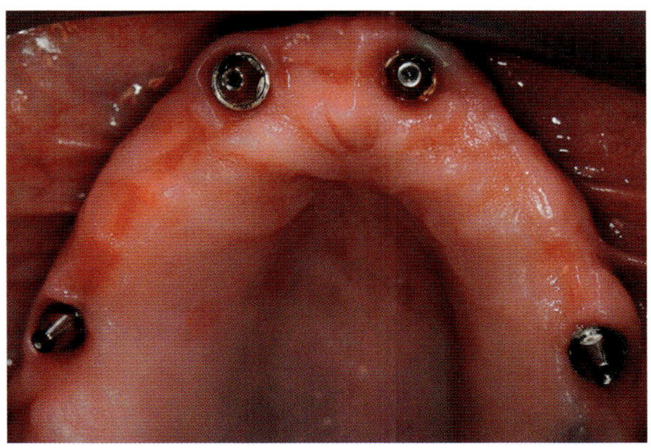

Fig 6.2 - Clinical occlusal image of edentulous maxilla treated with four implants inserted according to an angled implant surgical protocol. This implant placement greatly increased the anteroposterior spread when compared with that used in Fig 6.1. It provided significantly greater support for a fixed prosthesis than what would have been available with vertical implant placement as shown in Fig 6.1.

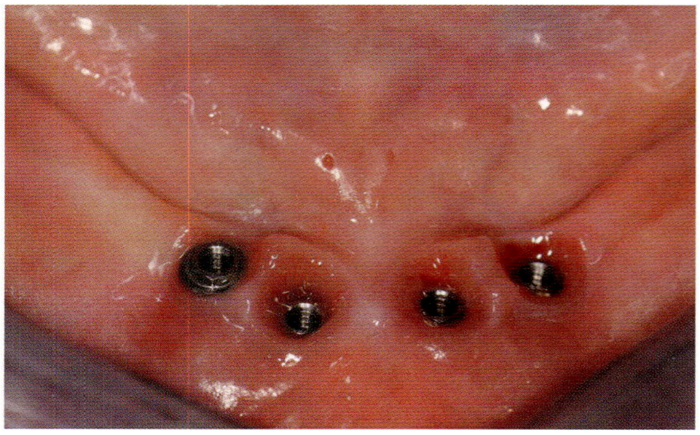

Fig 6.3 - Clinical occlusal image of four implants placed per the conventional Brånemark surgical protocol (interforaminal). The implants were placed vertically. In some clinical cases, the anatomical shape of the edentulous jaws does not provide for a satisfactory anteroposterior spread.

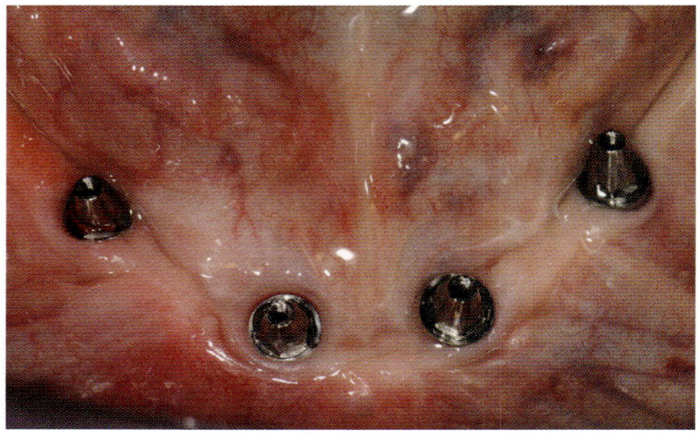

Fig 6.4 - Clinical occlusal image of four abutments in place on four mandibular implants placed according to an angled implant protocol. The distal implants were tilted distally but were still placed between the mental foramina. The anteroposterior spread of the implants was sufficient to provide satisfactory molar support for a full fixed prosthesis. The implant spread was optimized relative to the anteroposterior spread shown in Fig 6.3.

ANATOMICAL LIMITS

The two main anatomical limits routinely encountered with intraoral dental implants are: *(1)* the inferior alveolar neurovascular bundle and canal and *(2)* the maxillary sinus. Both of these structures must be respected during the surgical procedures associated with the use of angled implants. In cases of bone atrophy, angled implants may be the only treatment allowing for the insertion of sufficiently long implants with adequate primary stability that does not damage these important anatomical structures.

Inferior Alveolar Neurovascular Bundle and Canal

Usually, long implants cannot be inserted in distal positions in the posterior mandible because of the location of the mental foramen and nerve. Likewise, because the implants should emerge as distal as possible, care must be taken not to injure the inferior alveolar nerve, which is a terminal branch of the mandibular nerve (third branch of the trigeminal nerve). The mandibular nerve is a mixed nerve with sensory and motor roots. It exits the cranium through the foramen ovale between the external pterygoid and tensor veli palatini muscles. After the union of both nerve roots, the mandibular nerve separates into two collateral branches: laterally as the external pterygoid, and medially as the mandibular nerve. The mandibular nerve divides into two additional branches: The anterior branch supplies motor nerves to the masticatory muscles (masseteric, anterior and posterior deep temporal, internal pterygoid, and buccinator nerves); the posterior branch divides into auriculotemporal, lingual, and inferior

TABLE 6.2 - OUTCOMES OF CLINICAL STUDIESON ANGLED IMPLANTS

Author	Year of publication	Implant site location	Type of prosthesis	Time of load	# of Patients	# of inserted implants	# of failed implants	Implant survival rate	Prosthesis survival rate	Bone resorption (mm)	Follow-up (months)
Mattsson[1]	1999	PM	FFD	D	15	–	1	94.4%	100%	–	45
Krekmanov[2]	2000	PM - PJ	FFD	D	47	36 J 30 M	–	100% J 98% M	–	–	40 J 53 M
Krekmanov[3]	2000	M - J	PFD	D	–	75 M 86 J	4 M 0 J	94.7% M 100% J	–	–	12–123
Aparicio[4]	2001	PM	PFD	D	25	59 U 42 T	2 U 0 T	100% T 96.5% U	100%	0.92 U 1.21 T	21–87
Fortin[5]	2002	M	O	D	45	245	5	97%	100%	–	60
Malò[6]	2003	AJ	FFD	I	44	176	5	97.1%	100%	–	6
Malò[7]	2005	M	FFD	I	32	128	3	97.6%	–	0.9	12
Calandriello[8]	2005	PM	FFD PFD	I	18	60	1 U 1 T	96.7%	100%	0.82 U 0.34 T	12
Malò[9]	2006	M - J	FFD	I	56	189	2	98.1%	100%	1.2 +/- 0.7	12
Rosen[10]	2007	M	FFD	D	19	103	3	97%	100%	1.2	120
Capelli[11]	2007	M - J	FFD	I	65	342	5	97.6% M 100% J	100%	–	40
Testori[12]	2008	M	FFD	I	41	246	5	98.8%	100%	0.9±0.4 U 0.8±0.5 T	3–42
Francetti[13]	2008	AJ	FFD	I	62	248	0	100%	100%	–	6–43
Tealdo[14]	2008	M	FFD	I	21	64 U 47 T	3 U 5 T	95.3% U 89.4% T	100%	0.74 U 0.98 T	13–28
Agliardi[15]	2008	M	FFD	I	21	126	0	100%	100%	0.4 U 0.5 T	4–35

Legend: M: maxilla; J: jaw (mandible); A: anterior region; P: posterior region; FFD: full fixed denture; PFD: partial fixed denture; O: overdenture; D: delayed loading; I: immediate loading; U: upright; T: tilted alveolar nerves. The inferior alveolar nerve is a mixed nerve descending in a posterolateral position, with respect to the lingual nerve, between both pterygoid muscles. The inferior alveolar nerves exits at the lower border of the external pterygoid muscle. It then turns downward and laterally until it reaches the lingual surface of the mandible where it enters the mandibular foramen. After entering the mandibular foramen, the inferior alveolar nerve runs in the inferior alveolar canal until it exits at the level of the mental foramen. Here it divides into its two terminal branches, the mental and incisive nerves. In its intramandibular segment, the inferior alveolar nerve sends alveolar branches for innervation of the pulp and periodontal tissues of the molars, premolars, and sometimes even the canine teeth. Together with the buccinator and lingual nerves, the inferior alveolar nerve provides the innervation of the vestibular and lingual surfaces of the distal alveolar mucosa.

Three different morphologic types can be distinguished within the course of the inferior alveolar nerve:

- The nerve as a single structure is contained inside a single bony canal. Dental branches, generally short and direct, start from it (60% of cases)
- The nerve bundle is located much lower in the mandible, and dental branches are longer and more oblique than those found in the majority of people (39% of cases)
- Distally, the nerve divides into two large branches that innervate the posterior teeth while the main segment runs lower and goes to the mental foramen. A radiographic exam may show two mandibular canals (1% of cases)

In the anterior mandible, the mental foramen, the mental nerve, and the anterior loop of the inferior alveolar nerve must be taken into consideration. The most important characteristics of the mental foramen are its number, shape, dimensions, and location. The mental foramen is single in 94.5% of cases and double in another 2% to 5% of cases. In the remaining 0.5% to 1% of cases, there may be three or four foramina. Its variations may or may not be bilateral, and the diameters are variable. The mental foramen is elliptical in 65.5% to 82% of cases and rounded in the other 18% to 34.5%. Its dimensions are linked to the shape. If the foramen is elliptical, the horizontal axis (the major diameter) has an average dimension of 4 mm, and the vertical axis has an average dimension of 3.4 mm. If the foramen is round, its diameter ranges from 1.7 to 2 mm.

In adults, the position of the mental foramen in the vertical plane is about midway between the superior and inferior borders of the mandible, approximately 12 to 13 mm from either border. In elderly patients, the foramen can be in an extremely coronal position. In cases of severe residual atrophy, the foramen and the superior portion of the inferior alveolar canal may actually be open, and the nerve may be in direct contact with the intraoral tissues covering the edentulous ridge. In the sagittal plane, the mental foramen is located at the height of the roots of the second premolars in 43.5% of cases, between the first and second premolars in 20% to 28% of cases, and distally to the second premolar in 19% to 24% of cases. Various studies have reported that the inferior alveolar nerve can continue its infrabony course beyond the mental foramen, forming a ring-shaped anterior loop. In this case, the nerve proceeds in a mesial direction for a short segment, and then loops backward toward the posterior mandible, where it forms a loop and exits the foramen. This occurs in about 92% to 96% of cases. According to direct measurements, the average total length of this loop is 7 mm (Fig 6.5).[16]

The surgical technique proposed by the authors for inserting mandibular angled implants uses a round bur in the projection of the mental foramen of the inferior alveolar nerve at the level of the bone crest. The osteotomy is made with a distomesial inclination with a drill 2 mm in diameter. To avoid the anterior loop of the alveolar nerve, the direction of the osteotomy will vary from one case to another. The goal of the osteotomy is to use the entire vertical height of the mandible to provide an implant of maximum length. After this portion of the osteotomy has been completed, the surgeon proceeds with the pilot drill and the 3-mm twist drill (Figs 6.6 to 6.10).

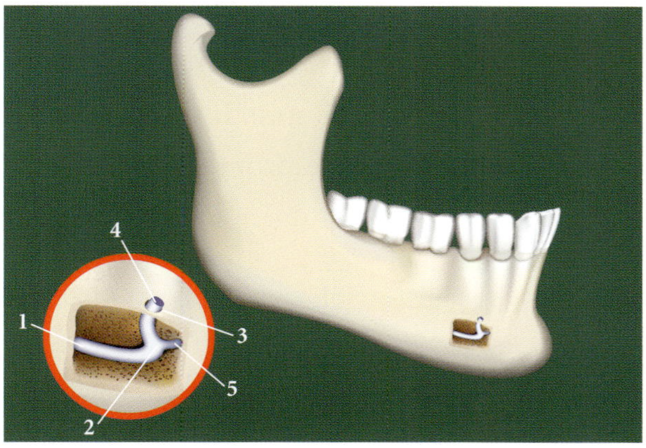

Fig 6.5 - Illustration of the anterior loop of the inferior alveolar nerve at the level of the mental foramen. The bone window permits observation of the inferior alveolar nerve (1), anterior loop (2), mental foramen (3), mental nerve (4), and incisive nerve (5).

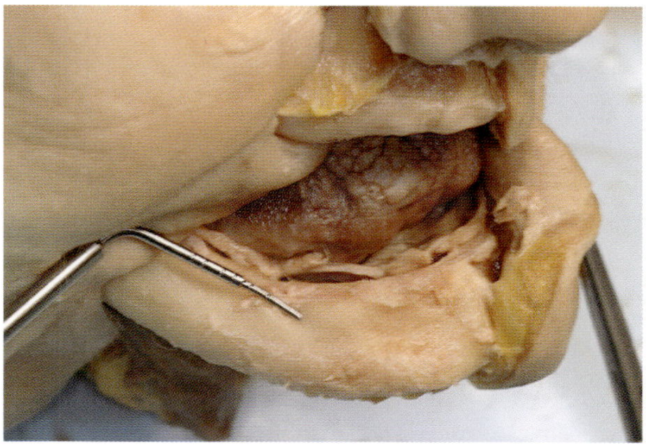

Fig 6.6 - A simulated insertion of a distomesially angled implant in a cadaver* mandible. The surgical probe approximated the position of an angled distomesial implant. On direct anatomical observations, the distance between the mesial border of the mental foramen and the most anterior margin of the inferior alveolar nerve loop was found to vary from 0.2 to 2.5 mm.

* The cadaver images were taken at the Department of Human Anatomy Chair Dr Gabriel Malka, University of Dijon, France.

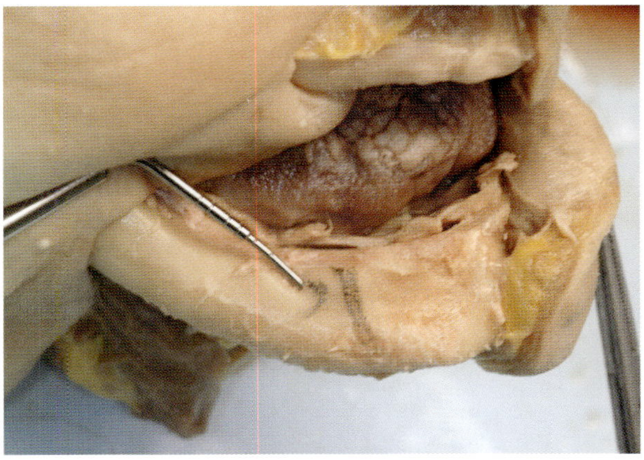

Fig 6.7 - Probing of the anterior loop of the inferior alveolar nerve in a cadaver mandible. Note that the probe has a rounded point. It is important for clinicians to identify the loop of the inferior alveolar nerve to identify the optimal implant position in the angled implant placement protocol.

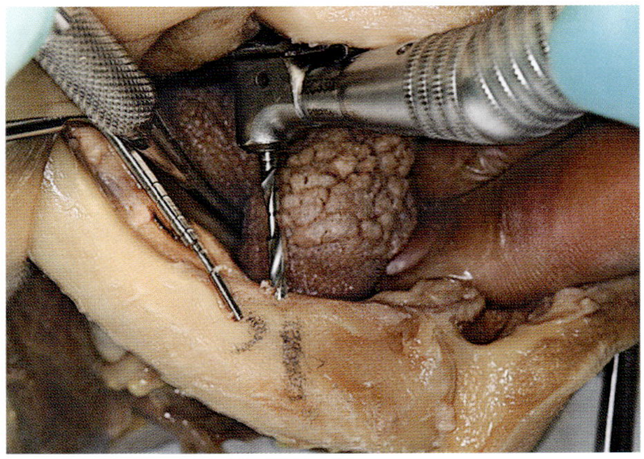

Fig 6.8 - An osteotomy preparation of the angled implant site in the right posterior mandible of a cadaver. It is important for clinicians to maintain the preestablished tilted orientation of approximately 45 degrees with respect to the superior border of the mandible.

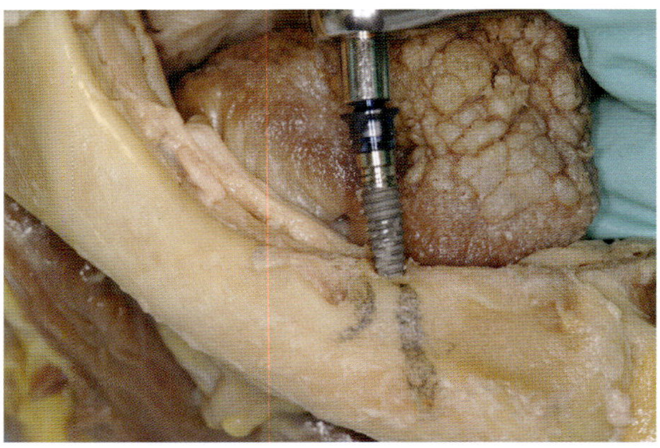

Fig 6.9 - Mandibular angled implant placement in a human cadaver. The occlusal emergence of the angled implant is as distal as possible. This implant orientation allows clinicians to use longer implants and reduces the length of prosthetic cantilevers without sacrificing the number of dental units in the prosthesis.

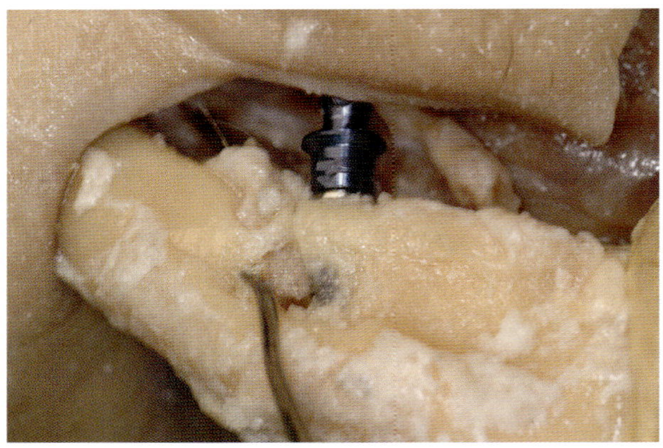

Fig 6.10 - A mandibular angled implant seated within the osteotomy in a human cadaver. The cortical bone was removed for didactic purposes. Mandibular angled implant placement is designed to place the distal implants without jeopardizing the integrity of the anterior loop of the inferior alveolar nerve.

Maxillary Sinus

In edentulous or partially edentulous maxillae, the maxillary sinus, also called the *Highmore antrum*, is the most important anatomical consideration for the insertion of distal angled implants that, as described in the surgical protocol, should emerge between the second premolar and first molar. The maxillary sinus is one of the largest paranasal cavities (ethmoid, frontal, and sphenoid sinuses), and typically, it occupies a large portion of the maxillary bones. The maxillary sinus starts developing between the second and third month in utero, with an evagination of the mucosa of the nasal cavity's lateral wall. In terms of pneumatization (increase in the volume of air contained in it), it completes its maturation process by the end of adolescence. In the course of life, the maxillary sinus can increase in volume subsequent to the loss of the maxillary posterior teeth.[17]

The sinus is a pyramid-shaped cavity, the base of which corresponds to the vertical lateral wall of the nose and the apex of which extends within the zygomatic ridge of the maxilla. The superior wall, or roof, of the maxillary sinus forms the base of the orbit, and the posterior wall protrudes onto the maxillary tuberosity, while the anterior wall is depressed at the level of the canine fossa (Fig 6.11).[18] The maxillary sinus communicates with the ipsilateral nasal cavity through a natural ostium located in an anterosuperior position on its medial surface, which drains through the medial meatus.[19] All paranasal sinuses communicate with the nasal cavity and, therefore, indirectly among themselves. Their main function is to humidify and heat the inspired air. They also decrease the weight of the facial bones, protect the cranial base from traumatic injury, provide thermal insulation to upper nervous centers, and influence phonation, acting as an indirect resonant cavity.[20,21]

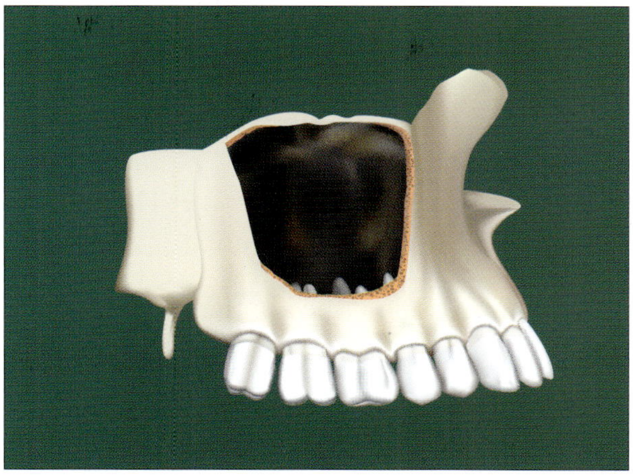

Fig 6.11 - Illustration of a right maxillary sinus.

The internal walls of the maxillary sinus are covered with a mucous membrane lined with columnar, pseudostratified, ciliated epithelium formed by basal cells, columnar cells, and chalice cells on the basal membrane. The thickness of subjacent lamina contains seromucous glands, especially proximate to the ostium. This sinus membrane normally ranges from 0.13 to 0.5 mm in thickness, but it can become thicker in the presence of sinusitis, in response to pathology or inflammation. The function of this membrane is to transport the mucus produced in its epithelial layer by numerous chalice cells and seromucous glands toward the sinus ostium and discharge it into the nasal cavity.[22] Since the sinus membrane is in direct contact with inspired air, it also serves as an immunologic barrier, although less so than nasal mucosa.

The average maxillary sinus has a volume of approximately 12 to 15 cm^3 (with wide variations, from 3.5 to 35.2 cm^3). The typical maxillary sinus is 36 to 45 mm in height, 38 to 45 mm in length, and 25 to 35 mm in width.[23,24]

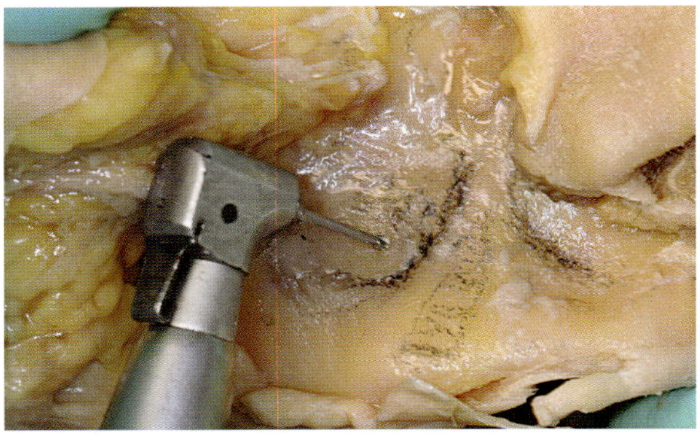

Fig 6.12 - Surgical protocol required for placement of angled maxillary implants in a cadaver. The anterior wall and the floor of the maxillary sinus, the floor of the nasal cavity, and the implant axis were identified with a blue marker. To do this clinically, a large full-thickness flap is needed to fully expose the lateral wall of the maxilla. A window is then prepared with a round bur to probe the anterior recess of the maxillary sinus.

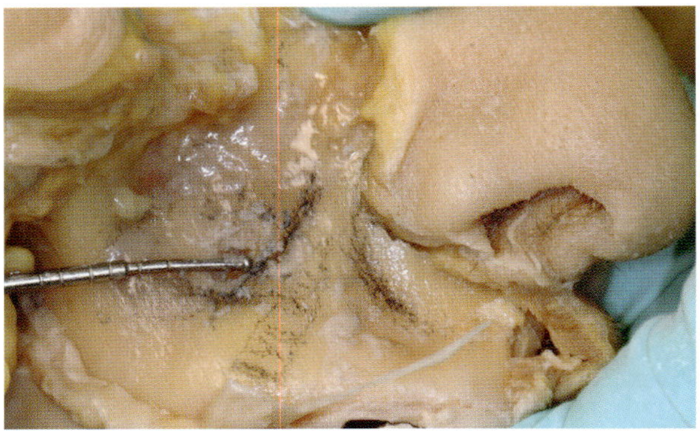

Fig 6.13 - Window prepared into the lateral wall of the maxillary sinus of a cadaver. The anterior recess of the sinus was identified with a surgical probe with a rounded point.

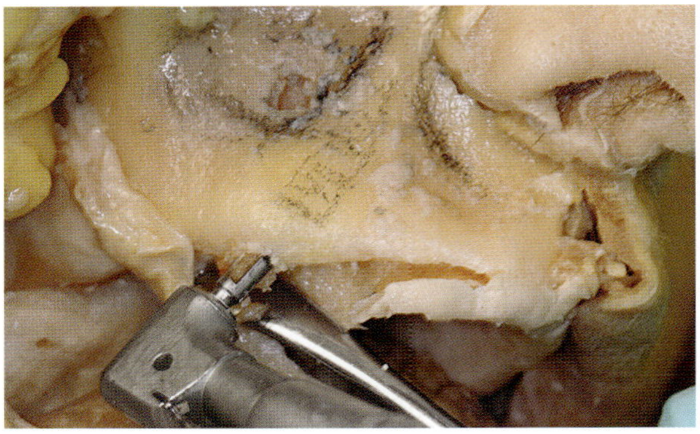

Fig 6.14 - Implant osteotomy for a maxillary implant in a cadaver. The osteotomy was prepared consistent with an angle of approximately 45 degrees; this orientation was parallel to the anterior wall of the maxillary sinus. The osteotomy was accomplished without violating the maxillary sinus.

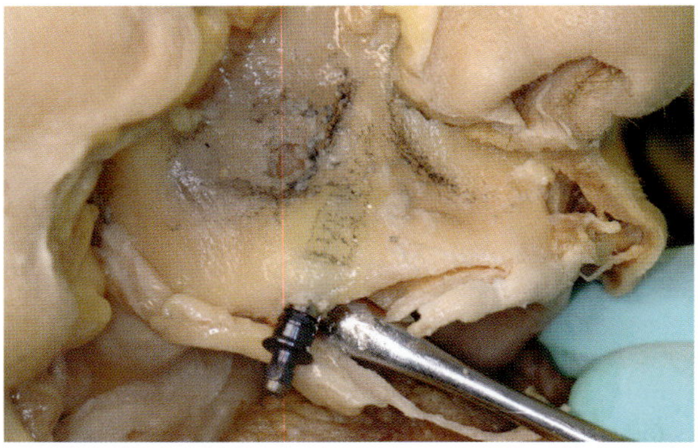

Fig 6.15 - Implant placement for an angled maxillary implant in a cadaver. This protocol eliminates the need for sinus grafting procedures such as a sinus elevation. This protocol permits the use of longer implants than would otherwise be used with vertical implant placement anterior to the sinus wall. The occlusal emergence of the angled implant is as distal as possible. The longer implants are placed into native bone.

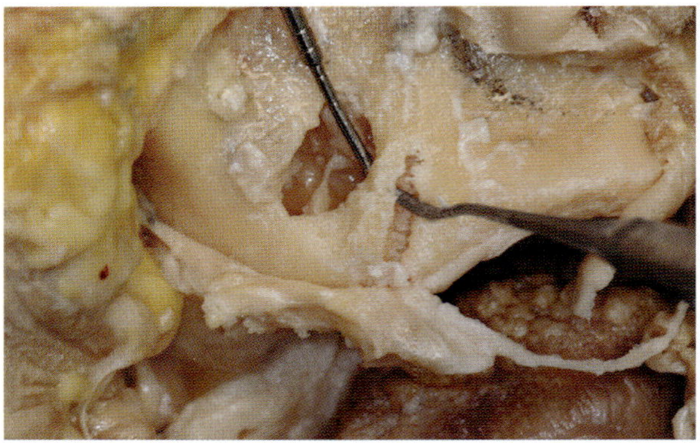

Fig 6.16 - Exposing the maxillary sinus in a cadaver. This was done for didactic purposes and proved that the maxillary sinus was not perforated during preparation of the angled implant osteotomy.

The dimensions of the antrum can vary significantly; its volume tends to increase with age because of the continuous resorption of its walls and the loss of maxillary posterior teeth. The entity and shape of such pneumatization can vary from person to person and even between the two opposing sinuses of the same patient.

In edentulous maxillae, the bone between the maxillary sinus and the alveolar crest tends to become remarkably thin and may decrease to thicknesses of 1 mm or less. This is thought to be caused by bone resorption of the alveolar crest, secondary to the absence or reduction of normal masticatory loads to the posterior maxilla.[25] Resorption and pneumatization of the sinus are related to the timing and duration of edentulism in posterior maxillae. Individuals with long-term edentulism do not generally have sufficient bone quantity for placement of dental endosseous implants, especially in the molar regions. This deficiency is probably the key factor making it necessary to elevate the sinus floor in anticipation of vertical dental implant placement or to insert angled implants in native bone.

In some surgical protocols, a bur in a contra-angle handpiece may be used to prepare a window into the lateral wall of the maxillary sinus in such a way as to allow the surgeon enough access to lift the sinus membrane and probe the anterior recess. In this way, once the morphology of the anterior wall of the sinus has been visualized, surgeons can more precisely determine the inclination of the osteotomy for optimal angled implant placement (Figs 6.12 to 6.16).

ANALYSIS OF LOAD TRANSMISSION USING IMPLANTS WITH DIFFERENT INCLINATIONS

In cases of maxillary full-arch treatment, the emergence of implants should be optimized relative to the implant restorative platforms of strategic abutments in conventional fixed prostheses, ie, canines and first molars. Such locations allow for optimal cross-arch stabilization, which is biomechanically favorable. It may not always be possible to place implants into these positions. Therefore, the use of vertical implants long enough to obtain high primary stability may be precluded.

To verify the biomechanical advantages associated with the use of angled implants, the Department of Prosthodontics at the University of Genoa developed a research protocol using finite element analysis to describe the stresses transmitted to alveolar bone with conventional vertical implants and angled implants submitted to occlusal loading.[26,27]

Finite element analysis is a computerized simulation that uses mathematic models to analyze the response of bodies to loads.[28,29] In this research, a human skull was scanned, and a mathematic maxillary model was developed (Fig 6.17). Within the computer model, screw-retained prostheses were screwed into four implants (4 mm in diameter and 13 to 18 mm in length).

Three tests were performed, each by simulating the insertion of the implants in both compact bone and trabecular bone. The value of elasticity given to each of the simulated elements was extrapolated using data available in the literature (Table 6.3).

Test 1: Single Implant

The first test consisted of simulating the insertion of a single maxillary molar implant with different inclinations: 0 degrees (implant inserted vertical to the occlusal plane), 15 degrees, 30 degrees, and 45 degrees (maximum implant inclination that can be corrected via angled abutments). The implants were submitted to axial loads of 150 N,[4,30] and the data were analyzed both in compact and trabecular bone.
The results indicated that stress levels at the peri-implant bone increased as implant inclination increased (Fig 6.18) (Table 6.4). The maximum stress reported in compact bone for a single implant was as follows:

- 10.6 MPa for the vertical implant (0 degrees)
- 18.9 MPa for the implant tilted 15 degrees
- 20.2 MPa for the implant tilted 30 degrees
- 25.0 MPa for the implant tilted 45 degrees

In the case of the vertical implant, the stress was not uniformly distributed along the entire surface of the peri-implant bone: the major concentration was limited to the first occlusal threads of the implant. In the other cases, the major stress concentrations were focused to the distal side of the implant. The maximum values were identified at the bottom of the first two threads.

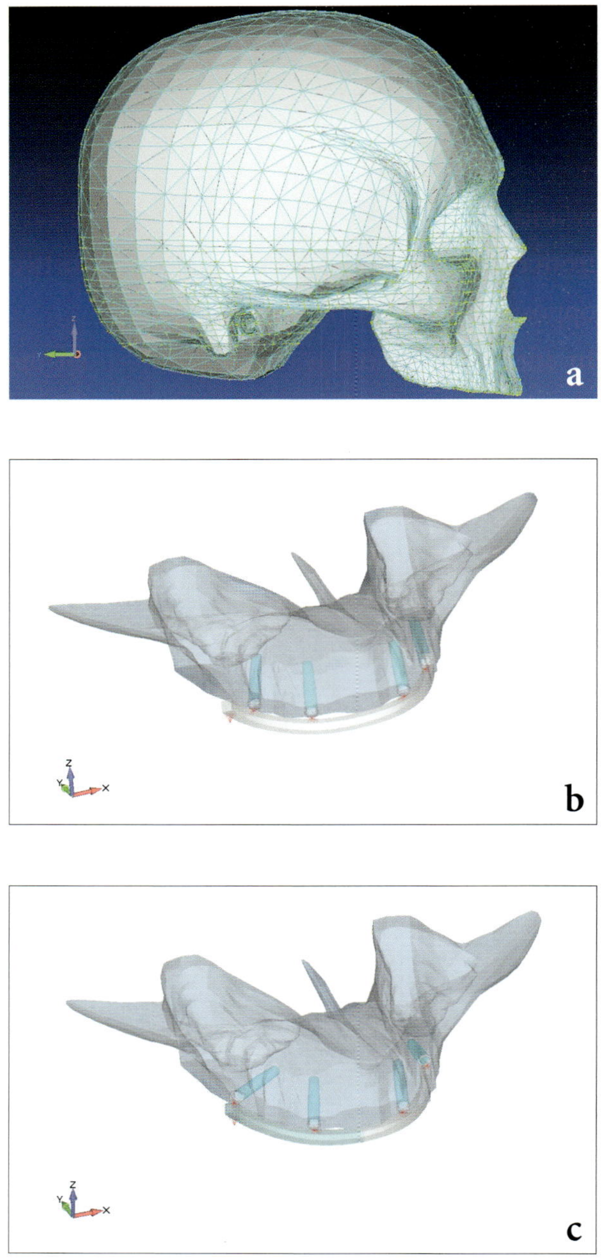

Figs 6.17 - *(a)* Illustration of a virtual model of a skull from three-dimensional radiographic images. *(b)* Three-dimensional reproduction of edentulous maxilla used in this finite element analysis research. This model simulated the insertion of four implants that would support a fixed prosthesis. The illustration depicts the vertical orientation of maxillary implants. *(c)* This illustration depicts the maxillary distal implants inclined at 45 degrees relative to occlusal planes.

TABLE 6.3 - MODULUS OF ELASTICITY AND POISSON RATIO OF MATERIALS USED IN THE VIRTUAL MODEL		
	Young Modulus (MPa)	**Poisson Ratio**
Titanium	103,400	0.3
Cortical bone	13,700	0.3
Trabecular bone	1,370	
Metal framework	210,000	

TABLE 6.4				
Inclination of a single implant (degrees)	**COMPACT BONE**		**TRABECULAR BONE**	
0	10.6 MPa	–	12.5 MPa	–
15	18.9 MPa	*+78.3%*	22.0 MPa	*+76.0%*
30	20.2 MPa	*+90.6%*	21.8 MPa	*+74.4%*
45	25.0 MPa	*+135.8%*	27.0 MPa	*+116.0%*

Table 6.4 - This table identifies the maximum values of stress recorded at the peri-implant bone for single implants submitted to a vertical load of 150 N. In italics, the percentage variation of recorded stress compared with the vertical implant is given.

Simulating the insertion of the implants into trabecular bone, higher values of stress were reported, and stress was more distributed along the surfaces of the implants (Fig 6.19). The maximum stress was reported at the level of the first thread with values close to the maximum reported at the level of the following threads.

The maximum stress values recorded for the single implant in trabecular bone were as follows:

- 12.5 MPa for the vertical implant (0 degrees)
- 22.0 MPa for the implant tilted 15 degrees
- 21.8 MPa for the implant tilted 30 degrees
- 27.0 MPa for the implant tilted 45 degrees

The slope of the curve representing the forces recorded in trabecular peri-implant bone was parallel to the slope of the curve representing the forces recorded in the presence of compact bone. However, the values were slightly higher with trabecular bone than with compact bone (Fig 6.20).

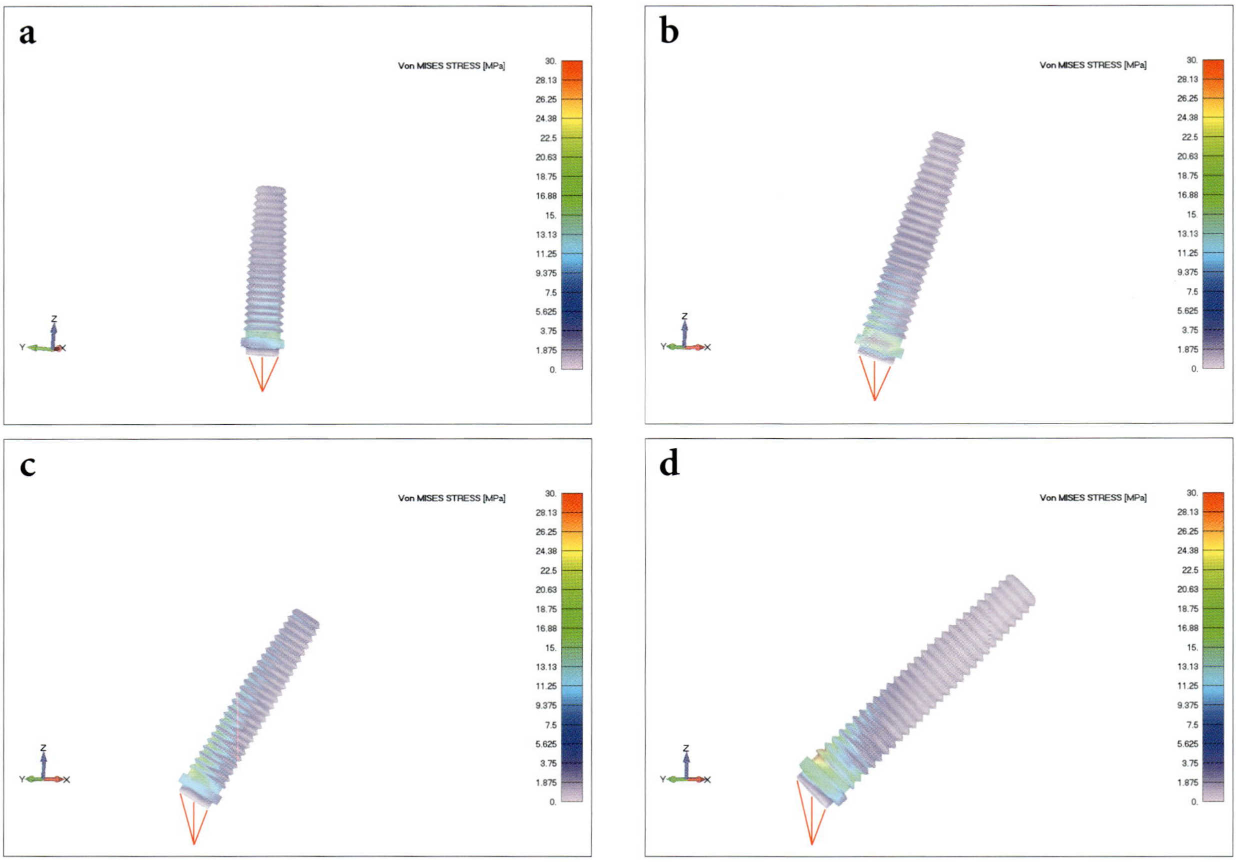

Figs 6.18 - Test 1. Simulation of stress distribution at the peri-implant bone with a vertical load of 150 N (*red lines*) on single implants inserted into compact bone with different degrees of inclination (relative to the vertical axis): 0 degrees *(a)*; 15 degrees *(b)*; 30 degrees *(c)*; 45 degrees *(d)*.

Test 2: Splinted Implants

The second test evaluated the distribution of loads in the peri-implant bone with four implants splinted together. In this virtual design, the implants were positioned in the maxilla and splinted with a framework that extended from the maxillary right first molar to the maxillary left first molar. Four different configurations were evaluated:

- The distal implants were positioned vertically in front of the anterior wall of the maxillary sinus according to the model of a Toronto-type fixed implant prosthesis. The framework was designed with a distal cantilever of 13 mm
- The distal implants were virtually angled by 15 degrees relative to the anterior wall of the maxillary sinus. The framework in this case had a distal cantilever of 9 mm
- The two distal implants were angled by 30 degrees with distal cantilevers of 5 mm

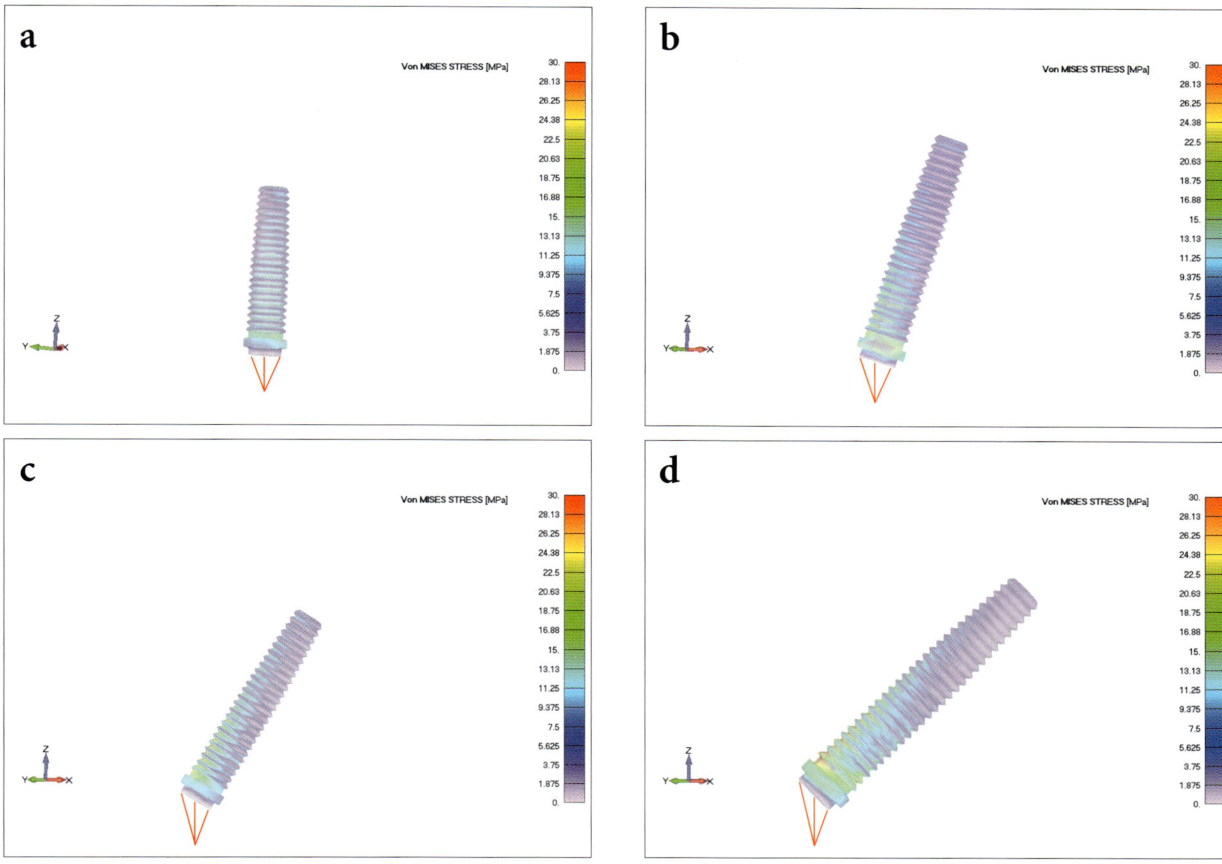

Figs 6.19 - Test 1. Simulation of stress distribution at the peri-implant bone with a vertical load of 150 N (*red lines*) on single implants inserted into trabecular bone with different degrees of inclination (relative to the sagittal plane): 0 degrees *(a)*; 15 degrees *(b)*; 30 degrees *(c)*; 45 degrees *(d)*.

- The two distal implants were angled by 45 degrees without a distal cantilever

A vertical load of 150 N was applied to the end of the bar–that is, in the most distal portion of the prosthetic cantilever. In this case, the stress in the peri-implant bone decreased with an increase of the inclination of the distal implant (Figs 6.21 to 6.26) (Table 6.5). The maximum stress values recorded in compact bone were for the vertical implant: 75.0 MPa for the distal fixture and 35.0 MPa for the mesial fixture. In the case of the distal angled implant, with the tilted implant inclined by 45 degrees, the maximum stresses were reduced to a value of 19.9 MPa for the distal fixture and 7.8 MPa for the mesial fixture.

Using the same loading conditions, the maximum stress values recorded in trabecular bone for the vertical distal implant were 68.6 MPa for the dis-

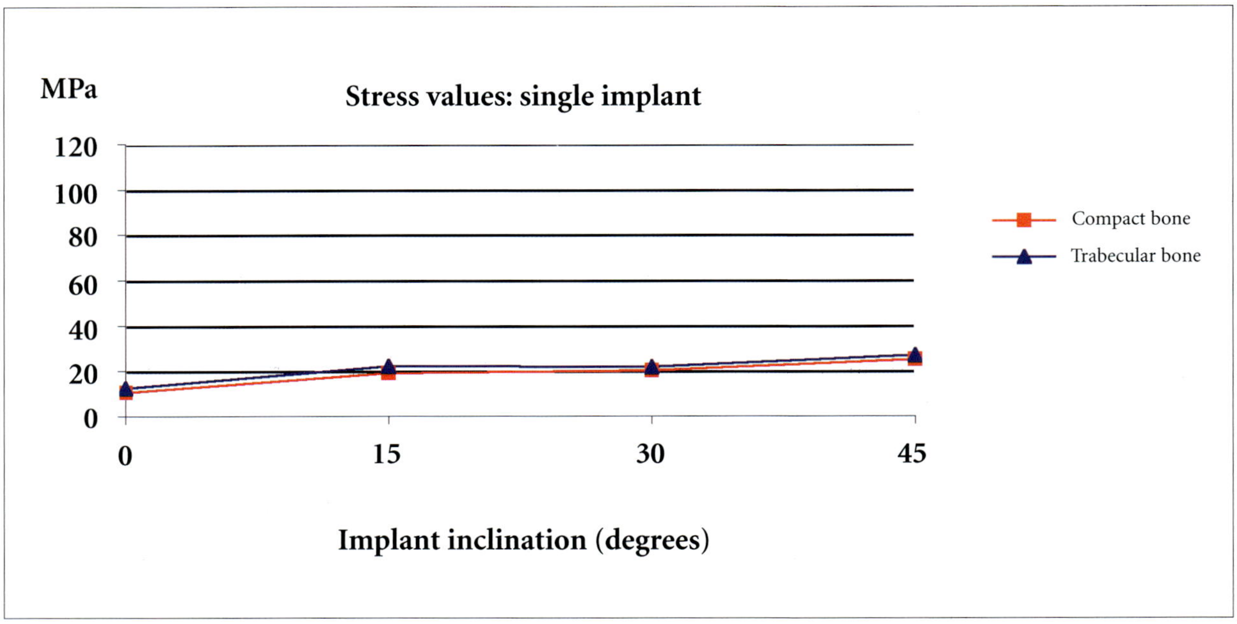

Fig 6.20 - This graph identifies the maximum stress values at the level of the peri-implant bone according to the inclination of a single implant. The x-axis identifies the degrees of implant inclination; the y-axis identifies the maximum stress values recorded. The stresses recorded for trabecular bone were slightly higher than the values recorded for compact bone.

tal fixture and 30.0 MPa for the mesial fixture. In the case of the distal angled implant, the maximum stresses were reduced to 15.5 MPa for the distal fixture and 5.7 MPa for the mesial fixture, with the distal implant tilted by 45 degrees.

Consistent with the results of test 1, in compact bone higher stresses were limited to the first three or four threads of the implant; in trabecular bone, the stresses were distributed along a greater number of threads until the apical portion of the implant was reached. Lower stresses were consistently recorded in trabecular bone.

Test 3: Stress of Metal Frameworks

The third test evaluated the stresses associated with metal frameworks supported by the distal vertical implant with a long cantilever (13 mm). The same test was conducted with the distal implant angled by 15, 30, or 45 degrees and with cantilevers of 9, 5, and 0 mm respectively. A 150-N vertical load was applied at the distal end of the framework. The point of maximum stress of the metal framework was at the level of the emergence of the distal implant. The precise location was at the junction of the framework and the

TABLE 6.5					
Inclination of distal implant (degrees)	**Length of distal cantilever (mm)**	**COMPACT BONE (MPa)**		**TRABECULAR BONE (MPa)**	
		Distal implant	**Mesial implant**	**Distal implant**	**Mesial implant**
0	13	75.0	35	68.6	30
15	9	65.3 *-12.9%*	28.6 *-18.3%*	56.8 *-17.2%*	24.5 *-18.3%*
30	5	39.4 *-47.5%*	16.6 *-52.6%*	31.0 *-54.8%*	13.7 *-54.3%*
45	0	19.9 *-73.5%*	7.8 *-77.7%*	15.5 *-77.4%*	5.7 *-81%*

Table 6.5 -Data of maximum values of Von Mises stress recorded at the bone-implant interface with a load of 150 Ncm on the distal end of the prosthetic cantilever. In italics, the percentage variation of recorded stress compared with the configuration with a vertical distal implant is given.

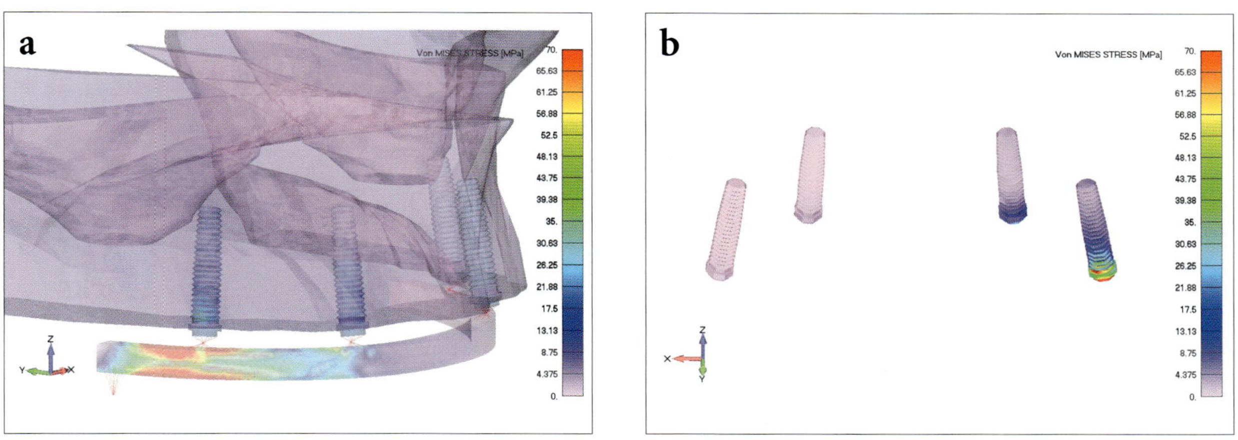

Fig 6.21 - Test 2. Simulation of the stress transmitted to the peri-implant bone interface with a load of 150 N on the right distal portion of the prosthetic cantilever on a vertical (relative to the occlusal plane) implant inserted into compact bone. The implants were splinted with a metal framework. *(a)* Right lateral view of the right maxilla. Application and transfer of the loads (*red lines*). *(b)* Views of the implants from a posterior view.

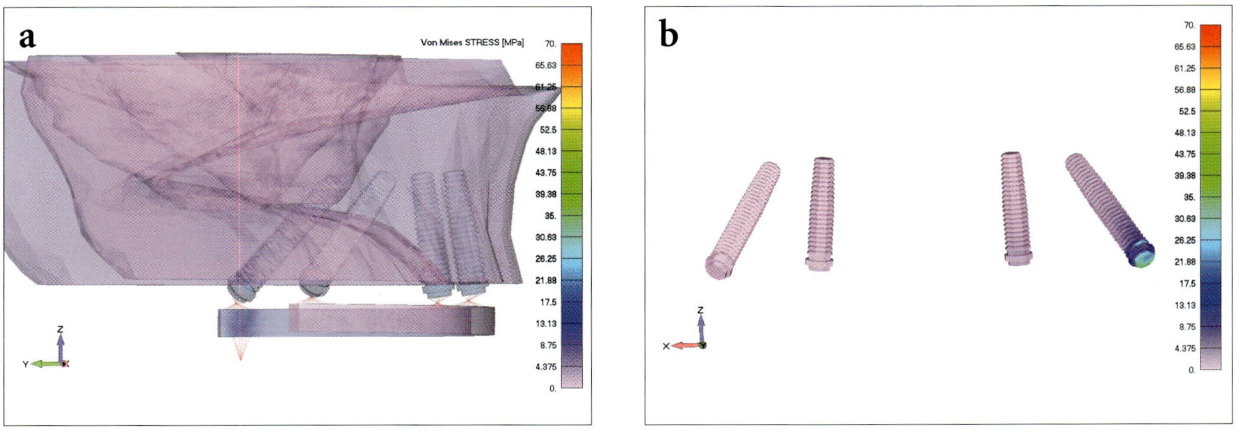

Fig 6.22 - Test 2. Simulation of the stress transmitted to the peri-implant compact bone with a load of 150 N on the right distal portion of the prosthetic framework. The implants were splinted with a metal framework. The distal implant was inclined by 45 degrees with respect to the occlusal plane. *(a)* Right lateral view of the right maxilla. The color scale reflects the Von Mises values and demonstrates lower stress than the analysis in Fig 6.21 (maximum value 19.9 MPa). *(b)* Detail of the implants from a posterior view. At the level of the anterior implant, stress was almost nonexistent.

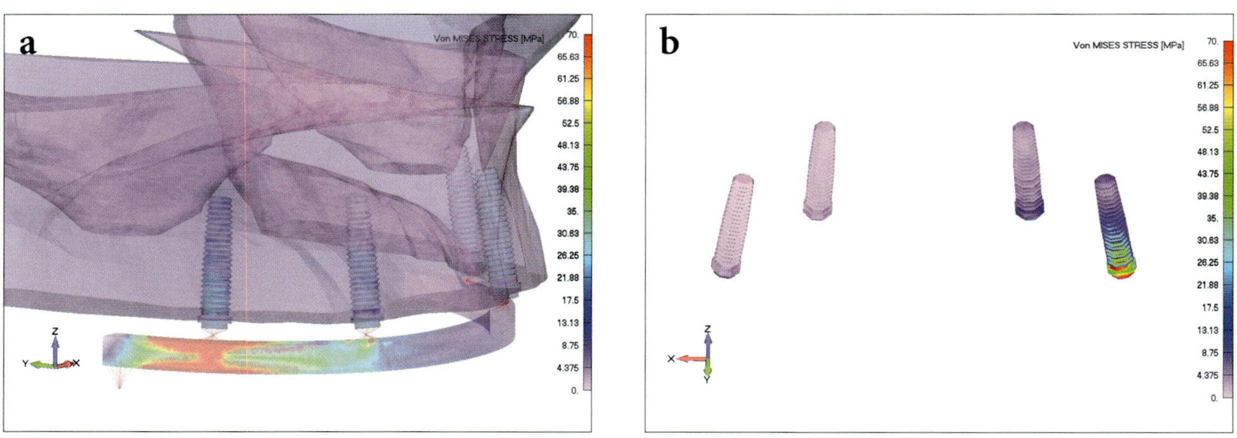

Fig 6.23 - Test 2. Simulation of the stress transmitted to the peri-implant trabecular bone with vertical (relative to the occlusal plane) implants. The implants were splinted with a metal framework. *(a)* Right lateral view. *(b)* Detail of the implants from a posterior view.

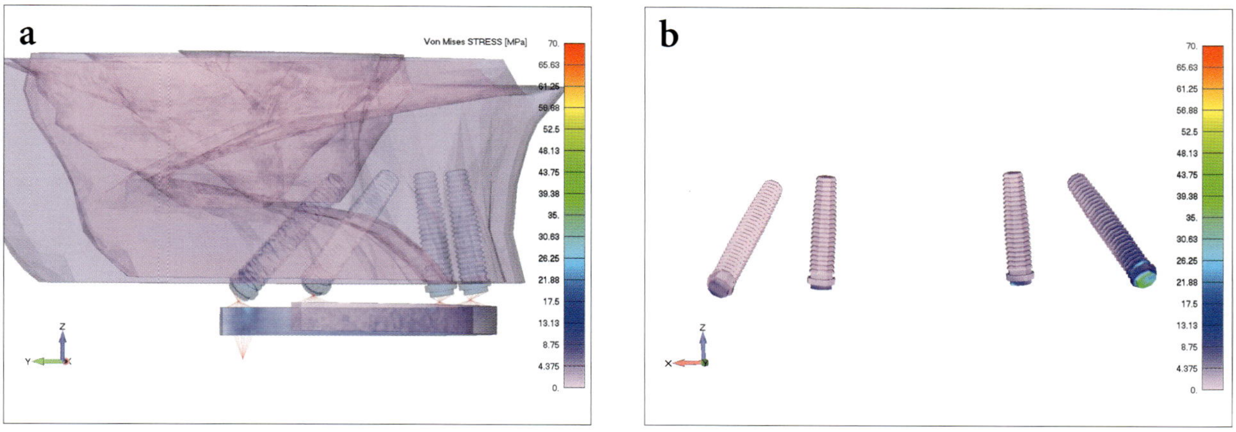

Fig 6.24 - Test 2. Simulation of stress transmitted to the peri-implant trabecular bone. The distal implants were inserted at inclinations of 45 degrees (relative to the occlusal plane). The implants were splinted with a metal framework. *(a)* The maximum stress recorded was 15.5 MPa. *(b)* Detail of the implants from a posterior view. The stress values were lower than those of the simulation in compact bone. The stress values around the anterior implant were virtually absent: 5.7 MPa.

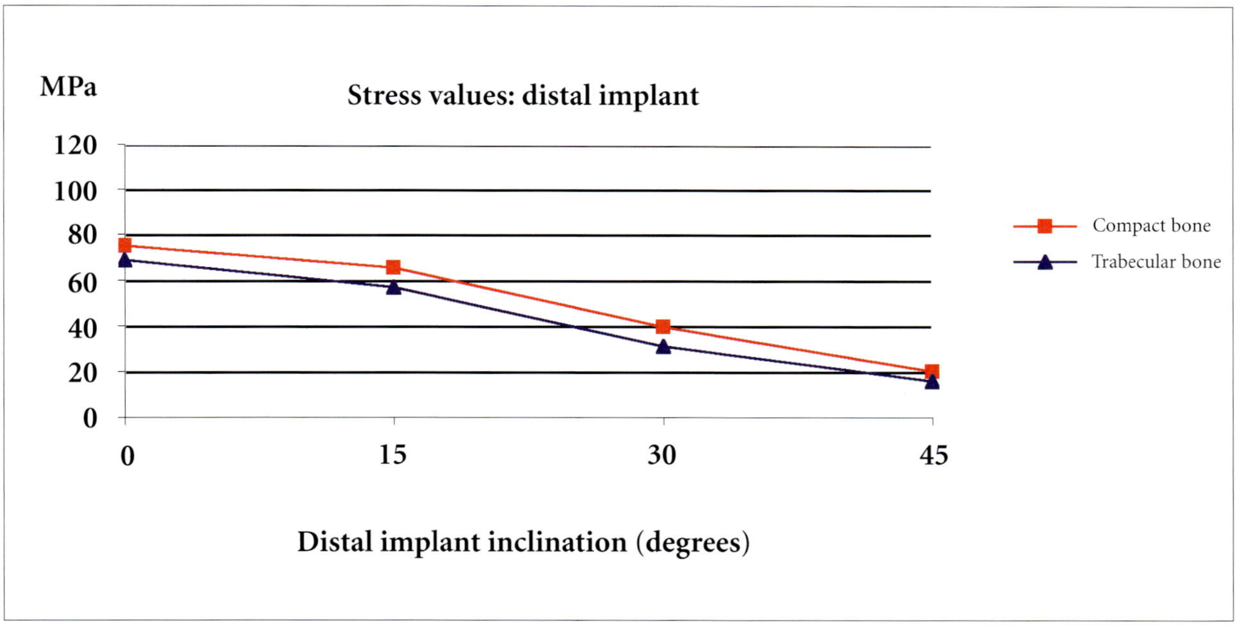

Fig 6.25 - This graph identifies the development of the maximum stress values at the level of the peri-implant bone in the distal implant relative to the inclination of the implant. The x-axis recorded the implant inclination in degrees; the y-coordinates recorded the maximum stress values. The values recorded in trabecular bone were slightly lower than those recorded in compact bone; both curves were relatively parallel.

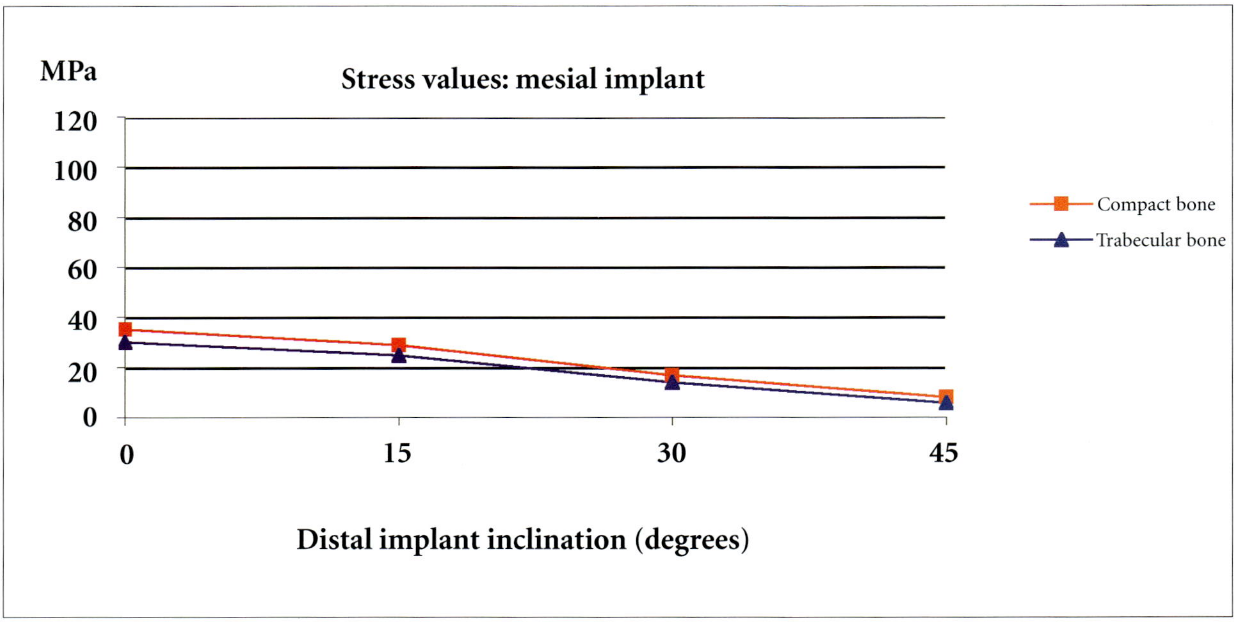

Fig 6.26 - This graph identifies the development of the maximum stress values at the level of the peri-implant bone of the vertical mesial implant relative to the inclination of the distal implant. The x-axis recorded the inclination degrees of the distal implant; the y-axis recorded the maximum values of stress. The values recorded in trabecular bone were slightly lower than those recorded in compact bone.

distal implant where the bar, at a point of resistance that acted as a fulcrum, tended to bend. As with the preceding tests, the stresses at the level of the metal framework decreased with increased inclinations of the distal implant. This occurred for implants placed into compact and trabecular bone (Figs 6.27 and 6.28) (Table 6.6).

The maximum stress value recorded on the framework in the presence of compact bone was 95.0 MPa for the distal vertical implant; it was reduced to 13.7 MPa for the distal angled implant with the 45-degree inclination. For the implants inserted into trabecular bone, the maximum recorded stress value was 103.9 MPa for the distal vertical implant; it was reduced to 16.3 MPa for the distal angled implant with the 45-degree inclination. In this case as well, the slope of the curve representing the forces recorded at the peri-implant trabecular bone is parallel to the slope of the curve of forces recorded in the presence of compact bone, but with higher values (Fig 6.29).

The results of this research contradicted the concept of placing splinted implants as vertical as possible per the original Brånemark protocol. Vertical implant placement was correct in the case of single implants, a situation where stress transmitted to the bone-implant complex increased with an increase in the inclination or tilting of the fixture.

This study proved that it was essential to reduce the lengths of distal cantilevers to obtain optimal distribution of stress in full-arch prosthetic treatment. Distal cantilevers, in the presence of vertical loads applied to the distal end of a prosthesis, result in unfavorable lever arms. If the goal of treatment is to design a prosthesis with minimal cantilevers and 10 to 12 masticatory units, it becomes necessary to accept the compromise of using distal angled implants. To eliminate or minimize a distal cantilever, a prosthesis could also be designed with short implants (less than 13 mm in length) in posterior maxillary segments that would support the distal portion of the prosthesis. This solution requires the use of at least six implants in edentulous maxillae, with a subsequent increase in costs. The use of short implants is not generally recommended for immediate loading in trabecular bone.

Stress at the level of the metal framework is reduced with reduction of the distal cantilever secondary to the insertion of a distal angled implant. Subsequently, this reduction also minimizes risks associated with the failure and fracture of prosthetic components.

In review, in the scope of full-arch fixed treatment and in the presence of both compact bone and trabecular bone, stresses recorded at the peri-implant bone and at the level of metal frameworks are lower in the presence of distal angled implants compared with values recorded in the presence of distal vertical implants. Vertically placed implants generally require the construction of relatively long, distal cantilevered segments to provide 10 to 12 masticatory units in a given prosthesis. Distal cantilevers put additional stresses on the distal implants.

TABLE 6.6

Distal implant inclination (degrees)	Length of distal cantilever (mm)	COMPACT BONE (MPa)		TRABECULAR BONE (MPa)	
0	13	95.0		103.9	
15	9	84.1	*-11.5%*	93.2	*-10.3%*
30	5	65.3	*-31.3%*	73.1	*-29.6%*
45	0	13.7	*-85.6%*	16.3	*-84.3%*

Table 6.6 - This table reports, in MPa, the maximum values of Von Mises stress recorded at the level of the metal framework with a load of 150 N on the distal end of the prosthetic cantilever. The percentage variation of stress recorded, compared with the orientation of the vertical distal implant, is in italics.

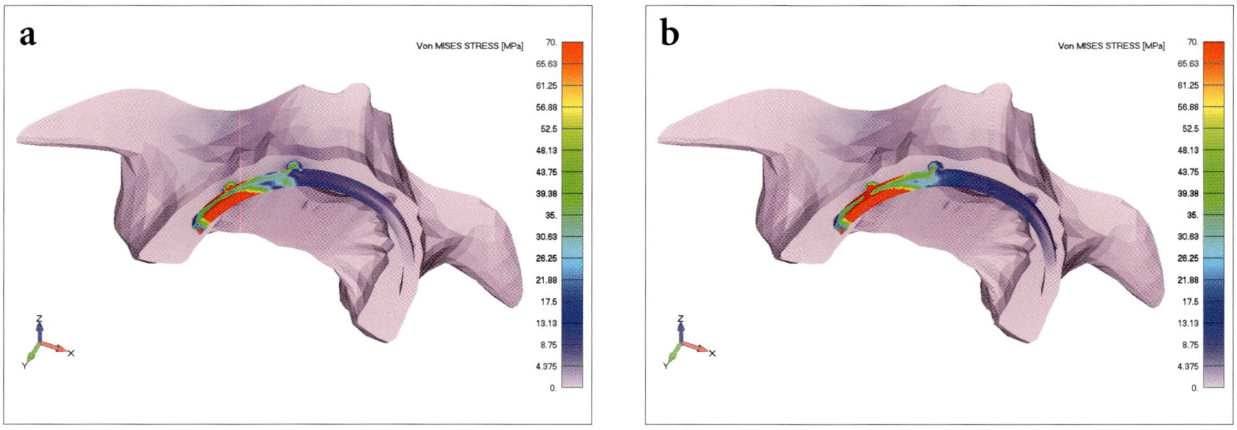

Fig 6.27 - Test 3. Simulation of stress recorded at the level of the metal framework used to splint the four implants. The implants were inserted vertically at the level of the occlusal plane in compact and trabecular bone. The distal cantilever was 13 mm. A vertical load of 150 N was applied at the right distal end of the bar. The point of highest stress was recorded at the distal implant where the bar tended to bend under load. *(a)* There was 95.0 MPa of stress recorded for implants inserted into compact bone. *(b)* There was 103.9 MPa of stress recorded for implants inserted into trabecular bone.

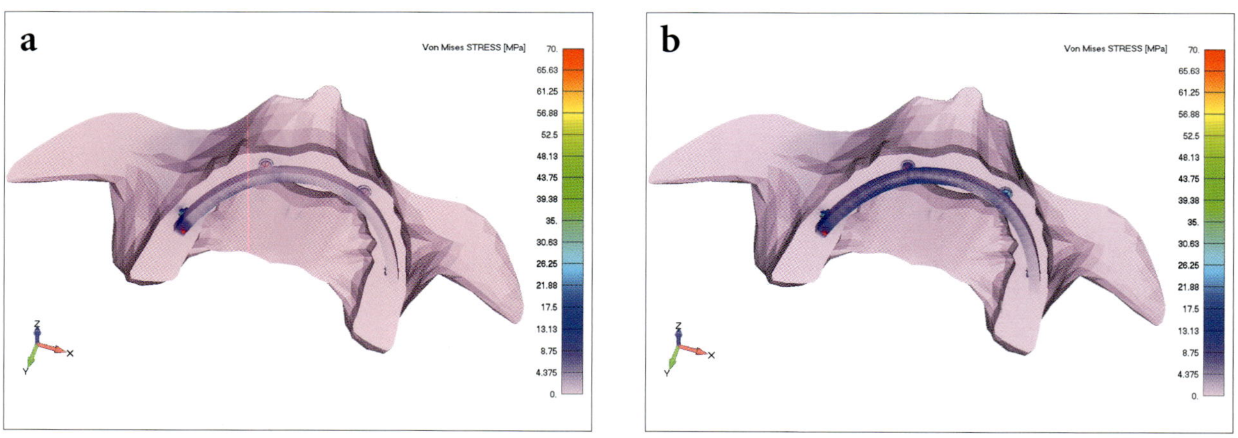

Fig 6.28 - Test 3. Simulation of the stress recorded at the level of the metal framework used to splint the four implants; the two distal implants were inclined 45 degrees relative to the occlusal plane. The distal cantilever was absent with the corresponding reduction of the lever arm that was present in Fig 6.27. *(a)* The stress values recorded for the metal framework decreased to 13.7 MPa for the implants placed into compact bone. *(b)* The stress values were 16.3 MPa for the implants placed into trabecular bone.

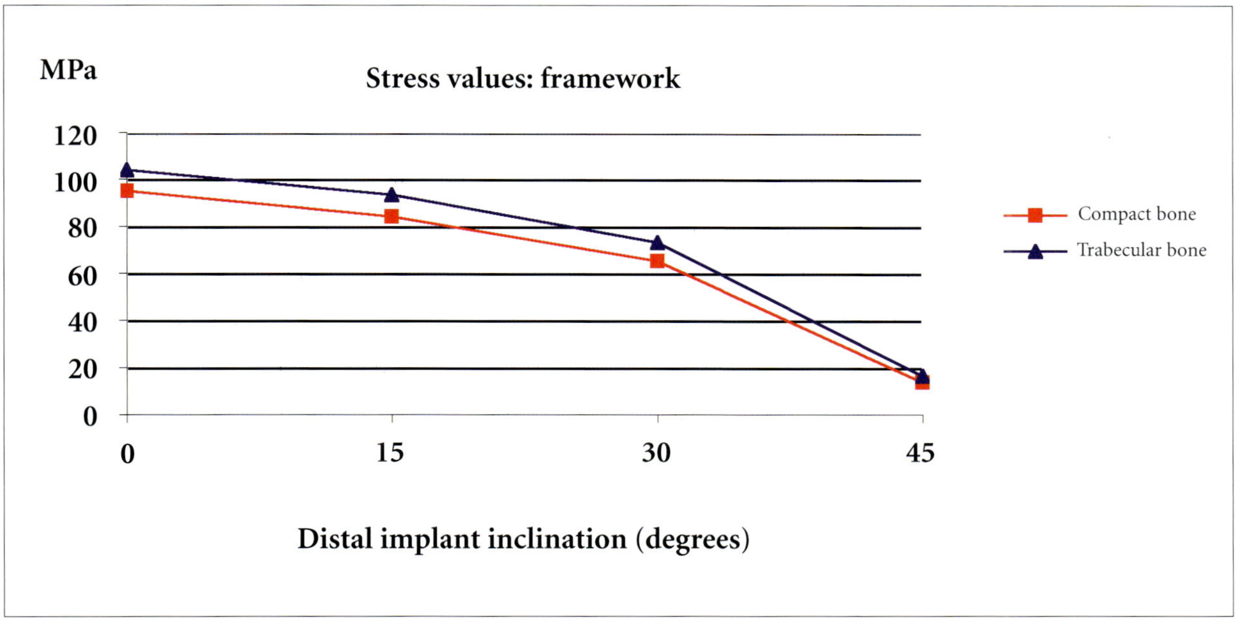

Fig 6.29 - This graph demonstrates the maximum stress values on the metal framework relative to the increase in inclination of the implants. The x-axis recorded the degrees of implant inclination; the y-axis recorded the maximum stress values. The values recorded in trabecular bone were higher than those recorded in compact bone. An increase in implant inclination (with reduction of the prosthetic cantilever) caused a reduction in stress values.

The protocol that calls for the use of angled implants allows for the insertion of longer distal implants than does the protocol that calls for the placement of vertical implants. Because longer implants result in increased bone-implant contact, they facilitate the achievement of implant primary stability–a mandatory prerequisite in immediate-loading protocols.

Finite element method studies are performed within computers and only simulate clinical situations. Biomechanical considerations realized from this type of study have proven helpful in increasing the clinical understanding of certain phenomena, especially stress within bone. The results of these studies should be taken into consideration during the planning of implant-prosthetic treatment. Within the limitations of this finite element analysis study, the use of distal tilted implants results in a reduction in stresses in the peri-implant bone and in metal frameworks secondary to cantilever length reduction and implant length increase. This treatment modality seems to be a valid therapeutic alternative to conventional maxillary fixed complete prostheses supported by vertical dental implants with posterior cantilevers.

REFERENCES

1. Mattsson T, Kondell PA, Gynther GW, Fredholm U, Bolin A. Implant treatment without bone grafting in severely resorbed edentulous maxillae. J Oral Maxillofac Surg 1999;57:281–287.
2. Krekmanov L, Kahn M, Rangert B, Lindstrom H. Tilting of posterior mandibular and maxillary implants for improved prosthesis support. Int J Oral Maxillofac Implants 2000;15:405–414.
3. Krekmanov L. Placement of posterior mandibular and maxillary implants in patients with severe bone deficiency: A clinical report of procedure. Int J Oral Maxillofac Implants 2000;15:722–730.
4. Aparicio C, Perales P, Rangert B. Tilted implants as an alternative to maxillary sinus grafting: A clinical, radiologic, and Periotest study. Clin Implant Dent Relat Res 2001;3:39–49.
5. Fortin Y, Sullivan RM, Rangert BR. The Marius implant bridge: Surgical and prosthetic rehabilitation for the completely edentulous upper jaw with moderate to severe resorption: A 5-year retrospective clinical study. Clin Implant Dent Relat Res 2002;4:69–77.
6. Maló P, Rangert B, Nobre M. "All-on-Four" immediate-function concept with Brånemark System implants for completely edentulous mandibles: A retrospective clinical study. Clin Implant Dent Relat Res 2003;5(suppl 1):2–9.
7. Maló P, Rangert B, Nobre M. All-on-4 immediate-function concept with Brånemark System implants for completely edentulous maxillae: A 1-year retrospective clinical study. Clin Implant Dent Relat Res 2005;7(suppl 1):88S–94S.
8. Calandriello R, Tomatis M. Simplified treatment of the atrophic posterior maxilla via immediate/early function and tilted implants: A prospective 1-year clinical study. Clin Implant Dent Relat Res 2005;7(suppl 1):1S–12S.
9. Maló P, Nobre Mde A, Petersson U, Wigren S. A pilot study of complete edentulous rehabilitation with immediate function using a new implant design: Case series. Clin Implant Dent Relat Res 2006;8:223–232.
10. Rosen A, Gynther G. Implant treatment without bone grafting in edentulous severely resorbed maxillas: A long-term follow-up study. J Oral Maxillofac Surg 2007;65:1010–1016.
11. Capelli M, Zuffetti F, Del Fabbro M, Testori T. Immediate rehabilitation of the completely edentulous jaw with fixed prostheses supported by either upright or tilted implants: A multicenter clinical study. Int J Oral Maxillofac Implants 2007;22: 639–644.
12. Testori T, Del Fabbro M, Capelli M, Zuffetti F, Francetti L, Weinstein RL. Immediate occlusal loading and tilted implants for the rehabilitation of the atrophic edentulous maxilla: 1-year interim results of a multicenter prospective study. Clin Oral Implants Res 2008;19:227–232.
13. Francetti L, Agliardi E, Testori T, Romeo D, Taschieri S, Del Fabbro M. Immediate rehabilitation of the mandible with fixed full prosthesis supported by axial and tilted implants: Interim results of a single cohort prospective study. Clin Implant Dent Relat Res 2008;10:255–265.
14. Tealdo T, Bevilacqua M, Pera F, et al. Immediate function with fixed implant-supported maxillary dentures: A 12-month pilot study. J Prosthet Dent 2008;99:351–360.
15. Agliardi EL, Francetti L, Romeo D, Taschieri S, Del Fabbro M. Immediate loading in the fully edentulous maxilla without bone grafting: The V-II-V technique. Minerva Stomatol 2008;57:251–263.
16. Franco M, Ferronato G (eds). Il Nervo Mandibolare in Odontoiatria. Padova: Frafin, 1996.
17. Van den Bergh JP, ten Bruggenkate CM, Disch FJ, Tuinzing DB. Anatomical aspects of sinus floor elevations. Clin Oral Implants Res 2000;11:256–265.
18. Lloyd DuBrul E (ed). Sicher's Oral anatomy. St Louis: Mosby, 1980.

19. May M, Sobol SM, Korzec K. The location of the maxillary os and its importance to the endoscopic sinus surgeon. Laryngoscope 1990;100:1037–1042.
20. Ritter FN. The Paranasal Sinuses. Anatomy and Surgical Technique. St Louis: Mosby, 1978.
21. Blanton PL, Biggs NL. Eighteen hundred years of controversy: The paranasal sinuses. Am J Anat 1969;124:135–147.
22. Stammberger H. Nasal and paranasal sinus endoscopy. A diagnostic and surgical approach to recurrent sinusitis. Endoscopy 1986;18:213-218.
23. Eckert-Mobius A. Maxillary sinusitis in children. Dtsch Stomatol 1954;4:170–177.
24. Uchida Y, Goto M, Katsuki T, Soejima Y. Measurement of maxillary sinus volume using computerized tomographic images. Int J Oral Maxillofac Implants 1998;13:811–818.
25. Cawood JI, Howell RA. A classification of the edentulous jaws. Int J Oral Maxillofac Surg 1988;17: 232–236.
26. Bevilacqua M, Tealdo T, Pera F, et al. Three-dimensional finite element analysis of load transmission using different implant inclinations and cantilever lengths. Int J Prosthodont 2008;21:539–542.
27. Bevilacqua M, Tealdo T, Menini M, et al. The influence of cantilever length and implant inclination on stress distribution in maxillary implant-supported fixed dentures. J Prosthet Dent 2011;105:5–13.
28. Geng JP, Tan KB, Liu GR. Application of finite element analysis in implant dentistry: A review of the literature. J Prosthet Dent 2001;85:585–598.
29. Papavasiliou G, Kamposiora P, Bayne SC, Felton DA. Three-dimensional finite element analysis of stress-distribution around single tooth implants as a function of bony support, prosthesis type, and loading during function. J Prosthet Dent 1996;76:633–640.
30. Brunski JB. Biomechanics. In: Worthington P, Lang BR, Rubenstein JE (eds). Osseointegration in Dentistry: An Overview, ed 2. Chicago: Quintessence, 2003:49–83.

CHAPTER 7

PROSTHETIC ABUTMENTS

COLUMBUS BRIDGE PROTOCOL	
SURGICAL PROTOCOL	**PROSTHETIC PROTOCOL**
External hex rough-surface implants	Screw-retained fixed prosthesis
Implant length ≥ 13 mm, Ø 4 mm	Plaster impression with pickup technique
Underprepared osteotomy	Rigid splinting with metal framework
Implant insertion torque ≥ 40 Ncm	Passive fit with the luting technique
Angled implants in native bone	Acrylic resin occlusal surfaces
Angled conical abutments	No distal cantilevers
No bone regenerative techniques	Immediate functional load 24–48 h after surgery

Table 7.1

At the beginning of the 1980s, the standard ad modum Brånemark[1] abutment was the only one available for prosthetic treatment and osseointegrated implants (Fig 7.1). These abutments, designed for transmucosal use, were often visible intraorally. Angle correction for implants nonoptimally placed was not possible because the abutments were straight, and the screw access openings of off-angle implants often compromised the final esthetics (Fig 7.2). Within the last 15 years, however, the number of abutment types available for clinical use in implant restorative dentistry has increased significantly.

Abutment selection is based on four clinical criteria:

- Available prosthetic space (affecting implant position)

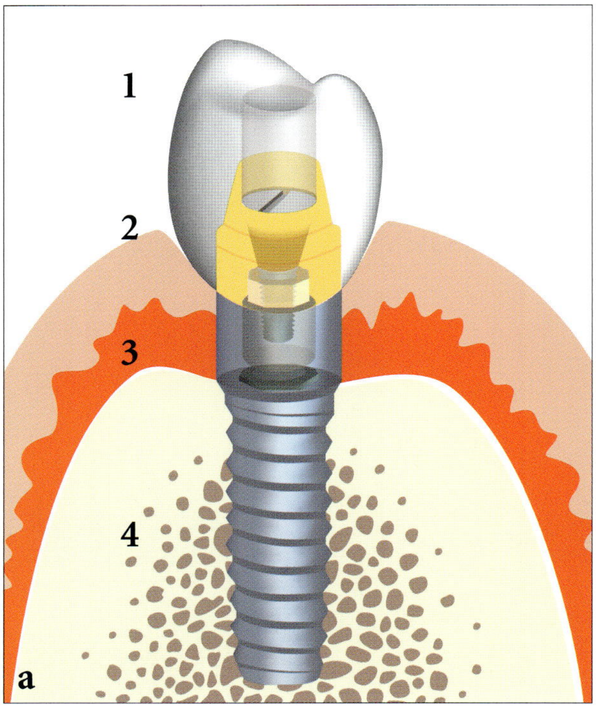

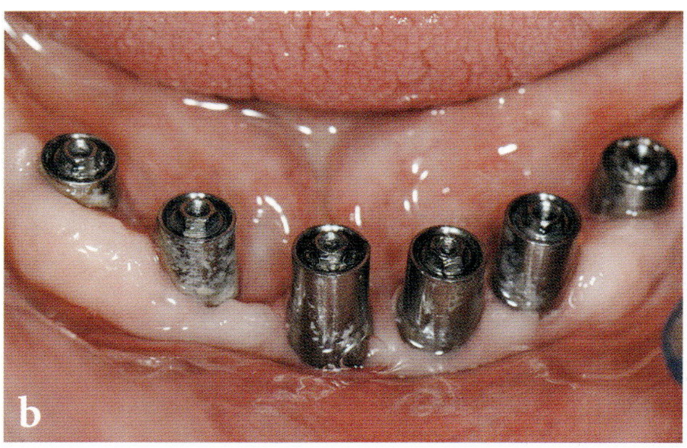

Fig 7.1 - *(a)* Illustration of a standard abutment of the Brånemark implant system. Artificial tooth (1); castable gold cylinder (2); standard abutment (3); implant (4). *(b)* Clinical labial image of six standard abutments placed on intraforaminal implants supporting a Toronto bridge.

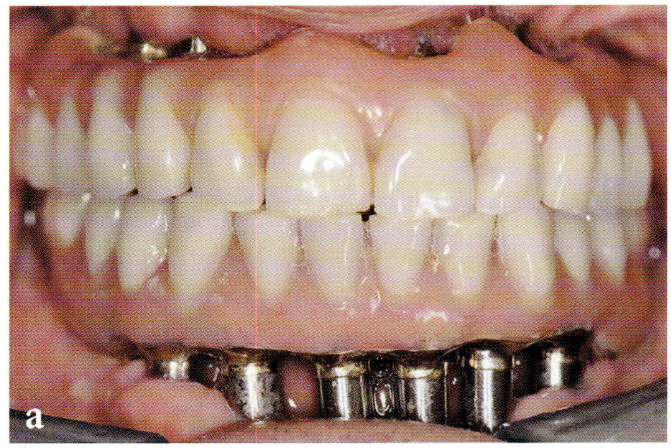

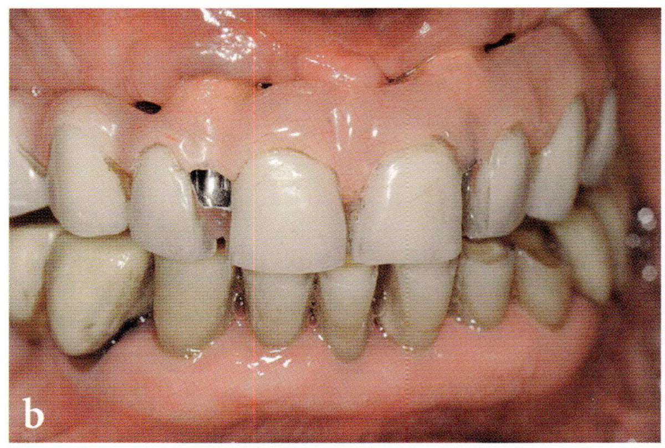

Fig 7.2 - *(a)* Clinical labial image of maxillary and mandibular fixed prostheses made per the original Brånemark protocol with standard abutments. These implants were placed vertically between the mental foramina. *(b)* Clinical labial image of a maxillary fixed prosthesis made per the original Brånemark protocol with standard abutments. Without angle correction, some screw access openings were visible and yielded unsatisfactory esthetic results.

- Presence of adjacent teeth or implants (affecting implant angulation)
- Vertical distance between the implant restorative platform and occlusal plane
- Vertical distance between the implant restorative platform and free margin of the peri-implant soft tissues (depth of the peri-implant sulcular tissues)

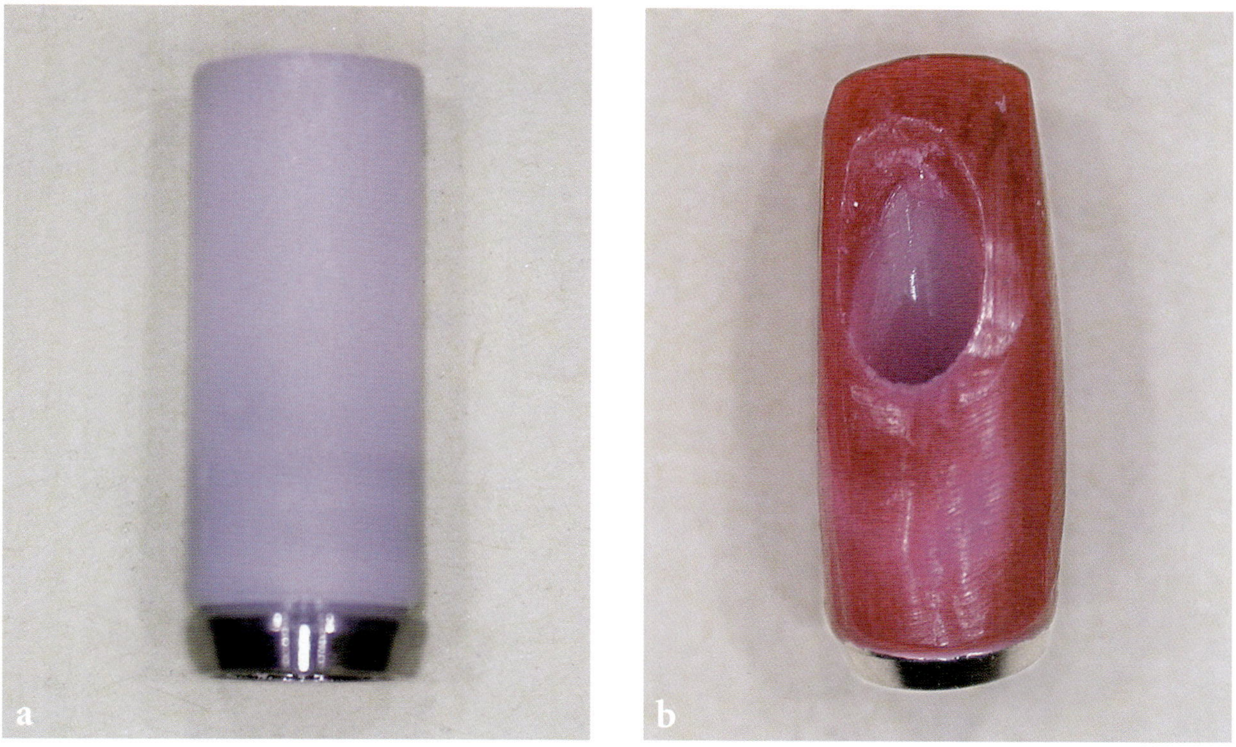

Fig 7.3 - *(a)* Laboratory image of a castable UCLA abutment as proposed by Lewis et al[2] in 1988. *(b)* Laboratory image of a waxed UCLA abutment designed for use as a custom-made screw-retained abutment.

Optimal treatment in esthetic areas generally calls for the restoration margin to be positioned 2 mm below the gingival margin.

In 1988, the introduction of the UCLA abutment for cemented implant restorations (Fig 7.3) allowed technicians and clinicians to develop significantly better esthetics than those obtained with standard abutments. Esthetics obtained with UCLA abutments were more similar to those of the natural dentition. The UCLA abutment, as proposed by Lewis et al,[2–4] consists of a castable cylinder with or without a gold alloy machined interface. In the latter design, the molten metal is cast directly to the machined gold alloy interface of the UCLA abutment (Fig 7.4).

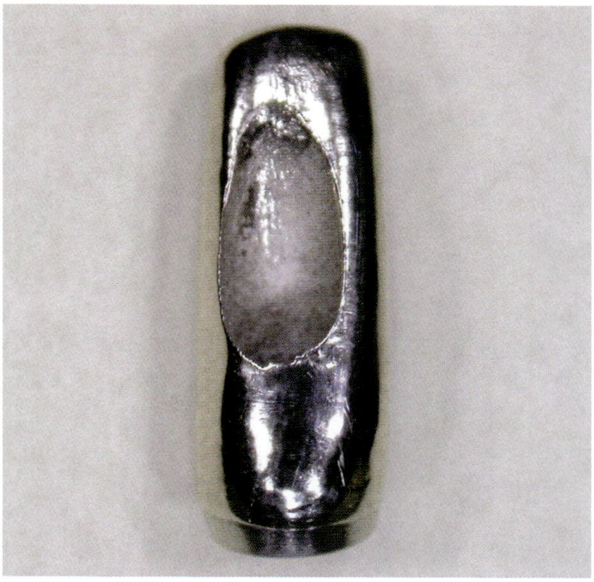

Fig 7.4 - Laboratory image of the cast custom UCLA abutment designed for use as a custom-made screw-retained abutment. The definitive crown will be cemented to this abutment.

UCLA abutments are mainly used for cement-retained implant restorations. Their development and refinement has assisted clinicians in avoiding supragingival metal margins, managing reduced interocclusal clearance in posterior quadrants, and correcting the alignment of nonparallel implants for splinted restorations or fixed partial dentures.

Cement-retained prostheses are contraindicated for full-arch fixed prostheses with immediate occlusal loading. Temporary cement is a risk factor that could compromise the maintenance of a rigid splinting of the implants. Rigidly splinting implants together is particularly important in the first stages of bone healing for attainment of osseointegration in immediate occlusal loading protocols, avoiding the risk of implant micromotion (physical inertia). Moreover, screw-retained prostheses allow for easy and nontraumatic removal of the prostheses for suture removal and management of prosthetic or surgical complications.[5,6]

SCREW-RETAINED PROSTHESES

Angled abutments for screw-retained prostheses were developed and made commercially available at the beginning of the 1990s. Angled abutments allowed for correction of nonoptimally placed implants with screw-retained prostheses because the location of the screw access hole openings could be changed from exiting through the facial surfaces of the artificial teeth to exiting through the palatal or occlusal surfaces of the artificial teeth (Fig 7.5).[7,8] Before the introduction of

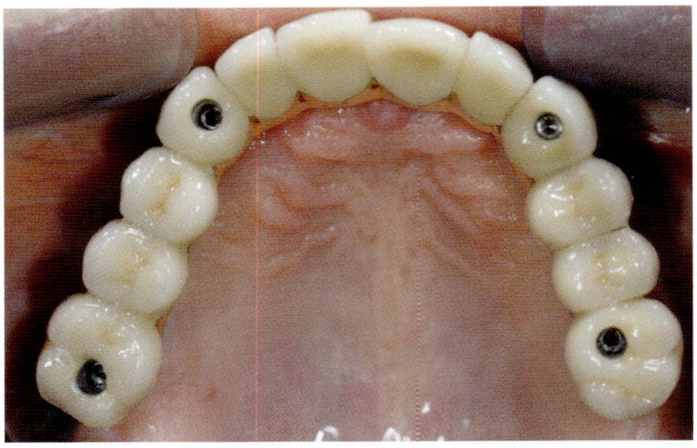

Fig 7.5 - Clinical occlusal view of a maxillary screw-retained prosthesis. Angled abutments were placed on the two anterior implants. These abutments corrected the labial inclination of the implants and allowed the clinician and laboratory technician to fabricate the prosthesis without compromising the esthetic results.

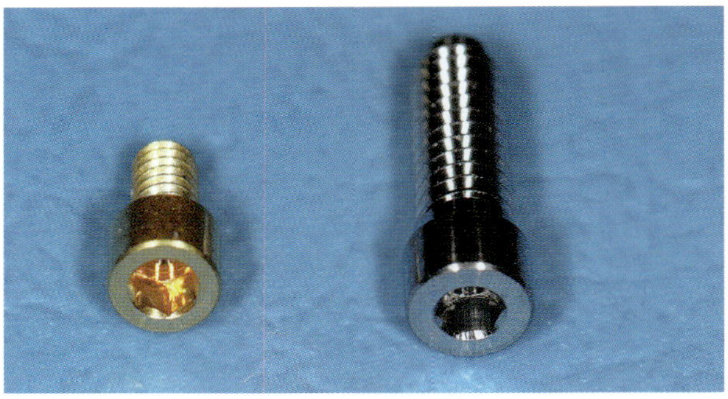

Fig 7.6 - A gold prosthetic (retaining) screw (*left*); a titanium abutment screw (*right*).

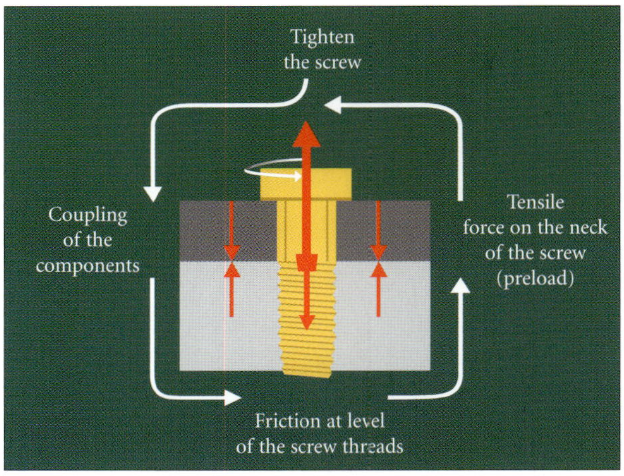

Fig 7.7 - Illustration describing the relationship between torque and friction within a screw-clamp system. This results in a tensile force defined as *preload*.

angled abutments, custom UCLA abutments were required to obtain optimal esthetics since the cemented crown restorations could cover the screw access openings in the abutments. The typical screw-retained prosthesis consists of an abutment with an abutment screw in titanium and a cylinder that is cast to or in the framework, and it is retained to the abutment with a (gold) retaining screw.

In a recent publication, Gervais and Wilson[9] highlighted the advantages that screw-retained prostheses offer clinicians over cement-retained prostheses. Screw-retained prostheses are easier to repair or replace in the event of failure within the mechanical components of the implant-prosthetic system. If a loss of osseointegration of one of the implants occurs, removal of a full-arch fixed prosthesis is much simpler with a screw-retained prosthesis. Also, more prosthetic complications have been reported in the medium to long term for implant restorations than for restorations on natural teeth, so the retrievability of screw-retained prostheses presents numerous benefits to clinicians and patients.[10]

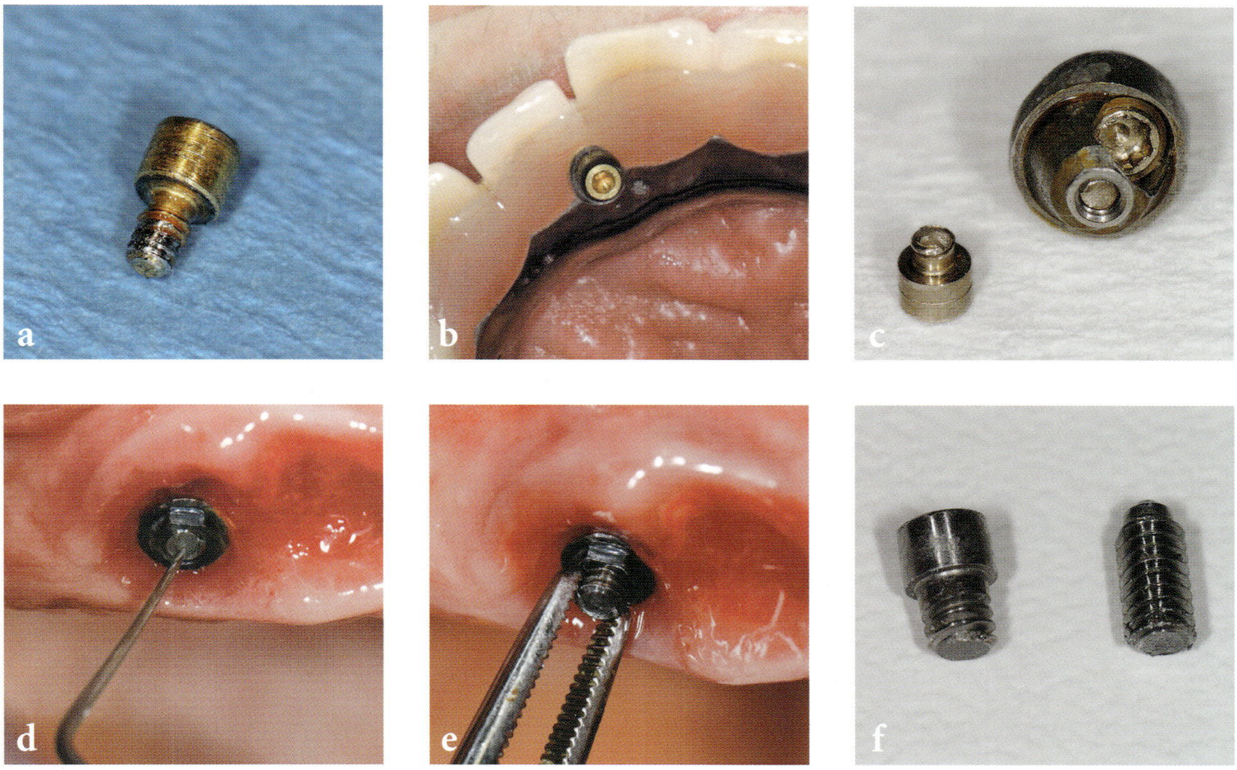

Fig 7.8 - *(a)* Clinical example of screw settling. *(b)* Clinical occlusal image of a maxillary full-arch fixed prosthesis with one gold prosthetic screw in place. *(c)* Laboratory image of fractured gold retaining screw. *(d)* Clinical image of a fractured abutment screw. The tip of a sharp explorer was used to unscrew the apical portion of the fractured screw that remained within the implant. *(e)* Clinical image of the apical portion of the fractured abutment screw in *d* as it was removed from the implant. *(f)* Laboratory close-up image of the fractured screw.

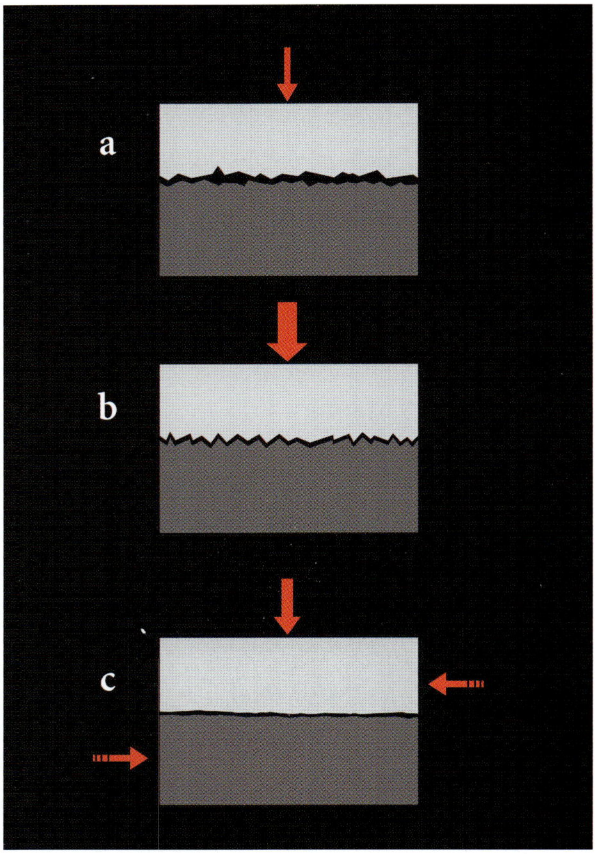

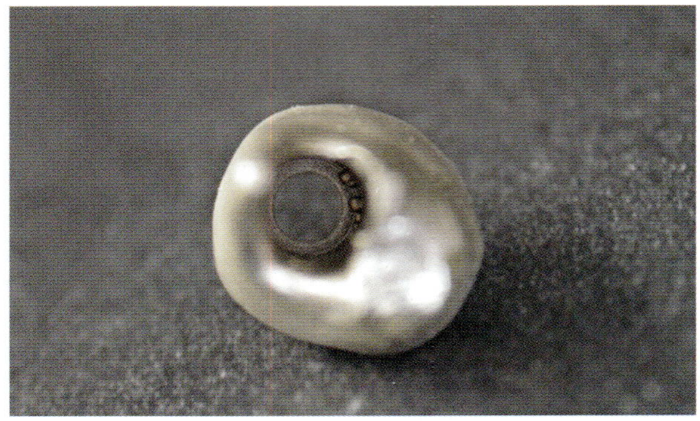

Fig 7.9 - (*left*) *(a)* Phenomenon of screw settling. Two opposing surfaces are placed in contact with the application of a light force (*thin vertical arrow*). *(b)* With increased loads (*thick vertical arrow*), there is a further reduction of the gap between the two surfaces. This interlocking is similar to point welding. *(c)* Micromovement caused by horizontal forces (*horizontal arrows*) round the unevenness of the interlock and reduce the preload (*thin vertical arrow*).

Fig 7.10 - (*top*) Laboratory image of the internal aspect of a UCLA custom abutment. Imperfections within the casting will likely cause incongruous adaptation between the screw and the abutment and lead to screw loosening.

Figure 7.6 illustrates the morphologic characteristics of a prosthetic gold retaining screw and a titanium abutment screw. Abutment screws are generally tightened from 20 to 30 Ncm, while prosthetic gold retaining screws are tightened to 10 Ncm. During screw tightening, a tensile force exerted onto the screw actually stretches the screw and results in the clamping force that holds the cylinder, abutment, and implant joints together. This phenomenon is known as *preload* (Fig 7.7).[11] Goheen et al[12] discussed the importance of applying the appropriate preload to screws to prevent them from becoming loose and jeopardizing the longevity of the implant restoration. Clinicians, without the aid of torque drivers or torque controllers, generate preloads that are generally 30% to 50% lower than those required by implant manufacturers.

Screw loosening may be a major complicating factor in implant dentistry, and its causes need to be investigated further. Screw loosening can occur because of insufficient tightening, inadequate design,[13–15] inappropriate constitutive material, and incongruous adaptation.

Screw settling (Figs 7.8 and 7.9) is a phenomenon secondary to deformation and flattening of the superficial microirregularities of the threads at the restoration interface. Screw settling may be

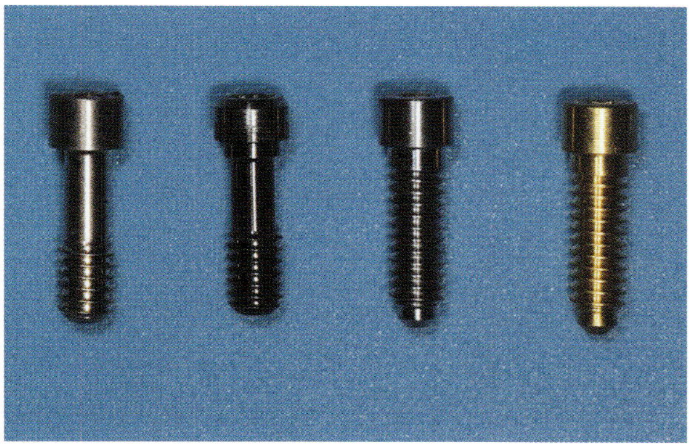

Fig 7.11 - Laboratory image of different types of abutment screws.

related to superficial irregularities (Fig 7.10), wear over time, type of material used, and functional loads.

The instability of the screw joint can affect prosthetic gold screws or abutment screws. For prosthetic gold screws, Kallus and Bessing[16] reported screw loosening percentages of 40% after 5 years in full-arch implant restorations; Ekfeldt et al[17] reported 43% after 3 years in single-unit implant restorations. Priest[18] reported 7.1% in complete-arch restorations and 14% in single-unit restorations after 10 years. Abutment screw loosening has been studied as well: Pjetursson and colleagues[10] reported that 5.8% of abutment screws become loose after 5 years in complete-arch implant restorations.

These results demonstrate that in the past, percentages of screw loosening were rather high. These percentages have been significantly reduced in recent years by improvements in the screw materials and modifications in the geometry of the screw heads. However, screw loosening and screw fracture are still accompanied by clinical complications such as plaque accumulation, malodor, fractured components, formation of granulation tissue, fistulae (see also Fig 14.32), and possible ingestion of the components.[19]

The stability of screw joints may be improved and maintained by taking into consideration characteristics of the screw (Fig 7.11), the prosthesis, and the individual patient. The use of new innovative technologies, such as gold plating, has helped screw joints maintain high preload values by reducing the amount of friction between the components. As friction decreases, preloads increase per the following formula:

$$\text{Preload} = \frac{\text{Tightening torque}}{\text{Friction}}$$

Prosthodontic laboratory procedures also play a key role in maintaining integrity of screw joints in implant prostheses. The laboratory must ensure:

- Quality and precision of the components
- Accurate mechanical adaptation
- Proper metallurgic characteristics of the framework (rigidity)
- Adequate occlusal morphology

Individual, clinical patient factors such as bone elasticity, excessive functional loads, and parafunctional habits, if adequately controlled, do not increase the instability of the system.

Patterson and Johns[20] state that tightening screws properly protects the screws and extends their longevity. The correct preload is not obtained with the first tightening. In fact, mastication and other functional loads cause a decrease in preload with a consequent need for retightening. Deformation occurs at three different points: under the screw head, between the cylinder and the abutment, and among the screw threads. Micromotion between any of these components, especially in the presence of flexible and thin frameworks, causes further reduction in preload values. Therefore, clinicians generally have to see patients with these types of frameworks more frequently for screw retightening so that they can reestablish optimal preloads to the screws and screw joints.

Rigid, properly fitting frameworks dramatically decrease the incidence of screw loosening and other prosthetic complications. In the Columbus Bridge Protocol, optimal framework design, especially in the presence of only four implant abutments, is essential for the long-term success of full-arch screw-retained prostheses. It is evident that the maintenance of balance over time, in terms of accurate adaptation and fit between implant components, is linked to factors such as quality of the components, correct use of the components, and quality of the prosthodontic bridge (Fig 7.12). Long-term success can be guaranteed if screw loosening is checked with regular follow-up. Screw tightening or substitution has to be taken in consideration in every recall.

ANGLED CONICAL ABUTMENTS

Based on these concepts, the protocol adopted for the Columbus Bridge Protocol uses screw-retained prostheses with machined angled conical abutments.[21,22] External hex implant connections are preferred over internal implant con-

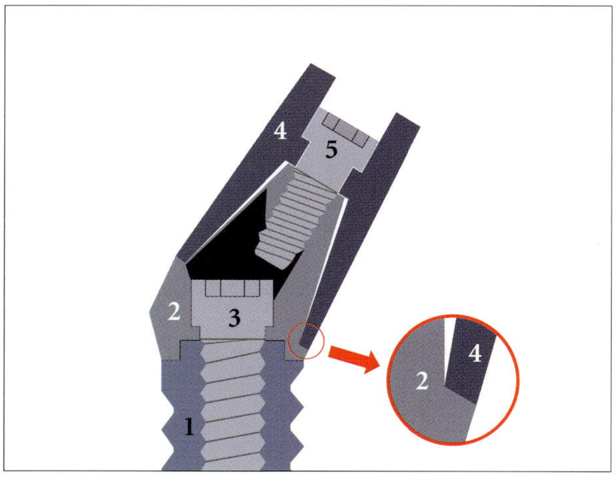

Fig 7.12 - Illustration of the fit among various components. Implant (1); angled abutment (2); abutment screw (3); titanium cylinder (4); prosthetic (retaining) screw (5).

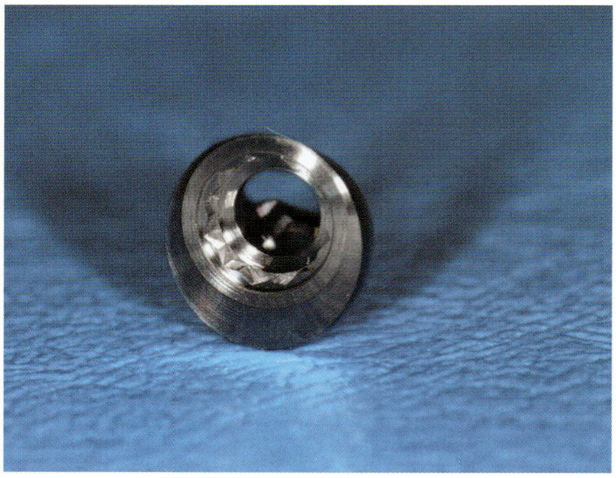

Fig 7.13 - Laboratory image of the restorative platform of an angled conical abutment. This connection is designed as a 12-point hex (dodecagon) that fits onto the external hex of an implant.

nections. The external implant-abutment connection is the most widely supported and referenced type of implant-abutment connection. External hexagonal implant-abutment connections offer multiple advantages in full-arch treatment:

- The use of pickup impressions in the presence of nonparallel implants
- Greater ease in choosing the optimal orientation of angled conical abutments for screw-retained prostheses
- A wide choice of machined abutment types

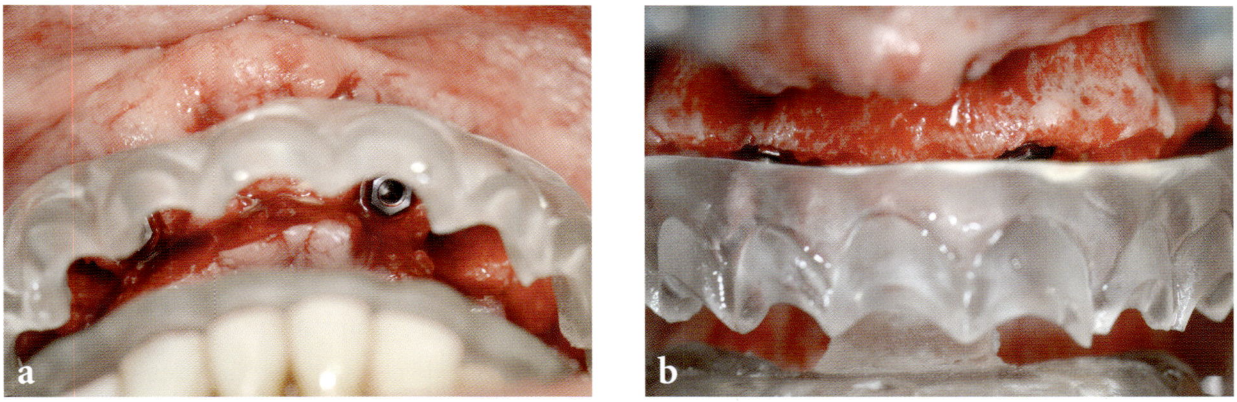

Fig 7.14 - *(a)* Clinical occlusal image of a surgical-prosthetic guide in place. One maxillary external hex implant is visible in the left maxillary central incisor site. Angled conical abutments may be placed in any one of 12 different positions on the external hexagon implant connection. *(b)* Clinical labial image with the surgical-prosthetic template in place. It is possible to correct the implant axis by placing the angled conical abutment optimally so that the screw access opening is not visible.

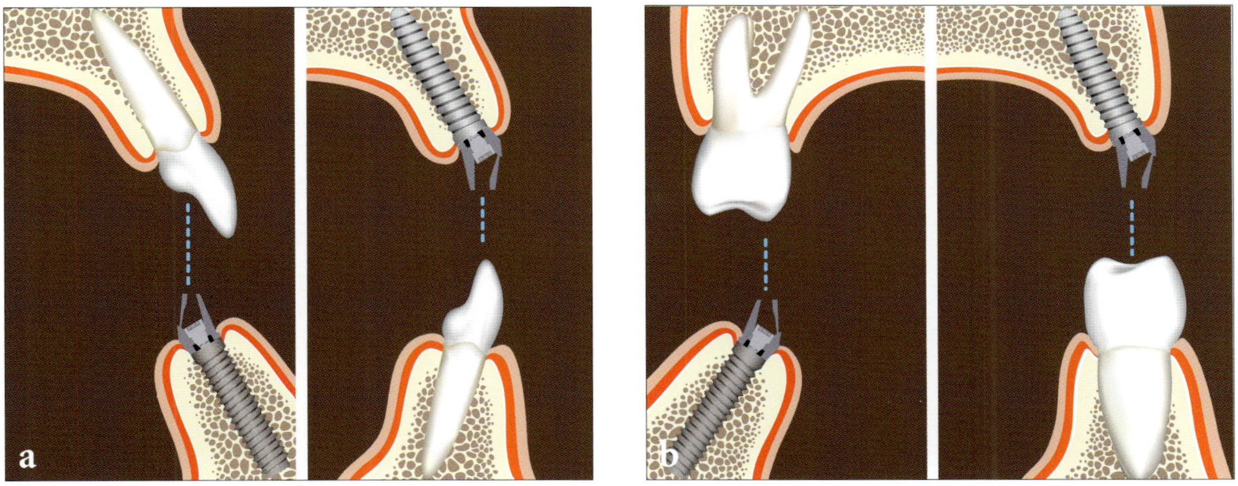

Fig 7.15 - *(a)* Sagittal plane illustration of projecting screw access openings for angled abutments relative to the opposing dentition. The screw access openings for mandibular screw-retained prostheses should coincide with the cingula of the maxillary anterior teeth. The screw access openings for maxillary screw-retained prostheses should coincide with the incisal edges of the mandibular anterior teeth. *(b)* Frontal plane illustration of projecting screw access openings for angled abutments relative to the occlusal surfaces of the opposing dentition. The projection of the screw access opening of angulated abutments for posterior implant restorations should coincide with the palatal cusps of the maxillary posterior teeth and with the central fossa of the mandibular posterior teeth.

Machined conical abutments are available with different emergence profiles, implant restorative platforms, and shoulder heights. The internal portion of the implant-abutment connection for angled conical abutments has 12 sides (Fig 7.13). This shape allows clinicians to place abutments on the hexagonal implant connections in one of 12 different orientations. Implant inclination can be corrected relative to the location of the screw access opening in the prosthesis on the basis of the surgical-prosthetic template (Figs 7.14 and 7.15). The need to use abutments with different angle corrections is secondary to the diverse clinical situations that may arise intraoperatively after implant placement. Four purposes support the use of angled conical abutments:

1. *Quadrilateral support achievement.* To receive adequate mechanical support, implants must be inserted with a distal tilt to enhance the anteroposterior spread of the bridge and avoid cantilever. Angle corrections that place the screw access openings within the palatal and occlusal surfaces of the anterior and posterior teeth, respectively, require the use of angled abutments of various degrees (17, 25, 30, or 45 degrees) (Fig 7.16).
2. *Use of long implants in cancellous bone.* The presence of sinus and nasal cavities necessitate the use of angled implants to allow the use of long implants in atrophic maxillae. Longer implants are more stable than shorter implants, especially in the presence of poor-quality bone (Figs 7.17 to 7.19).
3. *Insertion of implants in native bone.* The insertion of angled implants can avoid postextraction bone defects in native host bone, attaining the requisite high insertion torque values for immediate occlusal loading (Fig 7.20).
4. *Prosthetic correction of unfavorable jaw relations.* According to the intermaxillary discrepancy, jaw relation may be optimized with the use of angled conical abutments (Figs 7.21 to 7.24).

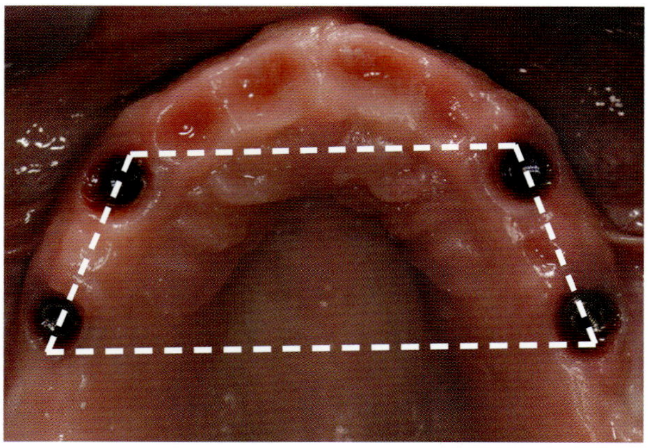

Fig 7.16 - Clinical maxillary occlusal image of four implants and abutments in place per the Columbus Bridge Protocol. The implants provide excellent quadrilateral support for a fixed prosthesis.

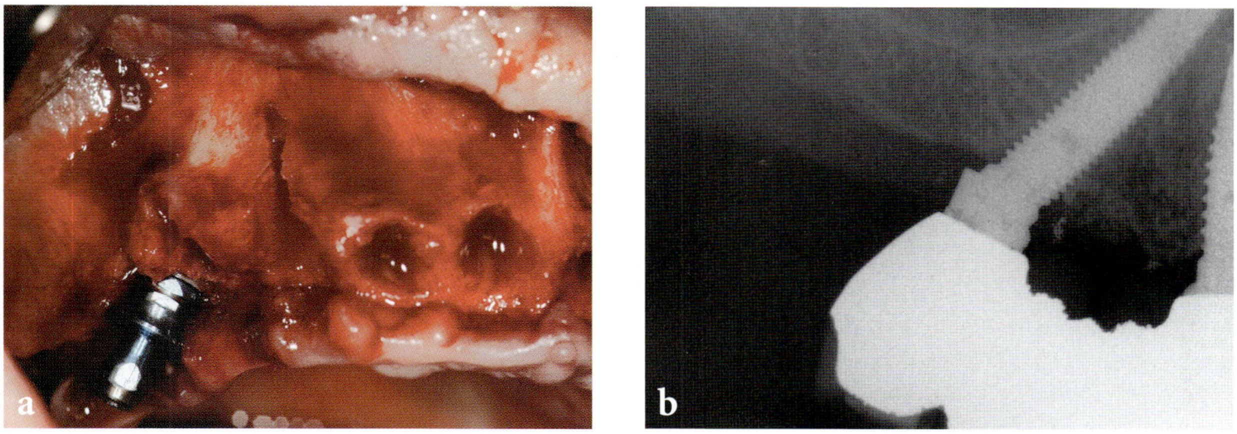

Fig 7.17 - *(a)* Clinical image of a left posterior maxillary segment with one angled implant near the anterior wall of the maxillary sinus cavity. Prosthetically, it was necessary to use an angled abutment to correct the implant axis. *(b)* Radiograph of an angled maxillary posterior implant that demonstrated an angled abutment and the immediate provisional prosthesis fabricated without a distal cantilevered segment. This provided a polygon of support and a favorable prognosis for the implants and the prosthesis.

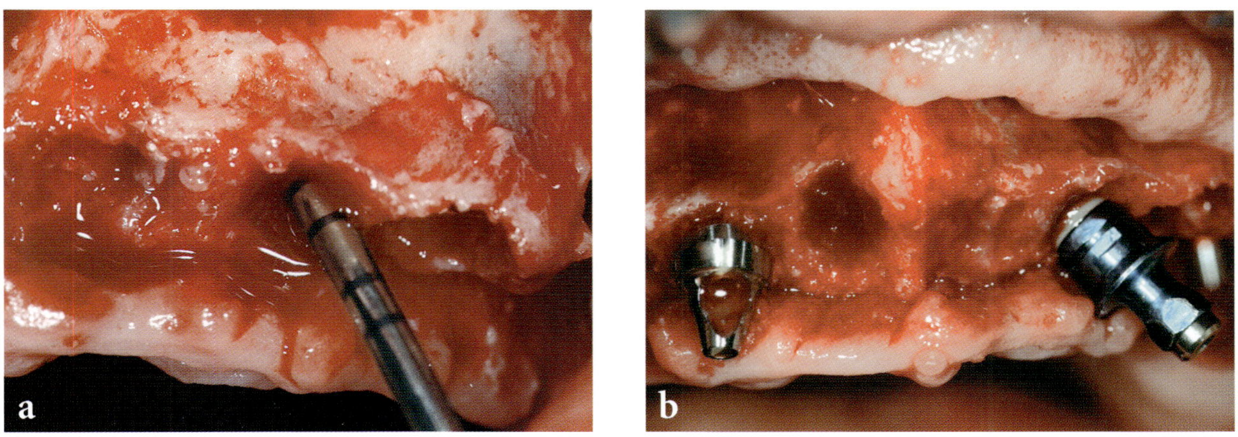

Fig 7.18 - *(a)* Clinical surgical image of an indicator probe in place after preparation of a tilted osteotomy in close proximity to the nasal cavity. *(b)* Clinical surgical image with the anterior angled implant in place.

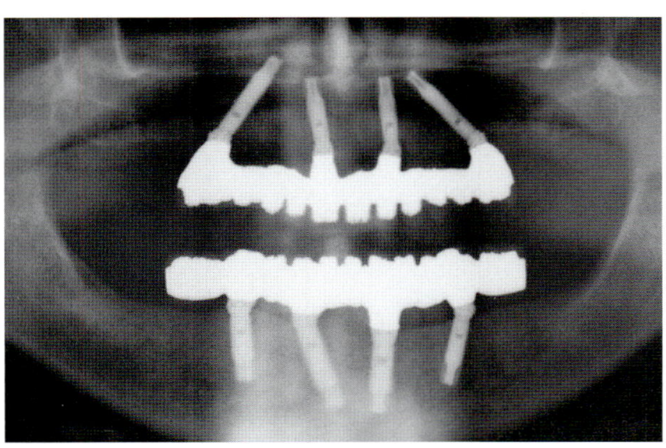

Fig 7.19 - Panoramic radiograph that illustrates a clinical example of implant treatment with maxillary and mandibular angled implants. The maxillary posterior angled implants were significantly longer than traditional vertical implants. The maxillary prosthesis was designed with a greater number of dental units, without cantilevers, than would otherwise have been used with vertical implants. This treatment also illustrates how the surgeon avoided the nasal cavities and bone grafting the maxillary sinus with the use of angled implants.

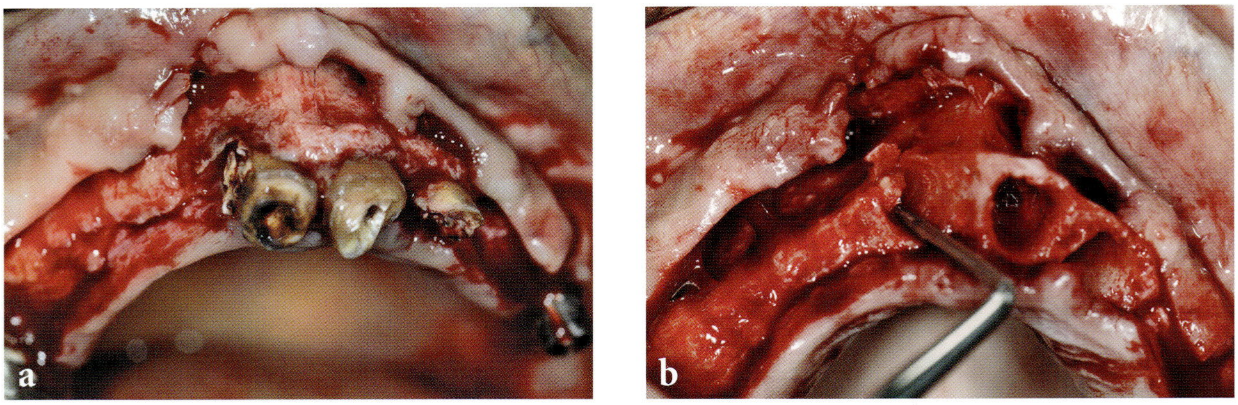

Fig 7.20 - *(a)* Clinical maxillary occlusal surgical image with three hopeless maxillary incisors in place. *(b)* Clinical maxillary occlusal image with a surgical probe in place demonstrating the distal orientation of the osteotomy in preparation for using an anterior angled implant. Long anterior angled implants may be used to take advantage of the remaining native bone and obtain high levels of implant primary stability.

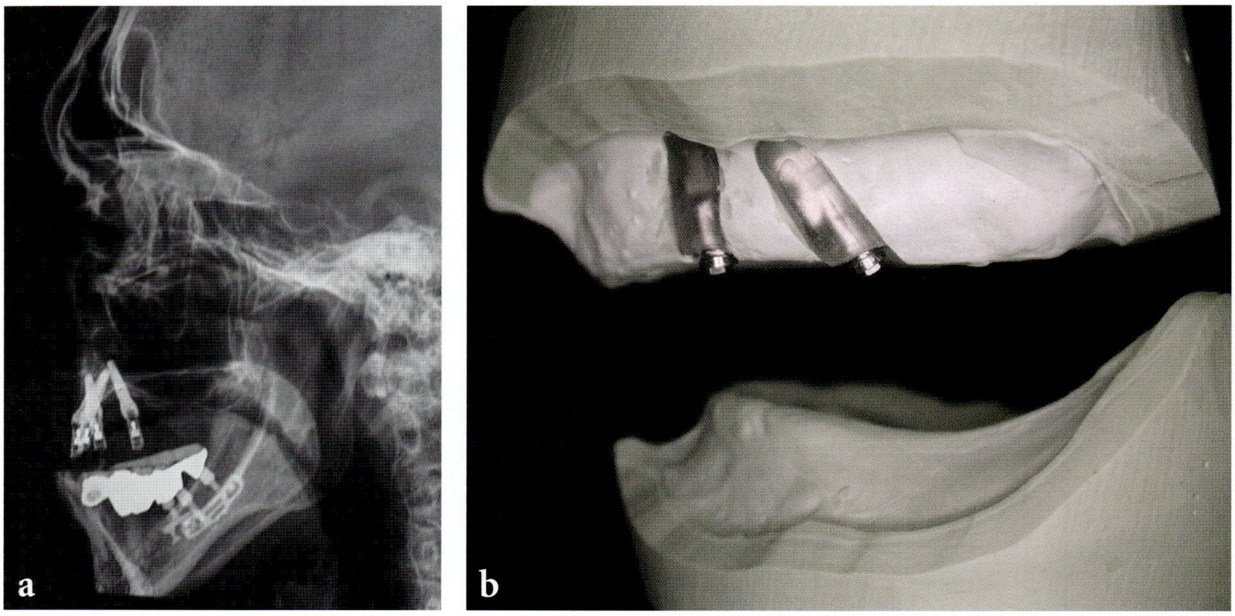

Fig 7.21 - *(a)* Lateral cephalometric radiograph that demonstrated an additional advantage associated with the use of angled implants and angled abutments to correct unfavorable jaw relationships. *(b)* Laboratory image of articulated master casts with laboratory analogs in place. The casts are used to simulate the implant treatment in an unfavorable jaw relationship.

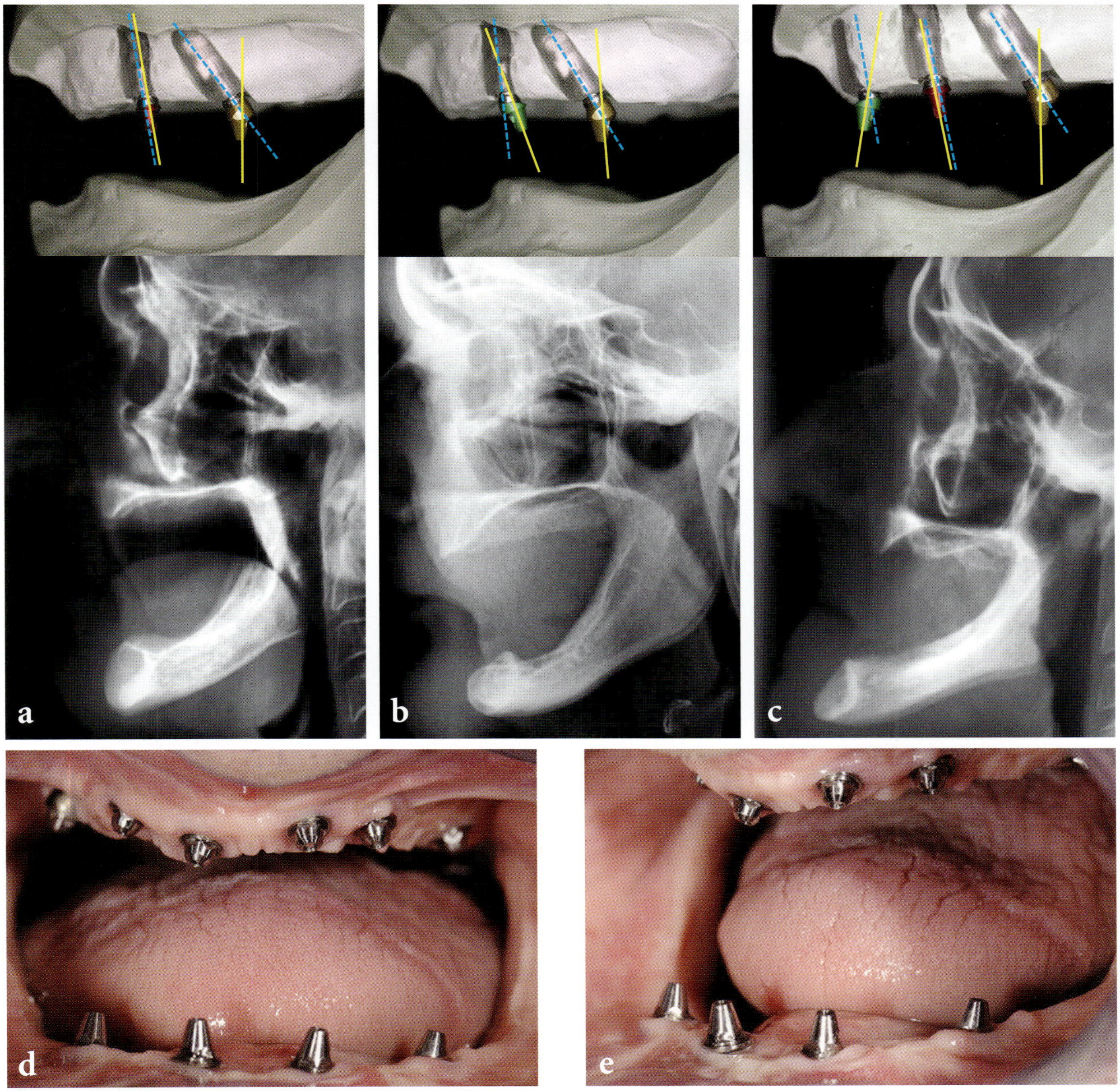

Fig 7.22 - This series of images demonstrates the use of angled abutments to manage unfavorable jaw relationships prosthetically, without orthognathic surgery. *(a to c)* Diagnostic images *(top)*; lateral cephalometric radiographs *(bottom)*; abutments: 0 degrees (*red*); 17 degrees (*green*); 30 degrees (*yellow*); implant axis (*dotted line*); corrected prosthetic axis (*continuous line*). *(a)* Class I jaw relationship: The mesial implant does not need angle correction and therefore was restored with a straight conical abutment; a 30-degree angled conical abutment in place on the distal implant. *(b)* Class II jaw relationship: A 17-degree angled conical abutment with distal direction in place on the mesial implant. *(c)* Class III jaw relationship: A 17-degree labially angled abutment in place on the most anterior implant. To reduce the biomechanical disadvantages associated with an anterior prosthetic cantilever, clinicians may place an additional implant in each anterior segment. *(d)* Clinical labial image of edentulous arches in Class III jaw relationship rehabilitated with implants. Four implants were inserted in the mandible and six in the maxilla. *(e)* Clinical lateral image of the same patient in the figure *d*. Labially angled abutments were placed on the anterior maxillary implants to reduce the disadvantages associated with the Class III jaw relationship.

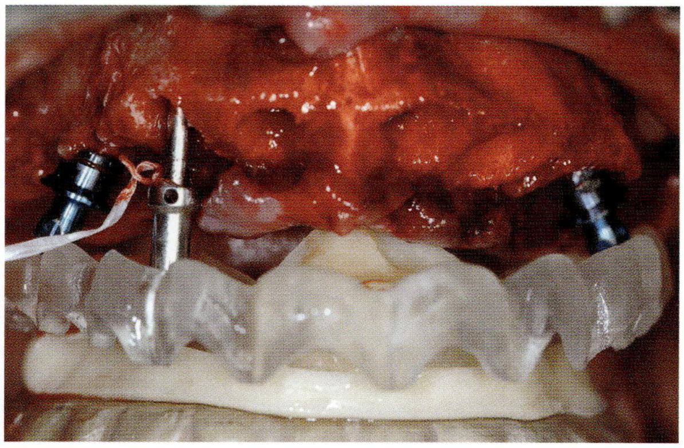

Fig 7.23 - Clinical surgical image with the surgical-prosthetic guide in place. Two distal, angled implants are in place posteriorly, and a directional indicator is in place in the right anterior implant. Per the Columbus Bridge Protocol, it is important to remember that angled abutments should comply with the morphology of the future provisional fixed prosthesis (as indicated by the surgical-prosthetic template). The specific design of the surgical-prosthetic template permits clinicians to correct spatial positioning of the angled implants with angled abutments.

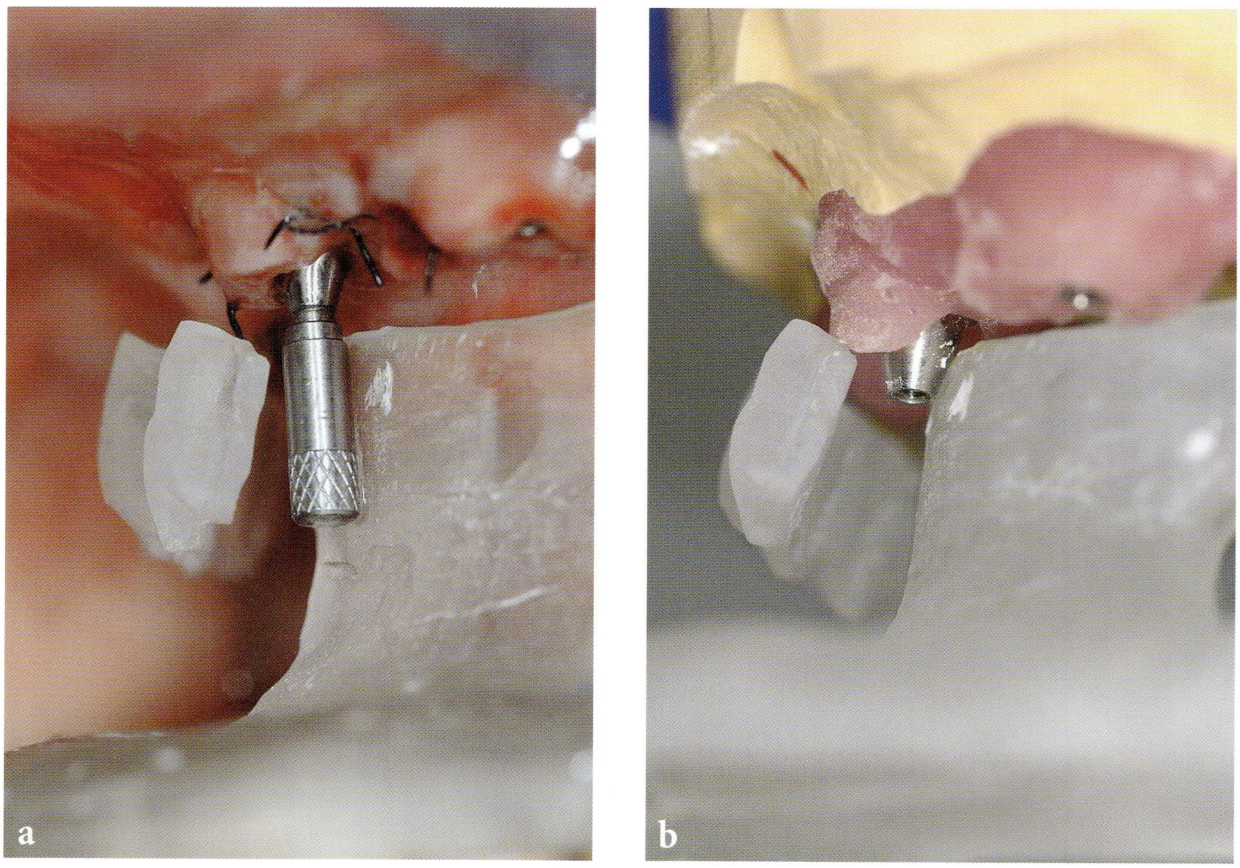

Fig 7.24 - *(a)* Clinical profile image of an anterior implant in place. A laboratory screw has been placed into the angled conical abutment that assisted the clinician in identifying the location of the screw access opening relative to the location of the teeth in the provisional prosthesis and in the opposing dentition. The surgical-prosthetic template was sectioned for illustrative purposes only. Notice the relationship between the laboratory screw and the facial surface of the surgical-prosthetic template. This precisely identified the location and profile of the artificial tooth within the provisional prosthesis. *(b)* Laboratory lateral image of the mounted maxillary cast with the surgical-prosthetic guide in place. The relationships noted clinically between the location of the angled abutment, the location of the screw access opening, and the facial surface of the surgical-prosthetic template also have been observed in the laboratory.

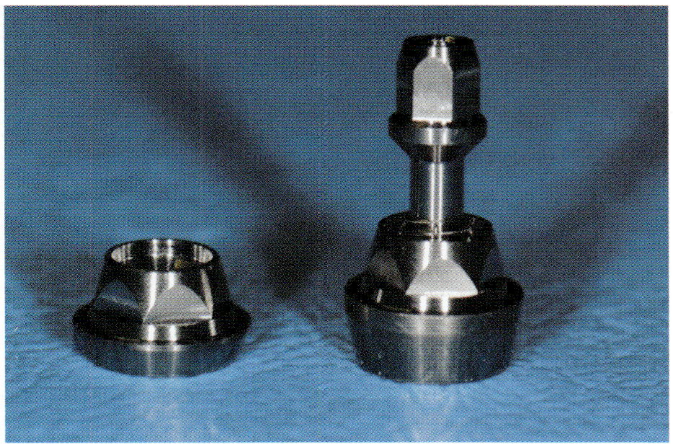

Fig 7.25 - A straight conical abutment (0 degrees) with a 1-mm shoulder (*left*); laboratory image of a straight conical abutment with a 3-mm shoulder and abutment screw (*right*).

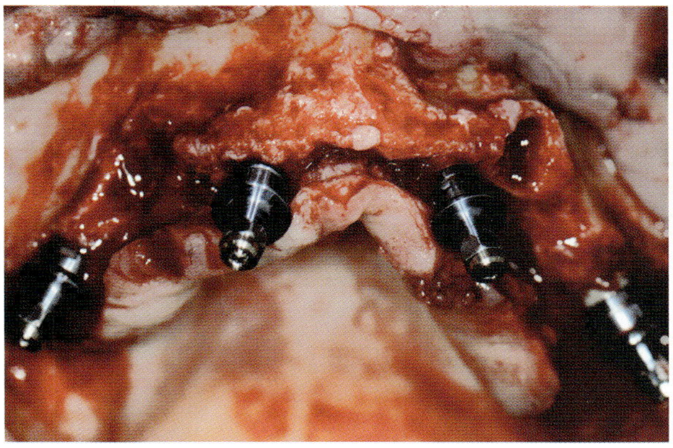

Fig 7.26 - Maxillary occlusal view with anterior implants to be rehabilitated with straight conical abutments (0 degrees).

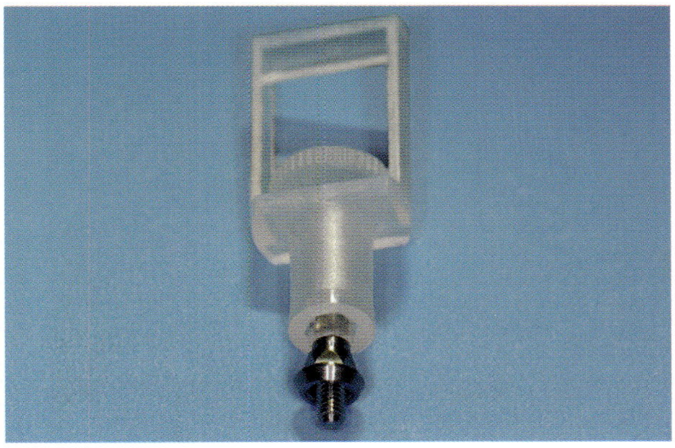

Fig 7.27 - A disposable manual abutment placement instrument for inserting a straight conical abutment (0 degrees).

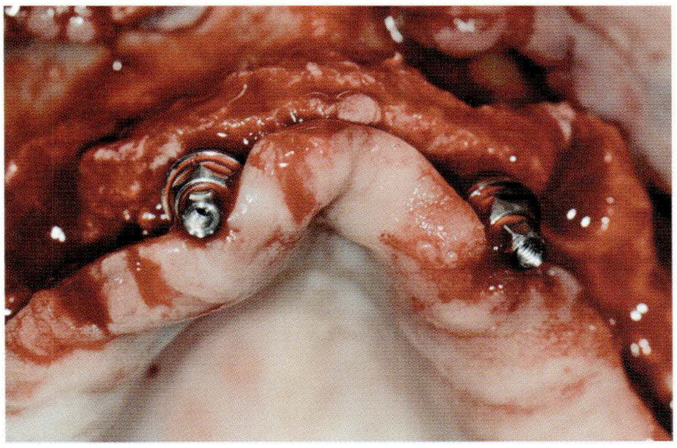

Fig 7.28 - Maxillary occlusal image of the patient in Fig. 1.14. Two straight conical abutments in place on maxillary anterior implants.

Images from the authors' clinical practice are presented here to illustrate some of the benefits associated with conical abutments (Figs 7.25 to 7.46). The 45-degree conical abutment is regarded as the prosthetic element of choice only in situations where severe atrophy requires the insertion of an implant with an inclination equal to or greater than 45 degrees relative to the occlusal plane. In these cases, clinical and laboratory procedures must follow special precautions; therefore, 45-degree angled conical abutments are regarded as custom-made components by the implant manufacturer. When the implant axis and the resultant screw access openings fall inside the contours of the surgical-prosthetic template, angled abutments are not necessary, and a straight conical abutment can be used.

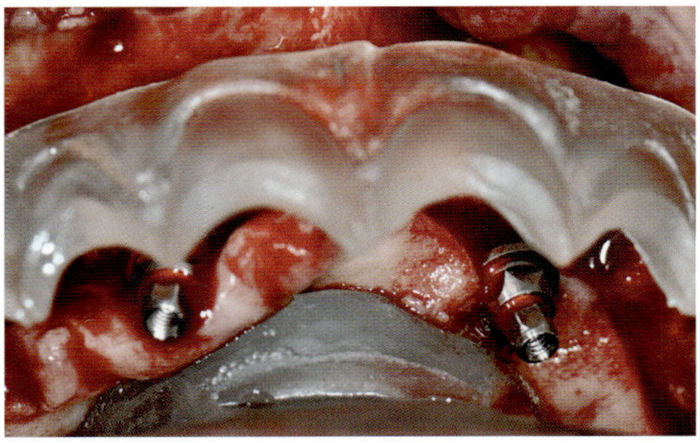

Fig 7.29 - Maxillary occlusal image of the patient in Fig 7.28. Two straight conical abutments in place on maxillary anterior implants. The locations of the screw access openings were controlled with the surgical-prosthetic template.

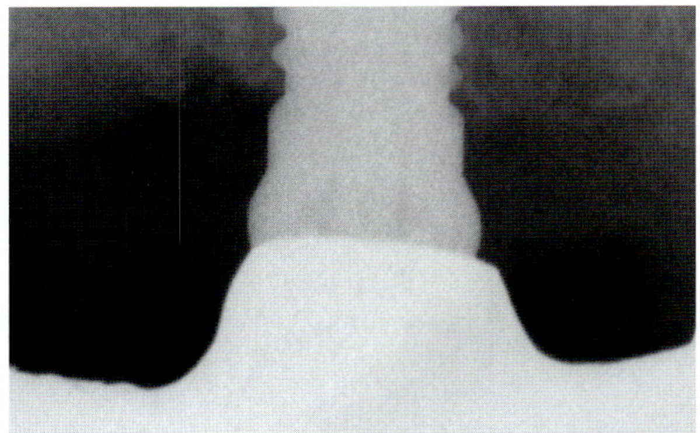

Fig 7.30 - Radiograph demonstrating an excellent fit between the framework and a straight conical abutment.

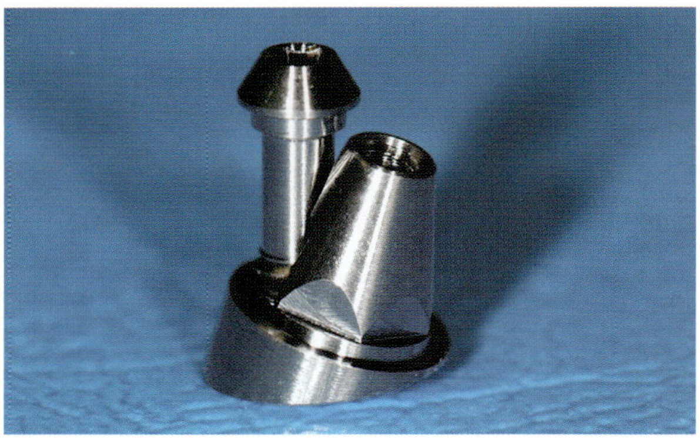

Fig 7.31 - A 17-degree angled conical abutment and abutment screw.

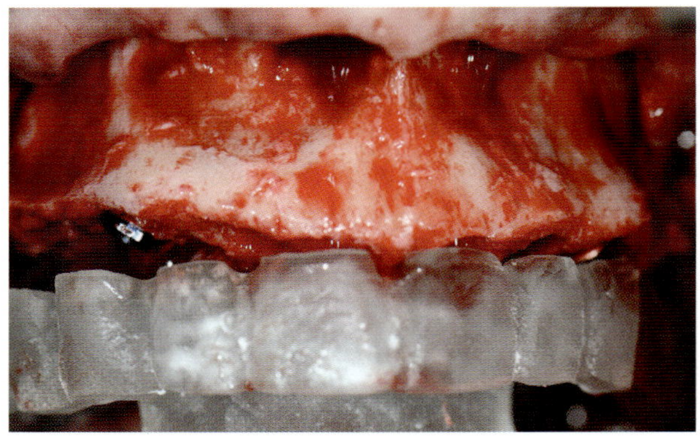

Fig 7.32 - Facial image with a surgical-prosthetic template in place. The locations of the implants were accomplished accurately using the surgical-prosthetic template.

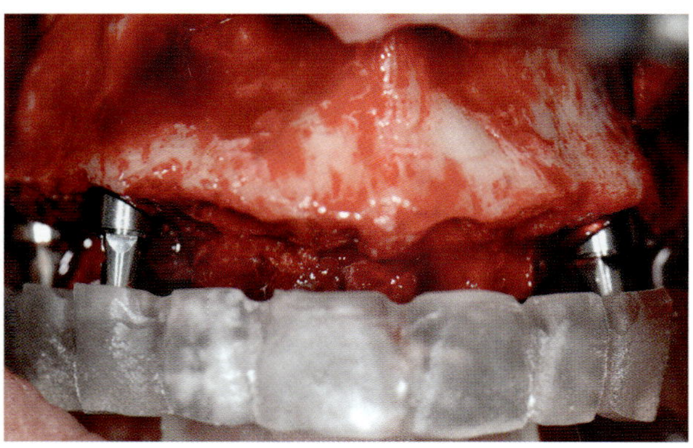

Fig 7.33 - Facial image of the patient in Fig 7.32 with a surgical-prosthetic template in place. The choice and the orientations of the 17-degree angled abutments were accomplished accurately using the surgical-prosthetic template.

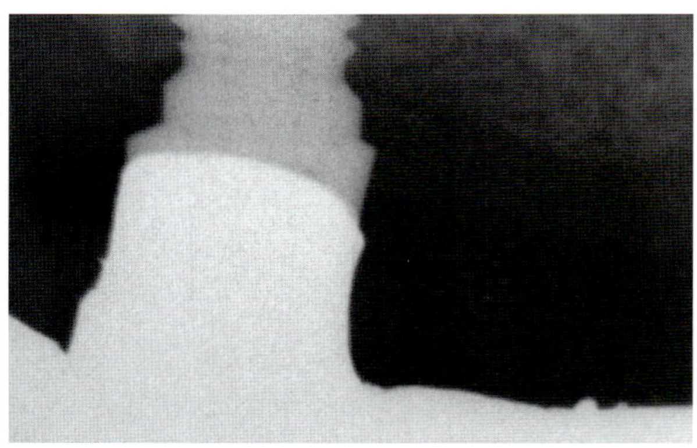

Fig 7.34 - Radiograph that demonstrated an excellent fit between the framework and an angled 17-degree conical abutment.

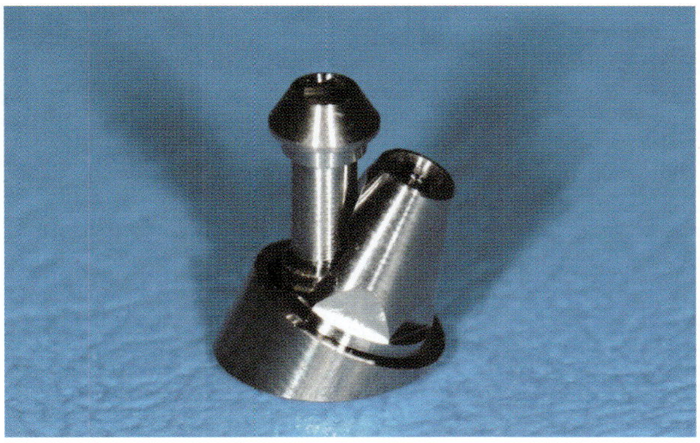

Fig 7.35 - A 25-degree angled conical abutment and abutment screw.

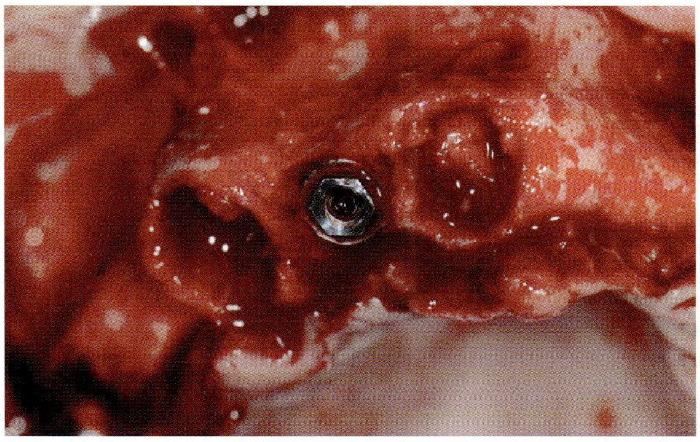

Fig 7.36 - Occlusal image immediately after implant placement. The location of the implant was accomplished accurately using the surgical-prosthetic template.

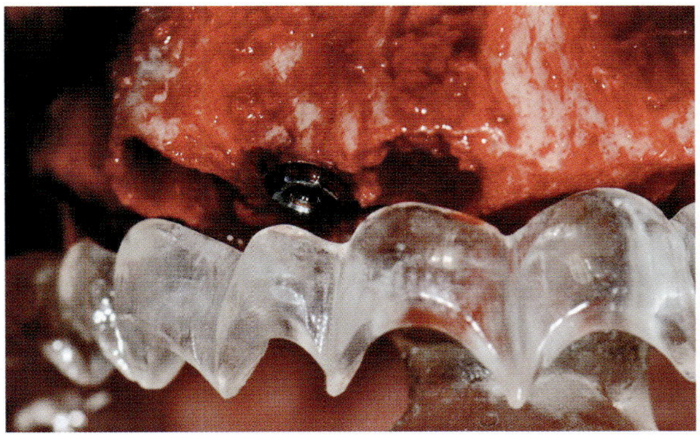

Fig 7.37 - Facial image of the patient in Fig 7.36 with a surgical-prosthetic template in place. The choice of the abutment has to be accomplished accurately by using the surgical-prosthetic template.

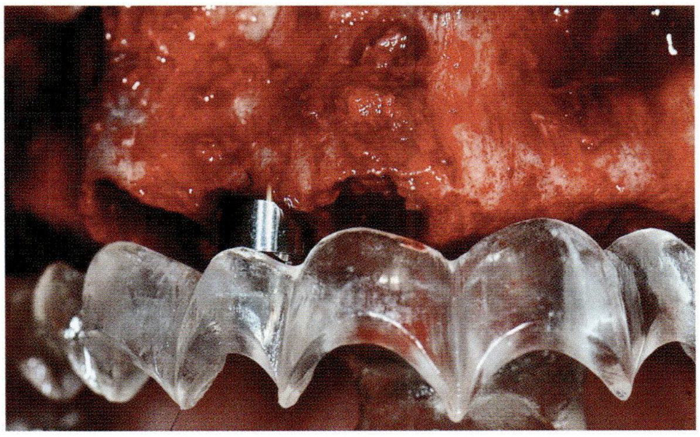

Fig 7.38 - Same view with abutment in place. The orientation of the 25-degree angled abutment were accomplished accurately using the surgical-prosthetic template.

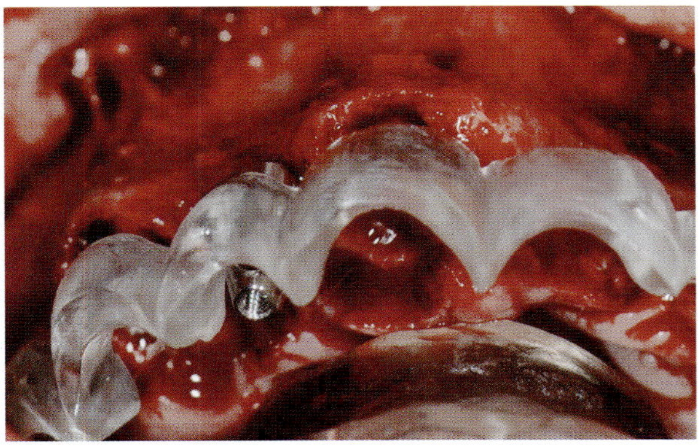

Fig 7.39 - Occlusal image of the patient in Fig 7.36 with a surgical-prosthetic template and abutment in place. The screw access opening was located palatal to the labial surfaces of the teeth in the surgical-prosthetic template.

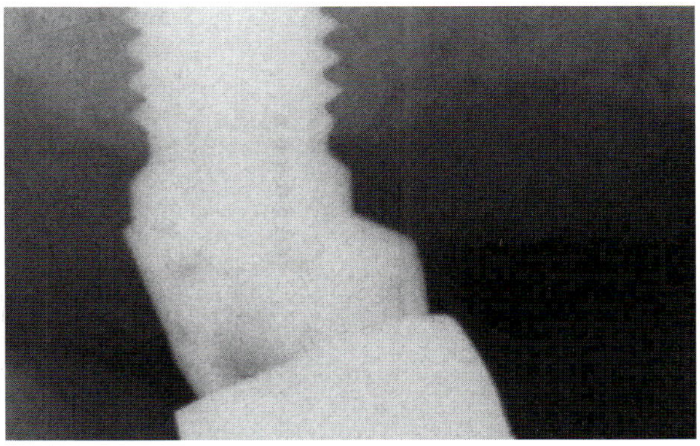

Fig 7.40 - Radiograph that demonstrated an excellent fit between the framework and an angled 25-degree conical abutment.

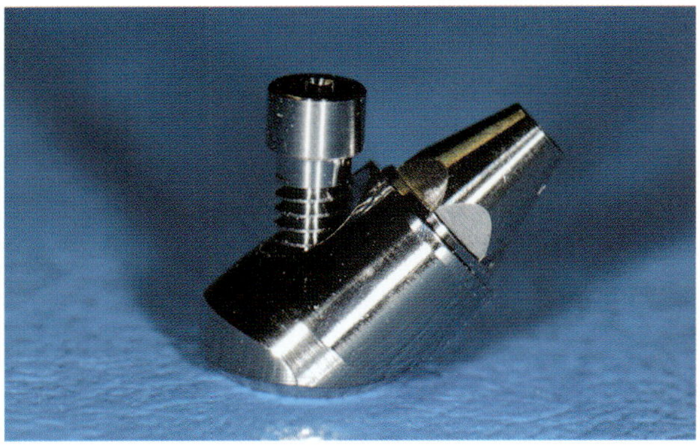

Fig 7.41 - A custom-made 45-degree angled conical abutment and abutment screw.

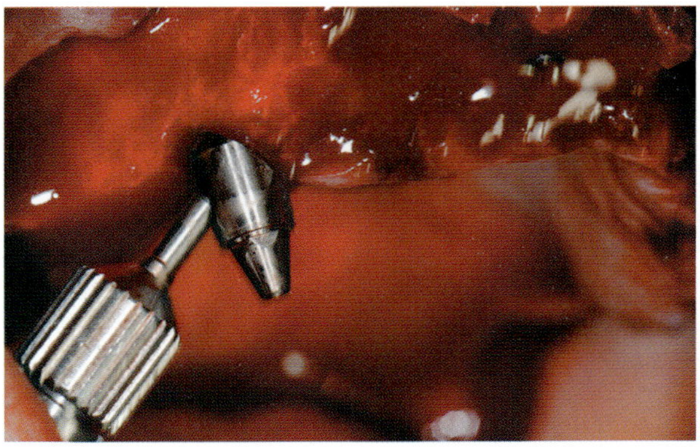

Fig 7.42 - Anterior image of a custom-made 45-degree angled conical abutment as it is placed.

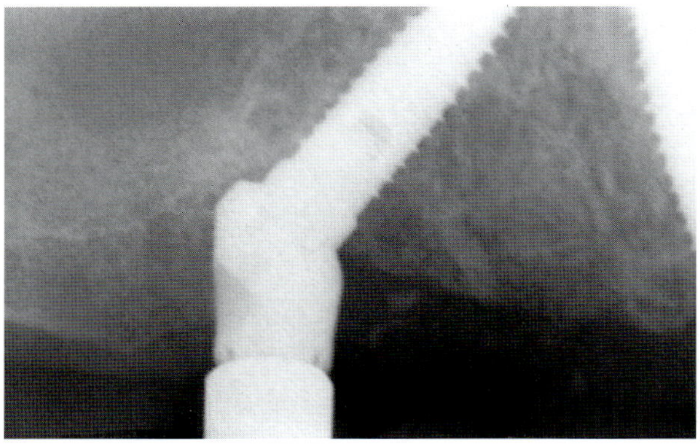

Fig 7.43 - Radiograph that demonstrated an excellent fit between the framework and the custom-made 45-degree angled conical abutment.

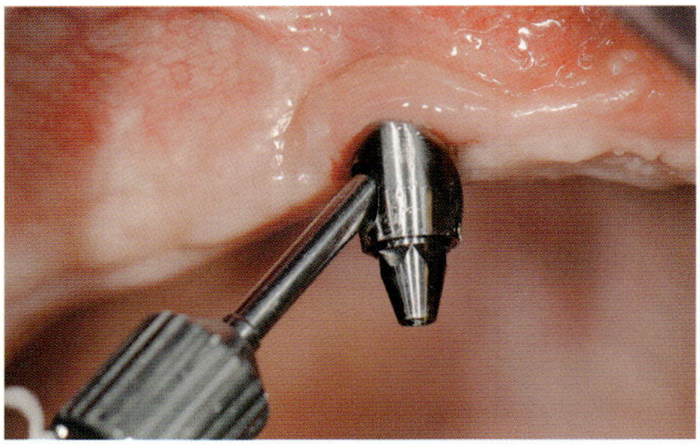

Fig 7.44 - Anterior image of the custom-made 45-degree angled conical abutment 24 months after placement. Note the health of the peri-implant soft tissues and the lack of inflammation.

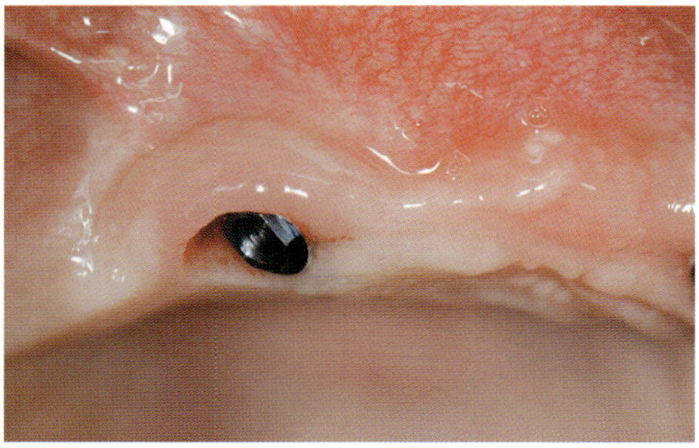

Fig 7.45 - Close-up occlusal image of the implant restorative platform of the implant in Fig 7-44. The implant was stable, and the peri-implant soft tissues demonstrated no signs of inflammation.

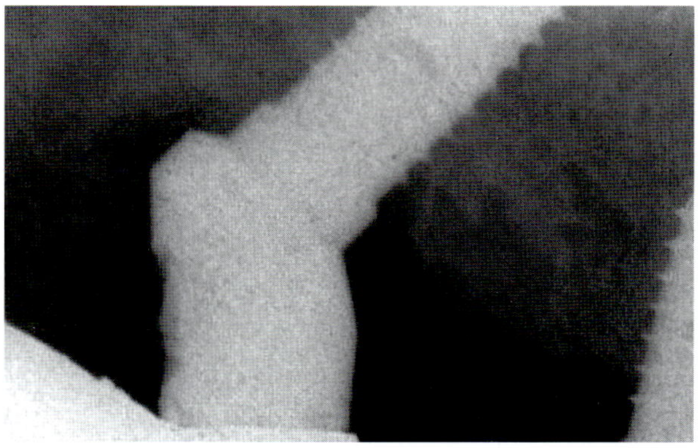

Fig 7.46 - Radiograph of the custom-made 45-degree angled conical abutment in Fig 7.43 after 24 months of function.

REFERENCES

1. Brånemark PI, Zarb GA, Albrektsson T (eds). Tissue Integrated Prostheses: Osseointegration in Clinical Dentistry. Chicago: Quintessence, 1985.
2. Lewis S, Beumer J, Hornburg W, Moy P. The "UCLA" abutment. Int J Oral Maxillofac Implants 1988;3:183–189.
3. Lewis SG, Beumer J, Perri GR, Hornburg WP. Single tooth implant supported restorations. Int J Oral Maxillofac Implants 1988;3:25–30.
4. Lewis S. An overview of Brånemark System restorative options. J Esthet Dent 1996;7:101–110.
5. Andersson B, Odman P, Carlsson L, Brånemark PI. A new Brånemark single tooth abutment. Handling and early clinical experiences. Int J Oral Maxillofac Implants 1992;7:105–111.
6. Mericske-Stern R, Grütter L, Rösch R, Mericske E. Clinical evaluation and prosthetic complications of single tooth replacements by non-submerged implants. Clin Oral Implants Res 2001;12:309–318.
7. Jorneus L. Screws and cylinders in the Nobelpharma implant system. Nobelpharma News 1987;1:7.
8. Esthetichone abutment-estetical restorations procedure. Technique booklet PRI 182 1991. Göteborg: Nobelpharma, 1991.
9. Gervais MJ, Wilson PR. A rationale for retrievability of fixed, implant-supported prostheses: A complication-based analyis. Int J Prosthodont 2007; 20:13–24.
10. Pjetursson BE, Tan K, Lang NP, Brägger U, Egger M, Zwahlen M. A systematic review of the survival and complication rates of fixed partial dentures (FPDs) after an observation period of at least 5 years. Clin Oral Implants Res 2004;15:667–676.
11. Duyck J, Van Oosterwyck H, Vander Sloten J, De Cooman M, Puers R, Naert I. Pre-load on oral implants after screw tightening fixed full prostheses: An in vivo study. J Oral Rehabil 2001;28: 226–233.
12. Goheen K, Vermilyea S, Vossoughi J, Agar JR. Torque generated by hand-held screwdrivers and mechanical torquing devices for osseointegrated implants. Int J Oral Maxillofac Implants 1994;9:149–155.
13. Skalak R. Biomechanical considerations in osseointegrated prostheses. J Prosthet Dent 1983;49: 843–848.
14. Rangert B, Jemt T, Jorneus L. Forces and moments on Brånemark implants. Int J Oral Maxillofac Implants 1989;4:241–247.
15. Kim Y, Oh TJ, Misch CE, Wang HL. Occlusal considerations in implant therapy: Clinical guidelines with biomechanical rationale. Clin Oral Implants Res 2005;16:26–35.
16. Kallus T, Bessing C. Loose gold screws frequently occur in full-arch fixed prostheses supported by osseointegrated implants after 5 years. Int J Oral Maxillofac Implants 1994;9:169–178.
17. Ekfeldt A, Carlsson GE, Börjesson G. Clinical evaluation of single-tooth restorations supported by osseointegrated implants: A retrospective study. Int J Oral Maxillofac Implants 1994;9:179–183.
18. Priest G. Single-tooth implants and their role in preserving remaining teeth: A 10-year survival study. Int J Oral Maxillofac Implants 1999;14: 181–188.
19. Goodacre CJ, Bernal G, Rungcharassaeng K, Kan JY. Clinical complications with implants and implant prostheses. J Prosthet Dent 2003;90: 121–132.
20. Patterson EA, Johns RB. Theoretical analysis of the fatigue life of fixture screws in osseointegrated dental implants. Int J Oral Maxillofac Implants 1992; 7:25–34.
21. Chee W, Felton DA, Johnson PF, Sullivan DY. Cemented versus screw retained prostheses: Which is better? Int J Oral Maxillofac Implants 1999; 14:137–141.
22. Michalakis KX, Hirayama H, Garefis PD. Cement-retained versus screw-retained implant restorations: A critical review. Int J Oral Maxillofac Implants 2003;18:719–728.

CHAPTER 8

DATA TRANSFER TO THE DENTAL LABORATORY

COLUMBUS BRIDGE PROTOCOL	
SURGICAL PROTOCOL	**PROSTHETIC PROTOCOL**
External hex rough-surface implants	Screw-retained fixed prosthesis
Implant length ≥ 13 mm, Ø 4 mm	Plaster impression with pickup technique
Underprepared osteotomy	Rigid splinting with metal framework
Implant insertion torque ≥ 40 Ncm	Passive fit with the luting technique
Angled implants in native bone	Acrylic resin occlusal surfaces
Angled conical abutments	No distal cantilevers
No bone regenerative techniques	Immediate functional load 24–48 h after surgery

Table 8.1

The prosthetic phase of the Columbus Bridge Protocol includes the fabrication and insertion of a fixed, provisional, full-arch screw-retained prosthesis within 24 to 48 hours of implant placement. In prosthodontic treatment, the accuracy of a given prosthesis is related to the precision and accuracy of the master cast.[1] Heckmann et al[2] state that in implant prosthodontics, 50% of the errors generally encountered relate to the techniques used in implant impression and cast construction. The remaining 50% of errors are generated by inaccurate laboratory procedures. The current dental literature does not present a consistent protocol or set of guidelines for laboratory procedures to produce accurate casts from intraoral impressions. Hsu et al[3] report that there were no statistically significant differences in master cast accuracy between those made from splinted impression copings and those made from unsplinted impression copings. Burawi and colleagues,[4] on the other hand, describe an intraoral impression technique in which unsplinted impression copings provided the most accurate master casts. Likewise, Kim et al[5] report that splinted impression coping techniques result in less precise master casts than with unsplinted impression techniques. However, the Kim team also notes that splinted impression coping techniques produced more accurate results in connecting laboratory analogs to the impression copings in the impression. Assif et al[6] also contribute to the discussion, concluding that rigid splinting of the impression copings is critical for the fabrication of master casts and, ultimately, for the development of the passive, accurate frameworks required in implant prosthodontics.

In implant prosthodontics, impressions may be made with one of the two following methods:

- *Indirect impression technique (transfer)*[7,8]: This technique calls for a closed impression tray. Transfer impression copings are placed onto the implants or abutments intraorally, and the impression is made in a standard impression tray. After the impression material sets, the impression is removed from the mouth. The transfer impression copings remain in place on the implants. They are then removed from the implants and attached to laboratory analogs, and the analog-impression coping complexes are reinserted into the impression. The impression is then boxed, and the master cast is poured.
- *Direct impression technique (pickup)*[9–11]: This technique calls for an open impression tray. Pick up impression copings are placed onto the implants or abutments intraorally, and the impression is taken with an open tray carved into the occlusal surface. The impression coping screws must be visible and accessible through the window in the open impression tray during and after the impression. After the impression material sets, the impression coping screws are unscrewed completely from the implants or abutments, and the impression is removed. The pick-up impression copings remain within the impression. Laboratory analogs are then attached to the restorative platforms of the impression copings, and the screws are tightened. The impression is boxed, and the master cast is poured.

In light of the literature reviewed in the previous paragraphs, the specific clinical procedures for impressions and jaw relation records for the Columbus Bridge Protocol are described below.

IMPRESSION PROCEDURES

The Columbus Bridge Protocol uses pick up impression copings in open impression trays. With this protocol, conical abutment pick up impression copings are screwed into the conical abutments prior to flap closure (Fig 8.1). The impression coping–abutment interfaces are flat; therefore, clinicians can be certain that if the impression copings are completely seated on the abutments, the impression copings will accurately record the positions of the abutments. Once the impression copings have been screwed onto the abutments, the flaps are closed with interrupted sutures (Fig 8.2). Closing the flaps in this fashion prevents impression material from contacting the osseous tissues during the impression procedure.

BOX 8.1 - PHYSICAL AND MECHANICAL FEATURES OF THE IMPRESSION PLASTER

- Setting expansion: < 0.02%
- Resistance to dry compression: 700 kg/cm^2
- Mixing ratio: 100 g powder to 33–34 mL water
- Mixing time: manual, 60 sec; mixer, 45 sec
- Working time: 2 min
- Initial setting time: 2–3 min
- Final setting time: 4 min

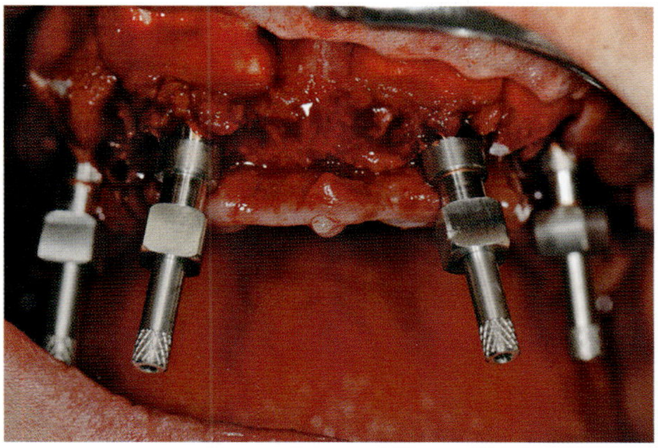

Fig 8.1 - Conical abutment pick up impression copings in place on conical abutments.

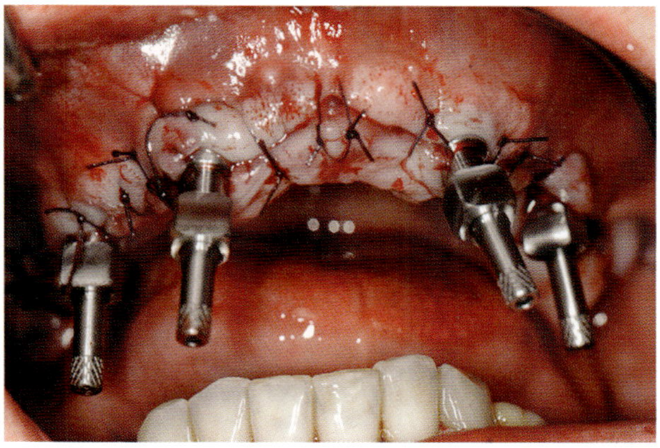

Fig 8.2 - After suturing the flaps closed around the impression copings.

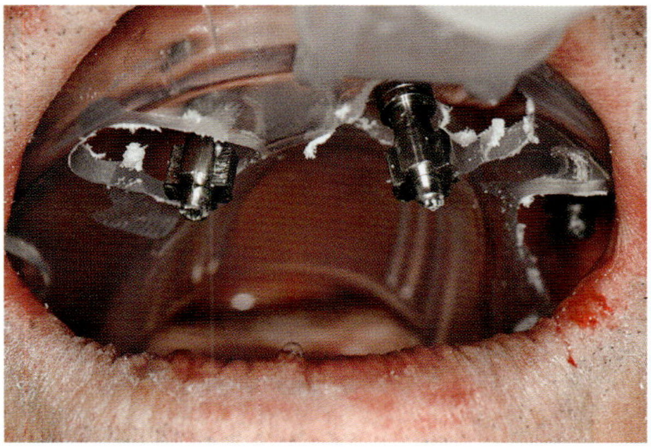

Fig 8.3 - The stock plastic impression tray in place. Windows were prepared in the occlusal surface of the tray to permit access to the impression coping screws per the pick up impression technique.

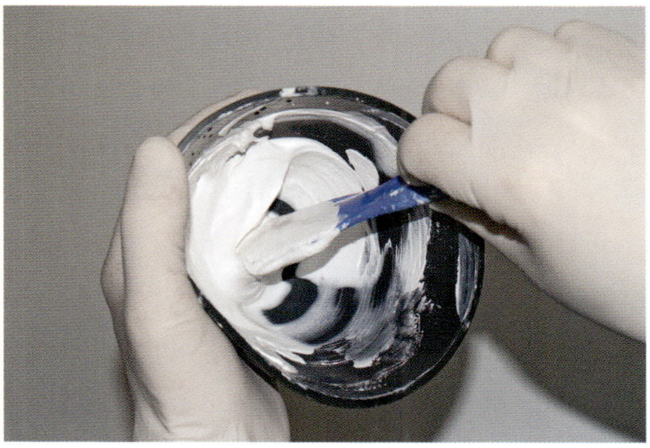

Fig 8.4 - Type III impression plaster mixing.

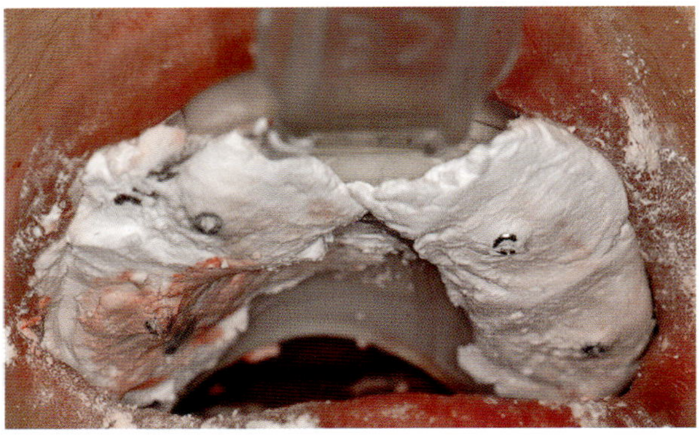

Fig 8.5 - The impression tray in place for the pick up impression. With the pickup impression technique, impression coping screws are visible through the windows of the impression tray.

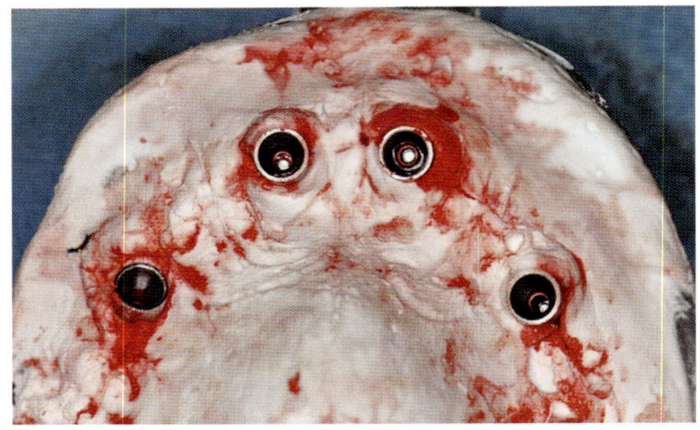

Fig 8.6 - The intaglio surface of the pick up impression. Note that the impression copings were completely surrounded by the impression plaster. The impression copings must be stable within the impression material.

The impression trays for this protocol are commercially available, clear stock plastic trays. Openings must be cut into the occlusal surfaces of the trays to allow access to the impression coping screws (Fig 8.3). Although some authors have stated that stock plastic impression trays are not rigid enough for implant impressions, the authors of the Columbus Bridge Protocol have found the trays to be sufficient because the impression material (plaster) provides the requisite rigidity for implant prosthodontics.[12] Furthermore, they believe the technique that splints impression copings to impression trays not to be as accurate as the pick up impression technique with impression plaster.[13–15] The material of choice for implant impressions in the Columbus Bridge Protocol is type III plaster (BF Plaster, DentalTorino) (Figs 8.4 to 8.6). Many variables can affect the ability of impression plaster to make an accurate impression (Box 8.1), yet both Assif et al[15] and Eid[16] have stated that its characteristics make it ideal for taking implant-abutment impressions to obtain precise-fitting implant prostheses. One important feature of impression plaster is that it is a low-expansion stone. Other favorable characteristics include its short setting time, rigidity, and accuracy, which make it the material of choice for use in edentulous patients.

Impression plasters have three negligible defects:

- Impression plaster sets with an exothermic chemical reaction that generates heat intraorally. In an in vitro study, Nissan and colleagues[17] report that plaster impression procedures increased the apical temperature of implants by up to 2°C and the cervical temperature by up to 10°C. To minimize this temperature change, the Nissan group recommends that clinicians decrease the volume of plaster used in each impression. However, this temperature increase may not be important because the setting time is relatively short, and in any case, it is negligible relative to the amount of heat generated during osteotomy preparation
- Impression plaster may tear the peri-implant

soft tissues if sutures have been inserted and become incorporated into the impression material prior to setting (Fig 8.7). To prevent this from happening, the sutures must be well tightened, the ends of the sutures must be cut over the knots to 2 to 3 mm, and the mucosa must be humid before making the impression

- Since impression plaster is a rigid material after setting, impression removal can be hampered or blocked by undercuts. However, in edentulous patients, the lack of teeth and gingival undercuts after flap suturing eliminates this inconvenience

Although other methods for rigidly splinting impression copings have been proposed in the literature, many do not perform well in the context of the Columbus Bridge Protocol. Among these methods, the use of autopolymerizing resins is undoubtedly the most frequently cited.[18–21] All resins contract with polymerization. This contraction may result in loss of the clinical accuracy needed for implant prosthodontics. Mojon et al[22] report shrinkage of up to 8% after 24 hours. Some clinicians have devised strategies to decrease or eliminate this factor.[23,24] Eighty percent of the volumetric shrinkage

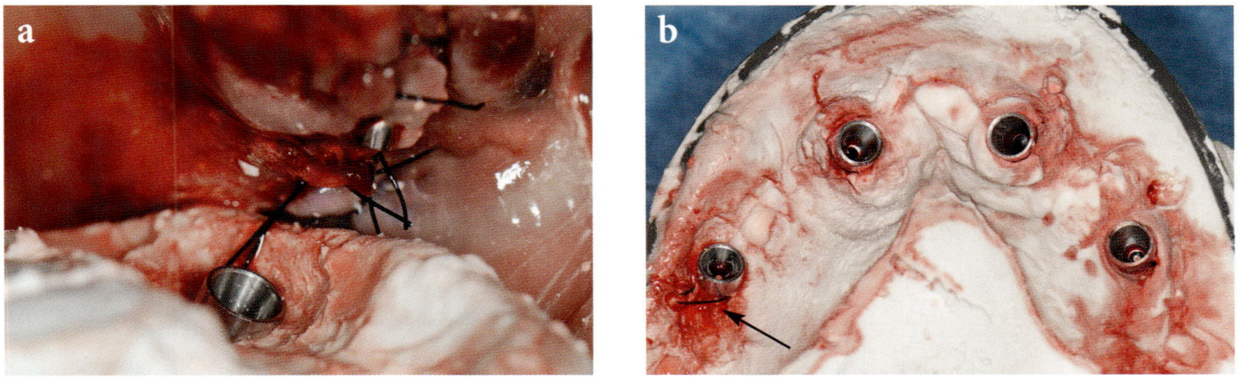

Fig 8.7 - *(a)* A torn suture that was retained within the plaster impression material. This was noted upon removal of the impression from the mouth. The suture was replaced. *(b)* The intaglio surface of the impression. The torn suture is visible in the impression material (*arrow*).

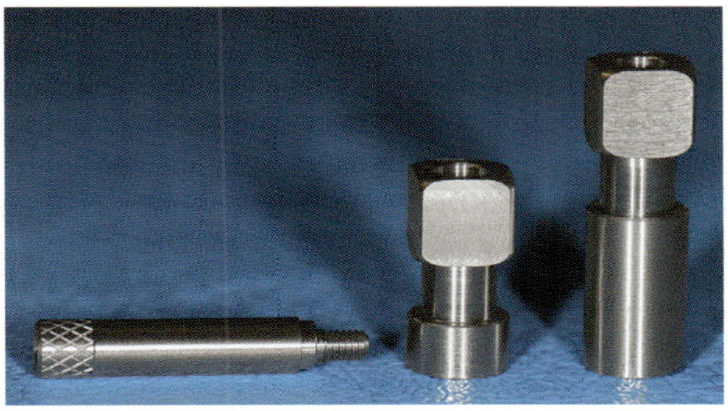

Fig 8.8 - Conical abutment pick up impression copings with the pin: standard size (*left*); tall size (*right*). In the Columbus Bridge Protocol, it has been noted that sometimes taller impression copings are easier and more predictable to pick up in the impression.

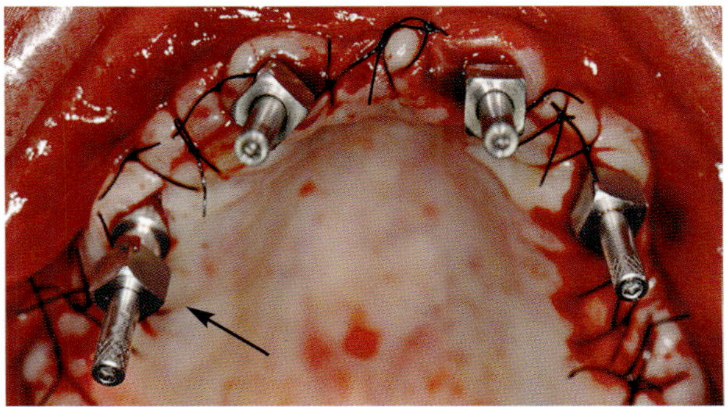

Fig 8.9 - A patient with conical abutment pick up impression copings in place on the conical abutments. A taller impression coping was used on the right distal abutment because of the increased thickness of the peri-implant soft tissues at this implant site (*arrow*).

associated with the set of autopolymerizing acrylic resins occurs during the first 17 minutes of polymerization. Cabral and Guedes[25] recommend that the resin be allowed to polymerize for at least 17 minutes, followed by sectioning the splinted impression copings and re-luting the sectioned segments together with additional resin. They state that this technique eliminates inaccuracies associated with the contraction of acrylic resin secondary to polymerization shrinkage. The complexity of this technique makes its use inadvisable in an immediate-loading protocol. In the Columbus Bridge Protocol, after the impression plaster has set, the impression tray is removed from the mouth, and the stability of the impression copings is evaluated clinically. If the impression copings are stable within the impression, the impression is sent to the dental laboratory for the cast to be poured (see Figs 14.43 and 14.44). Impression plaster differs significantly from elastomeric impression materials such as silicone and polyether in that it is not affected by the amount of time that elapses before the impression is poured.[26] The first laboratory step consists of screwing conical abutment analogs into the intaglio surfaces of the abutment impression copings (the pick up impression copings remain inside the impression). This portion of the procedure is technique sensitive because errors may be introduced into the three-dimensional positions of the analogs if the positions of any of the impression copings in the impression are altered while the analogs are being attached. In the case of deep peri-implant soft tissue sulcular depths around any of the implants, special abutment impression copings designed with taller vertical bodies (Figs

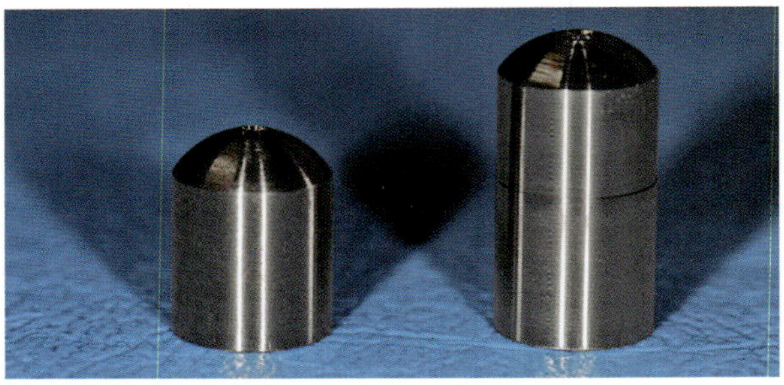

Fig 8.10 - Laboratory image of conical abutment healing caps: shorter (*left*); taller (*right*).

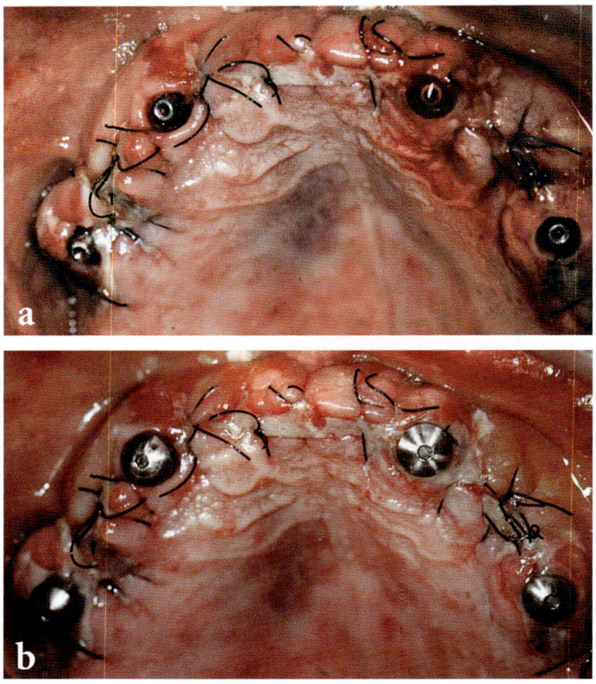

Fig 8.11 - *(a)* Maxillary occlusal image of a patient treated with the Columbus Bridge Protocol. The conical abutments are in place, and the wound has been closed with sutures. *(b)* Maxillary occlusal image of the patient in *a* with the healing caps in place. The patient is now ready for a jaw relation record.

8.8 and 8.9) should be used. These impression copings increase the amount of surface area of the copings, resulting in better retention inside the impression material and, therefore, in higher reliability of the intraoral impression (see chapter 16). After the impression is removed from the intraoral abutments, healing caps are screwed onto the abutments

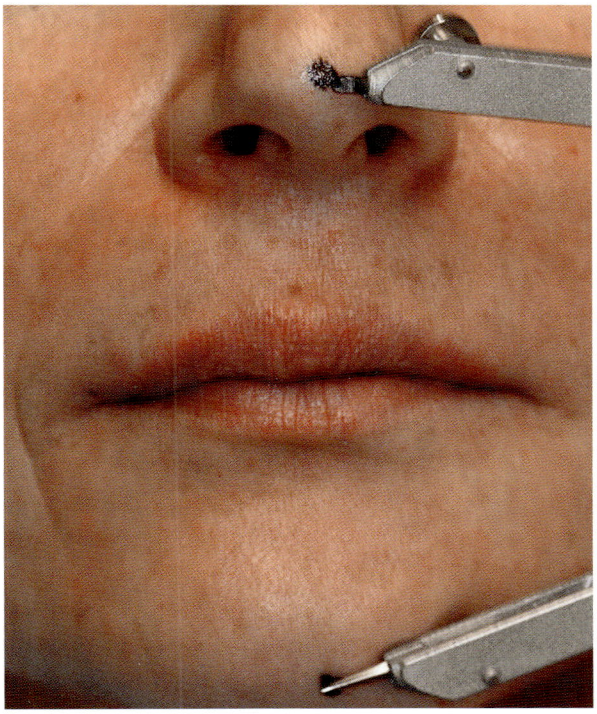

Fig 8.12 - Extraoral image of a patient at the preselected vertical dimension of occlusion (preoperative). Two cutaneous midline reference points were selected: one superior to and one inferior to the intraoral opening (pronasale and pogonion). This vertical dimension will be maintained throughout the clinical procedure.

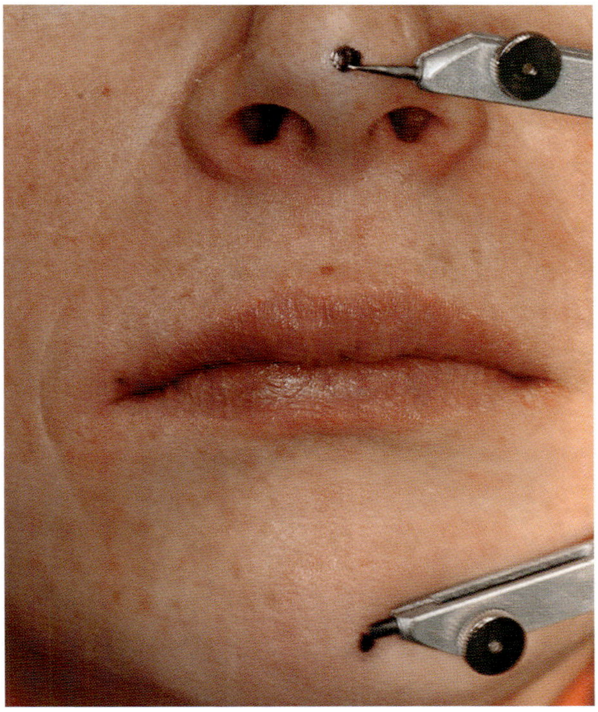

Fig 8.13 - Extraoral image of the patient in Fig 8.12 (postoperative). The vertical dimension of occlusion between the two cutaneous midline reference points was maintained by the wax record.

to prevent the peri-implant soft tissues from collapsing and obscuring the abutments. Healing caps for conical abutments are available in different heights and are selected according to the peri-implant sulcular depths (Figs 8.10 and 8.11). The healing caps must be visible since the jaw relation records are made with the healing caps in place (see chapter 16).

JAW RELATION RECORD PROCEDURES

Jaw relation records are made using the clinical techniques outlined in chapter 3 for the diagnostic phase. The patient's mandible is guided into the centric relation position at the proper vertical

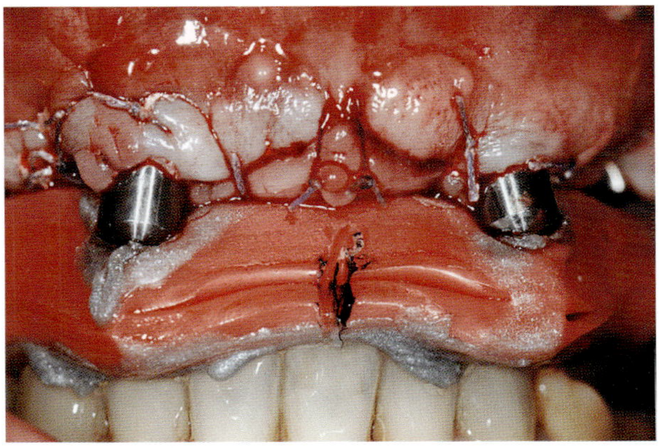

Fig 8.14 - Anterior image of the patient in Fig 8-13 with the wax record maintaining the proper vertical dimension of occlusion.

dimension of occlusion. This position is selected according to preextraction and clinical data.

Prior to the extractions, the vertical dimension can be measured with a caliper and recorded in millimeters (Fig 8.12). The preoperative vertical dimension is reevaluated immediately after the surgical phase (Figs 8.13 and 8.14).

Research for the optimal maxillomandibular relationship in the horizontal plane includes the definition of centric relation. The use of the mandibular position in centric relation is justified by the impossibility of using any dental landmarks associated with the position of maximal intercuspation (centric occlusion) because all of these landmarks have been removed secondary to the extractions of the remaining natural teeth. Clinically, manual manipulation is used for recording centric relation in the Columbus Bridge Protocol.

Both Dawson's bimanual manipulation technique and McCollum's gnathion (chin point) technique are preferred over the central bearing point technique because *(1)* they require less invasive clinical techniques immediately after the operation and *(2)* they are sufficiently reliable for the construction of the provisional prosthesis. In Dawson's bimanual manipulation technique, four fingers of each hand are placed onto the lower borders of the mandible bilaterally; the thumbs are placed onto the mandibular symphysis. The clinician then gently manipulates the mandible into centric relation (posterior movement) with the thumbs while the fingers and hands gently exert pressure superiorly. McCollum's method consists of manipulating the mandible by pushing it posteriorly until a consistent path of closure is found. Through this manipulation, vector forces are applied to the temporomandibular joints, which act as a fulcrum, and the condyle is pushed toward the superior and rear walls of the glenoid fossa. This technique is generally used in fixed prosthodontics and in complete prosthodontics where record bases can be stabilized with the thumb and forefinger.

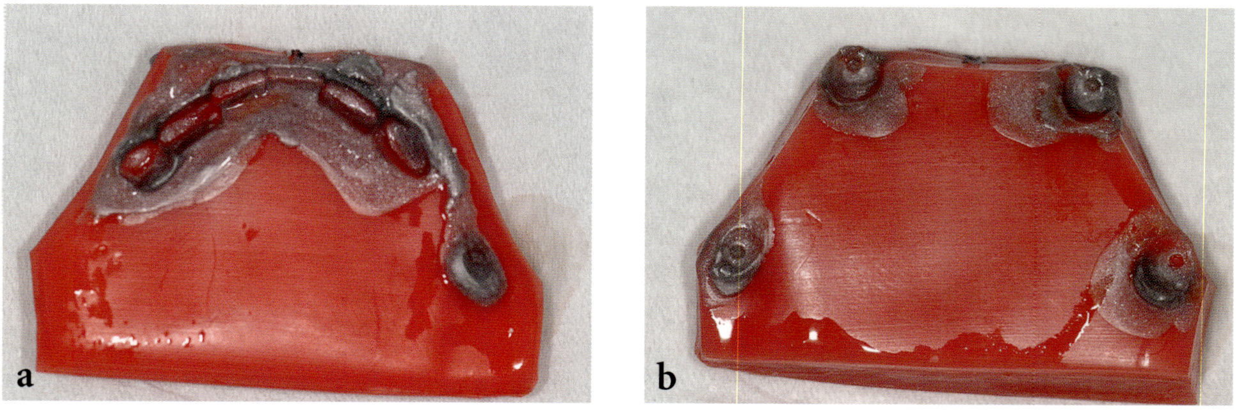

Fig 8.15 - The centric relation wax record that was made immediately after the surgical procedure. This wax record was relined with aluminous wax to improve the detail of the impression. *(a)* Inferior surface. *(b)* Superior surface.

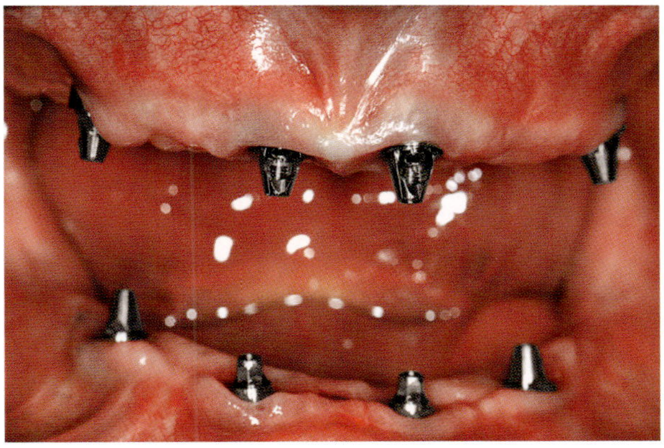

Fig 8.16 - A patient approximately 4 months after implant surgery. The provisional prostheses were removed. All of the implants and abutments were stable, and the soft tissues had matured and healed within normal limits. Treatment for the definitive prostheses will be consistent with conventional edentulous treatment regarding establishment of the optimal jaw relationship.

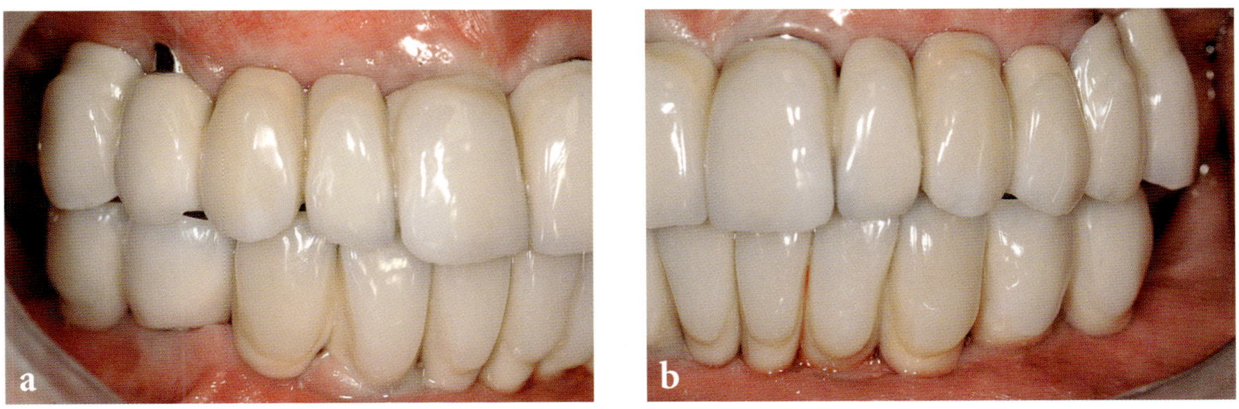

Fig 8.17 - Intraoral images of the patient of Fig. 8.16 with the definitive prostheses in place and the jaws in centric relation (terminal hinge position). These images were taken approximately 4 months after the surgical treatment was accomplished. *(a)* Right lateral view. *(b)* Left lateral view.

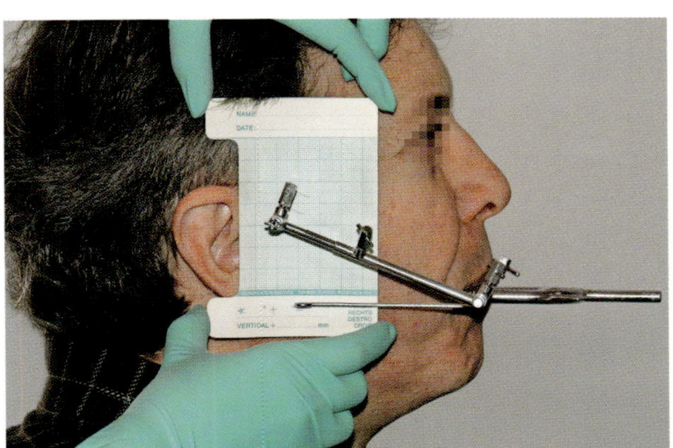

Fig 8.18 - Extraoral profile image with kinematic facebow in place to record and assess the hinge axes.

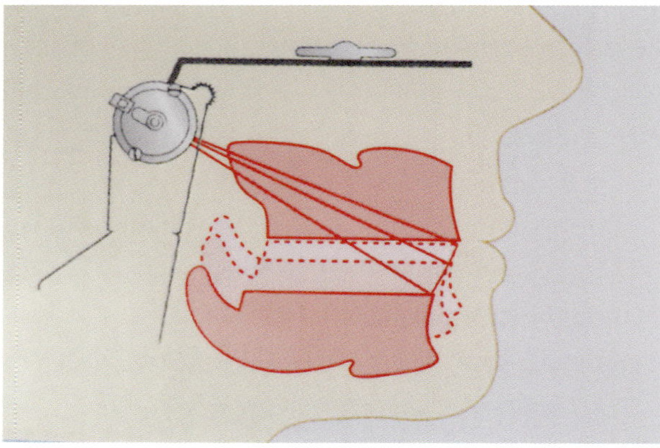

Fig 8.19 - Illustration that demonstrates the coincidental positions of the clinical terminal hinge axis and the laboratory terminal hinge axis on an articulator. Since both positions are coincidental, the vertical dimension of occlusion may be changed in the laboratory and accurately transferred to the patient. (*Reprinted from Preti and Gassino*[27] *with permission.*)

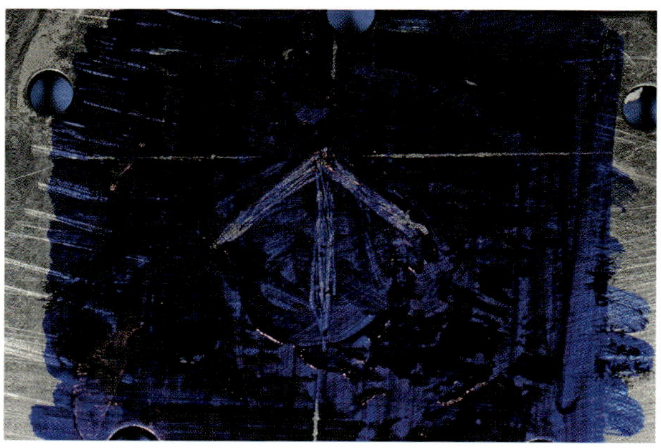

Fig 8.20 - Intraoral Gothic arch tracing for the centric jaw determination in the horizontal plane.

In the Columbus Bridge Protocol, jaw relation records require that the wax interocclusal record be rigidly attached to the healing caps while recording the positions of the teeth in the opposing jaw. The interocclusal record between the maxillary and mandibular jaws is obtained using the previously softened rigid positional wax wafer (X Hard Beauty Pink Wax, Miltex). Alminax wax (Kemdent) may be placed onto the occlusal surfaces of the wax wafer to obtain more accurate replications of the cusps of the teeth in the opposing jaw as well as the occlusal surfaces of the healing caps (Fig 8.15).

Accurate jaw relation records are necessary to accurately mount the casts on the articulator. The casts are mounted using a semi-adjustable articulator. The laboratory procedures are explained further in chapter 9.

Approximately 4 months after extraction, implant placement, and immediate occlusal loading, the patient is reevaluated for the definitive prostheses. These procedures are consistent with the traditional protocol for evaluating edentulous patients (Figs 8.16 and 8.17).[27] Jaw relation records for the definitive prostheses are made with the use of a transfer facial tracing that records the terminal hinge axis (Figs 8.18 and 8.19) and a Gothic arch tracing (Fig 8.20).

REFERENCES

1. Wise M. Fit of implant-supported fixed prostheses fabricated on master casts made from a dental stone and a dental plaster. J Prosthet Dent 2001;86:532–538.
2. Heckmann SM, Karl M, Wichmann MG, Winter W, Graef F, Taylor TD. Cement fixation and screw retention: Parameters of passive fit. An in vitro study of three-unit implant-supported fixed partial dentures. Clin Oral Implants Res 2004;15:466–473.
3. Hsu CC, Millstein PL, Stein RS. A comparative analysis of the accuracy of implant transfer techniques. J Prosthet Dent 1993;69:588–593.
4. Burawi G, Houston F, Byrne D, Claffey N. A comparison of the dimensional accuracy of the splinted and unsplinted impression techniques for the Bone-Lock implant system. J Prosthet Dent 1997;77:68–75.
5. Kim S, Nicholls JI, Han CH, Lee KW. Displacement of implant components from impressions to definitive casts. Int J Oral Maxillofac Implants 2006; 21:747–755.
6. Assif D, Fenton A, Zarb G, Schmitt A. Comparative accuracy of implant impression procedures. Int J Periodontics Restorative Dent 1992;12:112–121.
7. Herbst D, Nel JC, Driessen CH, Becker PJ. Evaluation of impression accuracy for osseointegrated implant supported superstructures. J Prosthet Dent 2000; 83:555–561.
8. Conrad HJ, Pesun IJ, DeLong R, Hodges JS. Accuracy of two impression techniques with angulated implants. J Prosthet Dent 2007;97:349–356.
9. Liou AD, Nicholls JI, Yuodelis RA, Brudvik JS. Accuracy of replacing three tapered transfer impression copings in two elastomeric impression materials. Int J Prosthodont 1993;6:377–383.
10. Barrett MG, de Rijk WG, Burgess JO. The accuracy of six impression techniques for osseointegrated implants. J Prosthodont 1993;2:75–82.
11. Lorenzoni M, Pertl C, Penkner K, Polansky R, Sedaj B, Wegscheider WA. Comparison of the transfer precision of three different impression materials in combination with transfer caps for the Frialit-2 system. J Oral Rehabil 2000;27:629–638.
12. Burns J, Palmer R, Howe L, Wilson R. Accuracy of open tray implant impressions: An in vitro comparison of stock versus custom trays. J Prosthet Dent 2003;89:250–255.
13. Assif D, Marshak B, Nissan J. A modified impression technique for implant-supported restoration. J Prosthet Dent 1994;71:589–591.
14. Assif D, Marshak B, Schmidt A. Accuracy of implant impression techniques. Int J Oral Maxillofac Implants 1996;11:216–222.
15. Assif D, Nissan J, Varsano I, Singer A. Accuracy of implant impression splinted techniques: Effect of splinting material. Int J Oral Maxillofac Implants 1999;14:885–888.
16. Eid N. An implant impression technique using a plaster splinting index combined with a silicone impression. J Prosthet Dent 2004;92:575–577.
17. Nissan J, Gross M, Ormianer Z, Barnea E, Assif D. Heat transfer of impression plasters to an implant-bone interface. Implant Dent 2006;15:83–88.
18. Naconecy MM, Teixeira ER, Shinkai RS, Frasca LC, Cervieri A. Evaluation of the accuracy of 3 transfer techniques for implant-supported prostheses with multiple abutments. Int J Oral Maxillofac Implants 2004;19:192–198.
19. Vigolo P, Majzoub Z, Cordioli G. Evaluation of the accuracy of three techniques used for multiple implant abutment impressions. J Prosthet Dent 2003;89:186–192.
20. Vigolo P, Fonzi F, Majzoub Z, Cordioli G. An evaluation of impression techniques for multiple internal connection implant prostheses. J Prosthet Dent 2004;92:470–476.
21. Assuncao WG, Filho HG, Zaniquelli O. Evaluation of transfer impressions for osseointegrated implants at various angulations. Implant Dent 2004;13:358–366.
22. Mojon P, Oberholzer JP, Meyer JM, Belser UC. Polymerization shrinkage of index and pattern acrylic resins. J Prosthet Dent 1990;64:684–688.
23. Carr AB, Master J. The accuracy of implant verification casts compared with casts produced from a rigid transfer coping technique. J Prosthodont 1996; 5:248–252.

24. Dumbrigue HB, Gurun DC, Javid NS. Prefabricated acrylic resin bars for splinting implant transfer copings. Prosthet Dent 2000;84:108–110.
25. Cabral LM, Guedes CG. Comparative analysis of 4 impression techniques for implants. Implant Dent 2007;16:187–194.
26. Holst S, Blatz MB, Bergler M, Goellner M, Wichmann M. Influence of impression material and time on the 3-dimensional accuracy of implant impressions. Quintessence Int 2007;38:67–73.
27. Preti G, Gassino G. Management of the edentulous patient: A biological approach. Berlin: Quintessence, 2008.

CHAPTER 9
LABORATORY PROCEDURES

COLUMBUS BRIDGE PROTOCOL	
SURGICAL PROTOCOL	**PROSTHETIC PROTOCOL**
External hex rough-surface implants	Screw-retained fixed prosthesis
Implant length ≥ 13 mm, Ø 4 mm	Plaster impression with pickup technique
Underprepared osteotomy	Rigid splinting with metal framework
Implant insertion torque ≥ 40 Ncm	Passive fit with the luting technique
Angled implants in native bone	Acrylic resin occlusal surfaces
Angled conical abutments	No distal cantilevers
No bone regenerative techniques	Immediate functional load 24–48 h after surgery

Table 9.1

After the clinical data have been recorded, fabrication of the fixed immediate provisional prosthesis commences with the development of the master cast and the accurate transfer of clinical information (jaw relation records, vertical dimension of occlusion, and facial midline) to the laboratory. Fabrication of the framework must be consistent with engineering principles. Specifically, the linear beam theory[1] should be followed to ensure that the full-arch fixed prosthesis will have sufficient rigidity and resistance to bending. It affirms that the rigidity of a beam is described by the following relationship:

$$\text{Inertia} = \frac{\text{width} \cdot \text{height}^3}{12}$$

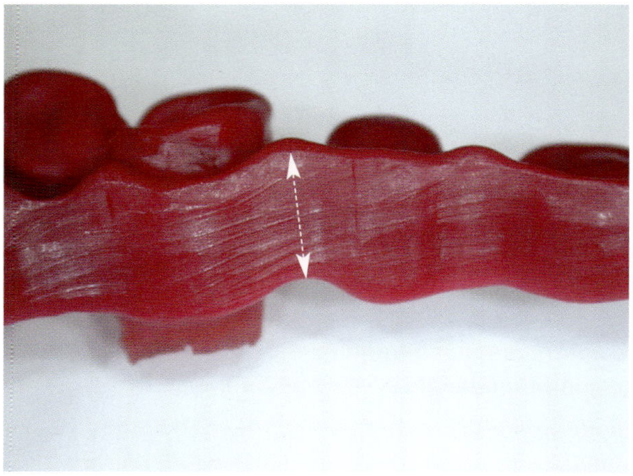

Fig 9.1 - Lateral image of the framework wax pattern with the vertical height of one of the rigid connectors indicated (*dashed arrow*).

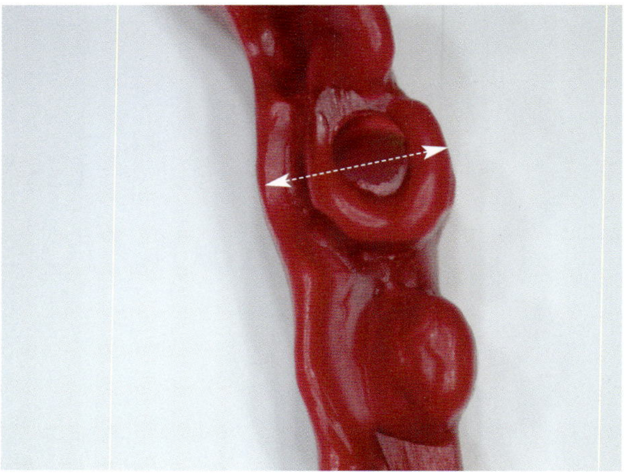

Fig 9.2 - Occlusal view of the framework wax pattern with the buccolingual width of the wax pattern indicated (*dashed arrow*).

- Doubling the height of the beam (framework) increases resistance to bending by a factor of 8 (Fig 9.1).
- Doubling the width of the beam (framework) increases the resistance to bending by a factor of 2 (Fig 9.2).

The authors have designed their prostheses according to these principles and the Columbus Bridge Protocol so that they include metal frameworks with sufficient height and thickness for optimal rigidity relative to the alloy used. Of the two parameters taken into consideration, the height of the framework plays a key role since it is connected to the framework resistance through a cubic relationship. The alloy must provide characteristics of rigidity and accuracy. The authors may choose a sufficiently rigid gold alloy or a palladium alloy. The latter is most commonly adapted for better rigidity together with good accuracy. The use of metal frameworks in this immediate-loading protocol helps in achieving a prosthesis with greater resistance to fracture than is possible with acrylic resin prostheses. Metal frameworks reduce the risk of fracture during osseointegration. Fractured prostheses require prosthetic intervention and could potentially compromise the long-term survival of the implants and prosthesis. It is important to note that the literature also reports high implant survival rates for maxillary all-acrylic resin prostheses (without metal substructures) used with full-arch immediate loading.[2,3]

In the Columbus Bridge Protocol, rigid frameworks are made to fit implants passively by means of a specific laboratory luting technique. Accuracy and rigidity of metal frameworks are fundamental prerequisites for the predictable osseointegration of implants that will be immediately loaded.[4] The Columbus Bridge Protocol calls for the insertion of a full-arch prosthesis within 24 to 48 hours of implant placement. Bergkvist[5] reported that this type of protocol was successful and found no significant differences between implant survival with an immediate-loading protocol within 24 to 48 hours of implant placement and a conventional nonloaded healing protocol. Bergkvist[5] also reported that using removable prostheses with unloaded or delayed loading may cause trauma at the level of the bone-implant interface by loading implants as they emerge from the peri-implant soft tissues. In a pilot study on full-arch maxillary immediate loading, Grunder[6] reported that five out of seven implant failures occurred in patients treated with an acrylic resin fixed provisional prosthesis without a metal framework.

In contrast, splinting implants with rigid prostheses immediately after implant placement seems to protect them from overloads.

PASSIVATION OF METAL FRAMEWORKS IN THE COLUMBUS BRIDGE PROTOCOL

In a literature review, Wee and colleagues[7] reviewed retrospective and prospective clinical studies regarding nonpassive adaptation of prosthetic frameworks on implant abutments. In particular, Wee's team wanted to understand whether the presence of prosthetic misfit could cause medium- to long-term biologic complications and/or late failures of implant restorations. They concluded that various factors prevented passive adaptation between implants and implant frameworks, even with the use of advanced techniques and protocols. Accurate and rigorous implant prosthetic procedures are recommended to obtain precise adaptation of implant prostheses to intraoral abutments or implants.

Nicholls[8–10] defined distortion resulting in prosthetic misfit as the "movement involving a single point (or a group of points) far from any originally specified reference position, so that permanent distortion was evident." In theory, the positional distortion of implant cylinders at every phase of prosthetic procedures may be summed to obtain a permanent distortion according to the equation of distortion (Fig 9.3). If the sum of this distortion equation equals zero, passive adaptation of the prosthesis to implant abutments is obtained.

Distortion Equation

Impression Procedure
+
Cast Construction
+
Fabrication of Wax Patterns
+
Construction of Framework
+
Construction of Prosthesis
+
Insertion of Prosthesis
↓
FINAL DISTORTION

Fig 9.3 - Distortion equation.

The following factors contribute to permanent distortion of implant prostheses during fabrication:

- Bone elasticity (mandibular treatment only)
- Arch curvature
- Impression technique
- Impression material
- Tolerances between intraoral abutments and impression copings
- Tolerances between impression copings and laboratory analogs
- Technique for fabricating master casts
- Tolerances between laboratory analogs and titanium cylinders
- Dimensional stability of acrylic resin/wax pattern used in fabricating metal frameworks
- Dimensional stability of cast frameworks
- Prosthesis shrinkage during the acrylic resin polymerization
- Tolerances between laboratory analogs and the cylinders in the finished prosthesis

Even though distortion caused by every factor can be clinically insignificant in itself, the sum of these potential errors may lead to distortions becoming

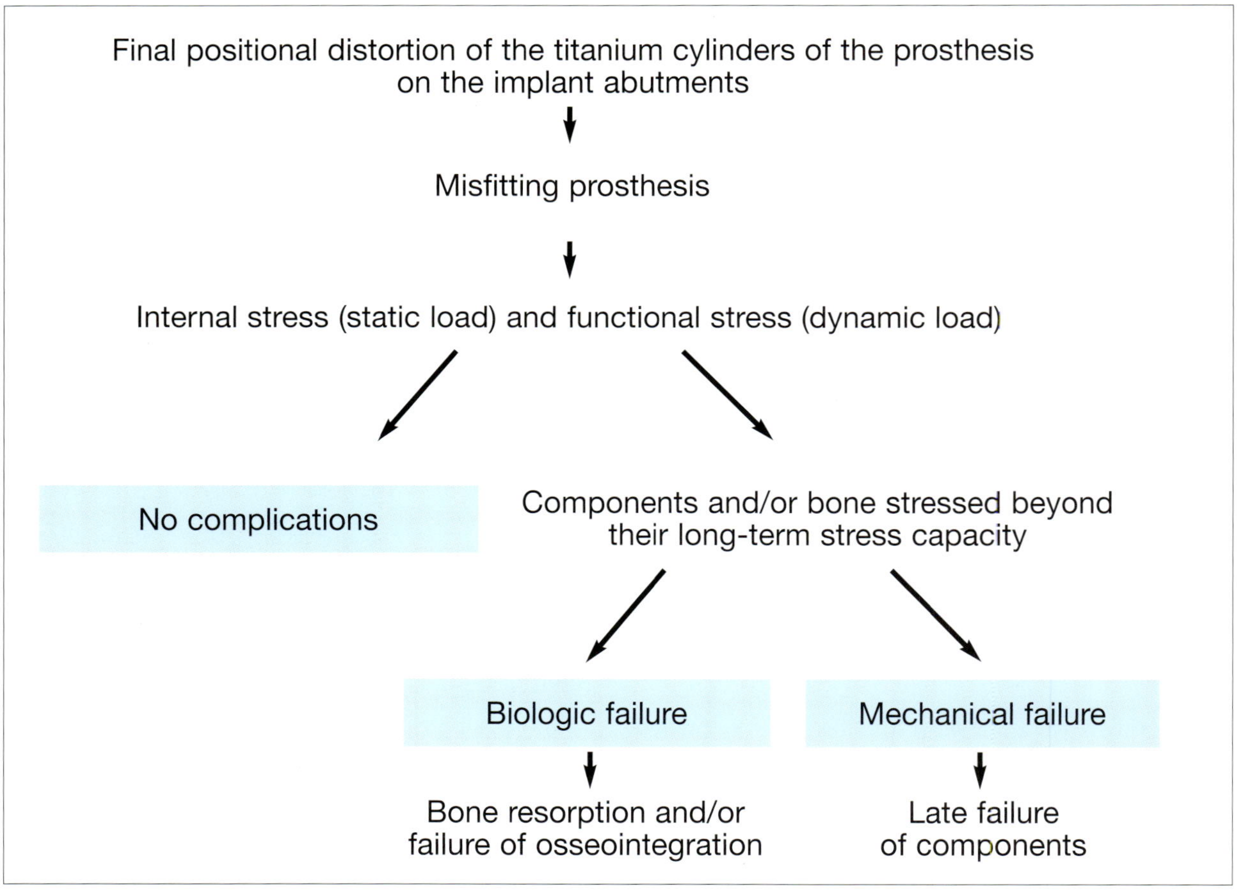

Fig 9.4 - Flow diagram of the correlation between distortion and potential biologic and mechanical failure of the implants.

clinically significant. This can be particularly dangerous during the first 2 to 3 weeks after an immediate-loading full-arch procedure when implant stability is purely mechanical in nature–that is, when implant stability is primarily related to the fit between the implants and the walls of the osteotomies. Relative to the distortions or limitations associated with the dental materials used, the functional misfit may be insignificant and tolerated by the entire system, or it may be significant and lead to biologic or mechanical complications (Fig 9.4). This, however, has not been demonstrated by the scientific literature.

Experimental results regarding passive framework fit in animals and in humans have led to conflicting conclusions. Kallus and Bessing[11] stated that late failure of implant prostheses may be caused by imprecisely fitting implant frameworks. Michaels et al[12] placed implants into rabbit tibias and then made ill-fitting implant frameworks. According to the report, there was evidence of bone remodeling around the implants, but the team found no significant clinical, radiographic, or histomorphometric evidence of implant failure. The Carr group[13] evaluated ill-fitting implant frameworks in primates. Using clinical, radiographic, and histomorphometric assessments, Carr et al concluded that ill-fitting implant frameworks actually improve bone quality, but they cautioned clinicians not to transfer these results to clinical situations since intraoral functional evaluations were not included in the study. Jemt and Book[14] performed an in vivo study where measurements of implant-prosthetic misfit and crestal bone level changes around maxillary implants were evaluated. They found no significant change in crestal bone levels due to prosthetic misfit and concluded that patients have a certain tolerance to ill-fitting frameworks.

Further long-term clinical trials are necessary to correlate ill-fitting frameworks and late implant component failures, as well as to quantify the amount of prosthetic adaptation necessary to prevent biologic and/or mechanical failures in implant prosthodontics. Nevertheless, it is prudent to make every effort to reduce stress in implant-framework connections and peri-implant bone. As such, the following procedures are commonly used to obtain accurate implant frameworks with a passive fit:

- Verified master casts
- Welded segments of conventional frameworks
- Spark erosion technology
- Computer-aided design/computer-assisted manufacture technology
- Laser-welded titanium frameworks
- Screw-retained frameworks cemented to restorative implant components

Verification of master casts with plaster indices of impression or temporary copings on master casts is feasible in delayed-loading protocols. In cases of delayed loading, plaster indices may be fabricated in the laboratory and tried in intraorally per the Sheffield one-screw test to verify that the laboratory analogs and implants occupy the same relative positions in space. Any verifications should be carried out prior to fabrication of the metal framework. As to other passivation techniques, several studies using different materials and different techniques have been published.[15–17] Cementing screw-retained frameworks to implant components, also defined as a *luting technique*, introduces an additional material between implant cylinders and cast frameworks. Gaps between frameworks and abutments are generally filled with resin cement. This technique has been shown to produce a strong framework. Clelland and van Putten[18] used a bone model to evaluate stresses generated by conventional, clinically acceptable screw-retained frameworks and screw-retained frameworks luted to prosthetic components with resin cement. They observed a statistically significant reduction in tension generated by the luted frameworks compared with those generated by traditional screw-retained frameworks. The luting technique requires the use of preformed components and was described for the first time by Voitik[19]; in the study, Voitik used a Kulzer abutment (Heraeus Kulzer). In an in vitro study and a clinical trial led by Stumpel and Quon,[20] the metal framework-abutment connection passivated by the luting technique was sufficiently strong to resist intraoral functional and parafunctional forces. Furthermore, in the event of cement failure, the luting technique can be repeated for a simple and rapid resolution of the problem.

Even if the concept of passive adaptation between implant frameworks and implant restorative components is desirable from a theoretical point of view, realization of completely passive adaptation is not yet clinically attainable. Currently, the worldwide dental community finds the term "clinically acceptable adaptation" to be relevant and accurate. Among the several methods identified above, the authors prefer to choose the most appropriate strategy to obtain the best possible adaptation. In the Columbus Bridge Protocol with immediate function within 24 hours of implant placement, the best clinically acceptable adaptation occurs when screw-retained frameworks are luted in the laboratory to some of the implant restorative components (luting technique).

TABLE 9.2 - CLINICAL METHODS TO ASSESS FRAMEWORK FIT

TECHNIQUE	AUTHOR	YEAR	DESCRIPTION
Radiographs	Hollender[22]	1980	Periapical radiographs can be used to detect misfit, maintaining the film as perpendicular as possible to the abutment-framework junction.
Disclosing materials	Loos[23]	1986	Disclosing materials (such as wax, elastomeric material, powder, spray or pressure-indicating paste) can be used at the fitting surfaces.
Finger pressure	Henry[24]	1987	Manual setting of the prosthesis with finger pressure applied alternately to one terminal abutment, then the other.
Sheffield test	Jemt[25]	1991	Also called *the one-screw test*. It calls for the tightening of a distal abutment screw without creating a gap between the other abutments and framework.
Tactile sensation	Rappold[26]	1992	Framework fit can be assessed by using a traditional dental explorer. Sensitivity is affected by the size of the explorer tip.
Screw resistance test	Jemt[27]	1994	This protocol involves tightening prosthetic screws while checking the resistance during the last half turn.
3D photogrammetric technique	Jemt[28]	1996	An accurate three-dimensional technique requiring special equipment. Information can be saved on a computer for further analysis.

EVALUATION OF FRAMEWORK FIT

Numerous methods have been proposed in the literature to evaluate implant framework fit (Table 9.2).[21] Per the Columbus Bridge Protocol, the authors prefer to use the Sheffield one-screw test to evaluate the fit or adaptation between metal implant frameworks and implant restorative components. This is performed first on the master cast in the laboratory and later intraorally by repeating the same procedure (Fig 9.5).

The one-screw test is performed on the cast by screwing a single retaining screw into the distalmost restorative cylinder on the framework and then evaluating if there is any discrepancy between the framework and the distalmost analog on the opposite side. The procedure is then

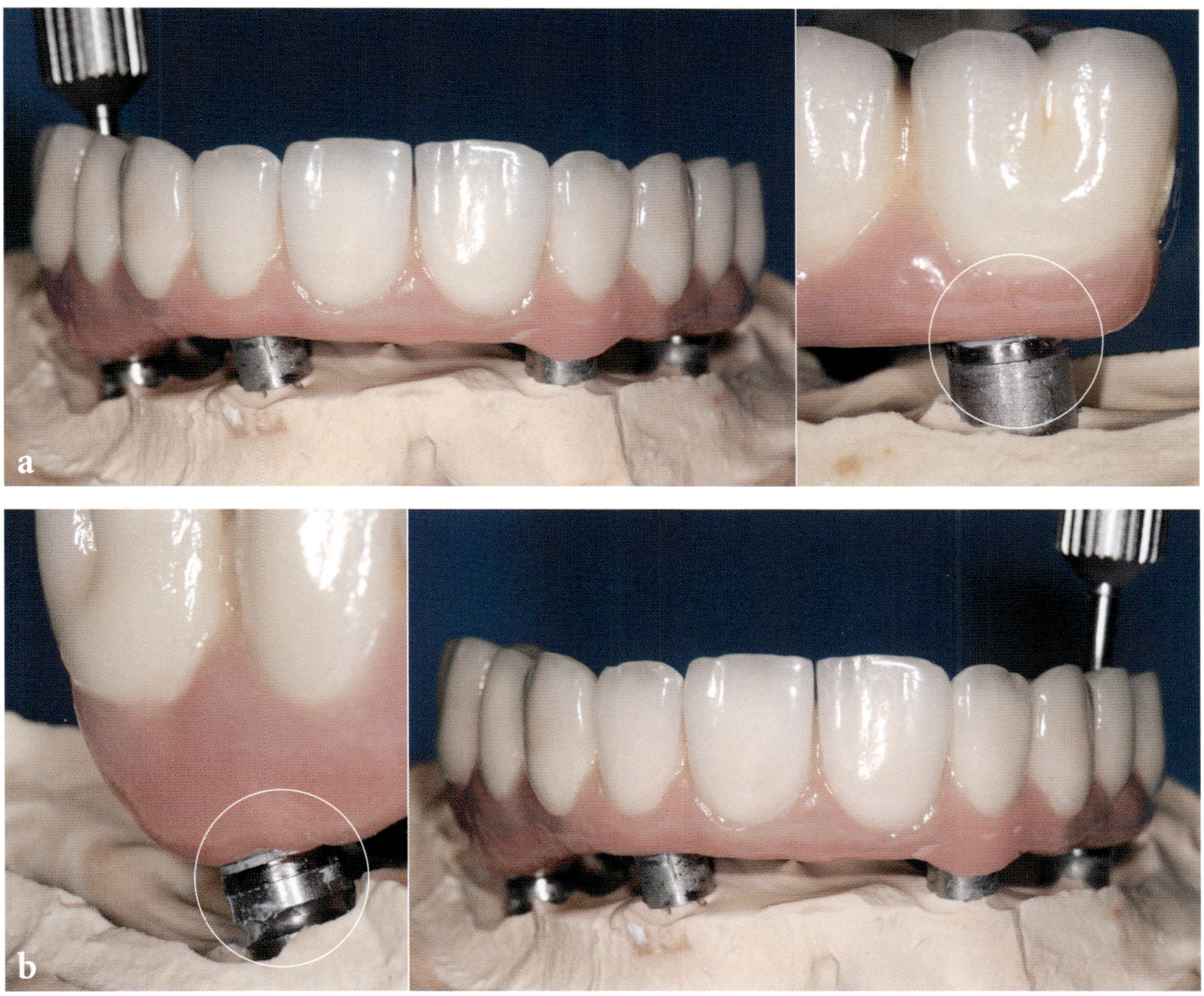

Fig 9.5 - The Sheffield one-screw test. *(a)* A left one-screw test. The screwdriver is in place in the left distal cylinder of the framework (*left*). The cylinder-abutment interface on the right side of the framework is intact; no space is seen between the implant components (*right*). *(b)* A right one-screw test. The screwdriver is in place in the right distal cylinder of the framework (*right*). The cylinder-abutment interface on the left side of the framework is intact; no space is seen between the implant components (*left*).

repeated on the other side. If no discrepancies are noted, it may be concluded that the framework fits passively on the restorative components, and the laboratory technician may proceed with the bridge delivery. The Columbus Bridge Protocol provides for a rigid plaster impression and passivation at the end of processing with a laboratory luting technique; discrepancies are rarely noticed, and no further procedures are generally necessary. If a discrepancy is present, it means that the fit of the prosthesis is unacceptable, and it needs to be remade. An investigation should be made to determine whether the discrepancy was caused by the impression or if the error occurred in the laboratory (Fig 9.6). The discrepancy is removed by repeating the luting technique directly in the mouth or on a new cast from a new impression. Research for clinically acceptable implant framework adaptation has indicated that passively fitting frameworks are required in immediate-loading protocols because tension in the system could be transferred to the bone-implant interface with negative effects. Ill-fitting frameworks could possibly exceed the threshold for micromotion (> 150 μm) established by Brunski.[29]

The Columbus Bridge Protocol uses only screw-retained components. In screw-retained prostheses, contact between implant and restorative components is flat. Satisfactory clinical fits are obtained when components fit along the entire circumference of each component. With cement-retained prostheses, ill-fitting components may be compensated for with cement. Ignoring prosthetic problems regarding ill-fitting components may lead to short-term and/or long-term failures. Ill-fitting components in delayed-loading protocols transmit static loads to the entire implant-prosthetic system as the screws are tightened. For immediate-loading procedures, such stress is delivered to the implant-bone interface.

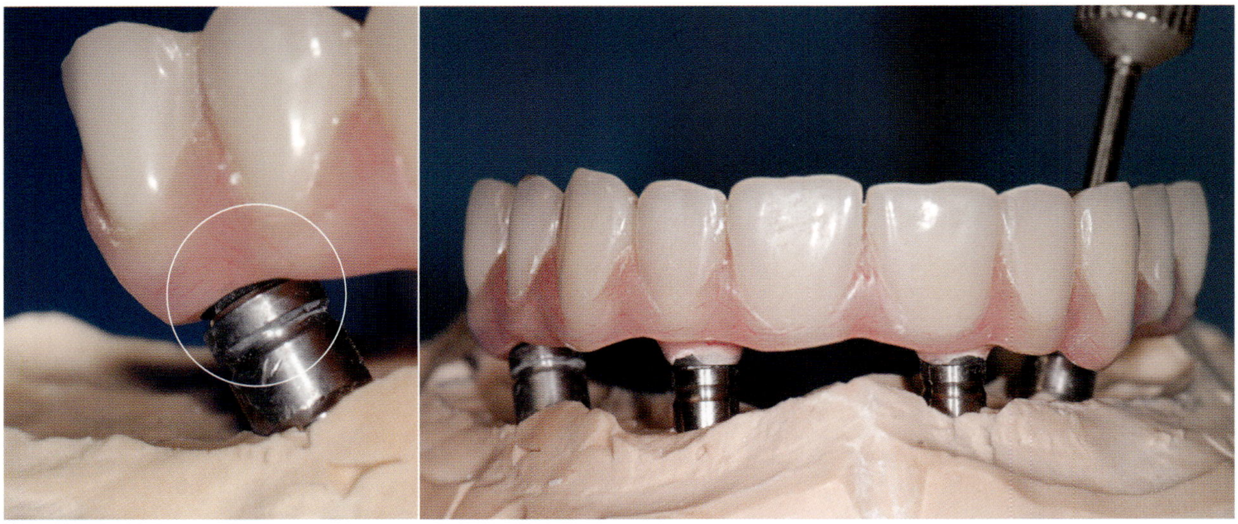

Fig 9.6 - A Sheffield one-screw test revealing a discrepancy. The screwdriver is in place in the right distal cylinder of the framework (*right image*). Space visible between the cylinder-abutment interface on the left side of the framework indicates that the framework is ill fitting (*left image*).

During masticatory function, static loads change into dynamic loads that are directly proportional to the level of the original prosthetic misfit between the prosthesis and implants. As previously discussed, the ideal situation is attained when each component used in the Columbus Bridge Protocol reaches a flat adaptation between the components during screw tightening. Three-dimensional imprecision may cause horizontal and vertical discrepancies between components and may produce compression and tension between the components.[30] The discrepancies most frequently noticed in the presence of prosthetic misfit can be classified as vertical or as horizontal discrepancies. *Vertical discrepancies* are defined as "gaps between abutments and cylinders within a framework in a vertical direction." The preload is transferred to the implant(s) and places the implant(s) under continuous tension. In immediate-loading protocols, this tension may cause implant stress with the potential loss of or lack of osseointegration (Fig 9.7). In cases of horizontal discrepancies, lateral discrepancies greater than 0.1 mm between a framework and implants cause the retaining screw(s) to bend when tightened. Laboratory procedures used in the fabrication of immediate prostheses per the Columbus Bridge Protocol are illustrated in the following pages (Figs 9.8 to 9.99).

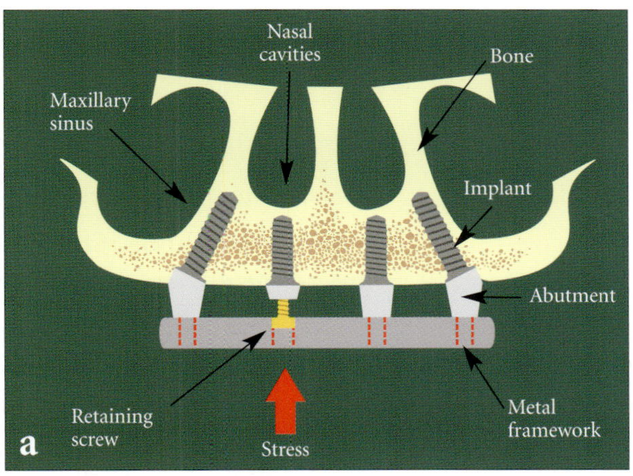

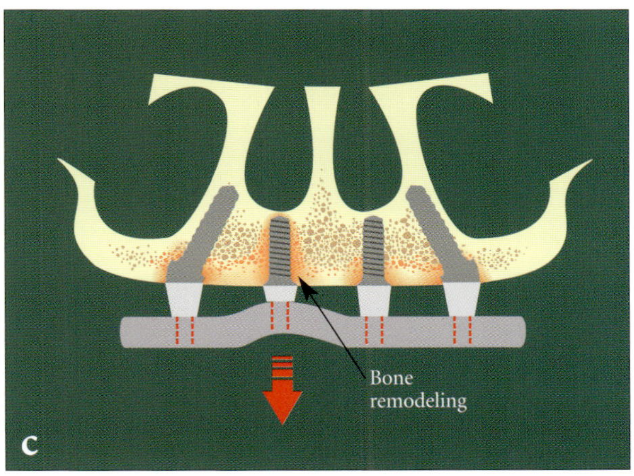

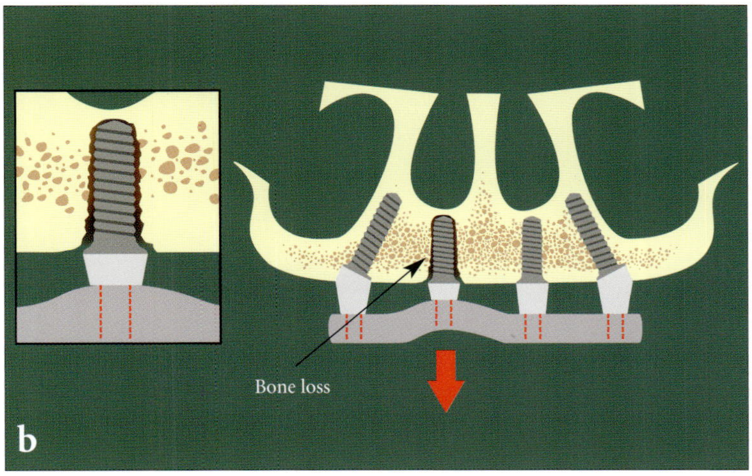

Fig 9.7 - Illustrations of distortion within misfitting prosthesis. *(a)* In the presence of a misfit between the metal framework and the abutments, tightening the retaining screw causes tension between the components. *(b)* In the case of immediate loading, the misfit can generate tensile forces that overcome implant primary stability and, ultimately, can result in loss of the implant. *(c)* In the case of delayed loading, the misfit may cause bone remodeling.

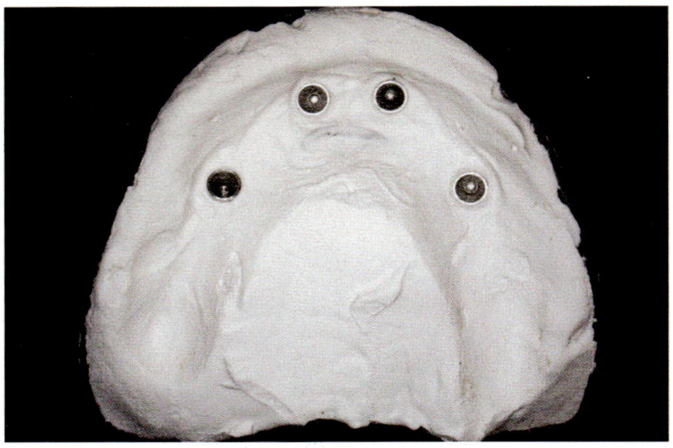

Fig 9.8 - Intaglio surface of the type III plaster impression sent to the laboratory.

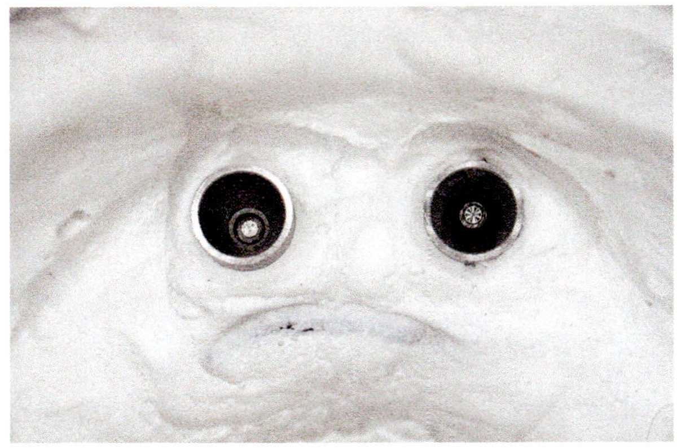

Fig 9.9 - Close-up image of the pick up abutment impression copings within the plaster impression. The impression copings must be evaluated for stability within the impression. This can be done chairside.

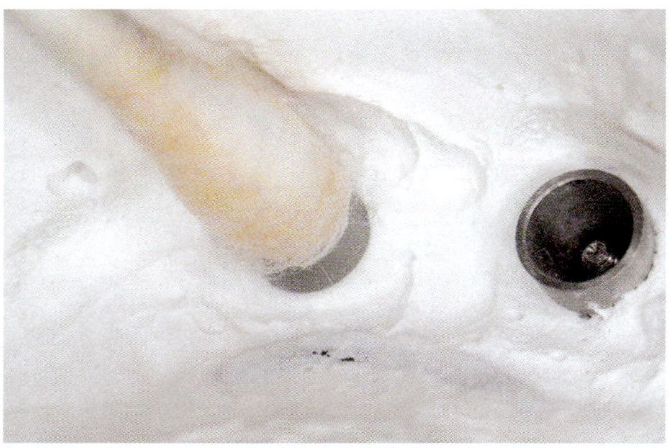

Fig 9.10 - The abutment restorative platform must be clean. A cotton swab wetted with alcohol may be used for this procedure.

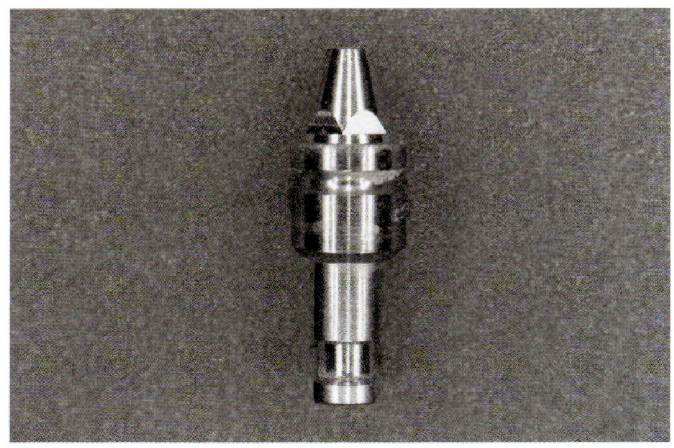

Fig 9.11 - A conical abutment laboratory analog. The analog will be screwed into the conical abutment impression coping within the impression.

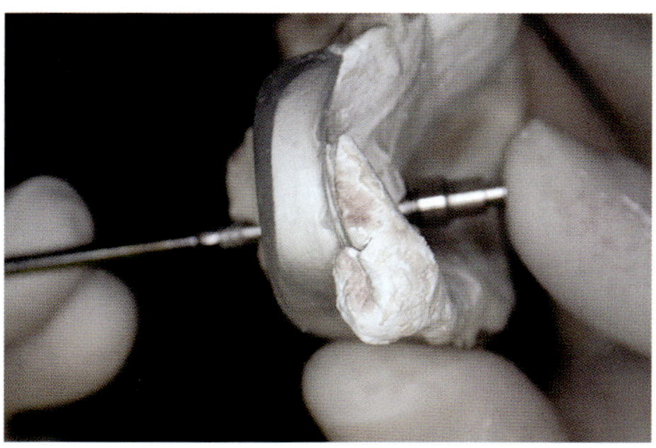

Fig 9.12 - The conical abutment analog must be secured into the impression coping while the impression screw is tightened.

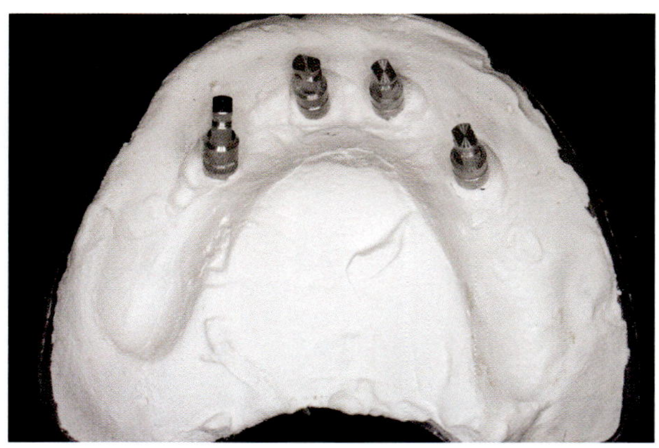

Fig 9.13 - Intaglio surface of the impression after all the conical abutment analogs are in place. Tightening the impression coping screws must be done carefully to avoid moving the impression copings within the impression. The rigid plaster impression material facilitates this procedure.

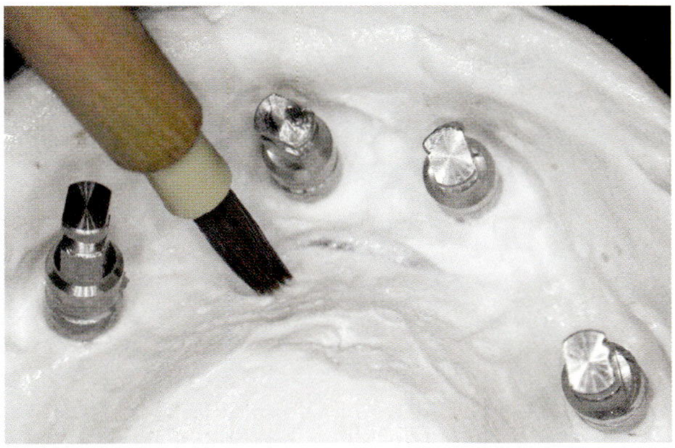

Fig 9.14 - Separating material being applied to the intaglio surface of the impression.

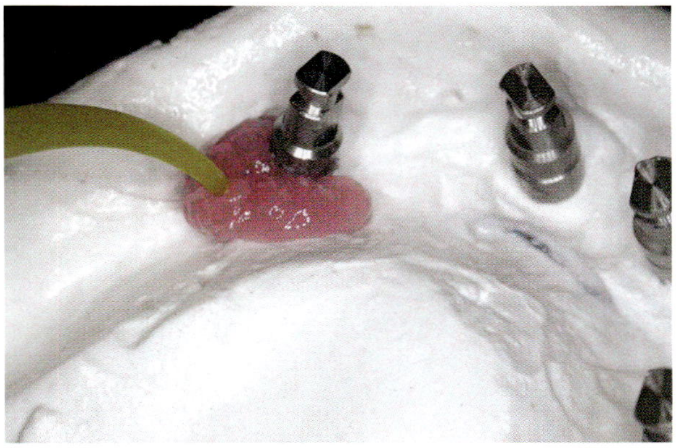

Fig 9.15 - Pink silicone material is injected around the conical abutment analog-impression coping junction prior to pouring the impression with dental stone.

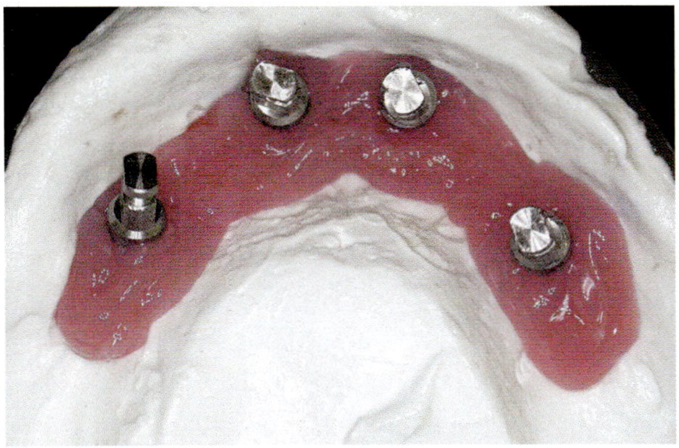

Fig 9.16 - Intaglio surface of the plaster impression after pink silicone was injected to reproduce the soft tissue.

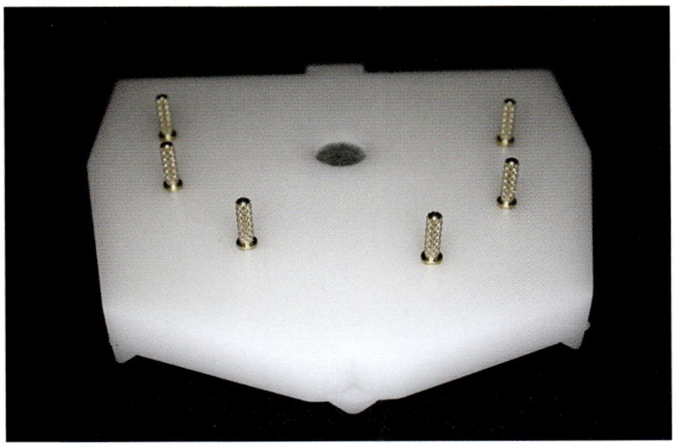

Fig 9.17 - Zeiser plates (Atlantic Zeiser) are used to make the base of the master cast.

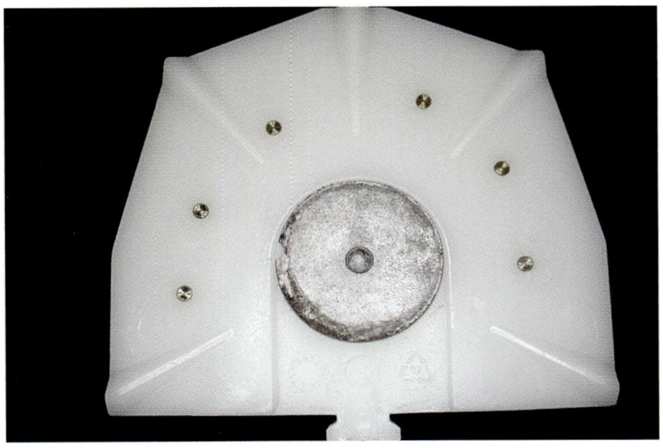

Fig 9.18 - The inferior surface of the Zeiser plate was manufactured with a magnet in the central portion. The magnet is used to connect the master cast to the articulator. The magnet facilitates quick removal and insertion of the mounting plate.

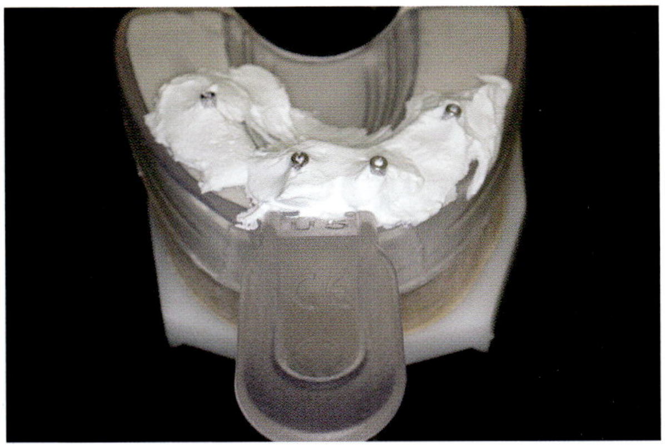

Fig 9.19 - The impression is poured in type IV dental stone per the manufacturer's instructions regarding the powder-to-liquid ratio.

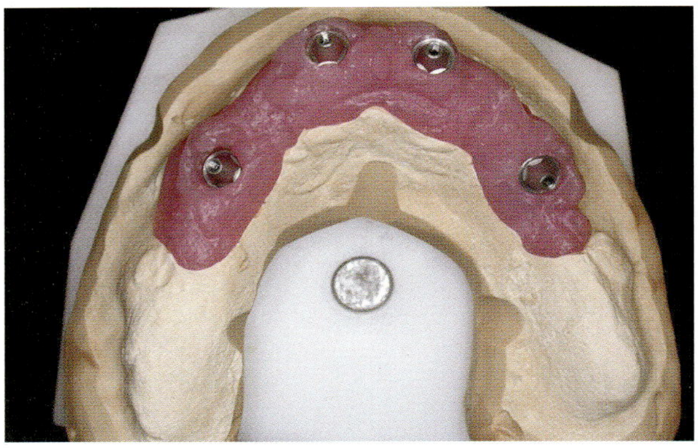

Fig 9.20 - Occlusal image of the master cast.

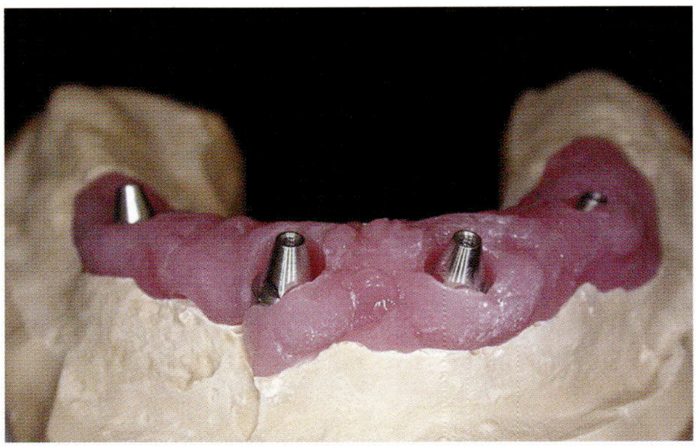

Fig 9.21 - Facial close-up image of the master cast.

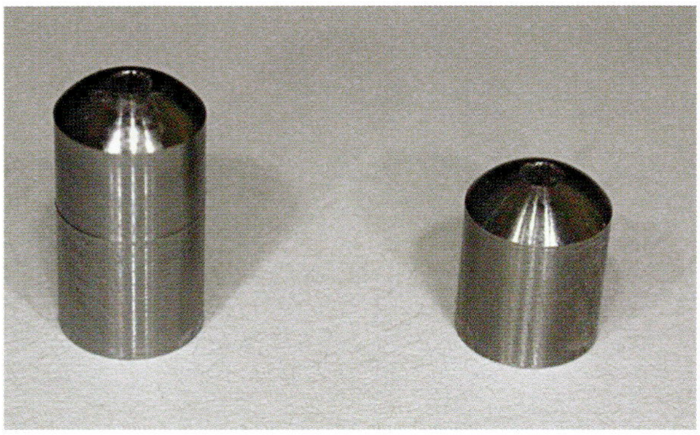

Fig 9.22 - The conical abutment healing caps. The healing caps used in the laboratory must duplicate the healing caps used intraorally during the jaw relation record.

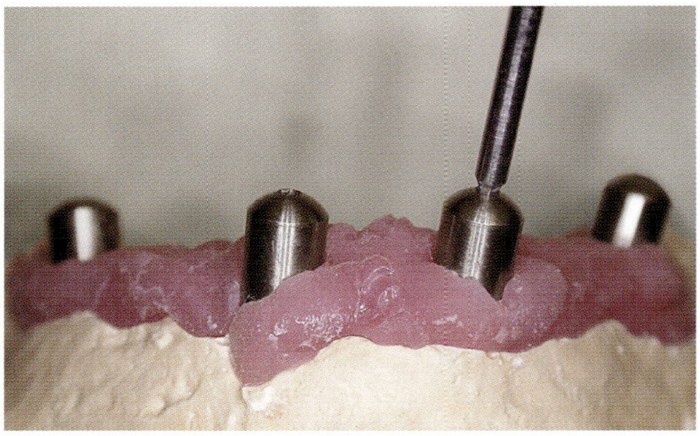

Fig 9.23 - The healing caps in place on the conical abutment analogs in the master cast. The healing caps are tightened with the large hex driver. The wax interocclusal record made in the mouth will fit onto the healing caps in the master cast.

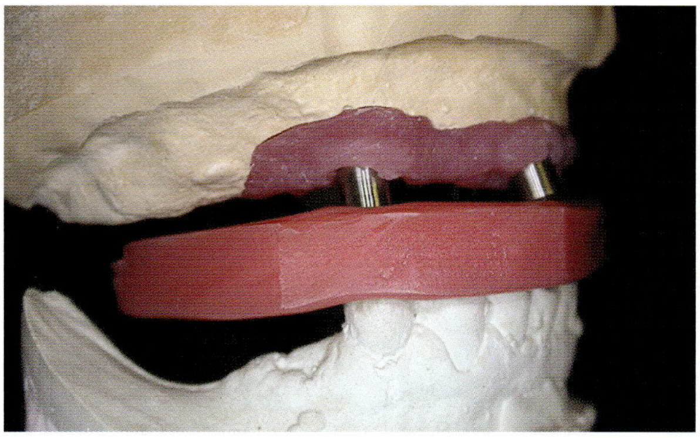

Fig 9.24 - Lateral image of the casts and wax interocclusal record in place. The wax interocclusal record fits precisely onto the healing caps on the conical abutment analogs in the master cast.

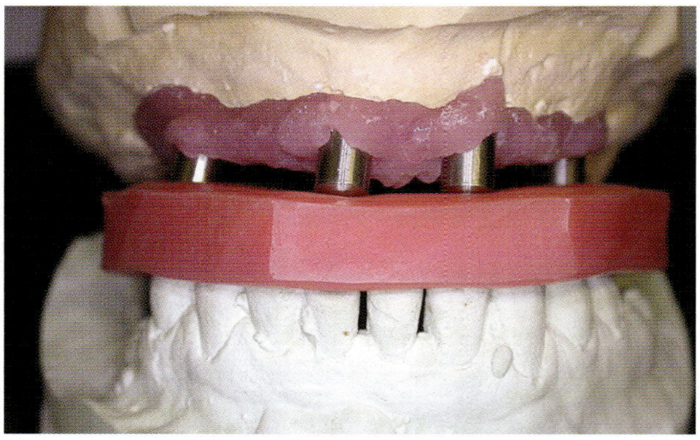

Fig 9.25 - Anterior image of the casts and wax interocclusal record in place. Prior to mounting the casts, the articulator is set to its medium values.

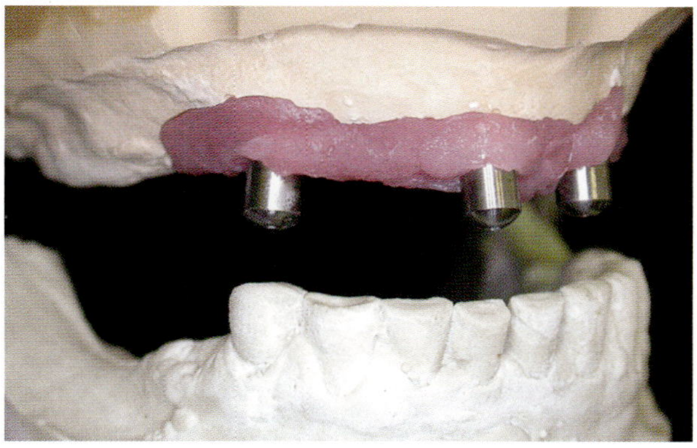

Fig 9.26 - Lateral view of the casts mounted in the articulator. The wax interocclusal record has been removed; the healing caps have remained in place on the conical abutment analogs.

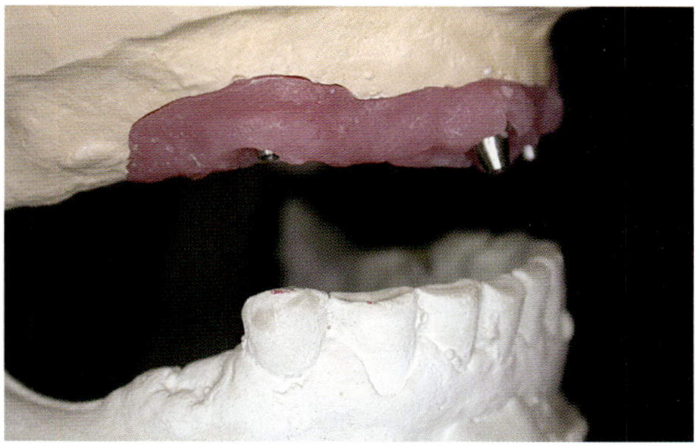

Fig 9.27 - Right lateral view of the casts mounted in the articulator. The healing caps have been removed from the conical abutment analogs. The restorative space can now be evaluated.

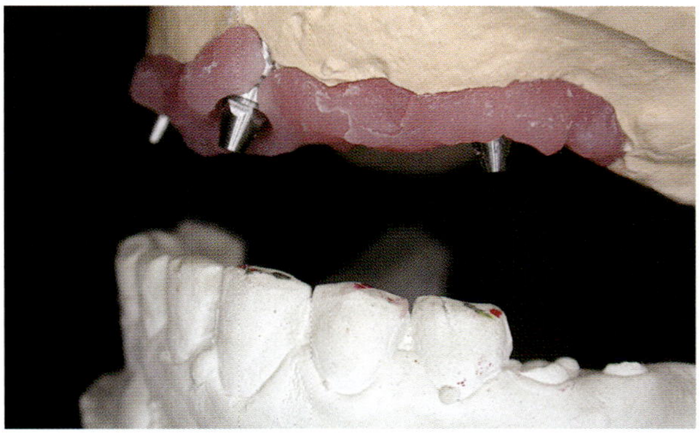

Fig 9.28 - Left lateral view of the casts mounted in the articulator. The healing caps have been removed from the conical abutment analogs. The restorative space can now be evaluated.

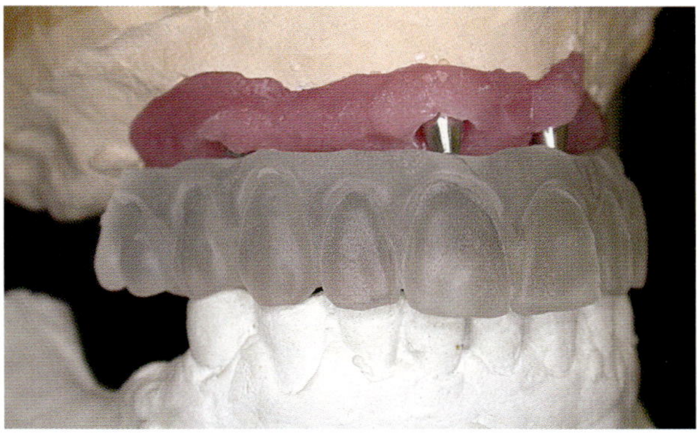

Fig 9.29 - Previously, the wax prosthesis was duplicated in clear acrylic resin. The occlusal surfaces of the resin prosthesis were positioned onto the occlusal surfaces of the opposing cast (see also Fig 3.33).

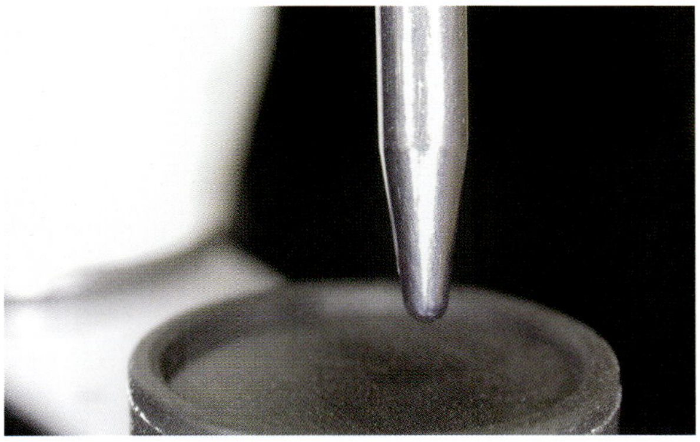

Fig 9.30 - Interferences between the resin duplicate prosthesis and the soft tissue replica in the master cast generally do not allow the incisal guide pin to touch the incisal guide table.

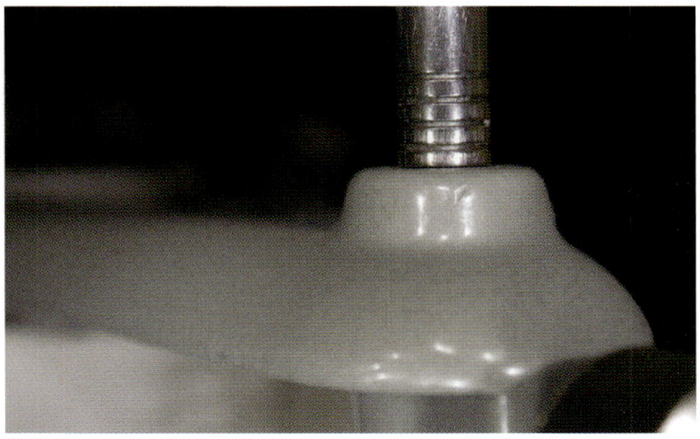

Fig 9.31 - The superior portion of the incisal guide pin indicates that the vertical dimension was increased from the original articulator mounting with the wax interocclusal record.

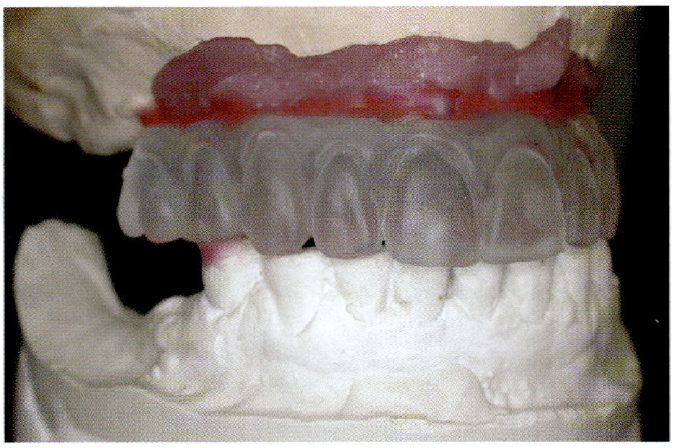

Fig 9.32 - The intaglio surface of the resin duplicate prosthesis is reduced by removing the interferences that prevented seating the duplicate prosthesis onto the cast.

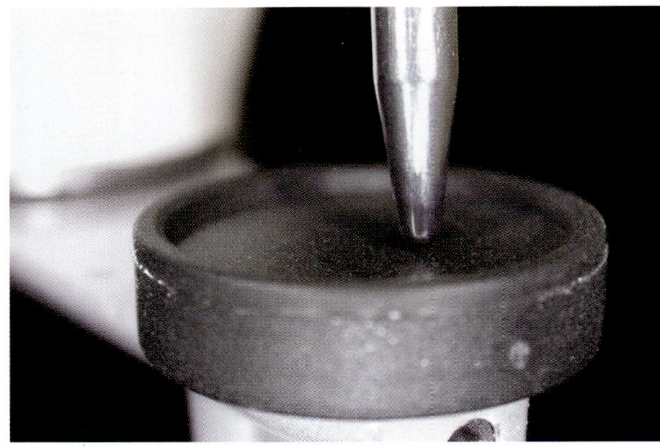

Fig 9.33 - After all the interferences are removed, the incisal guide pin touches the incisal guide table. The vertical dimension with the resin duplicate prosthesis is now consistent with the intraoral centric jaw relation record.

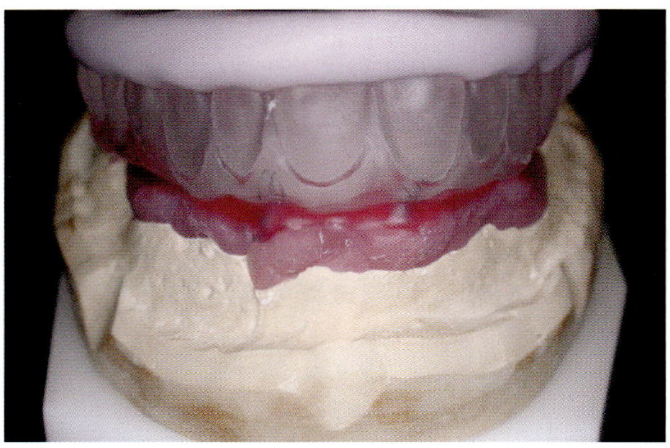

Fig 9.34 - After the resin duplicate prosthesis is fixed to the maxillary cast with wax. A palatal-occlusal index of the duplicate resin prosthesis was made.

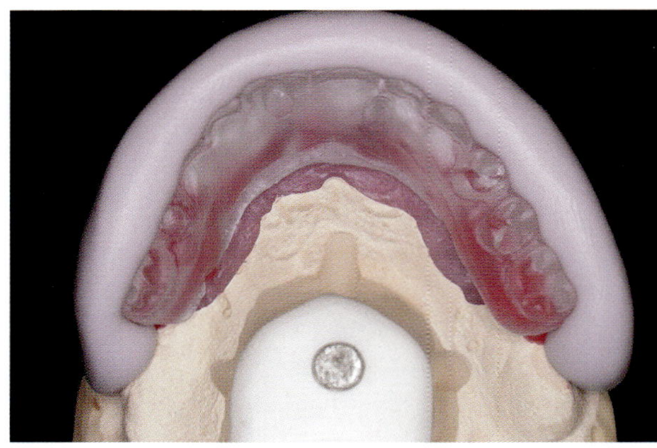

Fig 9.35 - Occlusal image of the facial silicone index made of the duplicate resin prosthesis in place on the maxillary cast.

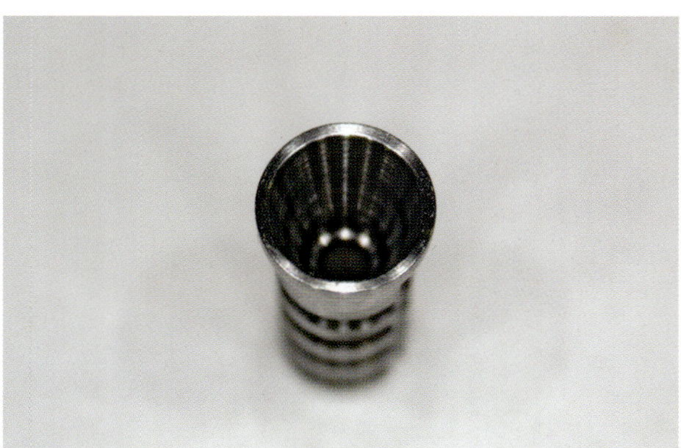

Fig 9.36 - Restorative interface of the titanium cylinder (TC) (Biomet 3i) used in the Columbus Bridge Protocol.

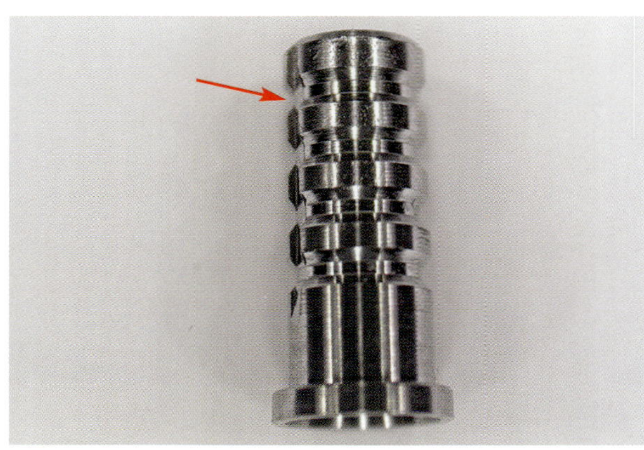

Fig 9.37 - The external surface of a titanium cylinder. One of the two opposing vertical grooves is indicated (*red arrow*).

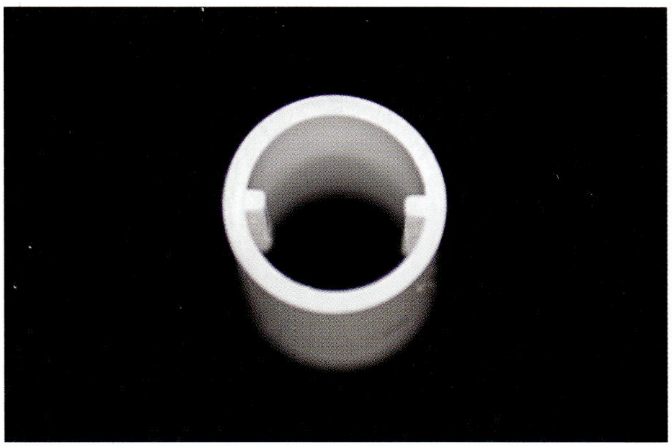

Fig 9.38 - The internal surface of the castable cap (CC). Two opposing vertical relief areas are visible within the castable cap.

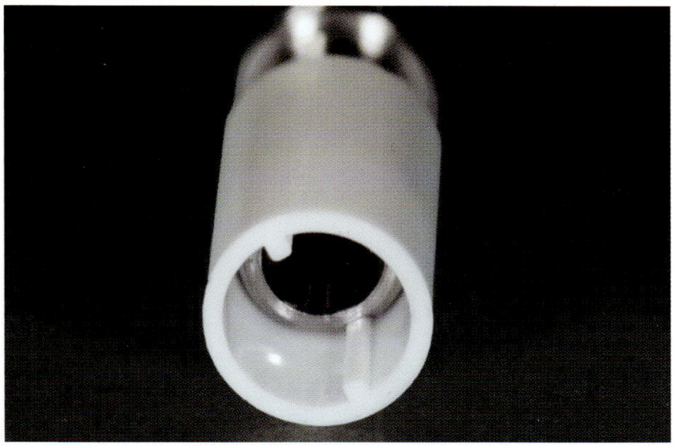

Fig 9.39 - The two vertical relief areas within the castable cap have been designed to prevent rotation between the titanium cylinder and the castable cap and to maintain a consistent space between the them.

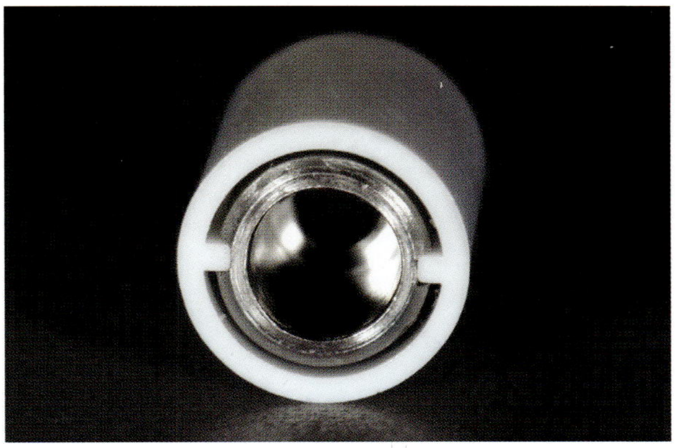

Fig 9.40 - Close-up image that demonstrates the 0.2-mm gap between the titanium cylinder and the castable cap. This is critical for the luting technique to occur without stress between the components.

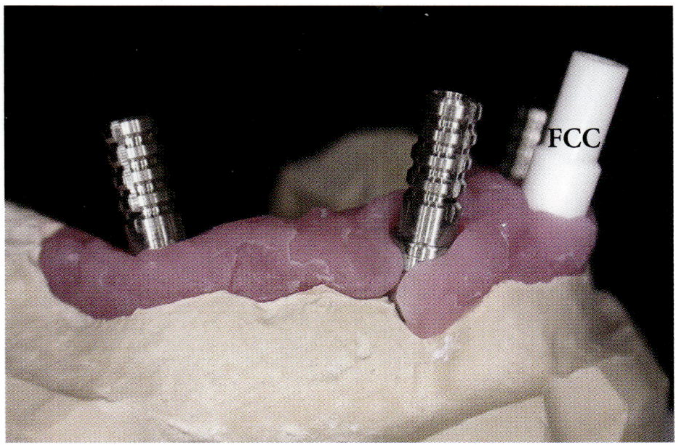

Fig 9.41 - The titanium cylinders were screwed into the analogs in the master cast. One full castable cylinder (FCC) is fitted to an analog to facilitate fabrication of a passively fitting implant framework.

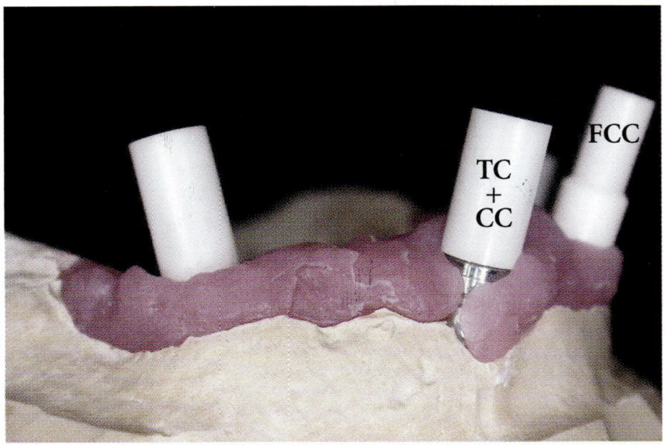

Fig 9.42 - The full castable cylinder (FCC) is chosen so that it is parallel to another titanium cylinder–castable cap assembly (TC + CC).

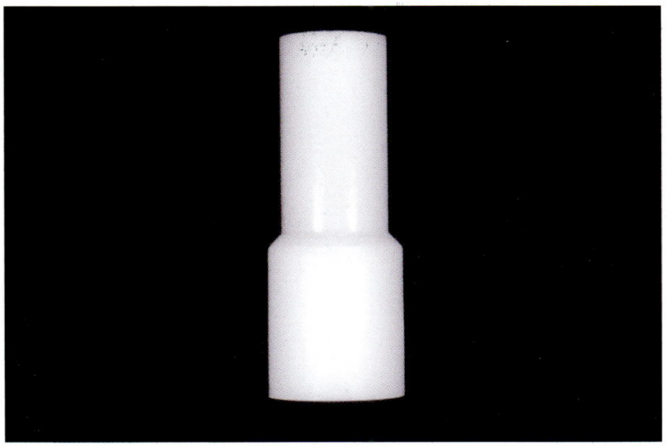

Fig 9.43 - Close-up image of the Full Castable Cylinder (FCC).

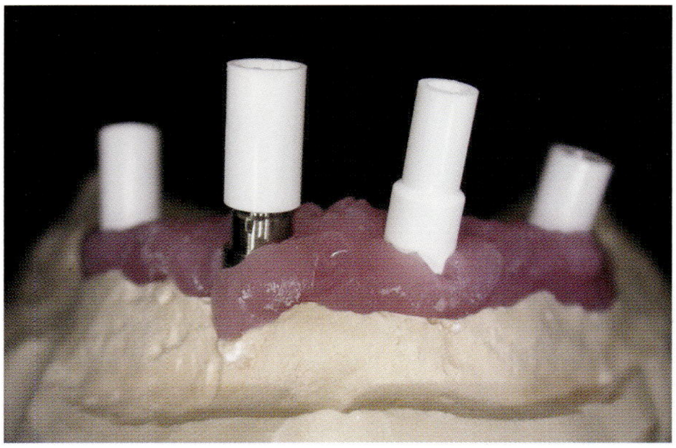

Fig 9.44 - The distal cylinders may not be completely parallel acording to the luting technique.

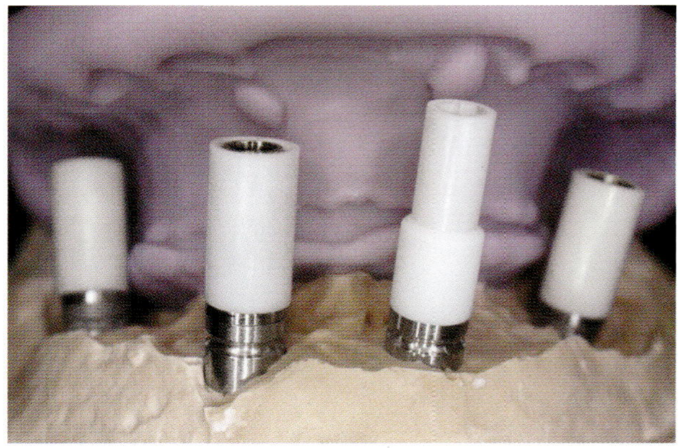

Fig 9.45 - Depending on the amount of available prosthetic space as determined by the palatal silicone index, the heights of the cylinders may be reduced.

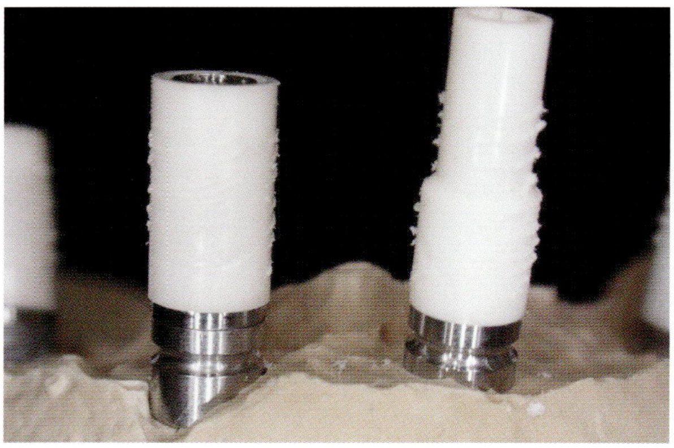

Fig 9.46 - The surfaces of the castable devices are roughened.

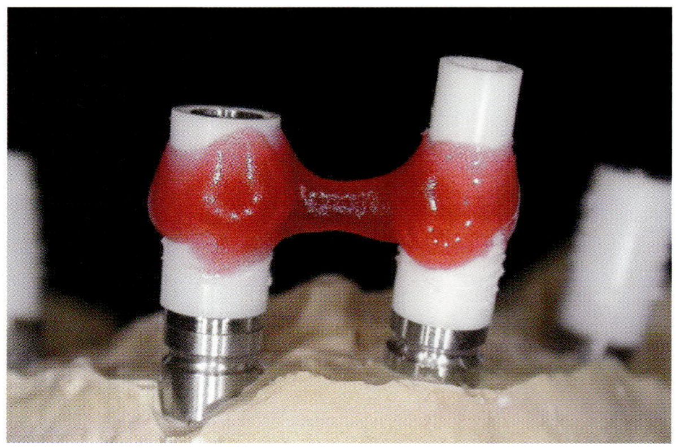

Fig 9.47 - The anterior castable devices are splinted together with a castable resin.

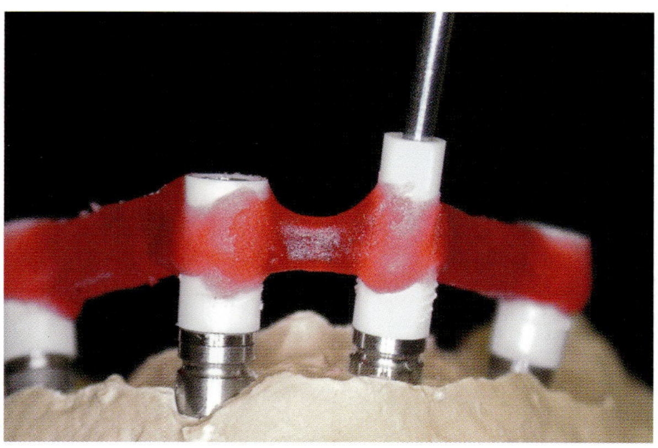

Fig 9.48 - After all the castable devices are splinted togheter with a castable resin.

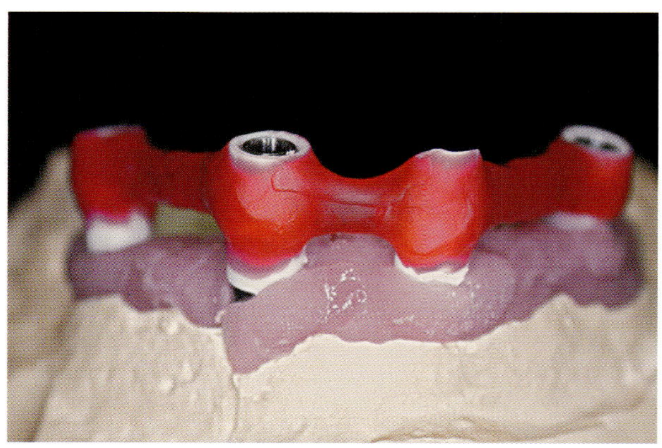

Fig 9.49 - The facial surfaces of the resin framework. The pattern may be modified with inlay wax to obtain the desired contours.

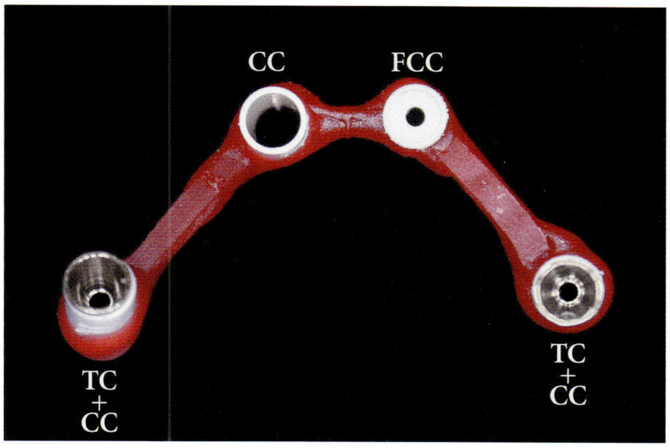

Fig 9.50 - The resin framework is unscrewed from the master cast. Note the distal nonparallel titanium cylinders inside the framework.

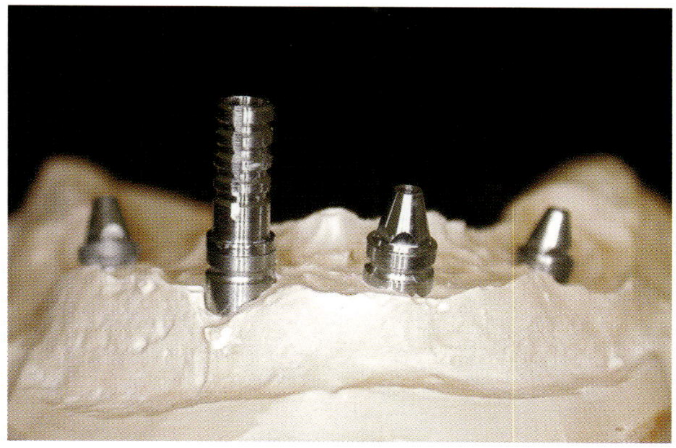

Fig 9.51 - The titanium cylinder in the maxillary left central incisor site. This titanium cylinder is parallel to the full castable cylinder and therefore does not interfere with insertion or removal of the framework resin pattern.

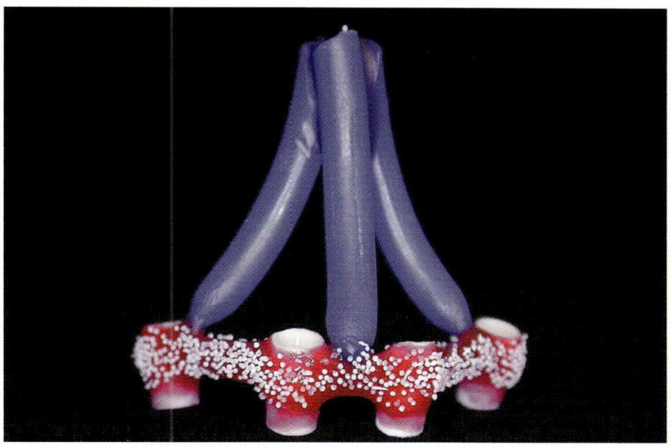

Fig 9.52 - The sprue design for the resin framework pattern. Micro-retention beads were applied to the resin pattern prior to spruing and investing.

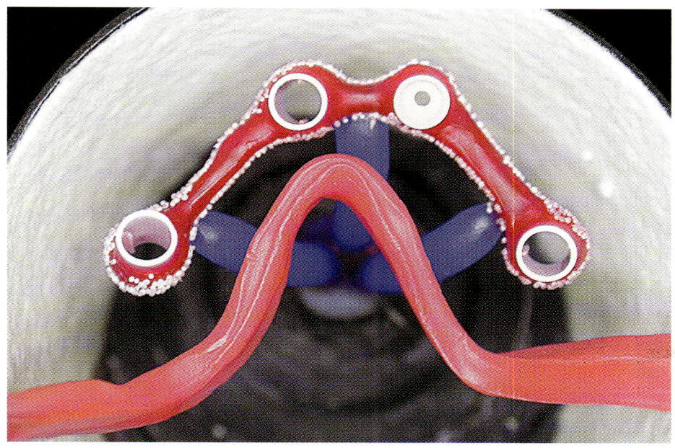

Fig 9.53 - The sprued resin pattern in the casting ring.

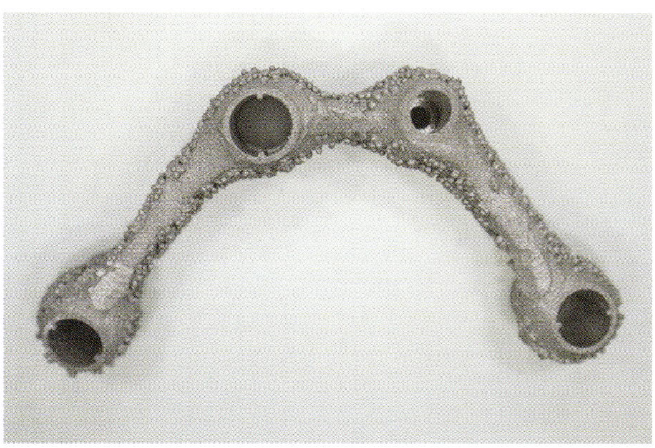

Fig 9.54 - The abutment restorative platforms of the casting. Note the opposing vertical relief areas in the casting corresponding to the relief areas within the castable cylinders.

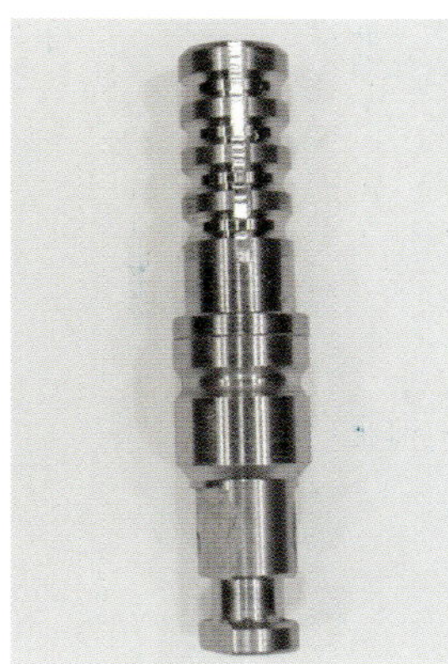

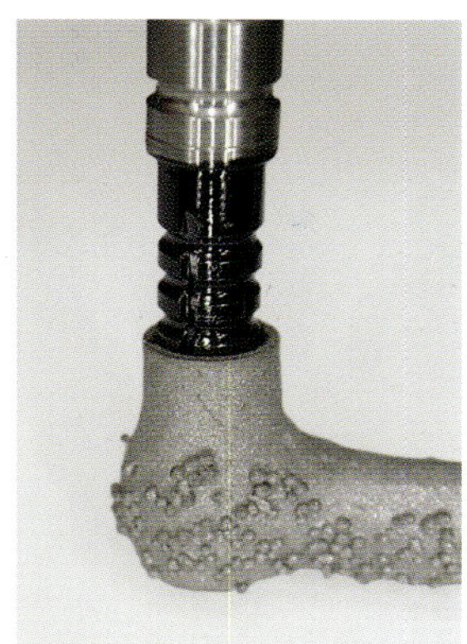

Figs 9.55 and 9.56 - A titanium cylinder in place on a conical abutment analog. The titanium cylinder is blackened with a black felt tip pen prior to being placed into the casting.

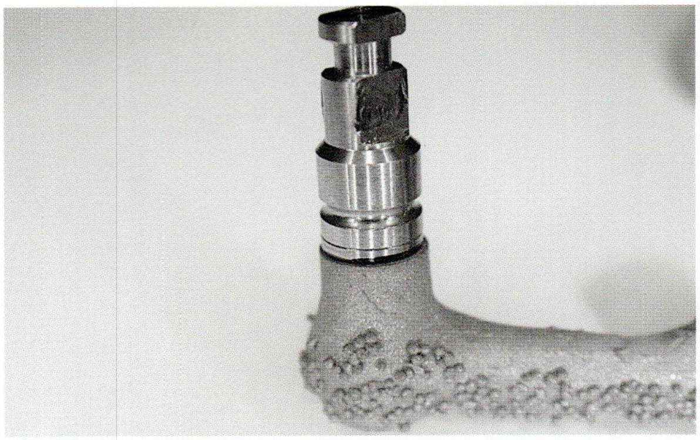

Fig 9.57 - Insertion of the titanium cylinder into the framework.

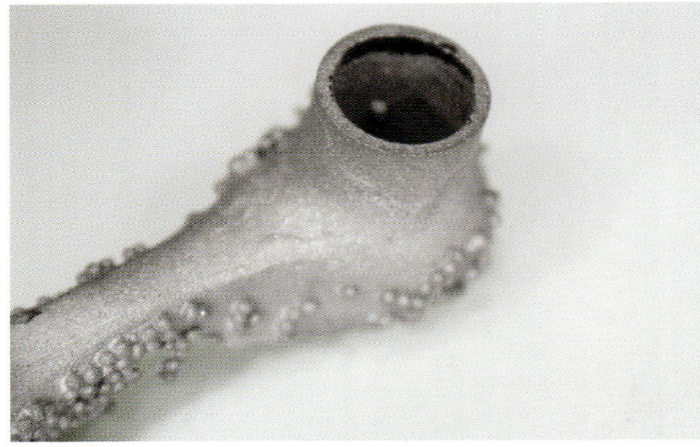

Fig 9.58 - The internal surface of the casting after the titanium cylinder is removed. Excess pressure markings are transferred from the cylinder to the internal surface of the casting.

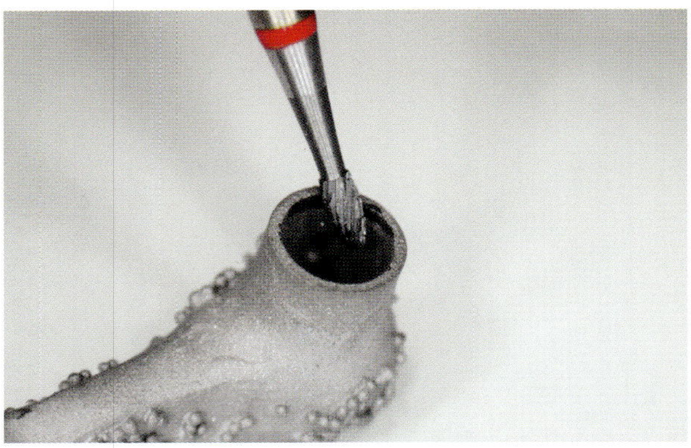

Fig 9.59 - The pressure spots are removed with a laboratory tungsten bur.

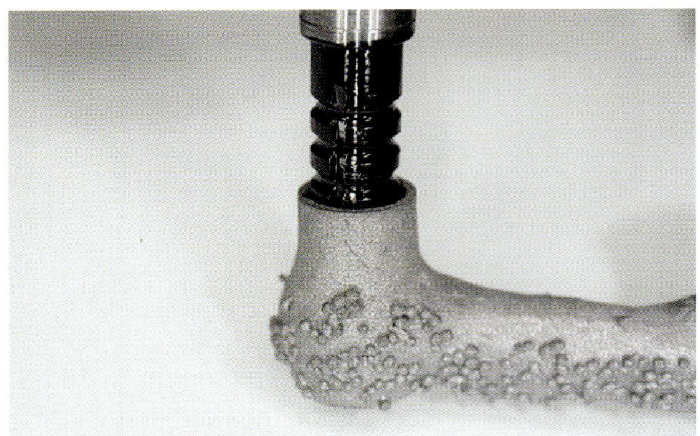

Fig 9.60 - The procedures illustrated in Figs 9-56 through 9-59 are repeated as needed so that the framework fits passively.

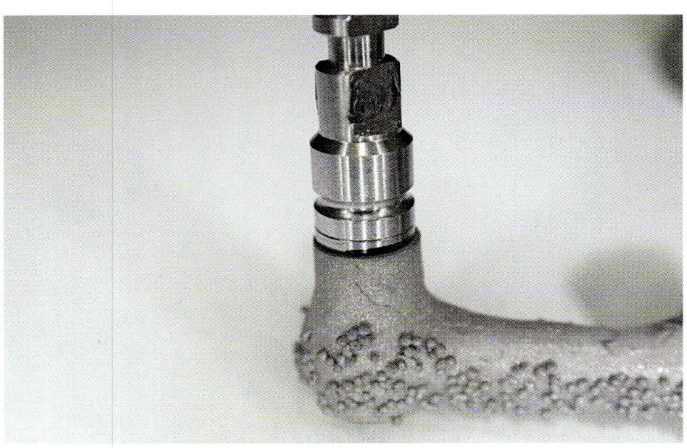

Fig 9.61 - The purpose of the laboratory adjustments is to obtain a frictional fit only on the two vertical relief portions of the casting.

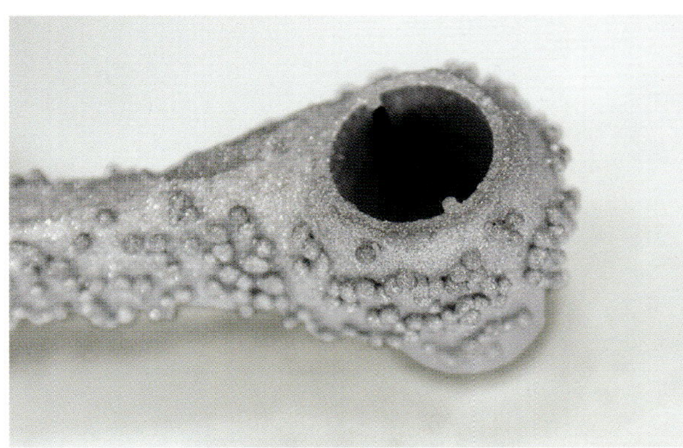

Fig 9.62 - Laboratory image of the internal surface of the casting. The only parts of the casting in contact with the titanium cylinder are the two vertical relief areas.

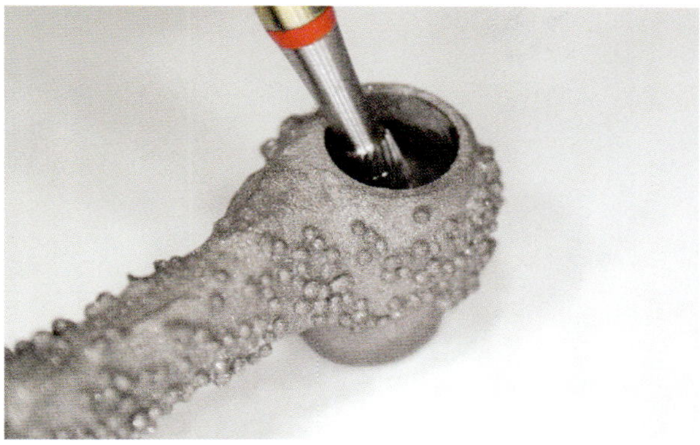

Fig 9.63 - After all of the adjustments have been made and only the vertical portions of the castings are in contact with the titanium cylinders, the vertical relief bars are removed.

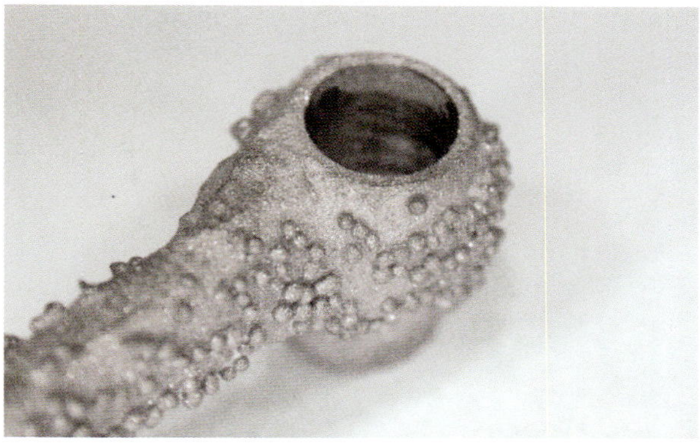

Fig 9.64 - Removal of the two vertical relief bars ensures that consistent relief of 0.2 mm has been obtained between the titanium cylinders and the framework.

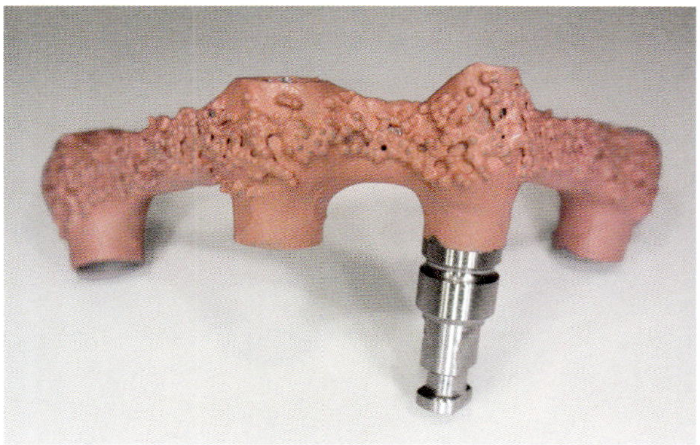

Fig 9.65 - The framework after it is opaqued.

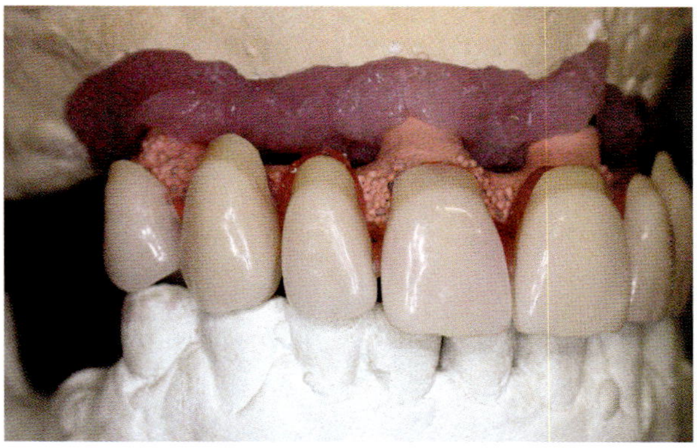

Fig 9.66 - Right lateral anterior view of the denture teeth set onto the framework in the mounted master cast. The denture teeth are set consistent with the location of the artificial teeth in the wax prosthesis using the silicone index that was previously made.

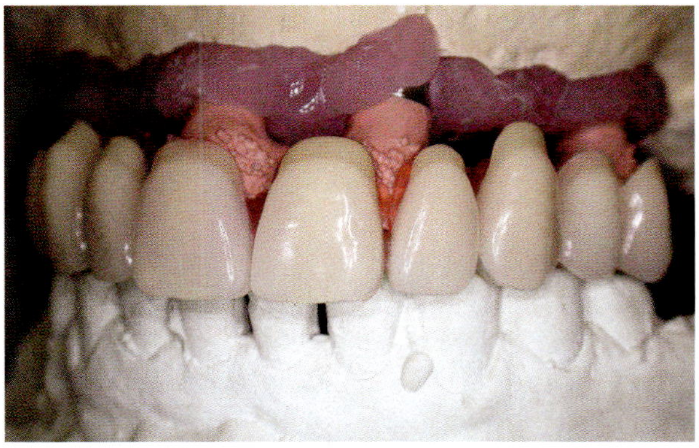

Fig 9.67 - Left lateral anterior view of the denture teeth set onto the framework in the mounted master cast.

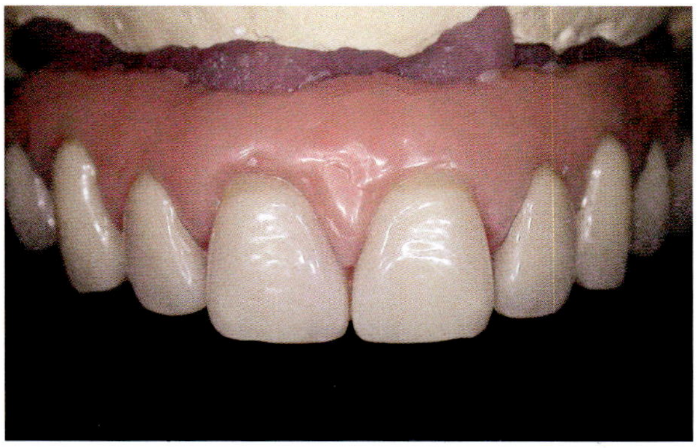

Fig 9.68 - The provisional wax implant prosthesis.

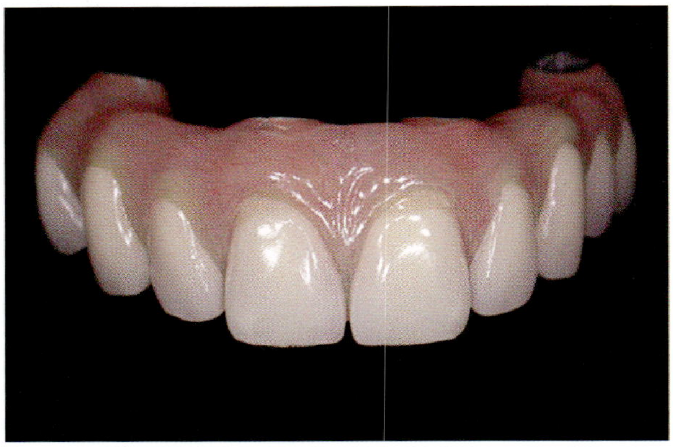

Fig 9.69 - The provisional implant prosthesis after it is finished and polished.

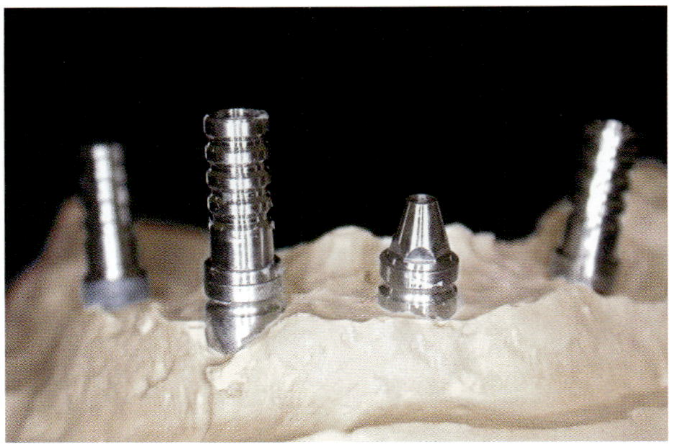

Fig 9.70 - Laboratory image that illustrates the beginning of the passivation process with the luting technique. Titanium cylinders are in place on the conical abutment analogs.

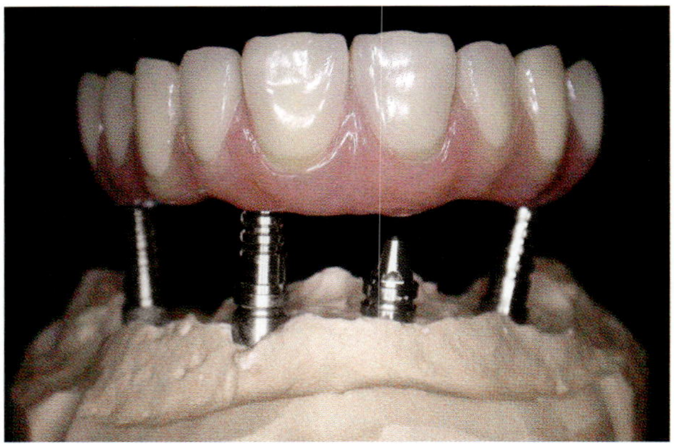

Fig 9.71 - The nonparallel orientation of the distal cylinders prevents the prosthesis from being simultaneously seated onto the three titanium cylinders.

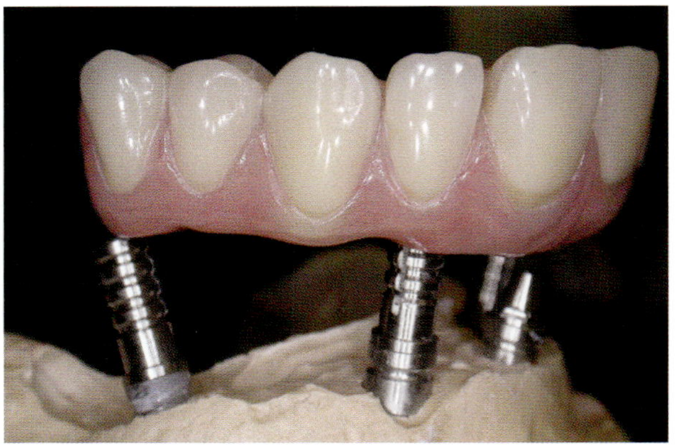

Fig 9.72 - Lateral image that demonstrates that the two cylinders on the patient's left side are actually divergent.

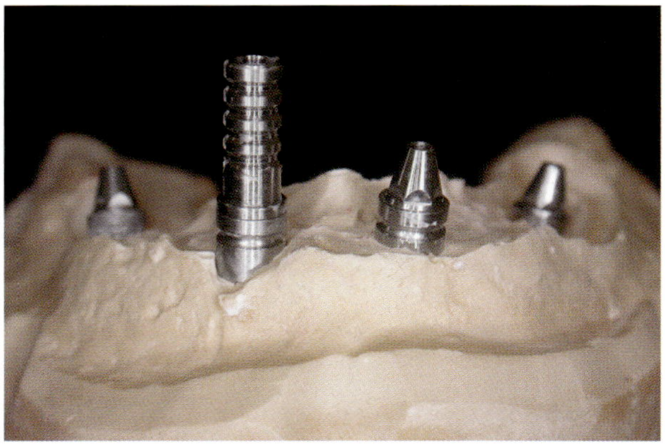

Fig 9.73 - Anterior image of the master cast after the nonparallel distal cylinders were removed from the conical abutment laboratory analogs. These were the cylinders that prevented the prosthesis from being seated on the cast.

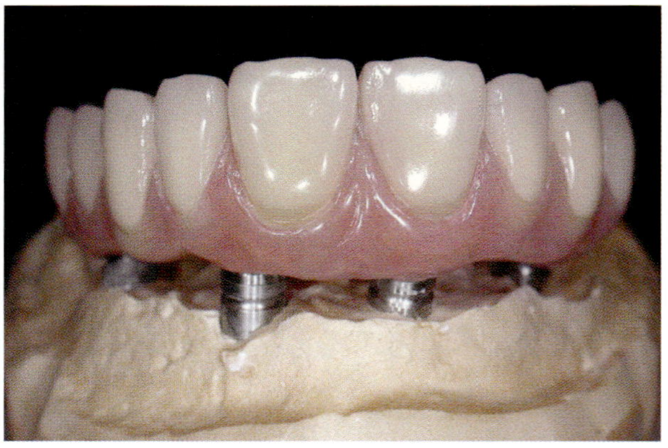

Fig 9.74 - Anterior image of the master cast after the nonparallel cylinders were removed from the conical abutment laboratory analogs. The prosthesis is completely seated on the titanium cylinder placed in the maxillary left central incisor implant site.

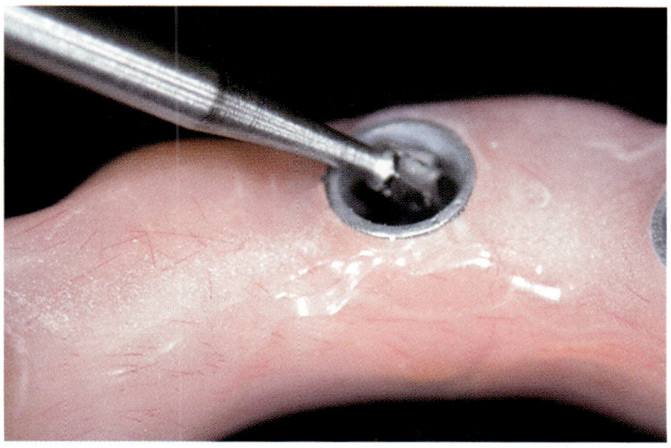

Fig 9.75 - The internal aspect of the metal framework; the internal surface was roughened with a round bur. This will improve cement retention between the titanium cylinder and the casting.

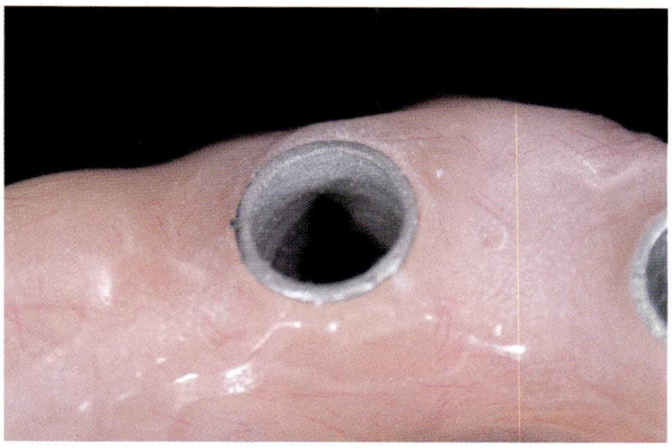

Fig 9.76 - The roughened internal surface of the metal framework.

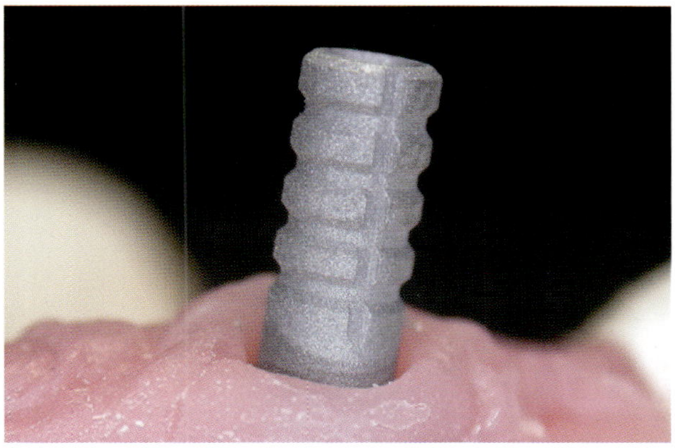

Fig 9.77 - The left mesial titanium cylinder after sandblasting. This will improve cement retention between the titanium cylinders and the casting.

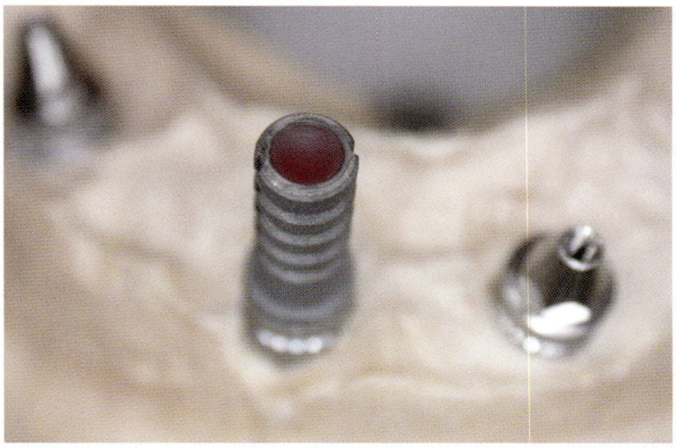

Fig 9.78 - Wax is placed into the screw access opening of the left mesial titanium cylinder.

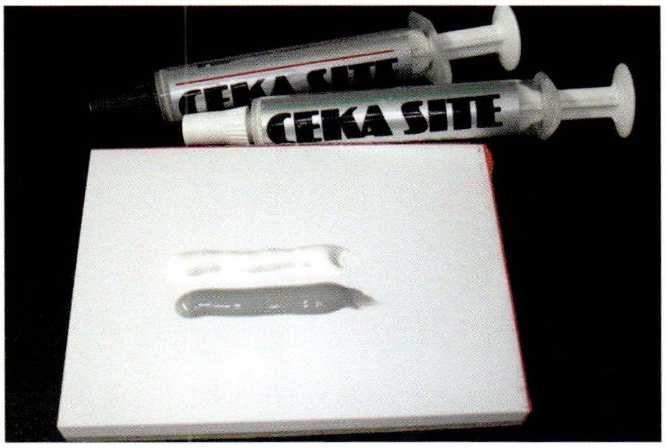

Fig 9.79 - Resin cement, mixed per the manufacturer's instructions, is the cement of choice for luting the titanium cylinder in the maxillary left central incisor site to the palladium alloy framework.

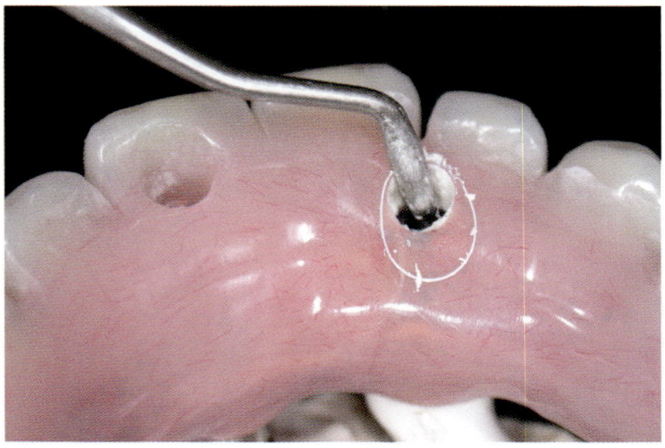

Fig 9.80 - The prosthesis is cemented to the titanium cylinder in the maxillary left central incisor implant site. Prior to the final set, the excess cement is removed from the prosthesis screw access opening to ensure access to the retaining screw.

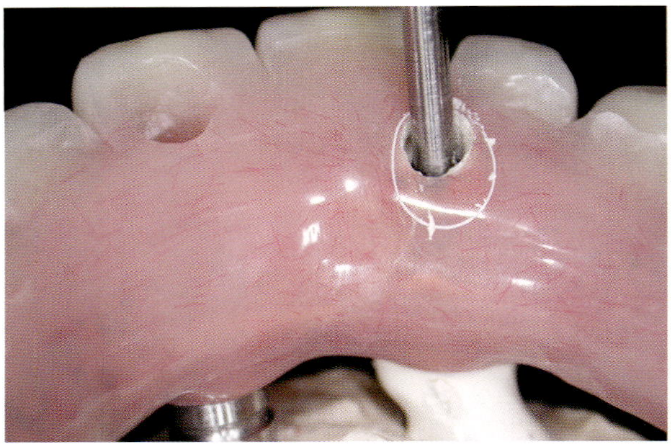

Fig 9.81 - The large hex driver used to remove the retaining screw at the maxillary left central incisor implant site.

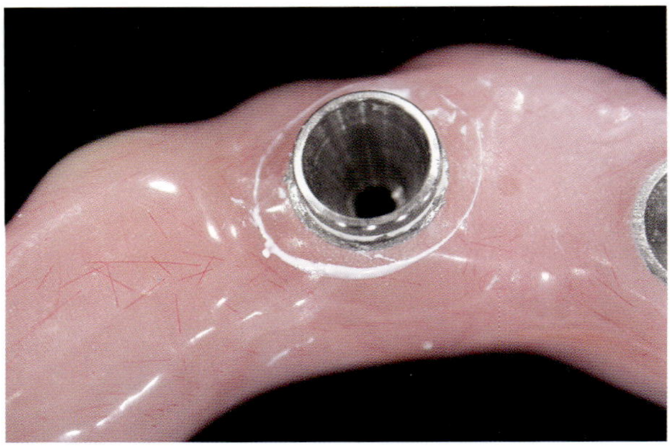

Fig 9.82 - Close-up image of the titanium cylinder–casting interface after luting passivation.

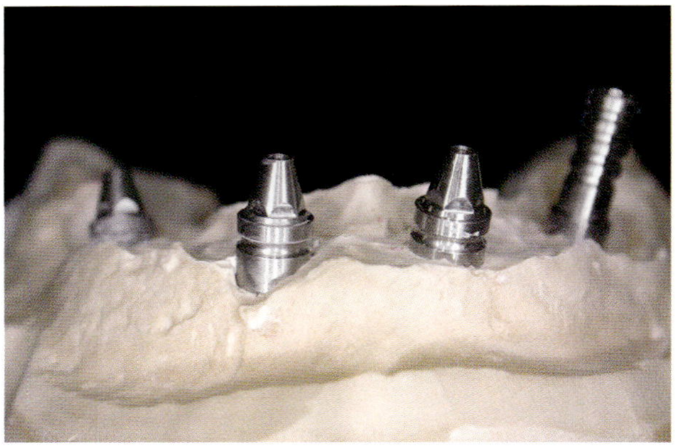

Fig 9.83 - The process illustrated in Figs 9.75 through 9.82 is repeated for the right distal titanium cylinder (maxillary right second premolar implant site).

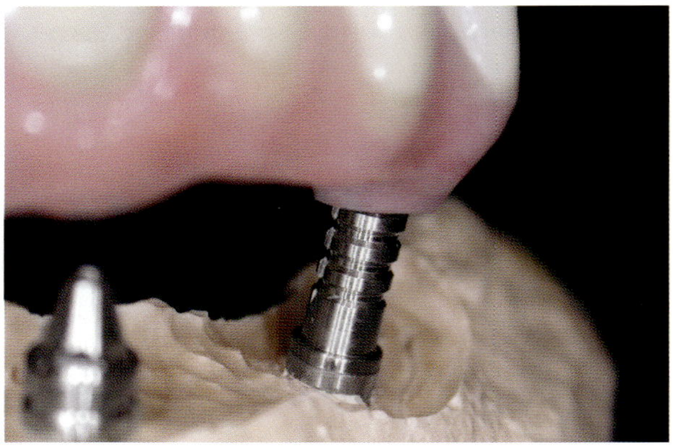

Fig 9.84 - The framework being seated onto the right distal titanium cylinder, cylinder three dimensional orientation.

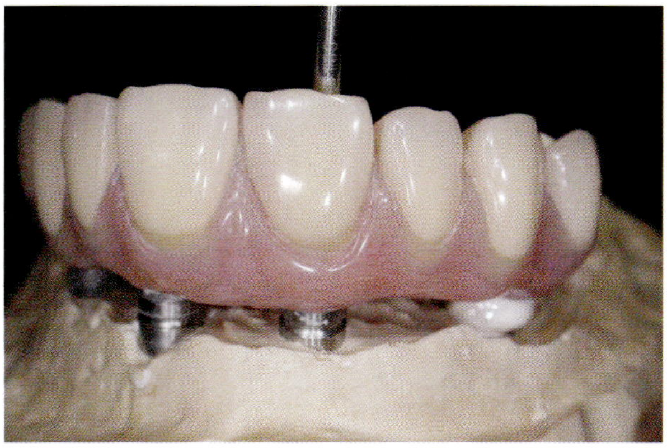

Fig 9.85 - The prosthesis in place on the analogs as the right distal titanium cylinder is being cemented to the casting. The prosthesis is retained to the anterior right implant site with a laboratory screw.

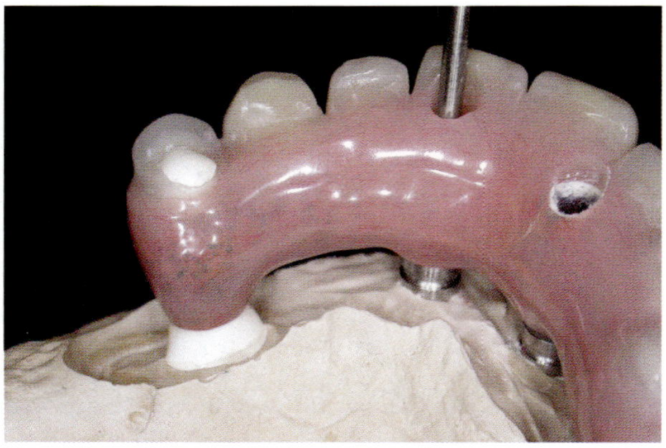

Fig 9.86 - Close-up image as the cement sets between the right distal titanium cylinder and the framework.

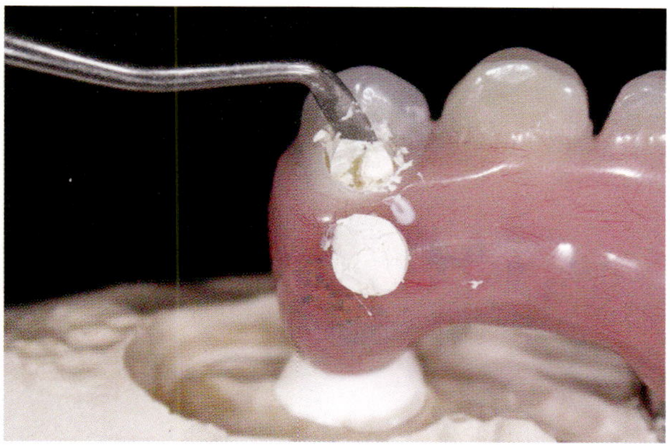

Fig 9.87 - The excess cement is removed after cementation.

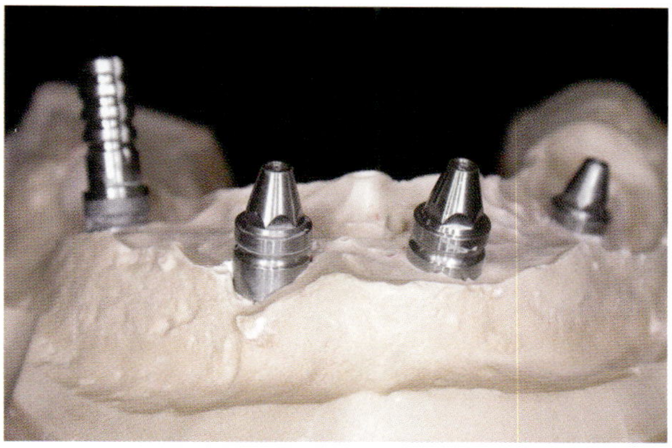

Fig 9.88 - The left distal titanium cylinder in place on the conical abutment laboratory analog prior to commencing the luting process.

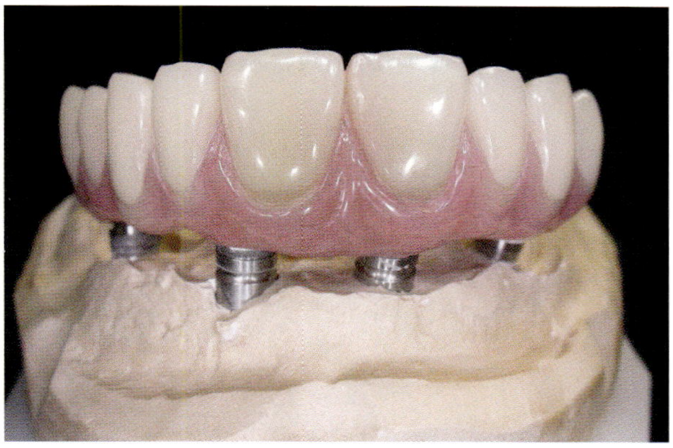

Fig 9.89 - The framework passively in place on the titanium cylinder in the maxillary left second premolar implant site.

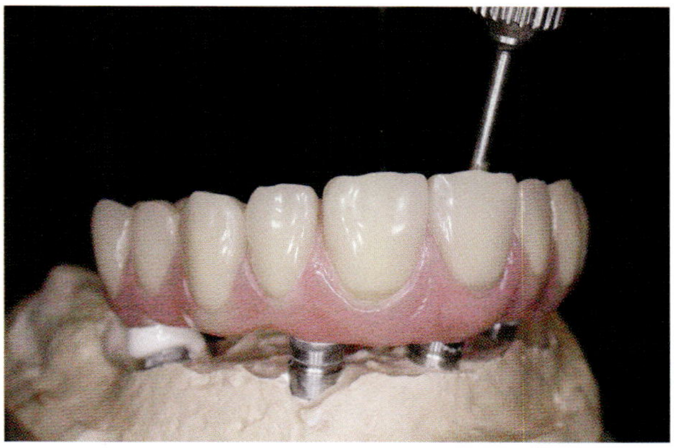

Fig 9.90 - The prosthesis in place on the analogs as the left distal titanium cylinder is being cemented to the casting. The prosthesis is retained to the anterior right implant with a laboratory screw.

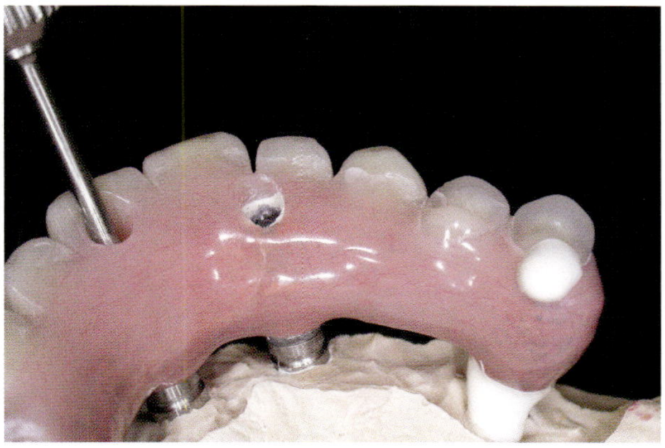

Fig 9.91 - Close-up image as the cement sets between the left distal titanium cylinder and the framework.

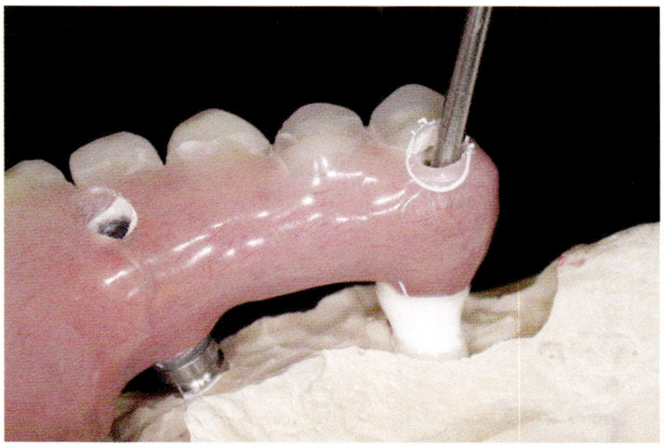

Fig 9.92 - The excess cement is removed after cementation.

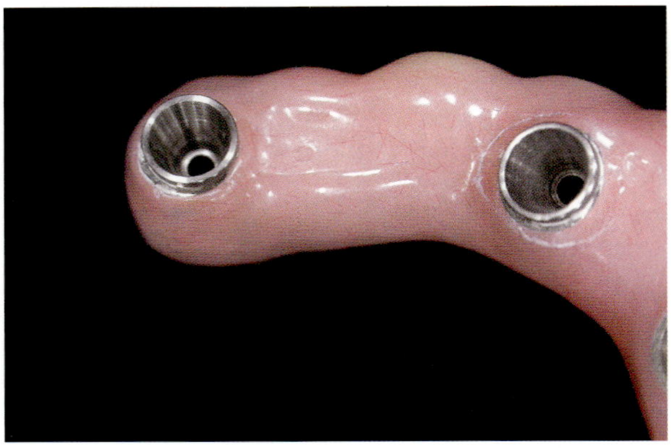

Fig 9.93 - The left intaglio surface of the fixed provisional prosthesis before final polishing.

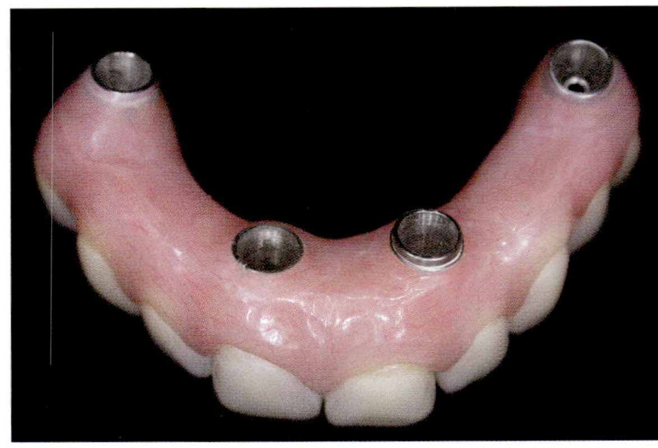

Fig 9.94 - The intaglio surface of the fixed screw-retained provisional prosthesis after final polishing.

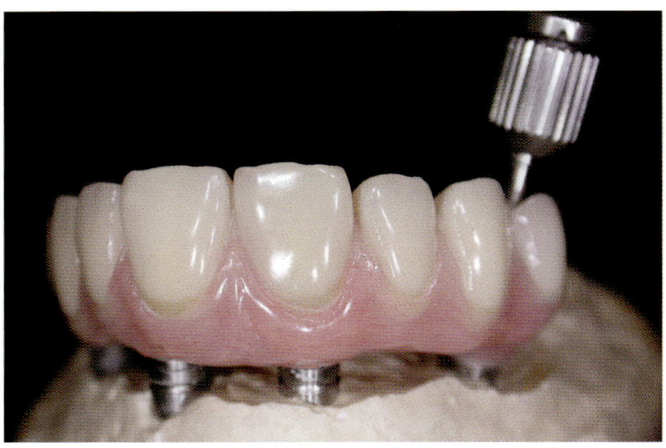

Fig 9.95 - Laboratory verification of the Sheffield one-screw test. A retaining screw is placed into the right distal screw access opening and hand tightened.

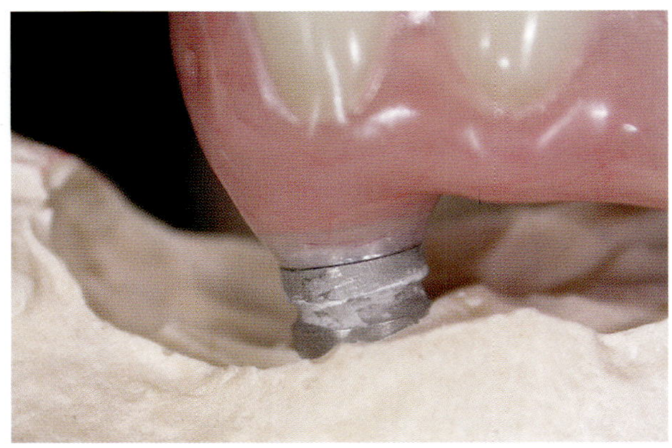

Fig 9.96 - Close-up of the cylinder-abutment interface on the patient's left side at the time Fig 9.95 was taken. Complete adaptation between the titanium cylinder in the framework and conical abutment laboratory analog is noted. This confirms that the prosthesis was completely and passively seated on the master cast.

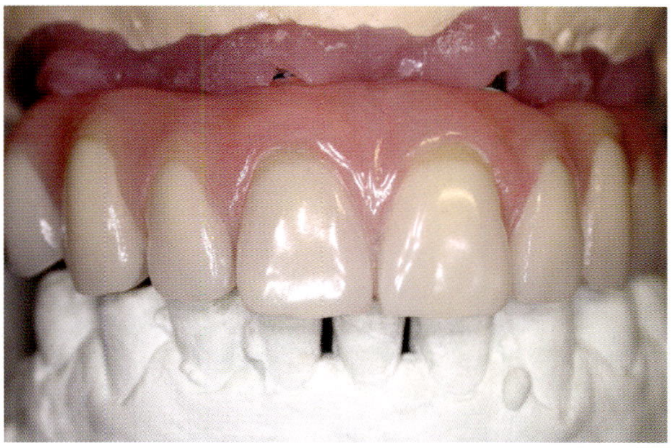

Fig 9.97 - Anterior view of the completed provisional prosthesis in place on the master cast in the articulator.

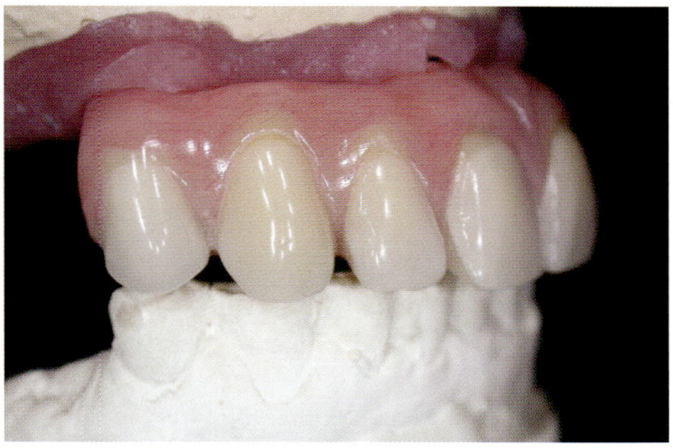

Fig 9.98 - Right posterior view of the completed provisional prosthesis in place on the master cast in the articulator.

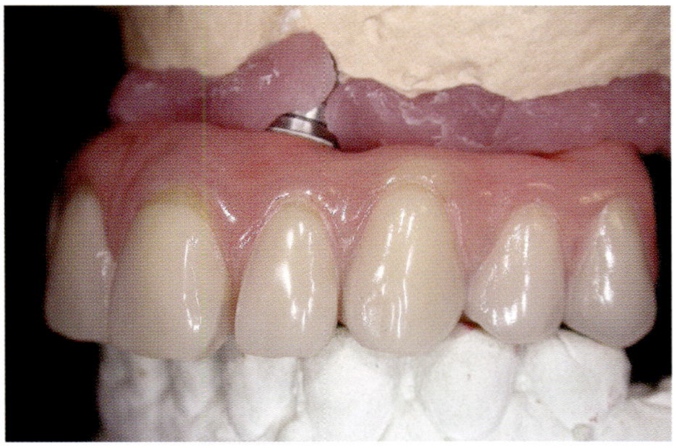

Fig 9.99 - Left posterior view of the completed provisional prosthesis in place on the master cast in the articulator.

REFERENCES

1. Timoshenko SP (ed). History of Strength of Materials. New York: Dover, 1983.
2. Maló P, Rangert B, Nobre M. All-on-4 immediate function concept with Brånemark System implants for completely edentulous maxillae: A 1-year retrospective clinical study. Clin Implant Dent Relat Res 2005;7(suppl 1):88S–94S.
3. Maló P, Nobre Mde A, Petersson U, Wigren S. A pilot study of complete edentulous rehabilitation with immediate function using a new implant design: Case series. Clin Implant Dent Relat Res 2006;8:223–232.
4. Brånemark PI, Engstrand P, Ohrnell LO, et al. Brånemark Novum: A new treatment concept for rehabilitation of the edentulous mandible. Preliminary results from a prospective clinical follow-up study. Clin Implant Dent Relat Res 1999;1:2–16.
5. Bergkvist G. Immediate loading of implants in the edentulous maxilla. Swed Dent J Suppl 2008;(196):10–75.
6. Grunder U. Immediate functional loading of immediate implants in edentulous arches: Two-year results. Int J Periodontics Restorative Dent 2001;21:545–551.
7. Wee AG, Aquilino SA, Schneider RL. Strategies to achieve fit in implant prosthodontics: A review of the literature. Int J Prosthodont 1999;12:167–178.
8. Nicholls JI. The measurement of distortion: Theoretical considerations. J Prosthet Dent 1977;37:578–586.
9. Nicholls JL. The measurement of distortion: Mathematical considerations. J Prosthet Dent 1978;39:339–343.
10. Nicholls JL. The measurement of distortion: Concluding remarks. J Prosthet Dent 1980;43:218–223.
11. Kallus T, Bessing C. Loose gold screws frequently occur in full-arch fixed prostheses supported by osseointegrated implants after 5 years. Int J Oral Maxillofac Implants 1994;9:169–178.
12. Michaels GC, Carr AB, Larsen PE. Effect of prosthetic superstructure accuracy on the osteointegrated implant bone interface. Oral Surg Oral Med Oral Pathol Oral Radiol Endod 1997;83:198–205.
13. Carr AB, Gerard DA, Larsen PE. The response of bone in primates around unloaded dental implants supporting prostheses with different levels of fit. J Prosthet Dent 1996;76:500–509.
14. Jemt T, Book K. Prosthesis misfit and marginal bone loss in edentulous implant patients. Int J Oral Maxillofac Implants 1996;11:620–625.
15. Jemt T, Bäck T, Petersson A. Precision of CNC-milled titanium frameworks for implant treatment in the edentulous jaw. Int J Prosthodont 1999;12:209–215.
16. Ortorp A, Linden B, Jemt T. Clinical experiences with laser-welded titanium frameworks supported by implants in the edentulous mandible: A 5-year follow-up study. Int J Prosthodont 1999;12:65–72.
17. Eisenmann E, Mokabberi A, Walter MH, Freesmeyer WB. Improving the fit of implant-supported superstructures using the spark erosion technique. Int J Oral Maxillofac Implants 2004;19:810–818.
18. Clelland NL, van Putten MC. Comparison of strains produced in a bone simulant between conventional cast and resin-luted implant frameworks. Int J Oral Maxillofac Implants 1997;12:793–799.
19. Voitik AJ. The Kulzer abutment luting; Kal technique. A direct assembly framework method for osseointegrated implant prostheses. Implant Soc 1991;2:11–14.
20. Stumpel LJ, Quon SJ. Adhesive abutment cylinder luting. J Prosthet Dent 1993;69:398–400.
21. Abduo J, Lyons K, Bennani V, Waddell N, Swain M. Fit of screw-retained fixed implant frameworks fabricated by different methods: A systematic review. Int J Prosthodont 2011;24:207–220.
22. Hollender L, Rockler B. Radiographic evaluation of osseointegrated implants of the jaws. Experimental study of the influence of radiographic techniques on the measurement of the relation between the implant and bone. Dentomaxillofac Radiol 1980;9:91–95.
23. Loos LG. A fixed prosthodontic technique for mandibular osseointegrated titanium implants. J Prosthet Dent. 1986;55:232–242.
24. Henry PJ. An alternative method for the production of accurate casts and occlusal records in osseointegrated implant rehabilitation. J Prosthet Dent 1987;58:694–697.
25. Jemt T. Failures and complications in 391 consecutively inserted fixed prostheses supported by Brånemark implants in edentulous jaws: A study of treatment from the time of prosthesis placement to the first annual checkup. Int J Oral Maxillofac Implants 1991;6:270–276.
26. Rappold AP, Ripps AH, Ireland EJ. Explorer sharpness as related to margin evaluations. Oper Dent 1992;17:2–6.
27. Jemt T. Fixed implant-supported prostheses in the edentulous maxilla. A five-year follow-up report. Clin Oral Implants Res 1994;5:142–147.
28. Jemt T. In vivo measurements of precision of fit involving implant-supported prostheses in the edentulous jaw. Int J Oral Maxillofac Implants 1996;11:151–158.
29. Brunski JB. Avoid pitfalls of overloading and micromotion of intraosseous implants. Dent Implantol Update 1993;4:77–81.
30. White G. Osseointegrated Dental Technology. London: Quintessence, 1993.

CHAPTER 10

CHOICE OF OCCLUSAL MATERIALS IN IMPLANT PROSTHODONTICS

COLUMBUS BRIDGE PROTOCOL	
SURGICAL PROTOCOL	**PROSTHETIC PROTOCOL**
External hex rough-surface implants	Screw-retained fixed prosthesis
Implant length ≥ 13 mm, Ø 4 mm	Plaster impression with pickup technique
Underprepared osteotomy	Rigid splinting with metal framework
Implant insertion torque ≥ 40 Ncm	Passive fit with the luting technique
Angled implants in native bone	Acrylic resin occlusal surfaces
Angled conical abutments	No distal cantilevers
No bone regenerative techniques	Immediate functional load 24–48 h after surgery

Table 10.1

Currently, the most widely used occlusal materials in implant prosthodontic treatment are ceramics, composite resins, and acrylic resins. When selecting occlusal materials for implant prosthodontics, several factors, including esthetics, abrasion resistance, fracture resistance, surface roughness, and ability to absorb occlusal forces, need to be considered by clinicians.

Ceramics are nonmetallic inorganic materials consisting of molecular chains with repeating crystalline structures. The various types of ceramic can be distinguished according to composition, firing temperature, and manufacturing process. Ceramics provide optimal esthetics–similar to the appearance of natural teeth–and higher abrasion resistance compared with resins. Furthermore, ceramic restorations exhibit low surface roughness and are less likely to accumulate plaque. The only disadvantage is that they can be quite rigid, with a lower fracture resistance compared with more elastic materials such as acrylic resin.[1,2]

Composite resins are restorative materials that consist of three parts: *(1)* a matrix (organic phase or basic resin); *(2)* a filler (dispersed inorganic phase); and *(3)* a bonding agent (intermediate phase connecting the matrix to the filler). In most cases, the matrix consists of bisphenol glycidyl methacrylate (bis-GMA; Bowen resin) or urethane dimethacrylate (UDMA). The resin monomers are capable of assembling the three-dimensional reticulated polymers (phenomenon of polymerization) when activated with physical (ultraviolet or visible light) or chemical methods. The fillers consist mainly of mineral particles dispersed throughout the matrix; fillers are manufactured with various shapes and dimensions. The quantity and dimensions of the fillers directly and significantly affect the esthetic and mechanical properties of the composite material. The bonding agent generally consists of silane.[3,4]

Composite resins have esthetic properties comparable to those of ceramic materials except that they are not as color-stable; composite resins are subject to intraoral discoloration. Composite resins have less abrasion resistance (even if remarkably improved in last generation composites[5-10]) than ceramic materials but possess higher fracture resistance due to a lower modulus of elasticity. The lower elastic modulus makes composite resins less fragile than ceramic materials and better enables them to absorb occlusal forces, which reduces the forces transmitted to the underlying structures (specifically, abutments and implants).[11,12]

Acrylic resins are resin materials that are not enriched with fillers. Acrylic resins have decreased esthetics compared with either ceramic materials or composite resins, and they have worse mechanical properties. Acrylic resins have significantly less resistance to abrasion, but are more elastic than ceramic materials or composite resins. These characteristics can be advantageous in implant prosthodontics, especially in cases of immediate loading, by reducing the stresses transmitted to peri-implant bone. Among other disadvantages it has been demonstrated that these resins attract bacterial adhesion and possess chromatic instability.[13]

The materials described above may be used in the fabrication of fixed partial prostheses with or without metal substructure support. Metal substructures provide less than optimal esthetic but improved mechanical properties.

Gold alloys are one of the various metals commonly used for implant frameworks, and in non-esthetic zones, they can be used without esthetic veneering materials. Gold alloy restorations include inlays, onlays, crowns, and fixed partial dentures. Gold alloys are metals with high corrosion and oxidation resistance. They have been classified into four distinct groups[14]: soft, medium, hard, and extra hard. Gold alloys offer multiple advantages:

- Modulus of elasticity and hardness similar to those of natural enamel[15]
- High biocompatibility
- High mechanical resistance
- High resistance to abrasion
- Low tendency to abrade the opposing dentition

The main limitation is their lack of esthetics; the gold color is often visible during speaking, smiling, or when resting.[13]

Increased esthetic demands by patients have led researchers to develop metal-free prostheses,[16] ie, prostheses made without metal substructures. One of the materials most recently developed for use as a rigid substructure in this type of prosthesis is zirconia, which offers excellent mechanical and esthetic properties for this purpose as well as high biocompatibility.[17,18] Zirconia is a ceramic material stabilized with yttrium oxide (Y_2O_3) to obtain high levels of molecular stability (yttrium tetragonal zirconia polycrystals).[19] When stress is applied to the surface of a zirconia restoration, the material undergoes a change in crystalline form, from tetragonal to monocline, which results in a 3% to 5% volumetric increase in the material.[16] This crystalline change decreases fracture propagation. Zirconia is not as esthetic as other ceramic materials used in dental restorations because it is opaque. Because its mechanical properties are similar to those of metals, however, zirconia can be used for abutments in implant and conventional fixed prosthodontics. Furthermore, less bacterial adhesion has been reported on zirconia than has been reported on titanium.[20,21]

The main characteristics of the materials described above are listed in Table 10.2.

TABLE 10.2

Characteristics	Zirconia	Ceramic	Gold alloy	Composite resin	Acrylic resin
Esthetics	high	high	low	medium	low
Abrasion coefficent	low	low	low	medium	high
Elasticity	low	low	medium	medium	high
Plaque accumulation	low	low	low	medium	high

Table 10.2 - Main characteristics of the most widely used restorative materials.

SHOCK ABSORPTION CAPACITY OF RESTORATIVE MATERIALS

The international literature has reported that the maintenance of osseointegration–and therefore the long-term survival of endosseous implants–is related to how occlusal loads are transmitted to implants during implant-prosthetic treatment.[22-27] In natural teeth, the periodontal ligament provides a semielastic connection between teeth and bone, absorbing loads applied to the teeth with a capacity called *shock absorption*. Because implants do not possess a periodontal ligament, when osseointegration occurs, implants achieve a direct bone-implant connection (ankylosis).[27,28] In implant prosthodontics, therefore, occlusal loads are transmitted directly from implants to peri-implant bone without an intermediate shock-absorbing medium.[29] Noxious microfractures in peri-implant bone[27] can be created with occlusal overload. As a result, it is particularly important to avoid overload to prevent damage to peri-implant bone.[30]

Many studies have focused on the effects of prosthetic restorative materials in absorbing occlusal stresses and in the long-term success of implant treatment.[22,27,29,31–48]

In the 1980s, engineer Richard Skalak,[29] a collaborator of Brånemark, emphasized the importance of using occlusal materials with shock-absorbing capacities in implant treatment. He stated that this would help to protect the bone from damages associated with occlusal overload. Shock-absorbing materials such as acrylic resin have a low elastic modulus, meaning that they are less rigid. These materials reduce the maximum value of forces transmitted through implants to bone by distributing the loads applied at the occlusal surface of the implant prosthesis over an extended period of time (Fig 10.1).

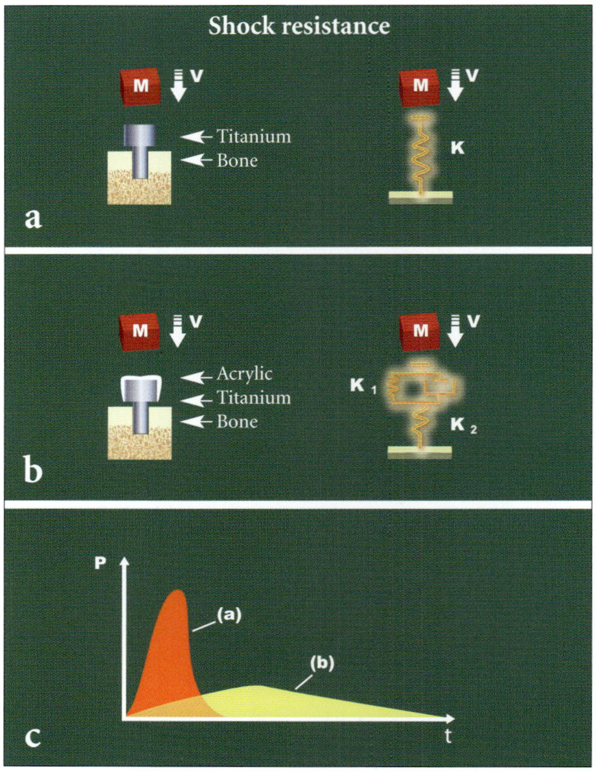

Fig 10.1 - *(a)* The impact of mass (M) at the speed (V) on a partial fixed prosthesis on one osseointegrated implant. The system acts as a rigid spring according to the Young modulus (K). *(b)* Acrylic resin has been added as a veneering material to the metal abutment. The resin interface responds as an elastic spring per the Young modulus (K_2). *(c)* A graph of force (P) over time (t) following impact. The impulse (*area beneath the curves*) is identical in the both cases (a, without acrylic resin; b, with acrylic resin), but the amount of force in the second case (b), with the acrylic resin veneer, was much lower. (Reprinted from Skalak[29] with permission).

Other authors have confirmed this theory with in vitro research, mainly performed with the finite elements method.[22,31–35]

A review of the literature over the last 15 years, however, demonstrated that many articles refute the existence of a relationship between prosthetic restorative material and transmission of stresses at the peri-implant level.[27,36–45] Some of these studies have used photoelastic models; some have used finite element analysis;[27,36,37] and still others have tested samples with Instron machines.[38] These studies have several limitations. They do not accurately reproduce the mandibular kinematics. Photoelastic models and finite element analysis are static and virtual tests, respectively. Instron machines perform intermittent movements in only a single plane. They do not replicate the same masticatory cycle that occurs clinically with mastication.

An experiment conducted on beagle dogs[39] did not show any clinical, radiographic, or histologic differences between peri-implant tissues surrounding prosthetic restorations made with composite resin versus those made with ceramic materials. However, this study did not control the amount of force exerted onto the implants, and dogs do not replicate human mastication. Other in vivo studies[40–42] have measured masticatory forces transmitted through various restorative materials without finding significant differences in the results.

This type of test requires that sensors and memory boards be applied intraorally, which raises several concerns. For instance, this type of testing may alter the masticatory cycles of the study participants and therefore may distort the results. Moreover, the technique is not conducive to studying humans over long experimental times, and the masticatory cycles are not identical. In addition, it is not possible to directly measure the forces transmitted to the bone-implant interface. Other authors,[43,44] without denying that ceramics and composite resins may provide different amounts of shock absorption, conclude that this does not result in clinically significant differences.

The above studies yielded inconsistent results and suggest that further research is necessary for clinicians and technicians to have a better understanding of forces, shock absorption, and impact on peri-implant bone.

Investigators at the University of Genoa[11,12] conducted an in vitro experiment to evaluate masticatory stresses transmitted through implants from prostheses made with different materials. The objective was to determine whether the stress transmitted by the implant prosthesis to the adjacent bone was higher in restorations made with zirconia or ceramic material versus restorations made with gold alloy, composite resin, or acrylic resin.

This investigation required the development of a mechatronic system—a "masticatory robot" that reproduced mandibular movements in three planes of space as well as the loads produced during mastication (Fig 10.2). The masticatory robot consists of a kinematic parallel structure to overcome the limits of the previously described research by re-creating in a laboratory setting reproducible mandibular movements in three dimensions and the loads exerted during mastication. Identical mandibular movements could be created for repeatability of the test. The amount of force transmitted to the peri-implant bone simulated around the implant was recorded and correlated with the type of occlusal material used in the prosthesis.

The robot was constructed in cooperation with Graal Tech Society of Genoa, Italy, and was financed by the Ministry of Instruction, University and Research in the scope of a Project of Research of National Interest (2002). The robot consists of an upper fixed portion that simulates the skull and maxilla; the inferior portion consists of a mobile robotic part, commonly called the *Stewart platform*, with parallel kinematic structure and six degrees of freedom. The robot was designed to reproduce functional mandibular movements commonly seen in normal masticatory function and to allow the execution of loading tests and stress on the material (Fig 10.3).

The mobile portion of the masticatory robot consists of a rigid upper body, or moving platform, which is connected to a fixed base by means of six identical kinematic legs arranged symmetrically to form two equilateral triangles on the fixed base. Every leg is equipped with universal joints at both ends, in parallel, that connect it to the fixed base and to the moving platform. Every leg consists of two steel cylinders connected by a cylindric joint. Linear motors adjust the upper and the lower bodies, which allow the leg lengths to vary independently of one another. By varying the lengths of the six legs, it is possible to vary the position

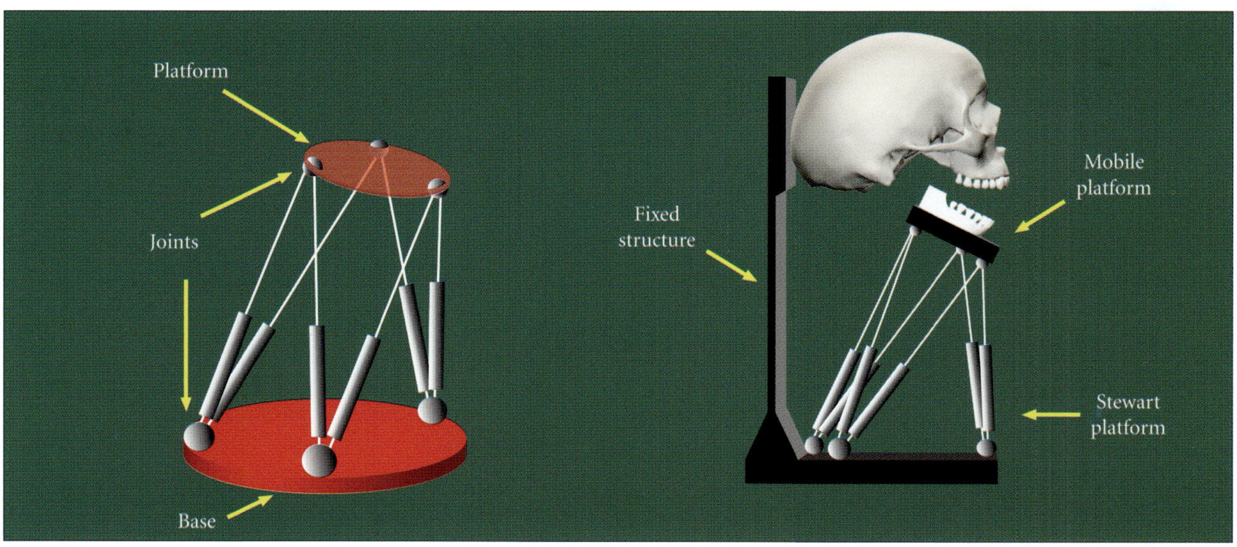

Fig 10.2 - Diagram of the masticatory robot.

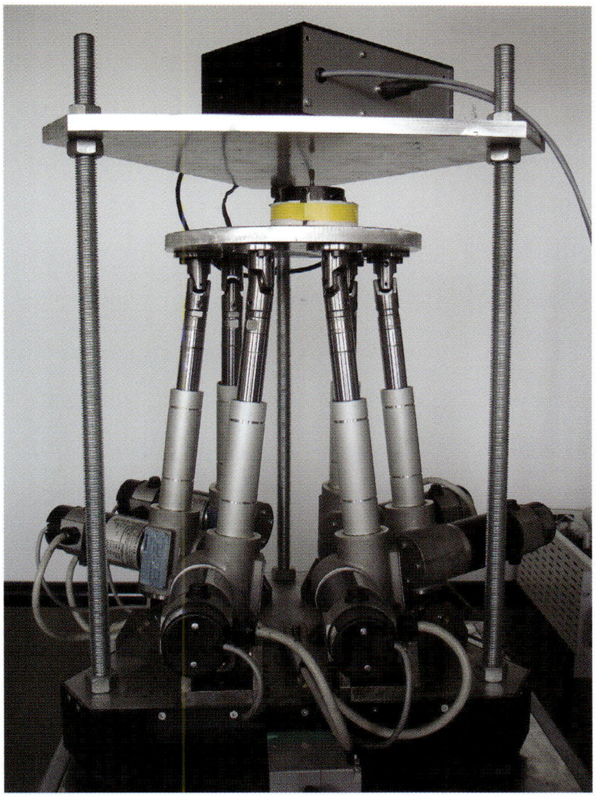

Fig 10.3 - The sensor-equipped masticatory robot.

and orientation of the platform with six degrees of freedom (three degrees of freedom in rotation; three degrees of freedom in translation). The movements are accurate to 0.1 mm. This system controls the movement of the platform but not the application of predefined loads. Loads are controlled indirectly by means of a sensor-equipped base that is fixed to the mobile platform (Fig 10.4). The sensors detect the amount of the forces transmitted to the x (laterolateral), y (anteroposterior), and z (vertical) axes.

A pin fixed to the base with the sensors (Fig 10.5) simulates the abutment-fixture complex and supports the test samples. Samples are stressed in the various planar directions. During the tests they occlude with the flat surface of the upper, fixed part of the robot.

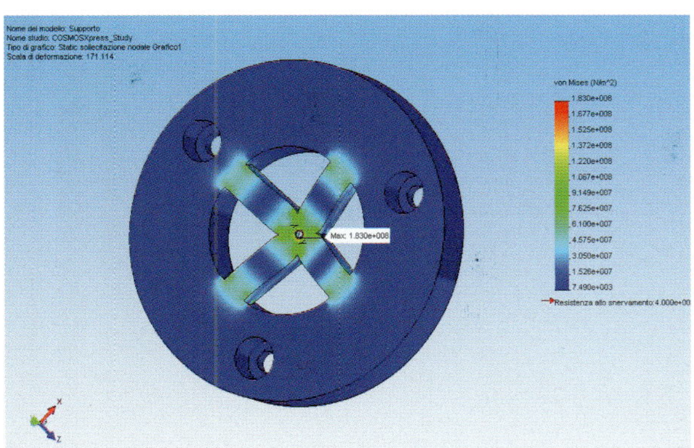

Fig 10.4 - Analysis of the behavior of the sensor-equipped base submitted to loads on the finished elements. The application of a force of 80 kg on the z-axis (vertical) on the support was simulated to visualize the consequent deformation. The image demonstrates the zone of maximum stress and verified the model near the maximum load applied.

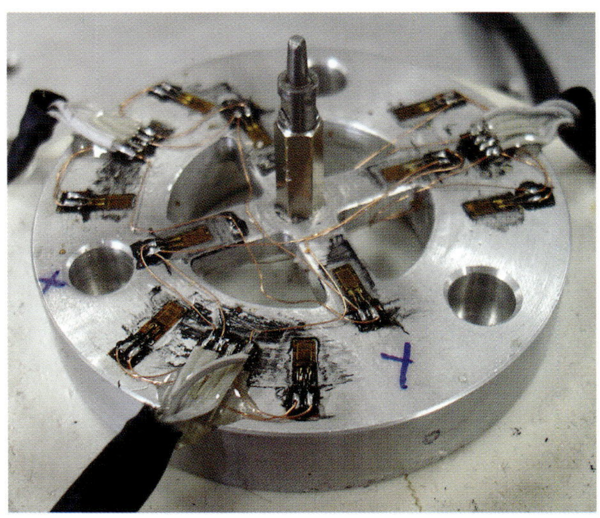

Fig 10.5 - The sensor-equipped base (simulating peri-implant bone) with a pin (simulating implant and abutment) supporting the sample crowns.

The base for the sensors has been designed with a computer-aided design/computer-assisted manufacture (CAD/CAM) program and underwent finite element analysis with the COSMOSXpress (SolidWorks). The finite element analysis was used to determine the position for placement of the strain gauges. The base can bear a maximum load of 80 kg on the vertical z axis without plastic deformation (see Fig 10.4).

This electromechanical system was connected to computers that send signals to the masticatory robot and allow the result to be visualized and recorded during the tests. The NI LabVIEW 5.0 program (National Instruments) was used for the tests. Prior to starting the tests, a baseline position was chosen (position zero) for the masticatory robot that defined the restoration and implant within the three planes of space. This step was consistently performed prior to any testing. This position was chosen because it allowed the transmission of loads inside a physiologic range of forces and would not damage the sensors in the base. The masticatory robot was programmed to perform a trajectory (Fig 10.6) traced according to the average displacement of the mandibular intraincisive point in three planes, as well as the mean velocity of every phase of the masticatory cycle for subjects in normal function, recorded with the aid of kinesiographic instruments.[49,50] This trajectory was repeated in all tests described in this study. The robot executed a masticatory cycle every 2 seconds.

The materials tested are reported in Table 10.3 and include the following:

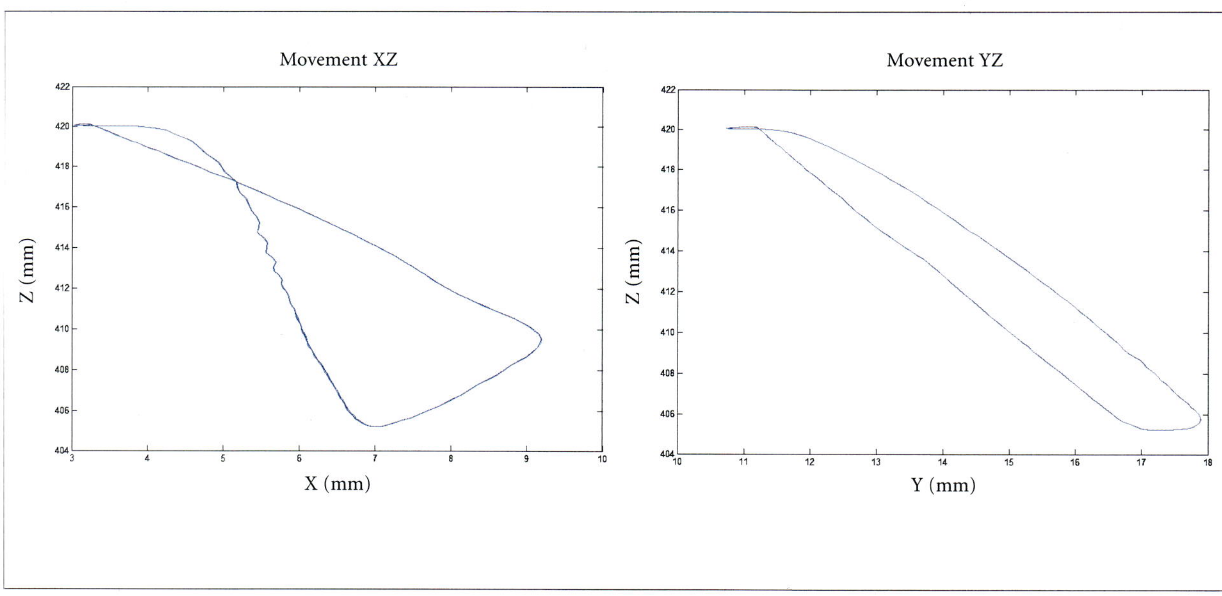

Fig 10.6 - Illustrations of the trajectory executed by the masticatory robot: frontal plane *(left)* and sagittal plane *(right)*.

- Zirconia with the occlusal surface restored with a ceramic material (Procera Zirconia and NobelRondo, Nobel Biocare)
- A glass ceramic (Empress 2, Ivoclar Vivadent)
- A gold alloy (Ney-Oro CB, Dentsply)
- Two composite resins:
  - Experience (DEI Italia)
  - Signum (Heraeus Kulzer)
- An acrylic resin (Easytemp 2, DEI Italia)

Two identical crowns were made for each material to be tested (Fig 10.7). One crown was to be used in the test; the second crown was to be used only if the first crown was damaged. The first sample crowns were made from glass ceramic (Empress 2). These samples were duplicated in different resin materials using the printing technique for photopolymerizable materials with transparent muffle,[51] which re-created the morphology of the original crown.

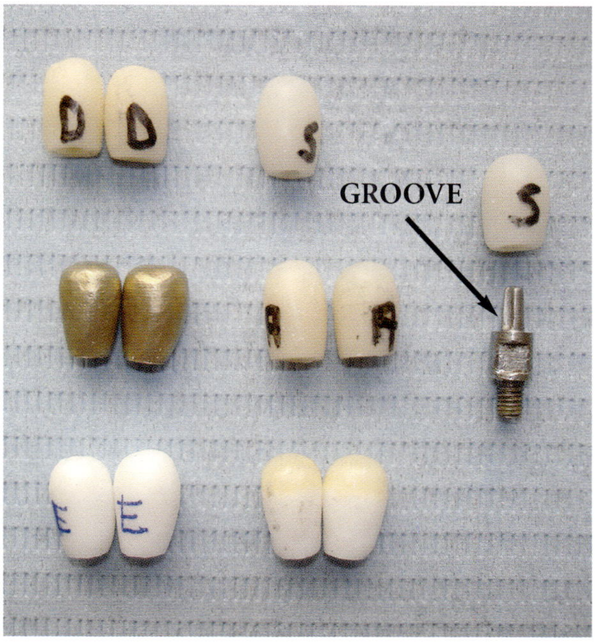

Fig 10.7 - Pin and sample crowns. The pin, which simulates the abutment-implant system, shows the groove that matches the ridge made on the inside of the samples, so that the crowns fit snugly onto the pin without possibility of rotation during the test phase.

TABLE 10.3 - MODULE OF ELASTICITY OF THE TESTED MATERIALS

Materials tested	Modulus of elasticity (MPa)
Procera Zirconia	210,000
Empress 2 glass ceramic	96,000
Ney-Oro CB gold alloy	77,000
Experience composite resin	13,000
Signum composite resin	3,500
Easytemp 2 acrylic resin	2,300

The zirconia crowns were duplicated with a CAD technique using the Procera Forte scanner (Nobel Biocare). The gold alloy crowns were made using the lost-wax casting technique and a silicone index for fabricating duplicate crowns. All of the test crowns were identical in size and shape.

The crowns were made with a morphology that permitted them to be inserted on the pin that simulated the abutment-fixture complex and were applied to the base with the sensors. A ridge that corresponded to a groove on the pin was created on the internal surface of the samples so that they were predictably and accurately placed without the possibility of rotation or other movements during the tests. The assembly of sensor, pin, and crown formed a single fixed structure that did not allow displacement among its components.

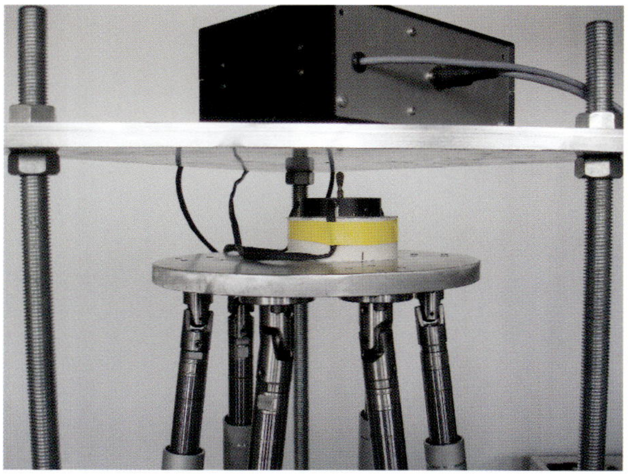

Fig 10.8 - Sample crown in occlusion with the upper flat surface of the masticatory robot.

To further minimize variables and limit the risk of accidental breakage of the crowns, a semispherical occlusal surface was chosen.

Every sample was marked on the basis of an alphabetic code. The operator who performed the tests did not know which material was being tested. A crown for each material was submitted to 350 masticatory cycles in the masticatory robot (approximately 10 minutes). The crown occluded with the flat surface of the upper fixed part of the masticatory robot (Fig 10.8). This testing apparatus evaluated vertical loads.

In review, a sample for each material was used with the same number of identical masticatory cycles and with the same starting conditions. The only variable was the material with which the crown was manufactured. A difference in the forces that were transmitted to the base of the pin depended exclusively on the capacity of deformation of the material (the modulus of elasticity). The measurements of the force transmitted were recorded by the sensor every 0.1 seconds. Twenty measurements were performed for each cycle of 2 seconds. The digitized signals were reproduced graphically with Matlab 6.1 (MathWorks).

For the statistical evaluation of the data, only the measurements recorded by the sensor on the vertical z axis were evaluated because with this type of test, where sample crowns occlude with flat surfaces, measurements taken on the two transverse axes (x and y) are not significant.

The Matlab 6.1 software program recorded the maximum peak force recorded for every masticatory cycle. The set of peaks measured at every test was submitted for statistical analysis using the StatView 5.0 program (SAS Institute). A comparison of the results is shown in Fig 10-9 and Table 10.4. When the crowns were evaluated from identical starting positions in contact with the flat upper part of the robot and performed the same number of identical masticatory cycles, the force transmitted on the vertical z axis through the pin and recorded at its base by the sensor was higher with zirconia crowns (average, 39.529 kg) and ceramic crowns (average, 30.127 kg) than with crowns made of gold alloy, composite resin, or acrylic resin. The gold alloy recorded an average force of 20.761 kg at the interface.

Among the composite resins, higher values were recorded for Experience (average, 17.491 kg) while Signum transmitted lower stresses at the peri-implant level (average, 9.510 kg).

Acrylic resin further reduced the loads transmitted to the simulated bone-implant interface (average, 2.471 kg).

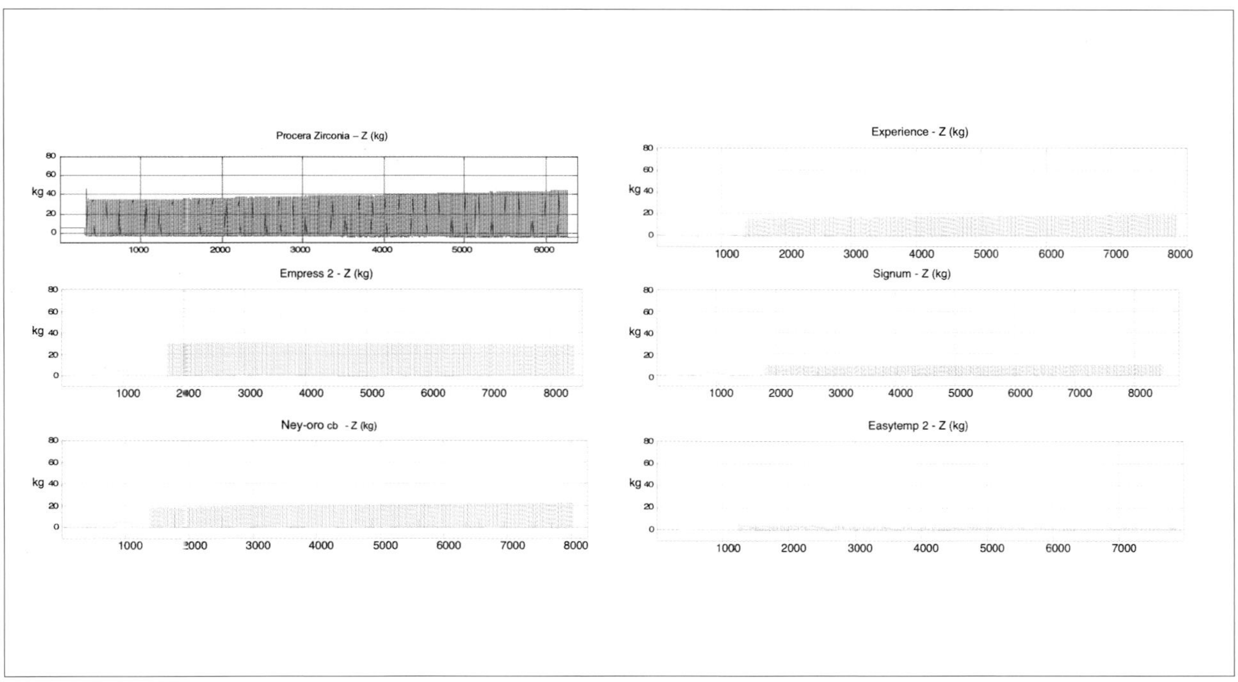

Fig 10.9 - Forces recorded on the vertical axis (z) from the pin to the sensorized base (simulating the peri-implant bone) during 350 masticatory cycles with the following restorative materials: Procera Zirconia, Empress 2 glass ceramic, Ney-Oro CB gold alloy, Experience composite resin, Signum composite resin, and Easytemp 2 acrylic resin. The x-coordinate reported the number of force samplings detected by the sensor.

Analysis of the slope of the curves representing the data (Fig 10.10) demonstrated that zirconia and ceramic yielded steeper peaks than did the other materials, and the maximum force was reached more rapidly. This was also demonstrated by Soumeire and Dejou[46] and is a further consequence of the different elastic modulus of the materials.

Table 10.4 shows that the highest stress values recorded on the vertical z axis were for the Procera zirconia crowns, followed in decreasing order by the ceramic, gold alloy, composite resin, and acrylic resin crowns. In this experiment, the masticatory robot always recorded that the values of forces transmitted to the simulated peri-implant bone were higher for crowns made with zirconia and ceramic than with gold alloy and composite or acrylic resins.

The ANOVA indicated a significant difference between forces transmitted using different materials. A multiple comparison among the samples was executed through the post hoc Scheffé test. Among the groups, every internal comparison was statistically significant with a P value < .0001 (Fig 10.11).

Several studies[22,29,31–35] have reported that the use of more elastic materials, opposed to the use of more rigid materials reduces the transmission of stresses in prosthetic restorations. This reduction has been reported as favorable for osseointegration of dental implants.

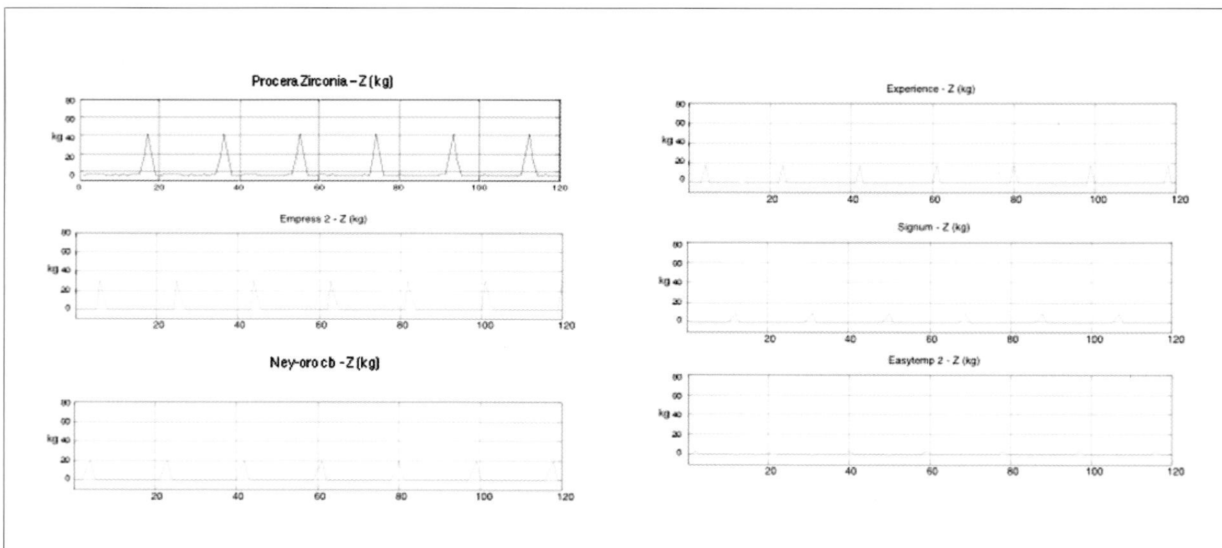

Fig 10.10 - Forces recorded during 12 seconds of chewing by the masticatory robot with the following restorative materials: Procera Zirconia, Empress 2 glass ceramic, Ney-Oro CB gold alloy, Experience composite resin, Signum composite resin, and Easytemp 2 acrylic resin. The x-coordinates reported the number of force samplings detected by the sensor.

TABLE 10.4 - MEAN STRESS VALUES ON THE VERTICAL Z AXIS				
Materials tested	**Average force (kg)**	**Standard deviation**	**Standard Error**	**Difference of force vs zirconia %**
Procera Zirconia	39.529	1.378	0.097	-
Empress 2	30.127	0.572	0.031	- 23.79
Ney-Oro CB	20.761	1.207	0.070	- 47.48
Experience	17.491	1.085	0.058	- 55.75
Signum	9.510	0.507	0.027	- 75.94
Easytemp 2	2.471	0.663	0.035	- 93.75

Table 10.4 - Comparison of mean maximum occlusal forces (in kg) recorded on the vertical axis. The last column reports the percentage difference of force compared to zirconia. Yellow, acrylic resin; orange, composite resin; red, gold alloy; purple, glass ceramic; blue, zirconia.

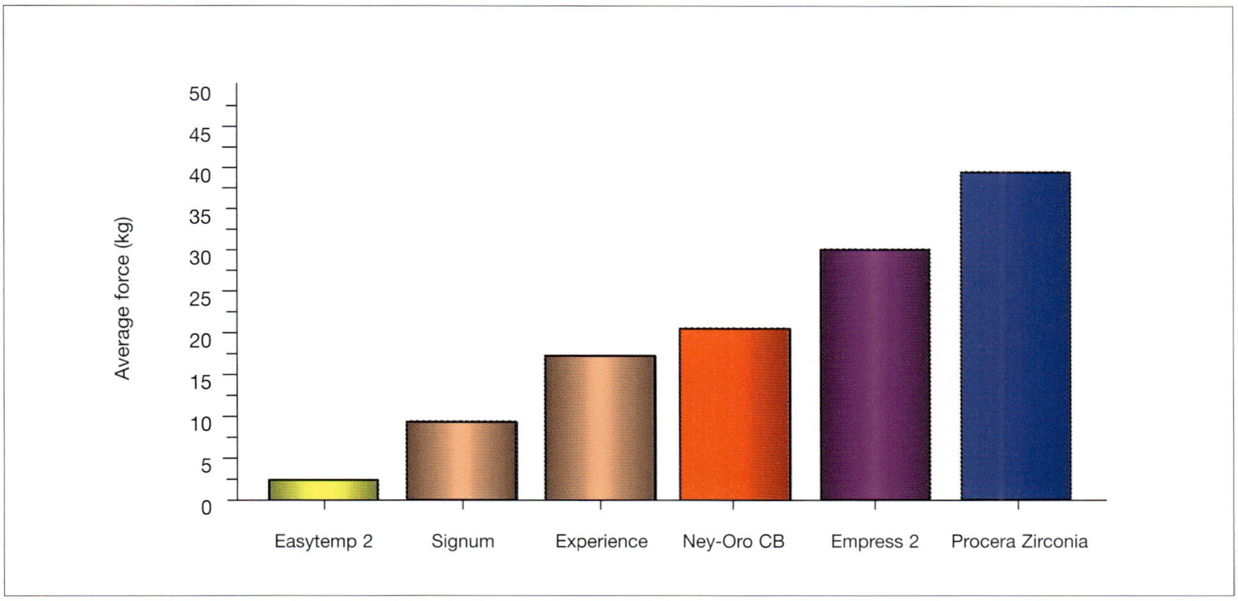

Fig 10.11 - The chart demonstrates the highest stress values on the vertical axis transmitted through the crowns. Acrylic resin demonstrated the best performance in reducing occlusal forces through the implant. Every internal comparison among the groups was statistically significant ($P < .0001$). Yellow, acrylic resin; orange, composite resin; red, gold alloy; purple, glass ceramic; blue, zirconia.

According to Hooke's law, the strain ε of an object is linearly proportional to the stress σ applied to it ($\varepsilon = \sigma/E$, where E is the elastic modulus)—that is, rigid materials (with greater elastic modulus) require greater forces for deformation to occur. The results of the experiments described in this chapter are consistent with this statement.

In this experiment, the acrylic resin crowns deformed to correspond to the shape of the opposing platform more quickly than did the other materials. Ceramic, in contrast, was more rigid. It adapted its form to the antagonist with more difficulty and had higher resistance to displacement. Therefore, to reach the position desired, a larger force had to be applied (with the robot) through the pin (simulating the fixture and abutments) to the base, where the force was recorded by sensors in the base (simulation of peri-implant bone).

Even if one acknowledges the shock-absorbing ability of acrylic and composite resins, Kohavi[47] points out that this characteristic, coupled with resins' minimal resistance to abrasion, could cause variations in the occlusal morphology of restorations and, therefore, in the creation of eccentric contacts.

However, it is the authors' opinion that the findings of the present research should be taken into consideration in clinical decision making, especially in clinical situations (such as immediate loading protocols) and in particularly unfavorable conditions (such as parafunctions) when implant loading needs to be limited.

The use of an acrylic resin occlusal material in provisional prostheses or a composite resin veneer in definitive prostheses is essential in such situations to reduce the risk of overload in a critical moment for the obtainment or maintenance of osseointegration.

The authors have drawn several conclusions from the research cited in this chapter:

- A functionally loaded zirconia or ceramic crown transmits greater stress to the implant abutment and the implant-bone interface than does a gold alloy or composite resin restoration. The stresses are noted to be even greater when compared with the stresses generated onto the abutment and implant-bone interface with acrylic resin restorations.
- Because of its lower elastic modulus, acrylic resin veneer has the capacity to absorb more of the occlusal forces that would otherwise be generated onto the implants.
- In implant-prosthodontic protocols, where improved prognoses and increased cumulative survival rates are the goals, the use of shock-absorbing occlusal surfaces is an additional clinical consideration in minimizing the transfer of occlusal loads to implants and is less likely to cause damages associated with occlusal overload.

- In this immediate occlusal loading protocol, the use of acrylic resin as occlusal material in the provisional prostheses is essential and fundamental to reduce the risk of overload prior to obtaining osseointegration.
- The selection of an occlusal material for the definitive prosthesis must be made:
  - Consistent with the amount of masticatory load the prosthesis will be subjected to
  - Dependent upon the nature of the opposing dentition
  - Dependent upon the strength of the muscles of mastication of individual patients
  - Consistent with the esthetic and biomechanical properties of the occlusal materials

REFERENCES

1. Pappalardo G. Porcellane o ceramica dentale. In: Pappalardo G (ed). Manuale di Materiali Dentari. Padova: Piccin, 1997:122–133.
2. Bertini F, Bagheri P, Grandini S. Intarsi estetici e faccette in ceramica. In: Grandini R, Rengo S, Strohmenger L (eds). Odontoiatria Restaurativa. Torino: UTET, 2004:411–436.
3. Pappalardo G. Materiali per otturazioni dentali. In: Pappalardo G (ed). Manuale di Materiali Dentari. Padova: Piccin 1997:163–240.
4. Grandini R, Bertini F, Giachetti P. Le resine composite. In: Grandini R, Rengo S, Strohmenger L (eds). Odontoiatria Restaurativa. Torino: UTET, 2004: 273–409.
5. Söderholm KJ, Richards ND. Wear resistance of composites: A solved problem? Gen Dent 1998;46:256–263.
6. Xu HH, Quinn JB, Giuseppetti AA, Eichmiller FC, Parry EE, Schumacher GE. Three-body wear of dental resin composites reinforced with silica-fused whiskers. Dent Mater 2004;20:220–227.
7. Turssi CP, Ferracane JL, Serra MC. Abrasive wear of resin composites as related to finishing and polishing procedures. Dent Mater 2005;21:641–648.
8. Turssi CP, Ferracane JL, Vogel K. Filler features and their effects on wear and degree of conversion of particulate dental resin composite. Biomaterials 2005;26:4932–4937.
9. Zeng J, Sato Y, Ohkubo C, Hosoi T. In vitro wear resistance of three types of composite resin denture teeth. J Prosthet Dent 2005;94:453–457.
10. Ferracane JL. Is the wear of dental composite still a clinical concern? Is there still a need for in vitro wear simulating devices? Dent Mater 2006;22: 689–692.
11. Conserva E, Menini M, Tealdo T, et al. Robotic chewing simulator for dental materials testing on a sensor-equipped implant setup. Int J Prosthodont 2008;21:501–508.
12. Conserva E, Menini M, Tealdo T, et al. The use of a masticatory robot to analyze the shock absorption capacity of different restorative materials for prosthetic implants: A preliminary report. Int J Prosthodont 2009;22:53–55.
13. Audenino G, Barone Monfrin S, Bassi F, et al. Edentulismo parziale. In: Preti G (ed). Riabilitazione Protesica. Torino: UTET, 2005:487–589.
14. Pappalardo G. Metalli e leghe. In: Pappalardo G (ed). Manuale di Materiali Dentari. Padova: Piccin, 1997:261–350.
15. Ekfeldt A. Incisal and occlusal tooth wear of some prosthodontic material. An epidemiological and clinical study. Swed Dent J Suppl 1989;65:1–62.
16. Raigrodski AJ. Contemporary materials and technologies for all-ceramic fixed partial denture: A review of the literature. J Prosthet Dent 2004; 92:557–562.
17. Manicone PF, Rossi Iommetti P, Raffaelli L, et al. Biological considerations of zirconia for dental devices. Int J Immunopathol Pharmacol 2007;20:9–12.
18. Manicone PF, Rossi Iommetti P, Raffaelli L. An overview of zirconia ceramics: Basic properties and clinical applications. J Dent 2007;35:819–826.
19. Denry I, Kelly JR. State of the art of zirconia for dental applications. Dent Mater 2008;24:299–307.
20. Rimondini L, Cerroni L, Carrassi A, Torricelli P. Bacterial colonization of zirconia ceramic surfaces: An in vitro and in vivo study. Int J Oral Maxillofac Implants 2002;17:793–798.
21. Scarano A, Piattelli M, Caputi S, Favero GA, Piattelli A. Bacterial adhesion on commercially pure titanium and zirconium oxide disks: An in vivo human study. J Periodontol 2004;75:292–296.
22. Juodzbalys G, Kubilius R, Eidukynas V, Raustia AM. Stress distribution in bone: Single-unit implant prostheses veneered with porcelain or a new composite material. Implant Dent 2005;14:166–175.
23. Barbier L, Vander Sloten J, Krzesinski G, Schepers E, Van Der Perre G. Finite element analysis of non-axial versus axial loading of oral implants in the mandible of dog. J Oral Rehabil 1998;25;847–858.

24. Cehreli M, Duyck J, De Cooman M, Puers R, Naert I. Implant design and interface force transfer. Clin Oral Implants Res 2004;15:249–257.
25. Isidor F. Histological evaluation of peri-implant bone at implants subjected to occlusal overload or plaque accumulation. Clin Oral Implants Res 1997;8:1–9.
26. Geng JP, Tan KB, Liu GR. Application of finite element analysis in implant dentistry: A review of the literature. J Prosthet Dent 2001;85:585–598.
27. Papavasiliou G, Kamposiora P, Bayne SC, Felton DA. Three-dimensional finite element analysis of stress-distribution around single tooth implants as a function of bony support, prosthesis type, and loading during function. J Prosthet Dent 1996; 76:633–640.
28. Brånemark PI, Hansson BO, Adell R, et al. Osseointegrated implants in the treatment of the edentulous jaw. Scand J Plast Reconstr Surg 1977;11:1–8.
29. Skalak R. Biomechanical considerations in osseointegrated prostheses. J Prosthet Dent 1983;49:843–848.
30. Gaggl A, Schultes G. Biomechanical properties in titanium implants with integrated maintenance free shock absorbing elements. Biomaterials 2001;22: 3061–3066.
31. Gracis SE, Nicholls JI, Chalupnik JD, Youdelis RA. Shock-absorbing behaviour of five restorative materials used on implants. Int J Prosthodont 1991;4:282–291.
32. Inan O, Kesim B. Evaluation of the effects of restorative materials used for occlusal surfaces of implant-supported prostheses on force distribution. Implant Dent 1999;8:311–316.
33. Çiftçi Y, Canay S. The effect of veneering materials on stress distribution in implant-supported fixed prosthetic restorations. Int J Oral Maxillofac Implants 2000;15:571–585.
34. Çiftçi Y, Canay S. Stress distribution on the metal framework of the implant-supported fixed prosthesis using different veneering materials. Int J Prosthodont 2001;14:406–411.
35. Sevimay M, Usumez A, Eskitascioglu G. The influence of various occlusal materials on stresses transferred to implant-supported prostheses and supporting bone: A three-dimensional finite-element study. J Biomed Mater Res 2005;73:140–147.
36. Sertgoz A. Finite element analysis study of the effect of superstructure material on stress distribution in an implant-supported fixed prosthesis. Int J Prosthodont 1997;10:19–27.
37. Wang TM, Leu LJ, Wang JS, Lin LD. Effects of prosthesis materials and prosthesis splinting on peri-implant bone stress around implants in poor-quality bone: A numeric analysis. Int J Oral Maxillofac Implants 2002;17:231–237.
38. Cibirka RM, Razzoog ME, Lang BR, Stohler CS. Determining the force absorption quotient for restorative materials used in implant occlusal surfaces. J Prosthet Dent 1992;67:361–364.
39. Hürzeler MB, Quiñones CR, Schüpbach P, Vlassis JM, Strub JR, Caffesse RG. Influence of the suprastructure on the peri-implant tissues in beagle dogs. Clin Oral Implants Res 1995;6:139–148.
40. Bassit R, Lindström H, Rangert B. In vivo registration of force development with ceramic and acrylic resin occlusal materials on implant-supported prostheses. Int J Oral Maxillofac Implants 2002;17: 17–23.
41. Hobkirk JA, Psarros KJ. The influence of occlusal surface material on peak masticatory forces using osseointegrated implant-supported prostheses. Int J Oral Maxillofac Implants 1992;7:345–352.
42. Wood MR, Vermilyea SG. A review of selected dental literature on evidence-based treatment planning for dental implants: Report of the Committee on Research in Fixed Prosthodontics of the Academy of Fixed Prosthodontics. J Prosthet Dent 2004;92: 447–462.
43. Naert I, Quirynen M, van Steenberghe D, Darius P. A six-year prosthodontic study of 509 consecutively inserted implants for the treatment of partial edentulism. J Prosthet Dent 1992;67:236–245.

44. Sahin S, Çehreli MC, Yalçin E. The influence of functional forces on the biomechanics of implant-supported prostheses–A review. J Dent 2002;30: 271–282.
45. Stegaroiu R, Khraisat A, Nomura S, Miyakawa O. Influence of superstructure materials on strain around an implant under 2 loading conditions: A technical investigation. Int J Oral Maxillofac Implants 2004;19:735–742.
46. Soumeire J, Dejou J. Shock absorbability of various restorative materials used on implants. J Oral Rehabil 1999;26:394–401.
47. Kohavi D. Complications in the tissue integrated prostheses components: Clinical and mechanical evaluation. J Oral Rehabil 1993;20:413–422.
48. Taylor TD, Wiens J, Carr A. Evidence-based considerations for removable prosthodontic and dental implant occlusion: A literature review. J Prosthet Dent 2005;94:555–560.
49. Mongini F, Tempia-Valenta G, Conserva E. Habitual mastication in dysfunction: A computer-based analysis. J Prosthet Dent 1989;61:484–494.
50. Mongini F, Conserva E, Tempia G. Analisi della masticazione in soggetti normali e disfunzionali. Dental Cadmos 1989;2:54–78.
51. Conserva E, Schembri D, Pagliari P. Composite flask: A new system for light-curing materials in prosthodontics. Presented at the 8th Meeting of the International College of Prosthodontists, Stockholm, Sweden, 1999.

CHAPTER 11

FULL-ARCH FIXED PROSTHETIC TREATMENT WITH REPLACEMENT OF SOFT TISSUES: THE TORONTO BRIDGE

This and the following chapter illustrate two clinical cases treated according to the Columbus Bridge Protocol. The treatments differ in regard to the replacement of the hard and soft tissues lost secondary to periodontal disease.

Background

A 54-year-old man in good health with multiple missing maxillary teeth had been treated with three fixed partial dentures supported by natural teeth. The prostheses had been constructed over the previous 10 years (Figs 11.1 to 11.6). The patient requested that treatment be nonremovable by design and accomplished as quickly as possible. He did not want to go through a treatment phase that included any type of transitional removable prosthesis.

Physical examination

The preoperative work-up was performed consistent with the steps outlined in Box 3.1 (see chapter 3). The physical examination included evaluation of periodontal pockets of the remaining teeth (average, > 5 mm), dental mobility (classes II and III), bleeding upon probing, furcations (grades II and III), and Plaque Index (Fig 11.7).

Radiographic examination

The radiographic examination consisted of a full series of periapical radiographs made with the parallel technique. The radiographs demonstrated generalized bone loss in excess of 66% around the roots (Fig 11.8).

Diagnosis

The maxillary dentition was diagnosed with advanced, generalized periodontal disease. All of the maxillary teeth were judged as hopeless.

Treatment plan

The decision was made to *(1)* extract all of the maxillary teeth, *(2)* recontour the maxillary alveolus as needed for implants, *(3)* place implants, and *(4)* fabricate an immediate provisional prosthesis with immediate occlusal loading.

Preliminary treatment

The first steps in treatment planning included identifying and recording the vertical dimension of occlusion (VDO) clinically and transferring the relationship to the dental laboratory with an articulator mounting. The accurate transfer of the jaw relationships is critical because the patient becomes edentulous during the surgical phase of treatment, so all landmarks associated with the maxillary teeth and maxillomandibular occlusal relationship are removed. The jaw relationship and VDO will be reconstructed with the provisional prosthesis.

The preoperative VDO was measured by placing dermographic pencil dots - one above and one below the occlusal plane - onto the patient's face. One was placed on the tip of the nose, the other one on the chin (Fig 11.9). Since the VDO was not going to be changed and the patient had a full complement of teeth, he was asked to close his teeth into the maximal intercuspal position (centric occlusion). The provisional fixed prosthesis would be made at this VDO.

Surgical-prosthetic template

Fifteen minutes prior to surgery, the surgical-prosthetic template was submerged in a cold sterilizing solution. It was rinsed with a sterile physiologic solution prior to its use. The intaglio surface of the maxillary portion of the template was made so that it was tissue-borne on both maxillary tuberosities (Fig 11.10). The intaglio surface of the mandibular portion of the surgical-prosthetic template fit directly onto the incisal and occlusal surfaces of the mandibular dentition (Fig 11.11). This design was critical to stabilize this template.

Surgical treatment

The patient was premedicated with an anxiolytic (diazepam) and an antibiotic medication (amoxicillin + clavulanic acid) per the protocol given in the chapter 17. Local anesthesia was obtained with 4% articaine and 1/100,000 epinephrine. The anesthetic was injected into the depths of the maxillary vestibules and the palatal portions of the maxilla.

The maxillary teeth were extracted prior to performing the full-thickness flaps. Care was taken to avoid fracturing the alveolar walls of the sockets (Fig 11.12). The extraction sockets were thoroughly curetted to remove granulation and/or infected tissues that remained after the tooth extractions (Fig 11.13).

A flap was made palatally through a crestal incision in the remaining maxillary tissues. A full-thickness flap was reflected to expose the alveolar crest and the palatal portion of the maxilla. The flap was fully reflected on the vestibular portion so that the surgeon had complete visualization of the osseous anatomy (Figs 11.14 and 11.15). The extensive flaps allowed optimal visualization of the entire surgical field and resulted in the complete removal of any remaining granulation tissue (Fig 11.16). In the case illustrated in this chapter, where the treatment plan called for fabrication of a prosthesis like the Toronto Bridge, implant locations were identified solely by the quantity of native bone available after tooth extraction. Per the Columbus Bridge Protocol, the distal implants were placed first. Both distal implants were placed parallel to the anterior walls of the maxillary sinuses. These positions were facilitated by identifying the anterior walls of the sinuses and reflecting the maxillary sinus membranes. Such positioning was facilitated by creating a small hole in the lateral wall of the maxillary sinus with a round bur mounted on a contra-angle dental handpiece. (Note: In Fig 11.17, the asterisk indicates the hole in the lateral wall of the sinus.) A blunt surgical probe was inserted, and the sinus membrane was reflected away from the bone. A tactile inspection of the anterior portion of the maxillary sinus was then conducted.

Once the direction and location of the anterior wall of the maxillary sinus was determined, a line was drawn with a sterile marker onto the lateral wall of the maxilla slightly anterior to the anterior wall of the sinus. This identified the correct, tilted angle for the osteotomy and implant placement. In this case it was possible to use distal implants with 18-mm lengths. An occlusal view of the maxilla demonstrates the impact that angulated implants can have on the development of optimal cross-arch stabilization for provisional and definitive prostheses (Fig 11.18). The cross-arch stabilization guarantees stability for the prostheses relative to displacing forces, especially horizontal loads, and also eliminates distal cantilevers in provisional prostheses (Fig 11.20). The benefits associated with elimination of distal cantilevers in provisional prostheses have been discussed in chapter 6. When a Toronto Bridge–type prosthesis is realized, all anterior implants do not have to be placed consistent with the location of the artificial teeth on the surgical-prosthetic template. They can be placed consistent with the amount and location of the native bone. However, placement of the anterior implants must avoid nasal cavities (Fig 11.19).

Prosthetic treatment

After the surgical phase was completed but prior to suturing, the prosthetic phase commenced. An anterior view of the fixtures demonstrated that the maxillary implants were nonparallel (Fig 11.21). The orientation of nonparallel implants may be corrected with the use of angulated abutments. The use of a laboratory-fabricated surgical-prosthetic template is critical for the optimal choice and orientation of the transmucosal angled abutments. The surgical-prosthetic template permits the surgeon to place the abutments relative to the locations of the teeth as determined by the preoperative clinical and laboratory procedures (Fig 11.22). The orientation of angulated abutments was decided upon such that the screw access openings exited from within the volume of the prosthesis and not through the labial or buccal surfaces of the prosthesis (Figs 11.23 and 11.24). With this protocol, the screw access openings exit the prosthesis palatal to the labial and buccal surfaces of the provisional and definitive prostheses.

Angulated conical abutments were placed onto the implants as follows:

- Three 25-degree angulated abutments with 2-mm shoulders
- One 17-degree angulated abutment with a 2-mm shoulder
- Abutment screws tightened with 20 Ncm of torque (Fig 11.25)

Pickup abutment impression

The Columbus Bridge Protocol calls for the use of pickup impression copings (Fig 11.26). Placement of the pickup impression copings was accomplished prior to suturing. This ensured that the clinician visualized all of the impression coping–abutment interfaces and that all of the impression copings were completely seated onto the abutments. Therefore, the clinician did not have to stop the clinical procedures to take radiographs to ensure that the impression copings were completely and accurately seated onto the abutments. The angulated abutments corrected the orientation of the nonparallel implants illustrated in Fig 11.21. For pickup impression copings to adequately retain impression material, the undercut areas of the copings must protrude at least 2 mm above the mucosa. Commercially available, disposable, stock plastic impression trays were used in this protocol. Holes were drilled into the occlusal surface of the maxillary impression tray that corresponded to the implant locations. The holes provided the clinician with the requisite access to the impression coping screws (Fig 11.27). In the Columbus Bridge Protocol, the impression material of choice is rapid-setting plaster with low volumetric expansion. The setting time for the plaster impression material used in this treatment was 2 to 3 minutes. Once the impression plaster had set, the impression coping screws were loosened, and the impression was removed. It was necessary to determine that the impression copings were stable within the impression to ensure that the impression was accurate (Fig 11.28). In this case, all of the impression copings were stable; if any of the impression copings had not been stable, the impression copings would have been removed from the impression and placed back onto the conical abutments, and the impression would have been repeated.

Jaw relation record

The next clinical step involved placement of the conical abutment healing caps onto the conical abutments. The occlusal surfaces of the healing caps have to be supragingival since they are used to make the jaw relation record. The jaw relation record was made using multiple layers of rigid baseplate wax warmed in water (60°C). The wax sheets were contoured consistent with the locations of the maxillary implants and the mandibular teeth. The patient's mandible was guided into centric relation (Fig 11.29), and the VDO was checked with extraoral calipers to make sure the preoperative VDO had been maintained (Fig 11.30). The interocclusal record was cooled with a spray of air and water and was then removed from the oral cavity. The superior and inferior surfaces of the jaw relation record were evaluated to guarantee that the indentations of the healing caps and mandibular teeth were recorded in wax (Figs 11.31 and 11.32). This type of interocclusal record has been proven to be sufficiently rigid and accurate, and it provides the clinician and dental laboratory technician with an accurate representation of the jaw relationships for the articulator mounting.

Provisional screw-retained prosthesis

Provisional prostheses made per the Columbus Bridge Protocol must possess the following properties:

- The frameworks must be cast of metal for rigidity, strength, and accurate fit.
- The provisional prostheses must fit passively onto the abutments. Passive fit is a function of the impression and laboratory techniques.
- The occlusal surface must be fabricated with commercially available acrylic resin denture teeth (Fig 11.33).

With this specific treatment, excellent cross-arch stabilization was achieved, the prosthesis consisted of 10 masticatory units (teeth), and there were no distal cantilevers. The access openings were contained within the occlusal and palatal surfaces of the prosthesis (Fig 11.34). Prior to delivering the prosthesis to the clinician, the dental laboratory technician verified that the prosthesis was fabricated without distortion and passed the Sheffield one-screw test on the master cast.

Prosthetic delivery

The prosthesis was delivered within 24 hours of the extractions and implant placement. The clinician removed the healing caps from the conical abutments; all of the conical abutments and implants were stable (Figs 11.35 and 11.36). The provisional prosthesis was then placed onto the conical abutments. The authors recommend that the prosthetic retaining screws be tightened diagonally opposite one another to allow the interimplant soft tissues to adapt gradually to the pressures of the intaglio surface of the prosthesis (Fig 11.37). The four gold retaining screws were tightened slowly and diagonally opposite from one another until the preload registered 10 Ncm. The occlusion was evaluated. Uniform occlusal contacts were obtained throughout the prosthesis; right and left working occlusions were designed for group function occlusion (Figs 11.38 and 11.39).

Intraoral radiographs taken with the Rinn paralleling technique demonstrated complete and accurate seating of the prosthesis to the abutments. The abutments were correctly placed on the implants. The radiographs also demonstrated the absence of distal cantilevers and the presence of the postextraction sockets. These radiographs also provided baseline information relative to the location of the crestal bone and its relationships to the implant restorative platforms at time 0. Baseline crestal bone levels were important to qualify the location of the crestal bone relative to the implants during follow-up (Figs 11.40 to 11.42).

In the Columbus Bridge Protocol, minimal facial swelling is usually present for 48 to 72 hours after surgery. Postoperative pain is generally well managed following the pharmacologic protocol presented in the chapter 17. The patient's postoperative condition was consistent with the usual course of events (Figs 11.43 and 11.44).

Removal of provisional prosthesis and sutures

The patient's first scheduled follow-up visit occurred approximately 1 week after the surgery and immediate occlusal loading. The intraoral tissues had healed nicely and were adapting to the contours of the fixed provisional prosthesis (Figs 11.45 and 11.46). The Columbus Bridge Protocol calls for removal of the provisional prosthesis 7 to 10 days after the operation to remove any remaining sutures from the surgical sites. This was accomplished at this first scheduled postoperative visit. Removal of the prosthesis allowed the clinician to evaluate all of the soft tissues and their adaptation to the implants and restorative components. Removal of the provisional prosthesis was possible only because the implants were placed with high insertion torque with high implant stability at the time of implant placement. High implant stability has proven to be critical to the long-term survival of endosseous implants subjected to immediate occlusal loading.

Figures 11.47 and 11.48 demonstrate how the insertion of an immediate fixed provisional prosthesis within 24 hours of implant placement guided the soft tissue contours during the initial healing process. This aspect is even more important in cases treated with the natural fixed bridge. The definitive screw-retained prosthetic treatment commenced 4 months after extraction, implant placement, and immediate occlusal loading with the provisional prosthesis. This time was necessary for soft tissue healing, soft tissue maturation, and osseointegration to occur (Figs 11.49 and 11.50). During this period, the patient was scheduled for hygiene follow-up appointments and occlusal evaluations to maintain optimal peri-implant soft tissue health and a uniform distribution of occlusal contacts throughout the prosthesis.

Design of the definitive impression and prosthesis

The provisional prosthesis was carefully evaluated regarding esthetics, phonetics, and function (Fig 11.51). It was judged to be satisfactory by the clinician and the patient, so few changes were planned for the definitive prosthesis (Fig 11.52). Nevertheless, the vestibular emergence of the prosthesis at the level of the maxillary left lateral incisor was reduced to help improve the phonetic results. Thus, for the definitive prosthesis it was necessary to make an implant-level impression of the maxillary left anterior implant. This provided the dental laboratory technician the possibility to develop an optimal, anatomical emergence profile for the abutment-implant interface in this area (Figs 11.53 and 11.54). The definitive impression was made with plaster and the pickup technique, similar to the procedure used for the provisional prosthesis. In this case, a pickup implant impression coping was used for the left maxillary anterior implant. The other three angulated conical abutments remained in place on the other implants. The nonparallel alignment of the left anterior implant relative to the other implants was visualized (Figs 11.55 to 11.58). The definitive impression was made, and a new master cast was poured. A new angulated conical abutment, in its most appropriate orientation (indicated by the arrow on the master cast in Fig 11.60), was chosen and placed onto the master cast in the dental laboratory (Figs 11.59 and 11.60). A new metal framework was waxed, cast, finished, and polished.

The esthetic veneering material in the gingival portion of the definitive prosthesis was made with composite resin (SR Adoro, Ivoclar Vivadent). The gingival contours of the definitive prosthesis were developed through cooperation between the clinician and the dental technician (Figs 11.61 to 11.63).

Delivery of the definitive, screw-retained prosthesis

At the delivery appointment for the definitive prosthesis, the preexisting provisional prosthesis was removed. The preexisting conical abutment was removed from the maxillary left anterior implant, and the new, 25-degree angulated conical abutment was placed onto the implant and tightened by hand. The definitive prosthesis was then placed onto the abutments to confirm that the new abutment was in its correct orientation, and the abutment screw was tightened to 20 Ncm with a torque driver (Figs 11.64 to 11.66).

The definitive, screw-retained fixed prosthesis was made with gold alloy and a composite resin veneering material. It was delivered 4 months after dental extractions, implant placement, and immediate occlusal loading and successfully reproduced the esthetic, phonetic, and functional aspects of the provisional prosthesis with minimal modifications. The anterior clinical view of the definitive fixed prosthesis demonstrated how the loss of supporting tissue secondary to advanced chronic periodontitis was anatomically replaced by the gingiva-colored artificial tissues of the Toronto Bridge–type prosthesis (Fig 11.67). This procedure confirmed the importance of presurgical treatment planning, appropriate treatment, and laboratory support.

It should be noted that two additional masticatory units were placed onto the definitive prosthesis because cantilevers can be fabricated on prostheses supported by osseointegrated implants. Thus, the definitive prosthesis included a total of 12 masticatory units instead of the 10 units that were present on the provisional prosthesis (Fig 11.68). At the delivery of the definitive prosthesis, periapical radiographs demonstrated the lack of peri-implant radiolucencies, excellent bone-implant contact, crestal bone levels at the location of the first implant threads, and bone remodeling of the extraction sockets (Figs 11.69 and 11.70).

The definitive prosthesis maintained the occlusal relationships that were present in the original provisional prosthesis, including stable centric occlusal contacts and group function occlusion in both the right and left working mandibular positions (Figs 11.71 and 11.72). In addition, it restored the correct harmony of the inferior third of the face and optimal masticatory function (Figs 11.73 to 11.75).

The Columbus Bridge Protocol completely satisfied this patient's requests. It avoided any type of removable provisional prosthesis postoperatively and provided a fixed provisional screw-retained prosthesis within 24 hours of a single surgical appointment. The patient's progress has been followed for 3 years. The 3-year radiographs demonstrate that crestal bone levels around the implants are stable compared with the bone levels visualized at time 0 (Figs 11.76 to 11.78). Clinically, the definitive prosthesis was still satisfactory in terms of esthetics, phonetics, and function (Figs 11.79 to 11.81).

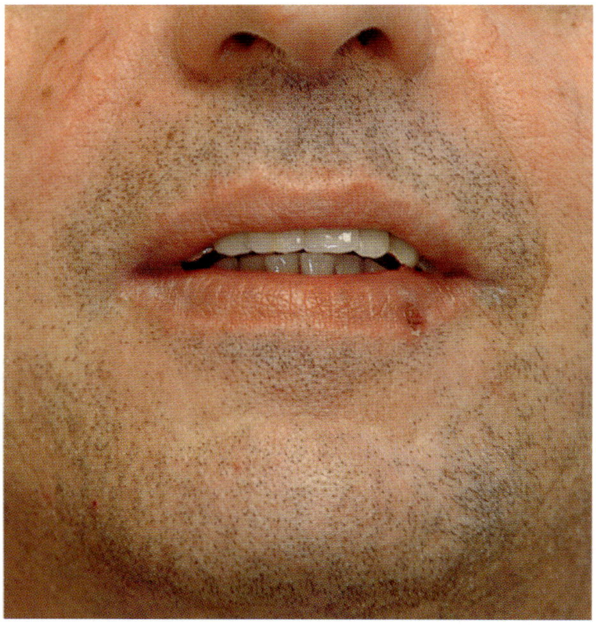

Fig 11.1

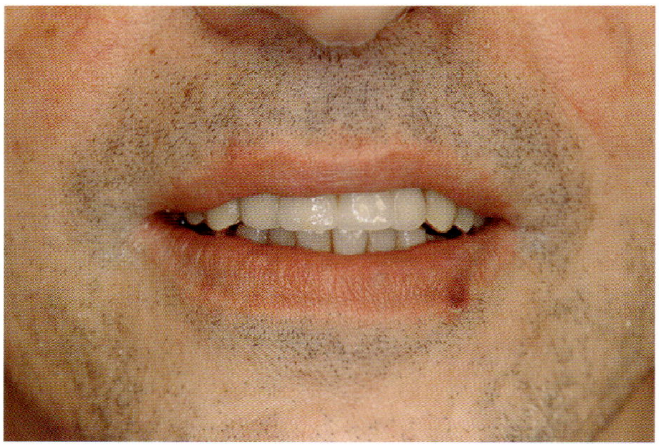

Fig 11.2

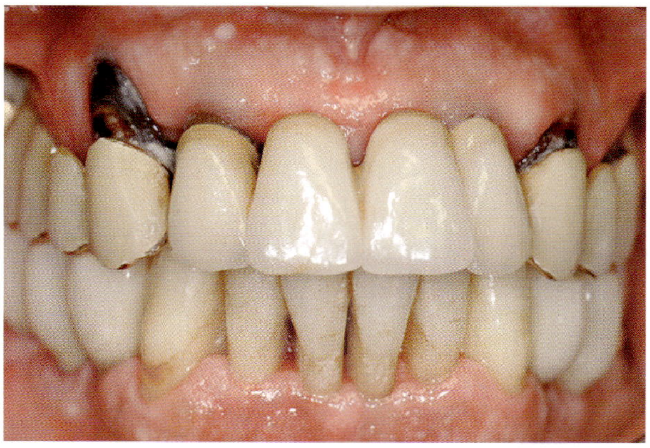

Fig 11.3

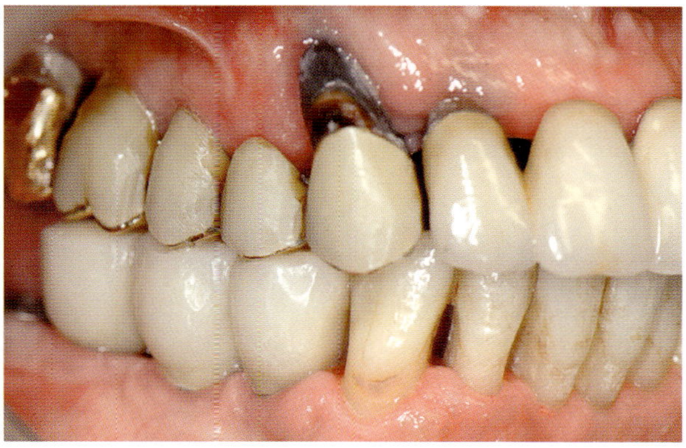

Fig 11.4

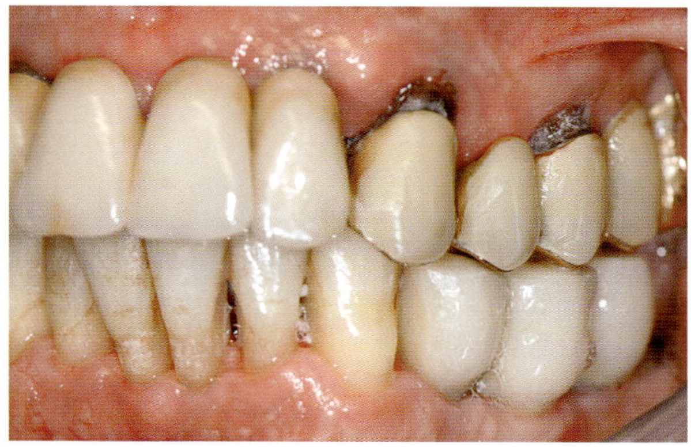

Fig 11.5

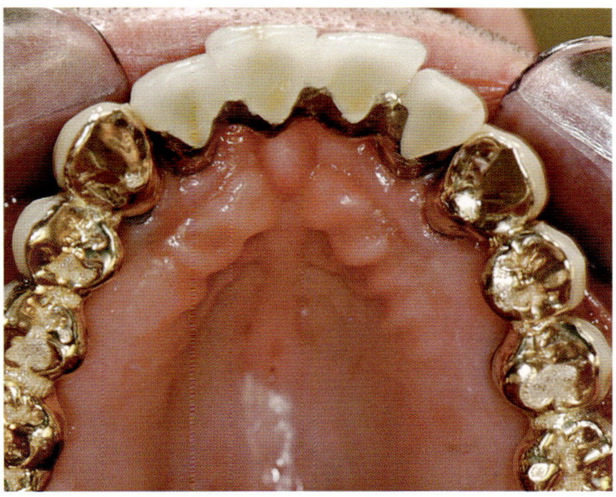

Fig 11.6

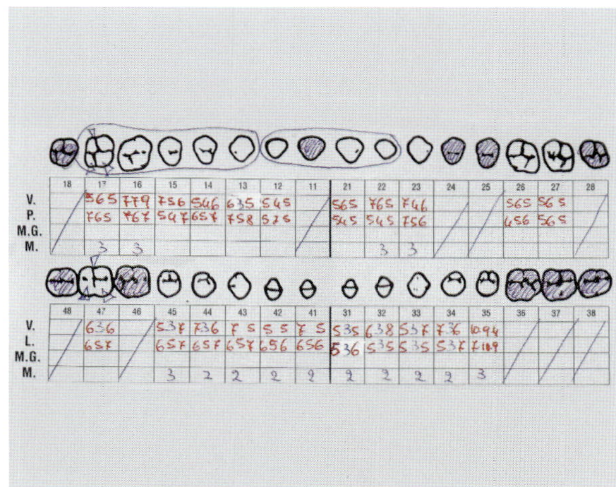

Fig 11.7

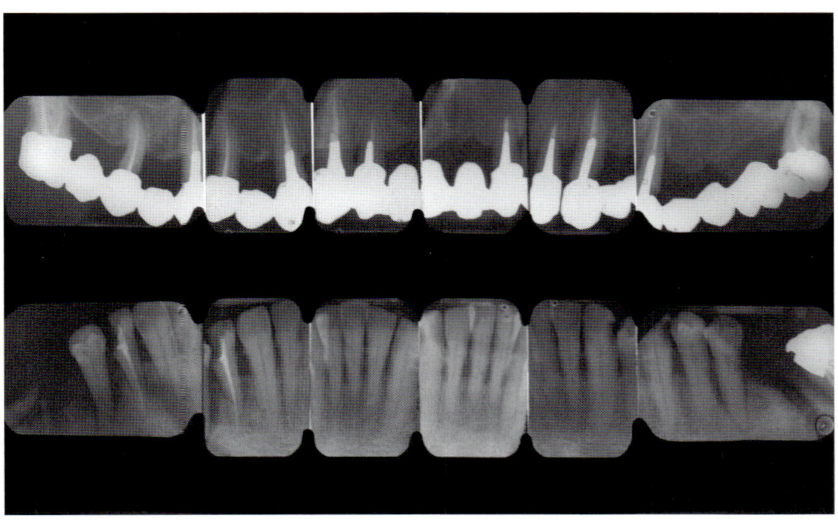

Fig 11.8

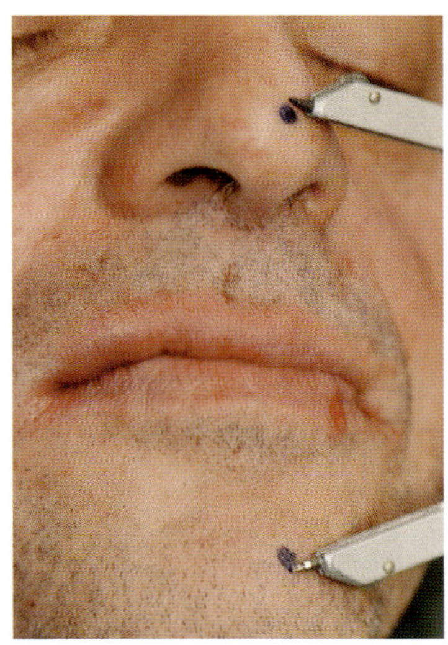

Fig 11.9

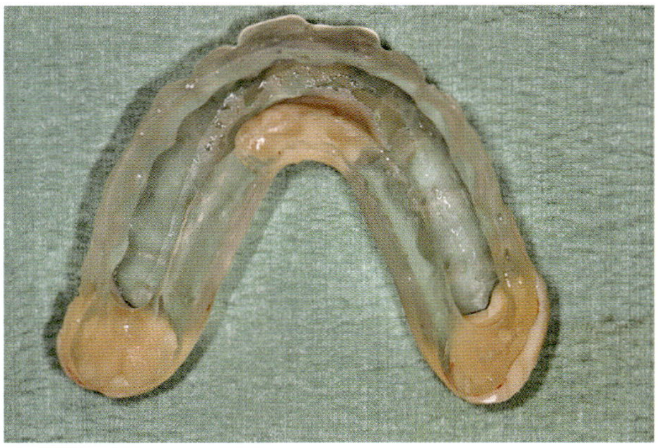

Fig 11.10

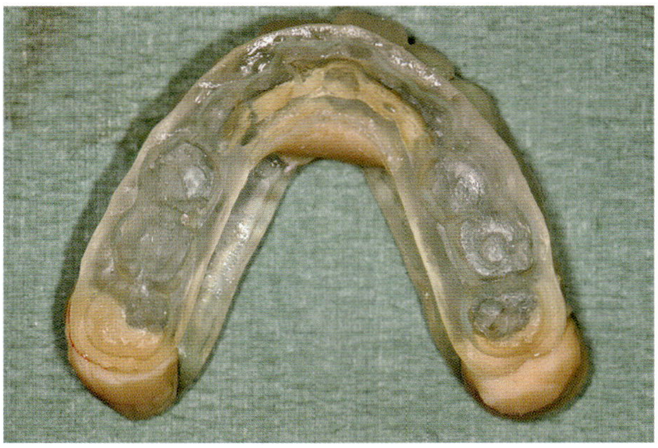

Fig 11.11

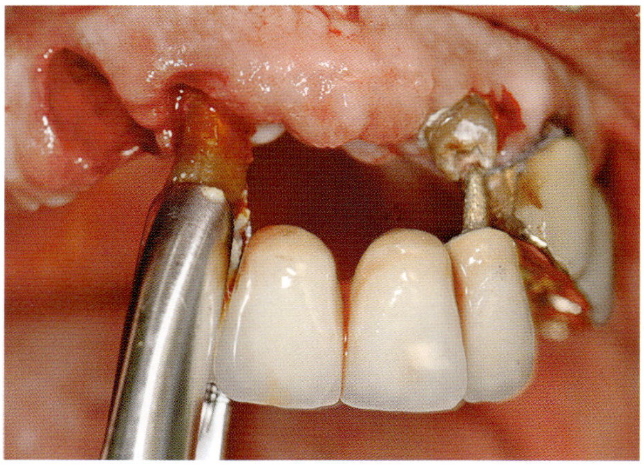

Fig 11.12

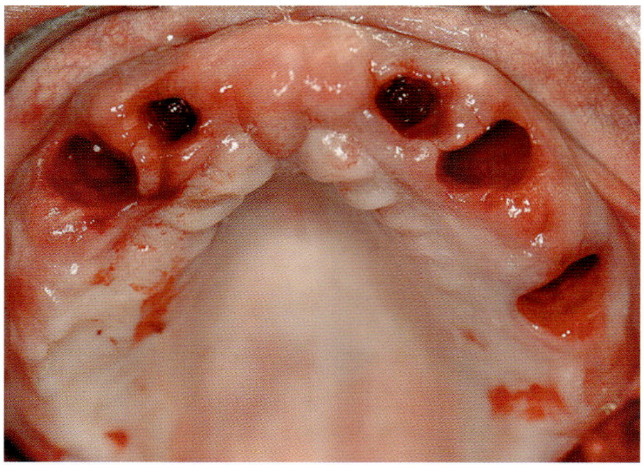

Fig 11.13

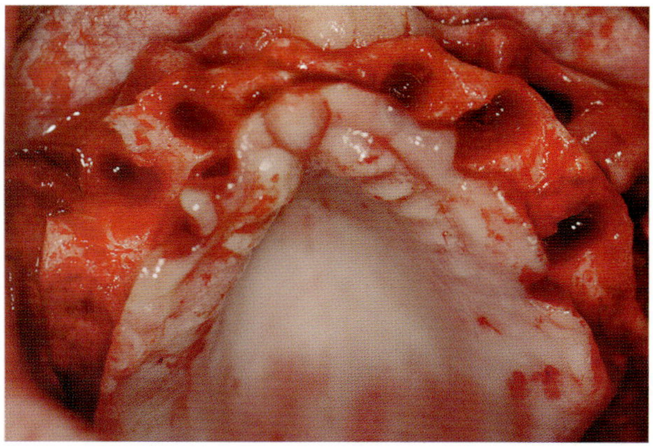

Fig 11.14

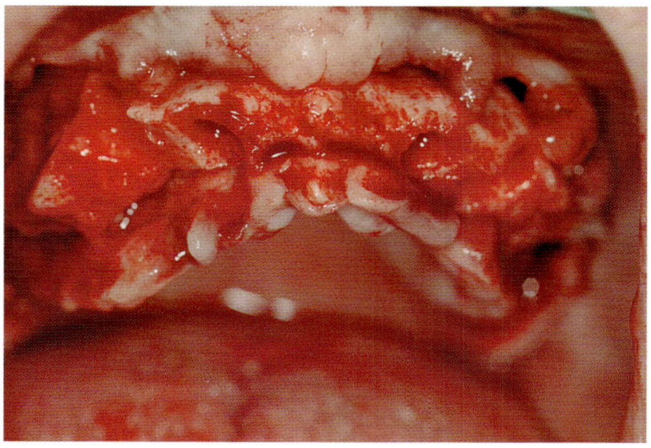

Fig 11.15

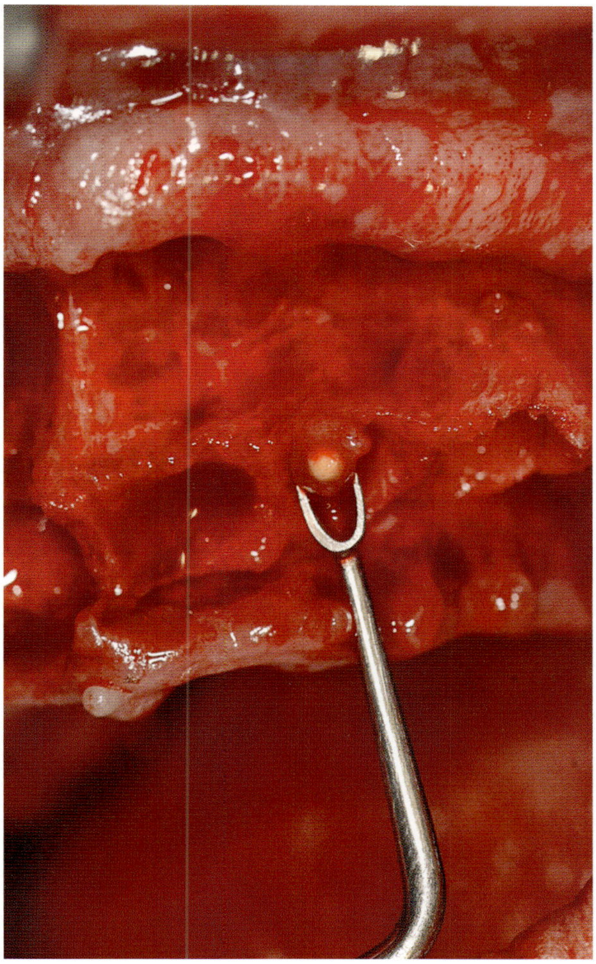

Fig 11.16

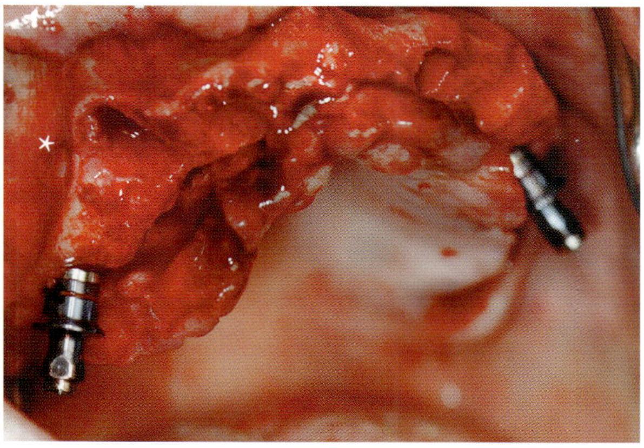

Fig 11.17

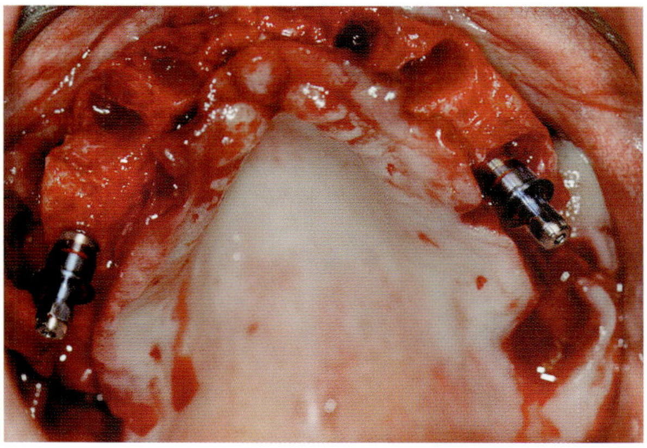

Fig 11.18

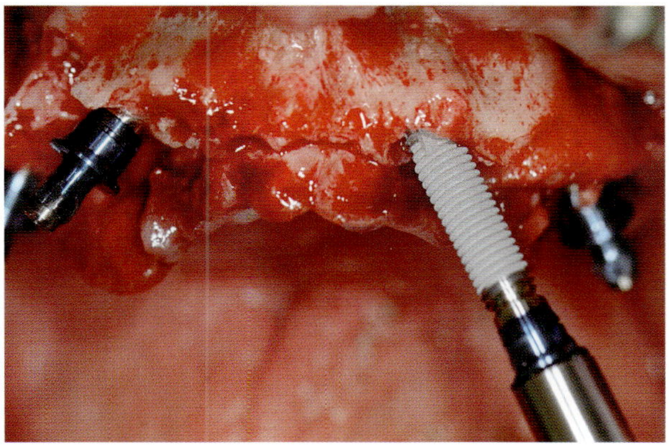

Fig 11.19

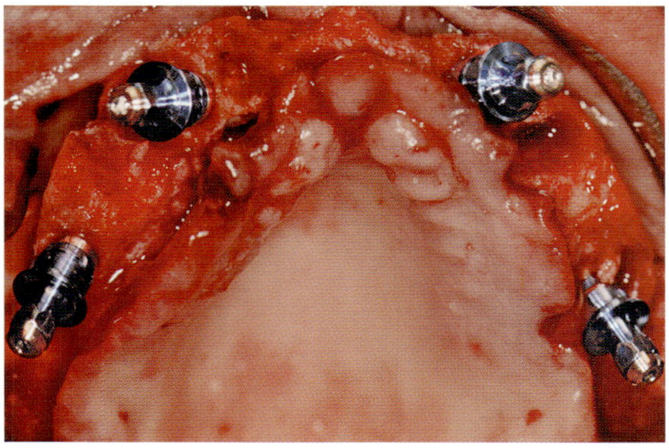

Fig 11.20

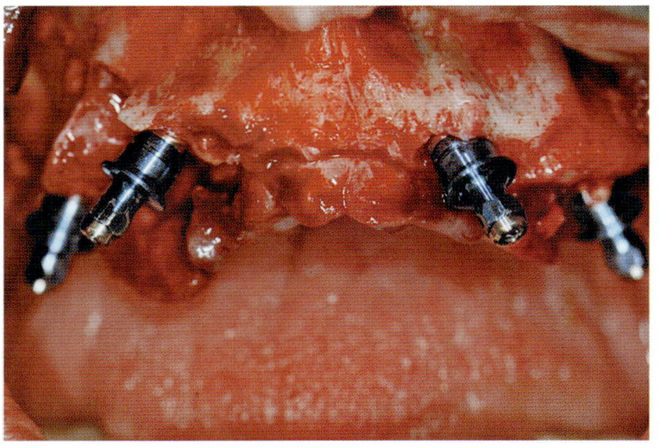

Fig 11.21

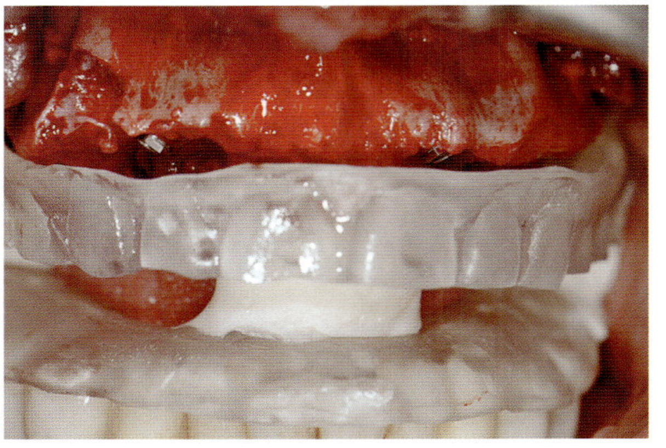

Fig 11.22

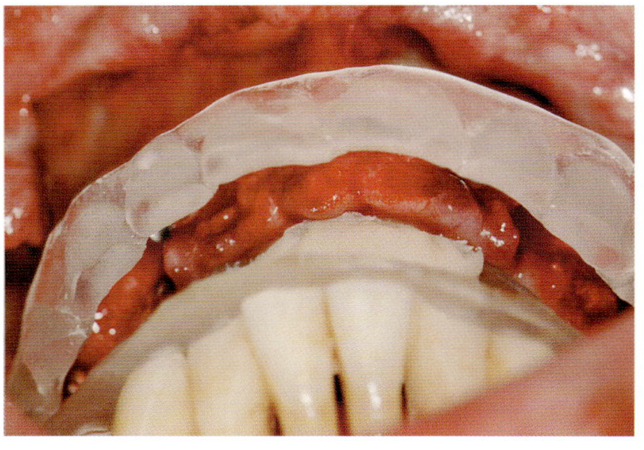

Fig 11.23

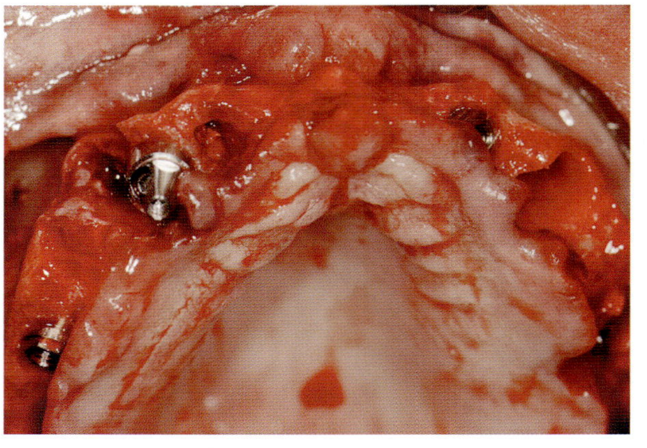

Fig 11.24

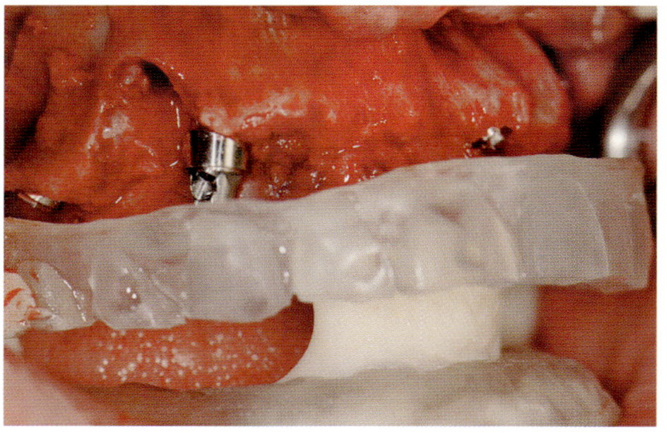

Fig 11.25

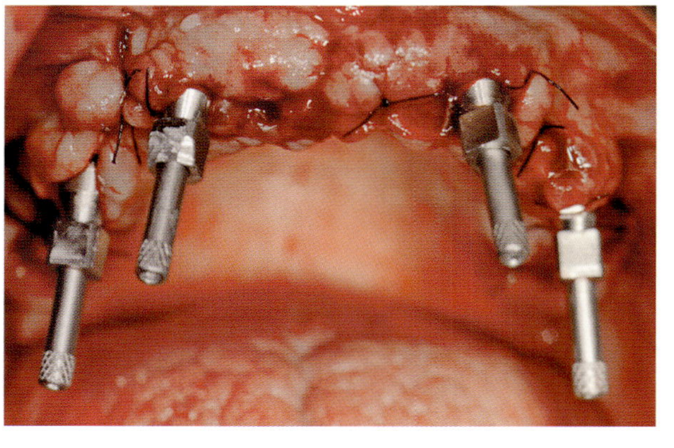

Fig 11.26

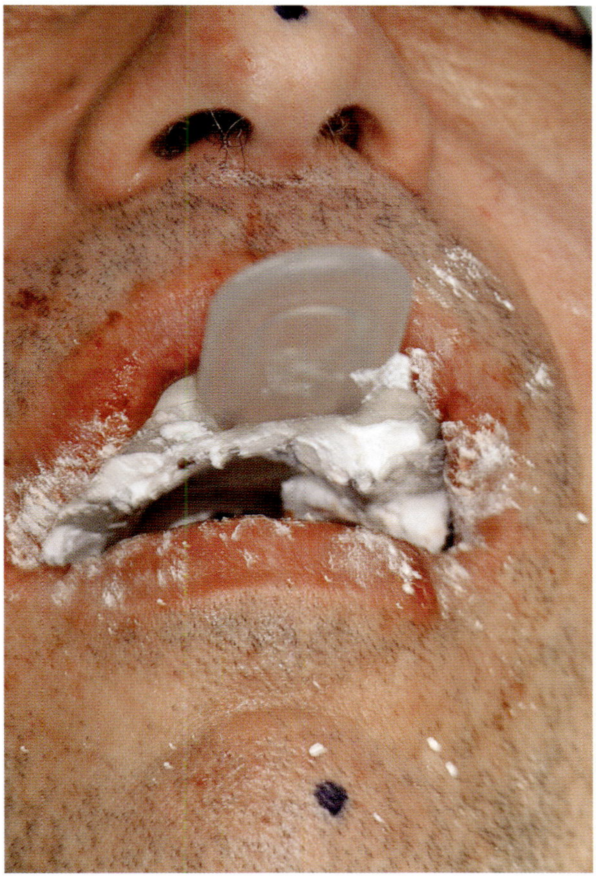

Fig 11.27

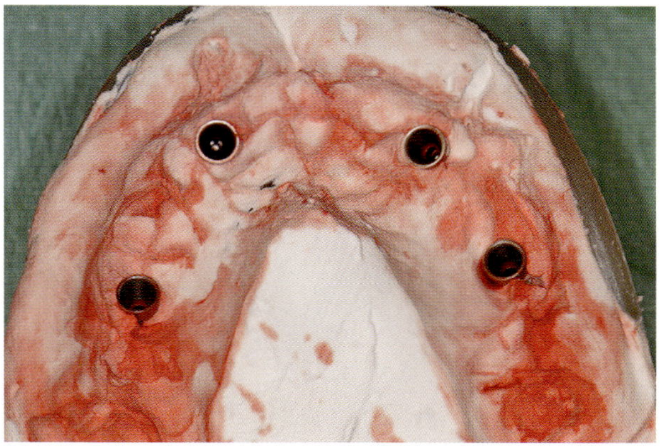

Fig 11.28

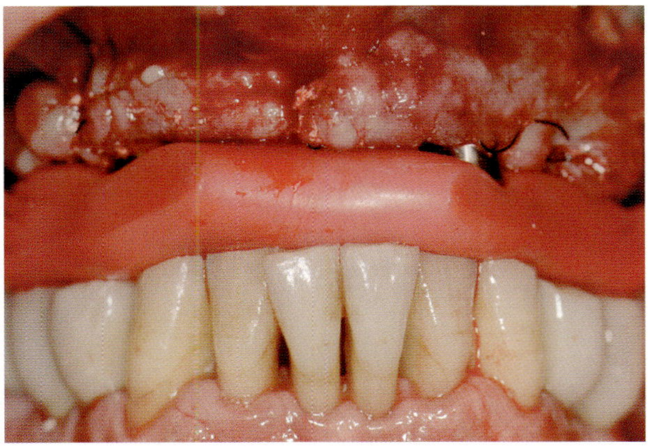

Fig 11.29

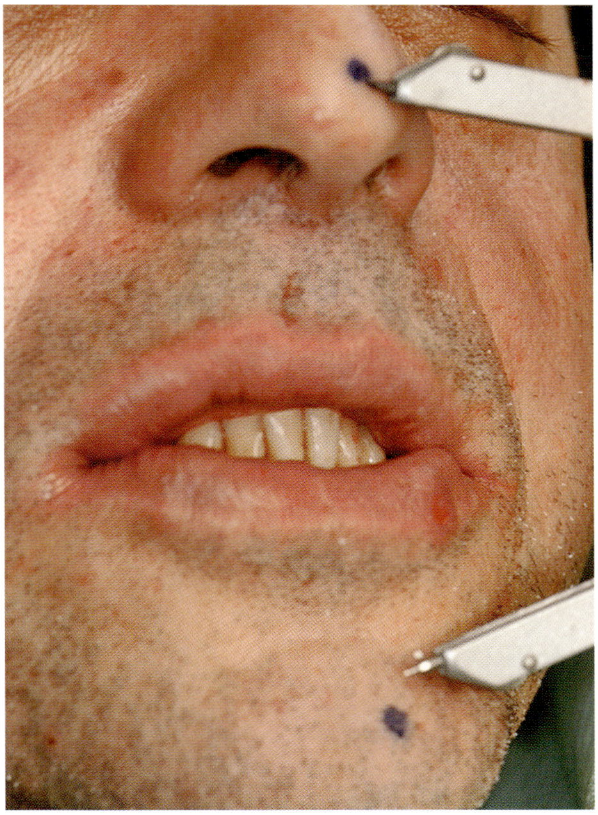

Fig 11.30

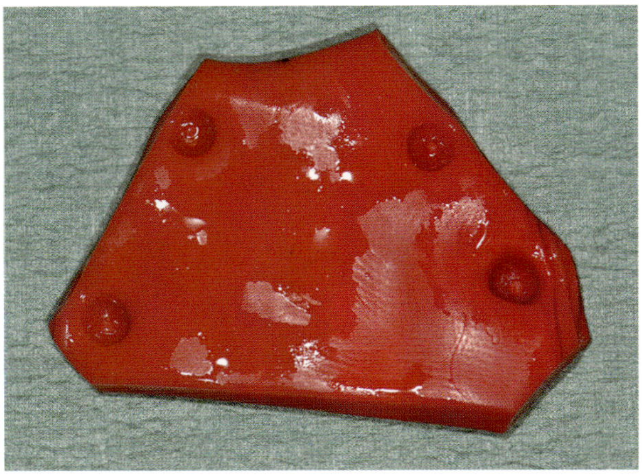

Fig 11.31

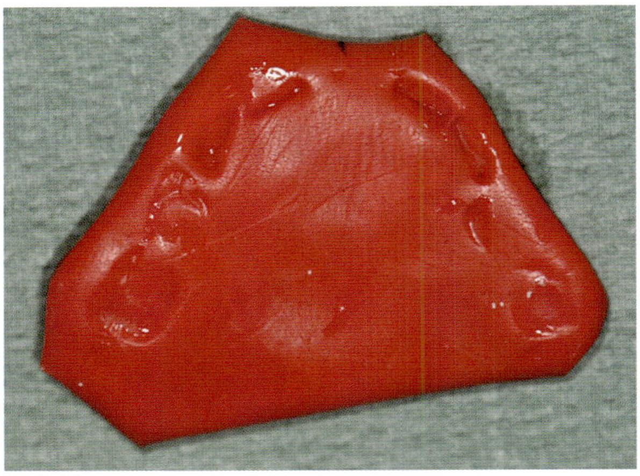

Fig 11.32

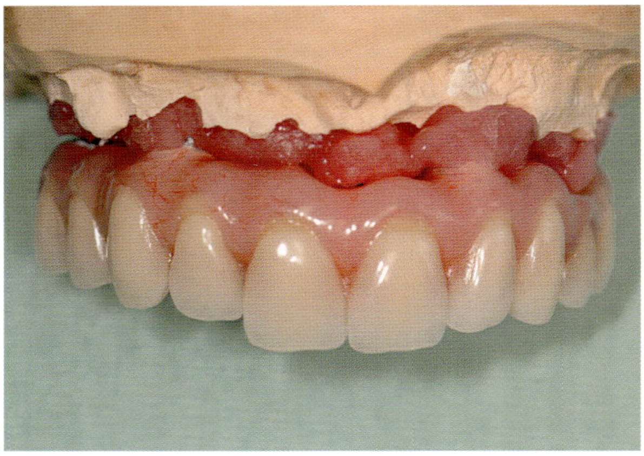

Fig 11.33

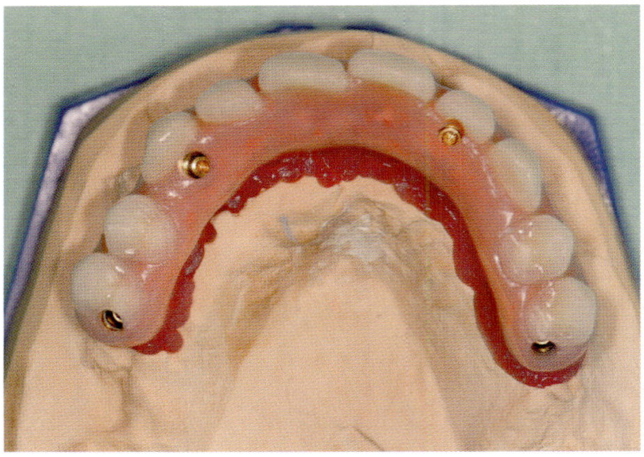

Fig 11.34

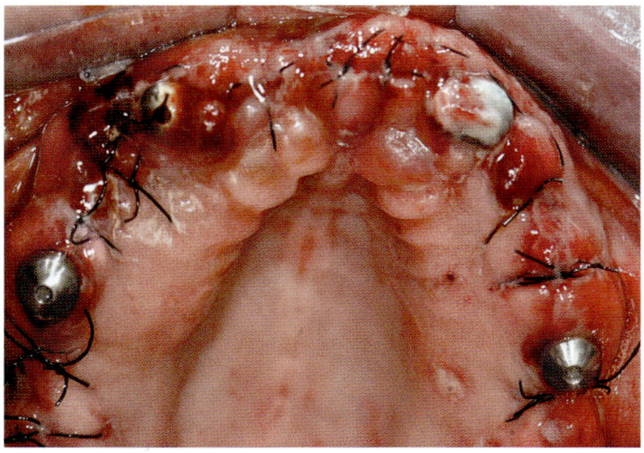

Fig 11.35

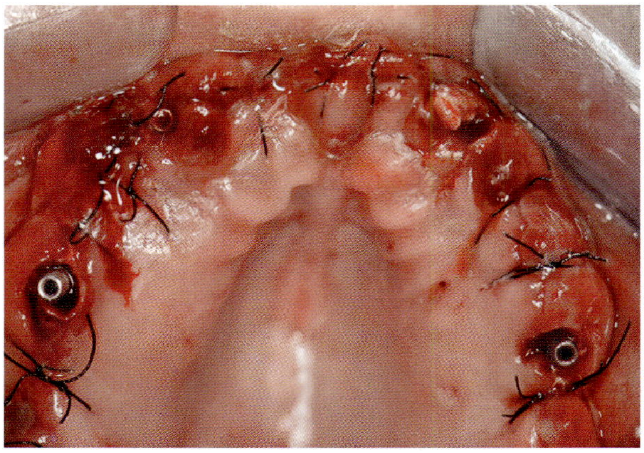

Fig 11.36

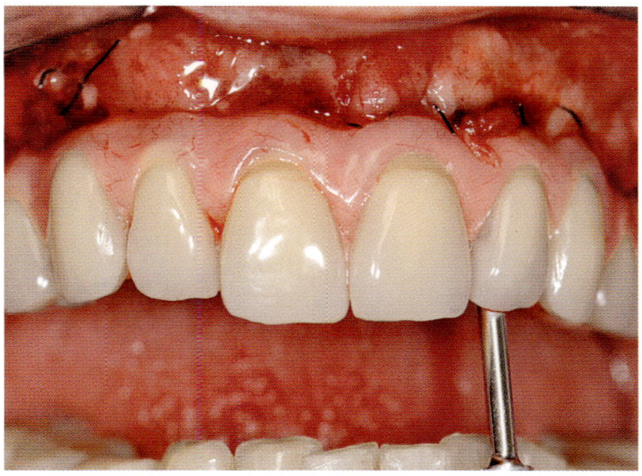

Fig 11.37

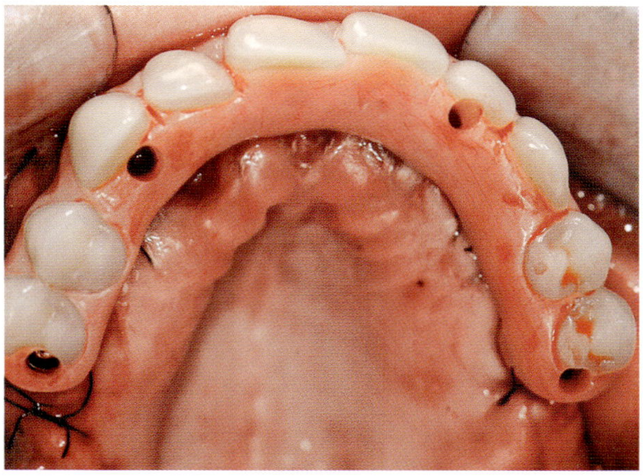

Fig 11.38

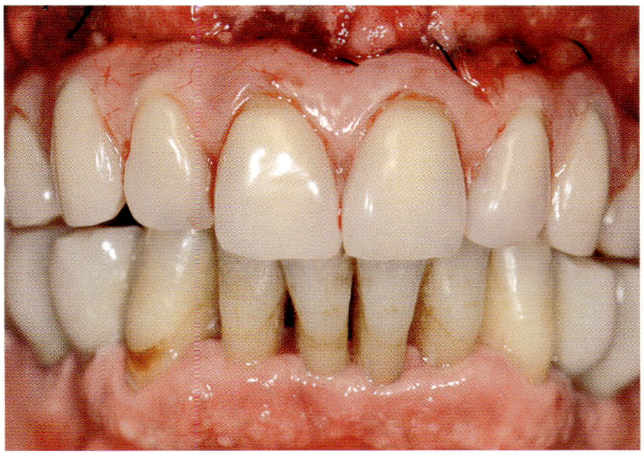

Fig 11.39

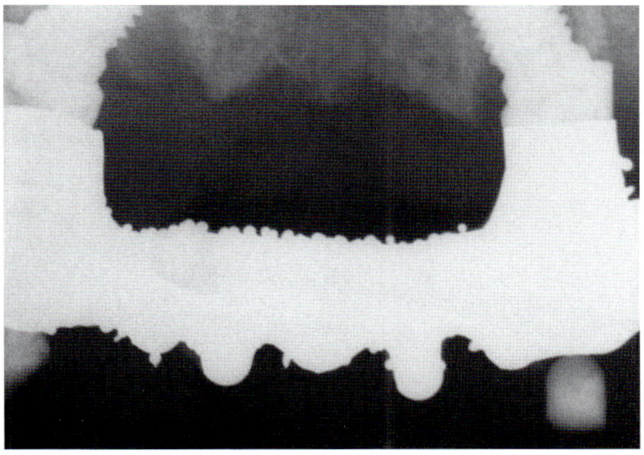

Fig 11.40

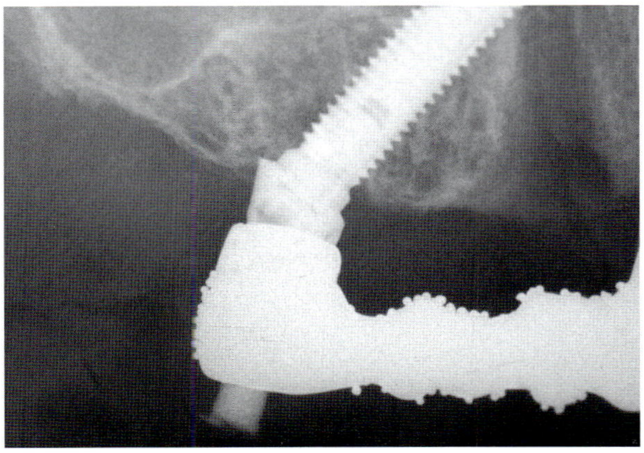

Fig 11.41

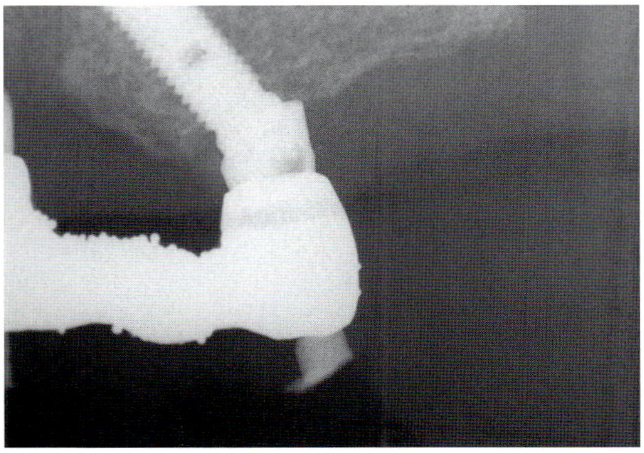

Fig 11.42

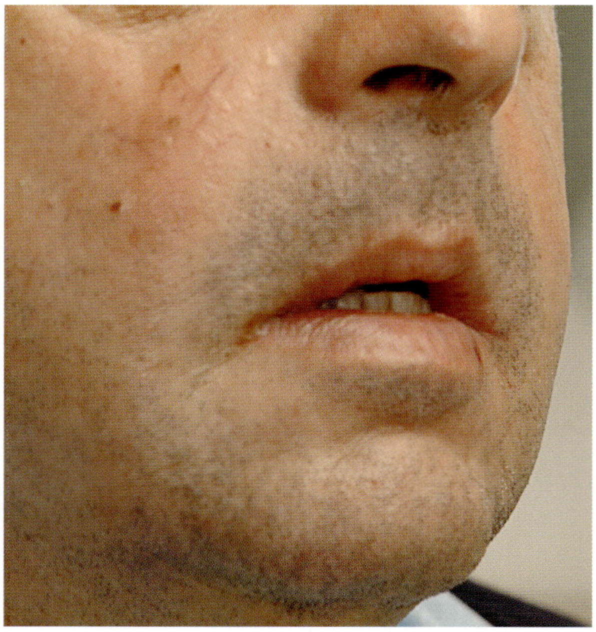

Fig 11.43

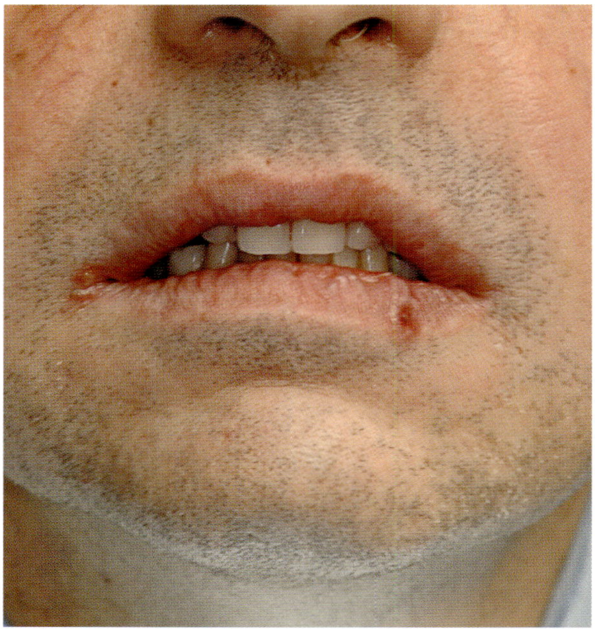

Fig 11.44

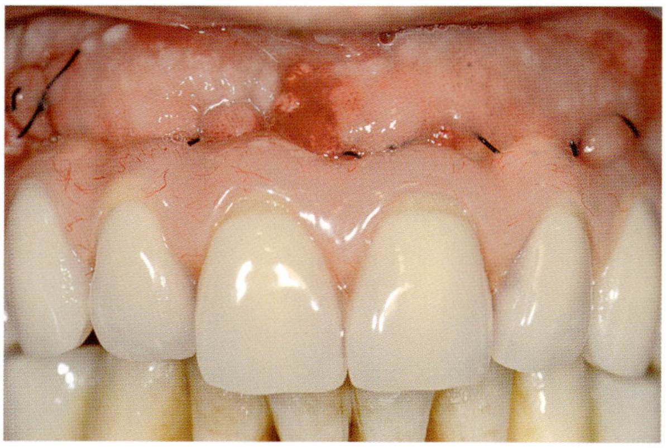

Fig 11.45

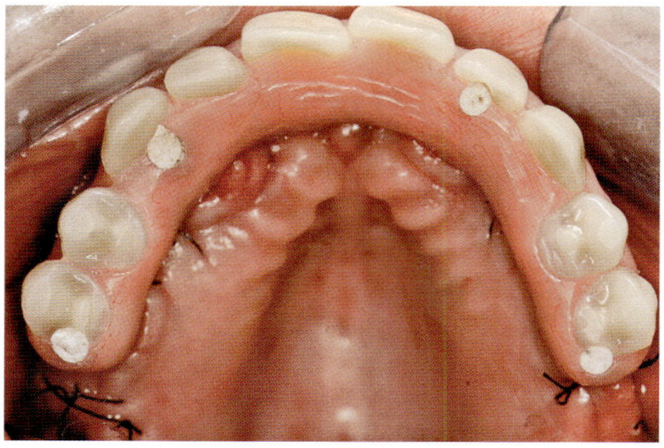

Fig 11.46

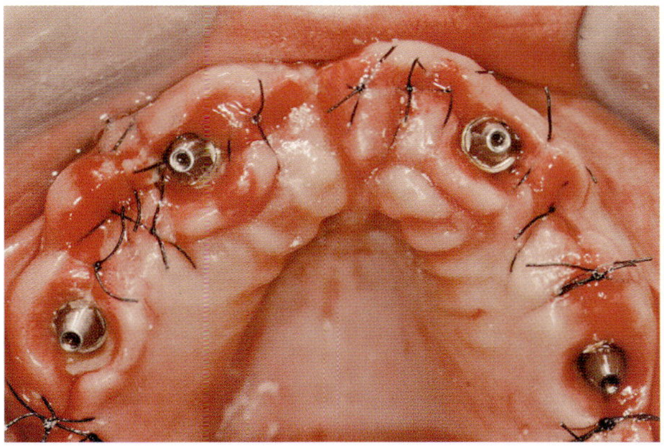

Fig 11.47

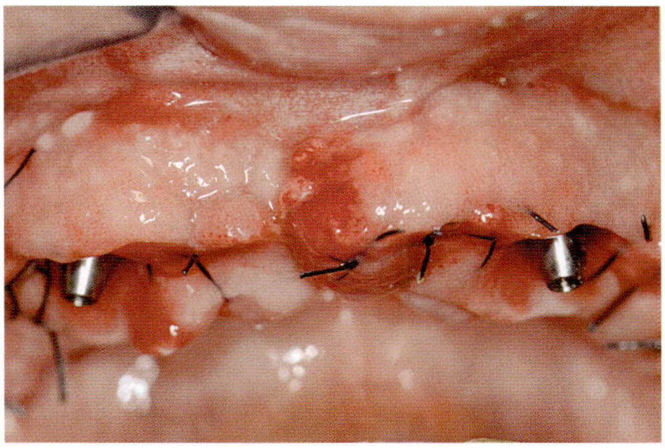

Fig 11.48

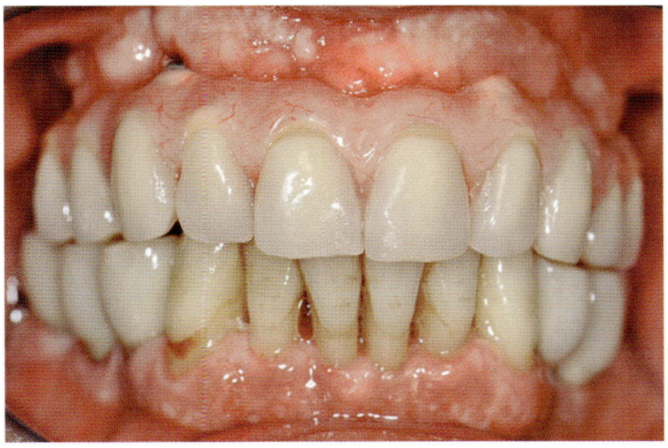

Fig 11.49

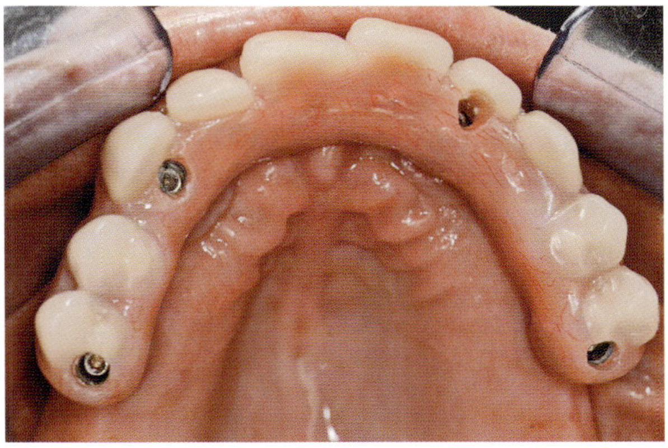

Fig 11.50

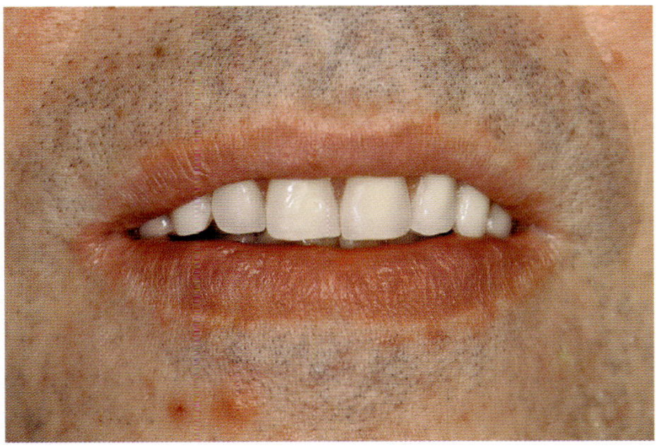

Fig 11.51

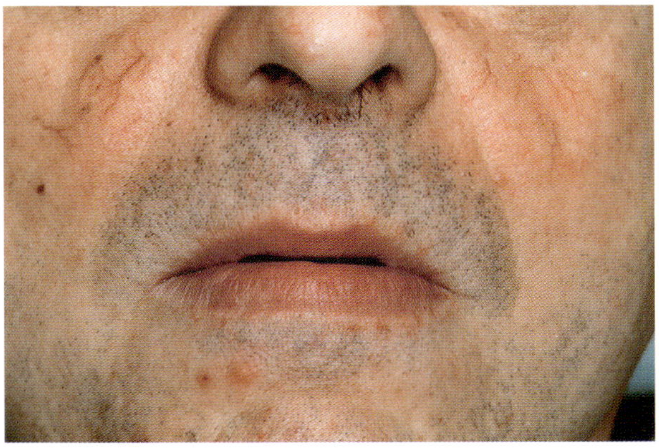

Fig 11.52

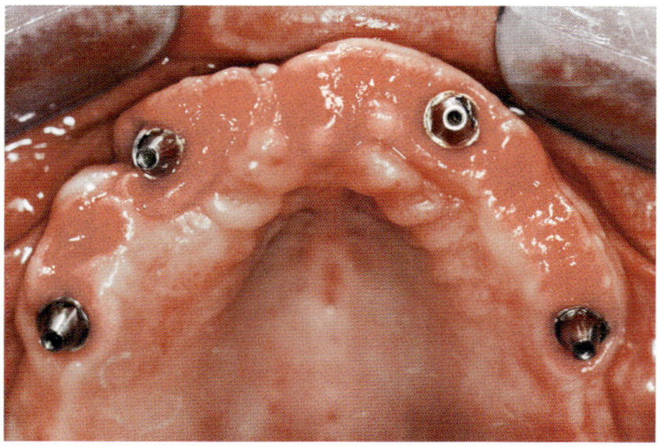

Fig 11.53

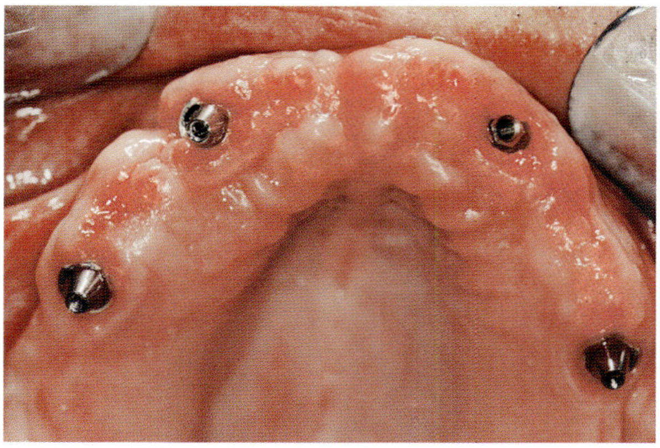

Fig 11.54

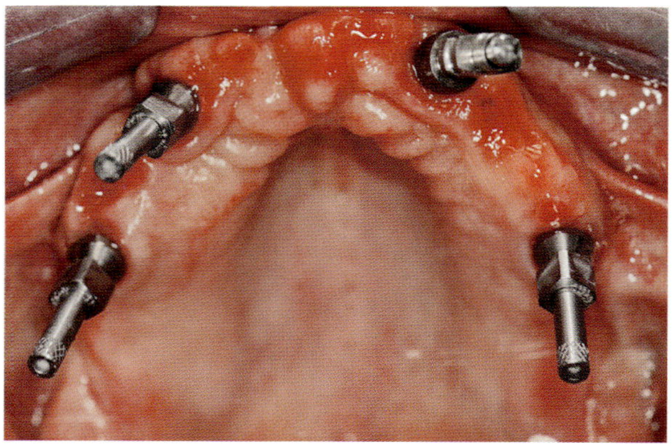

Fig 11.55

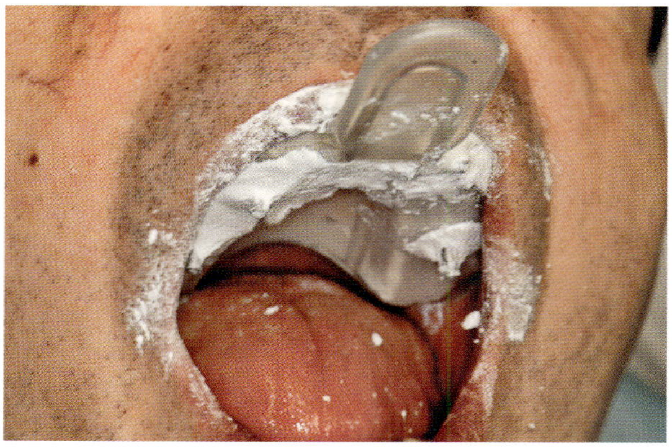

Fig 11.56

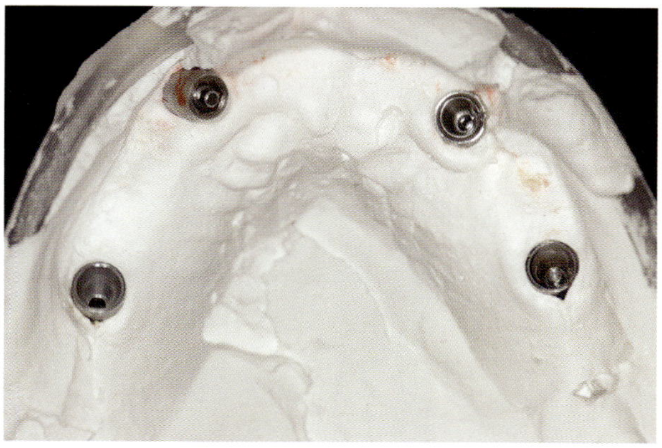

Fig 11.57

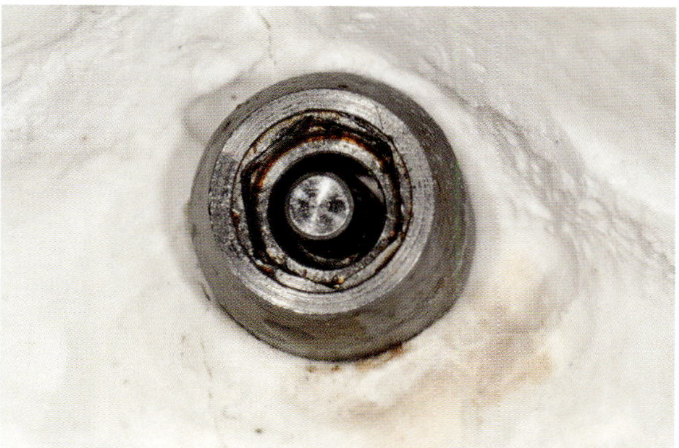

Fig 11.58

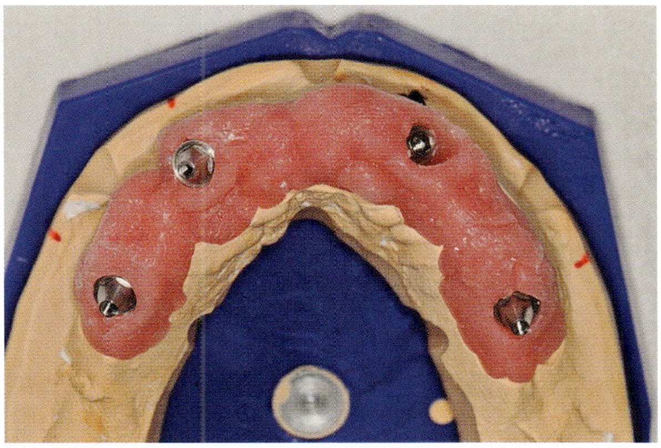

Fig 11.59

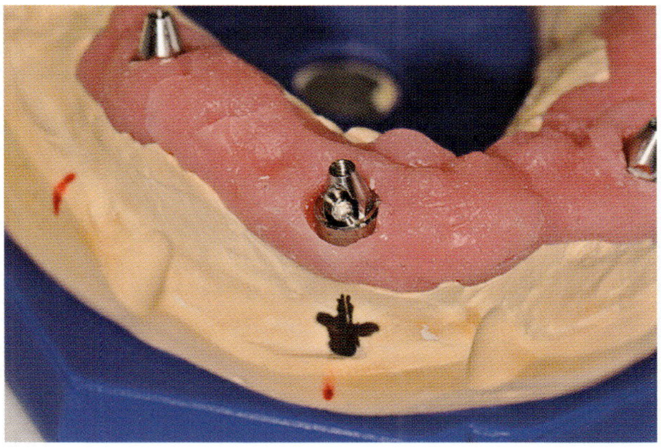

Fig 11.60

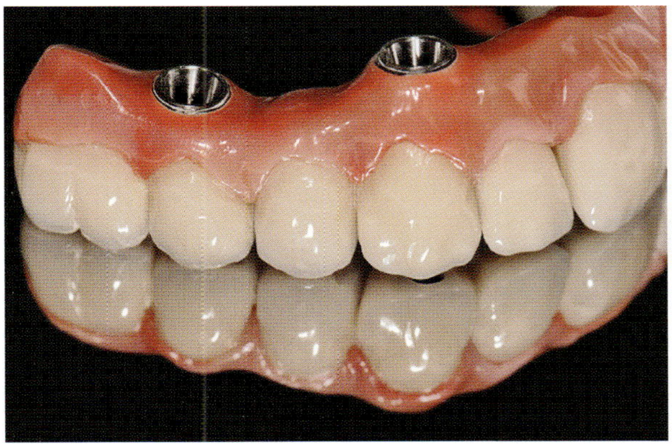

Fig 11.61

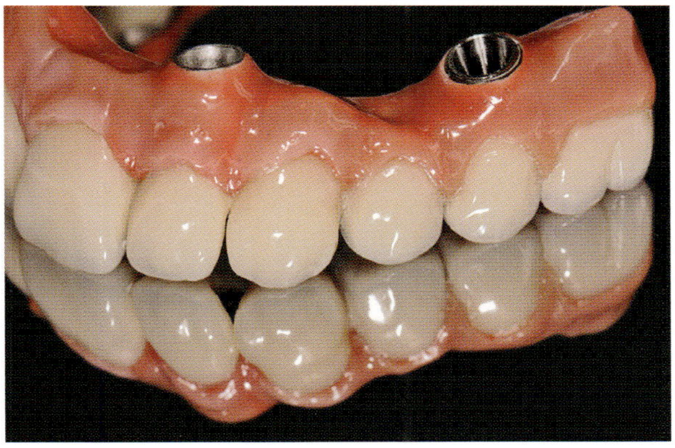

Fig 11.62

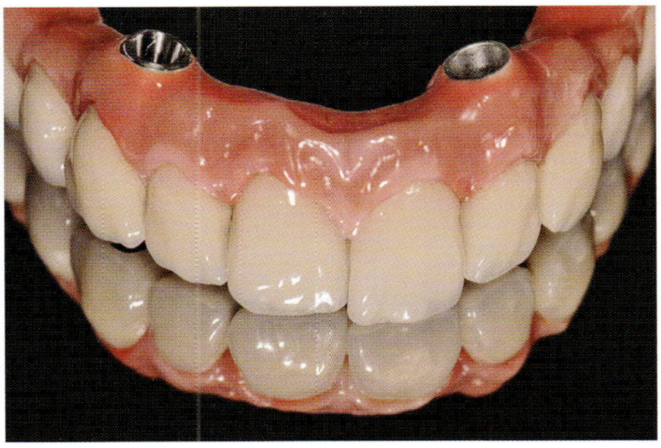

Fig 11.63

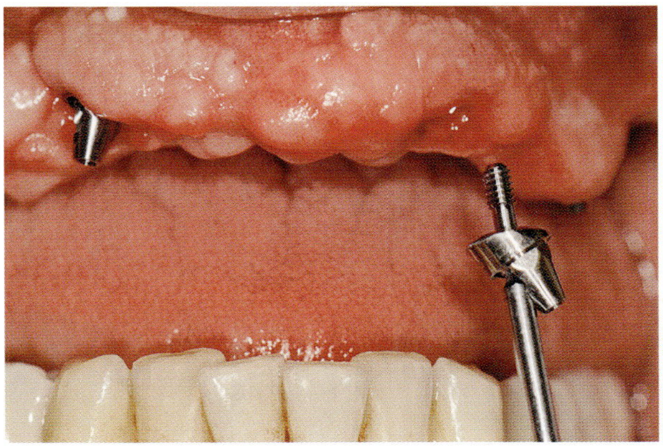

Fig 11.64

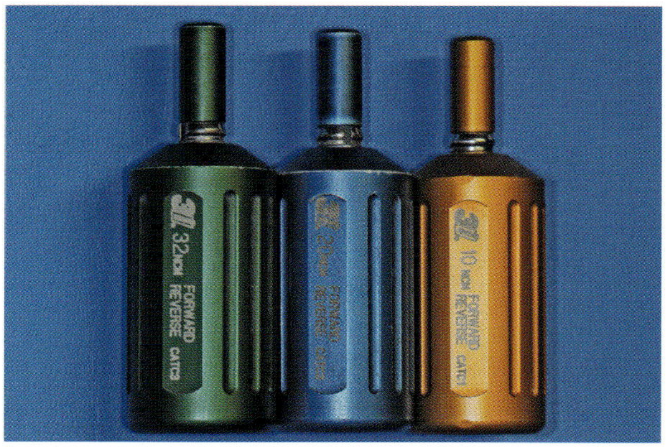

Fig 11.65

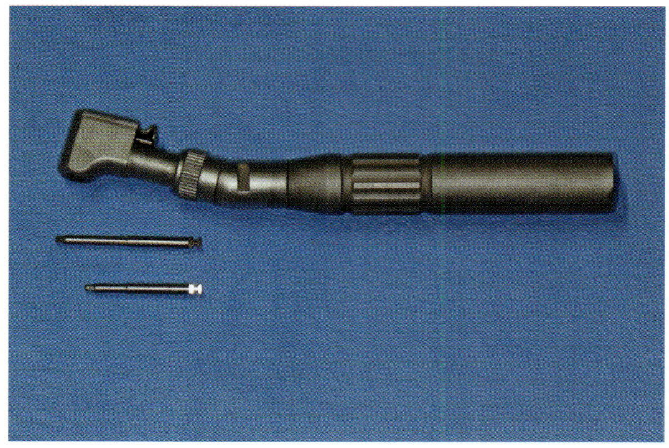

Fig 11.66

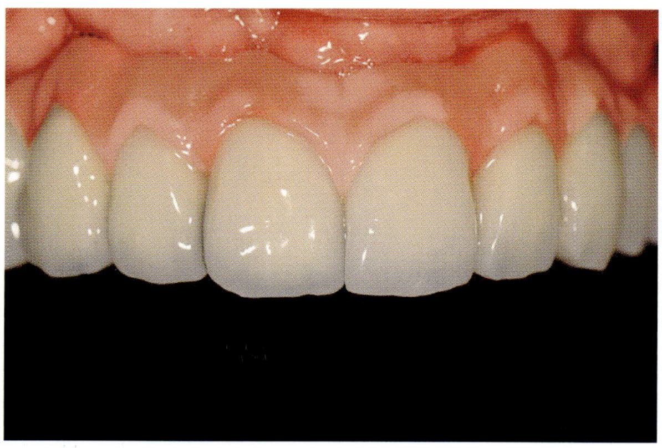

Fig 11.67

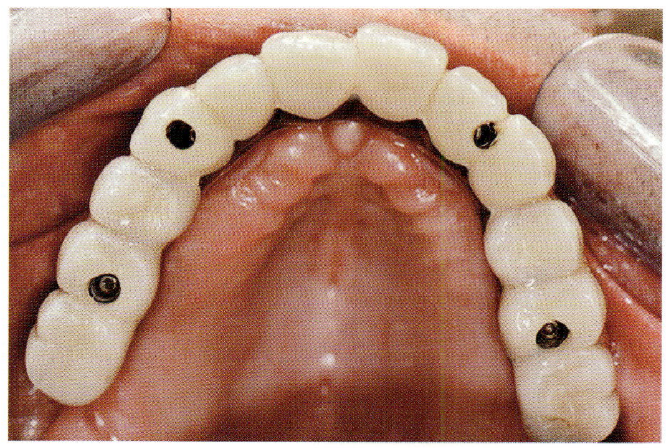

Fig. 11.68

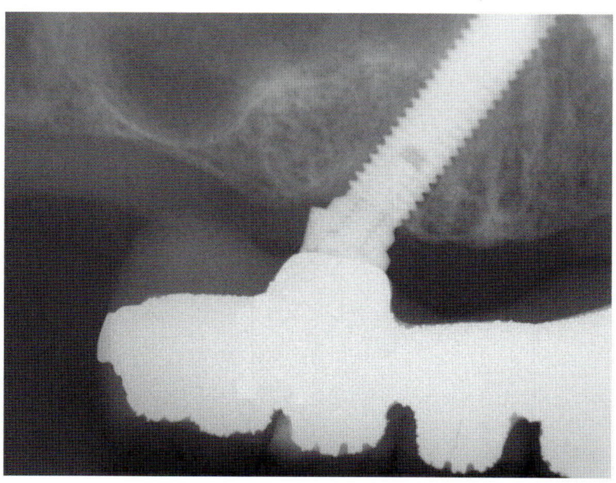

Fig 11.69

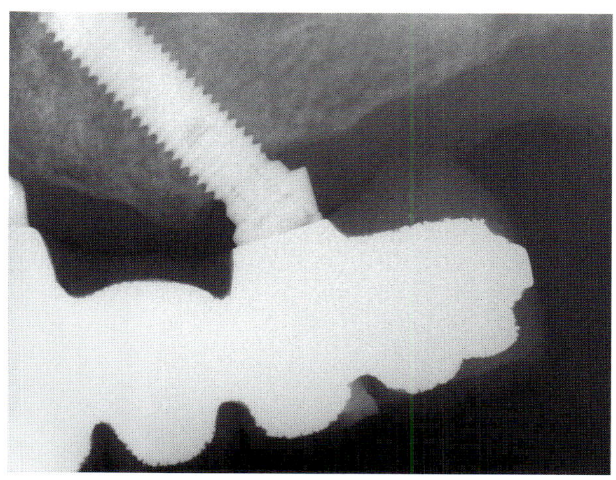

Fig 11.70

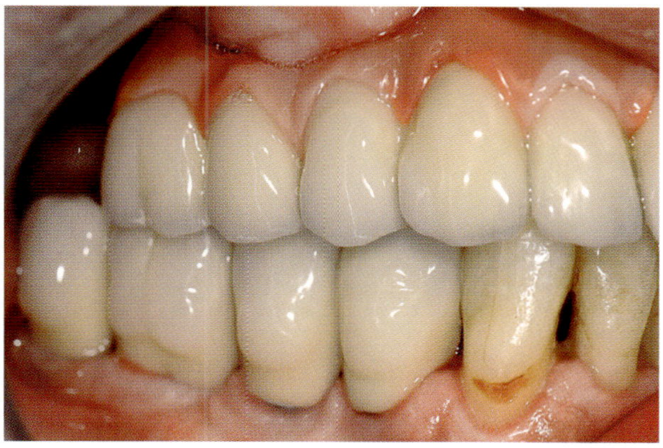

Fig 11.71

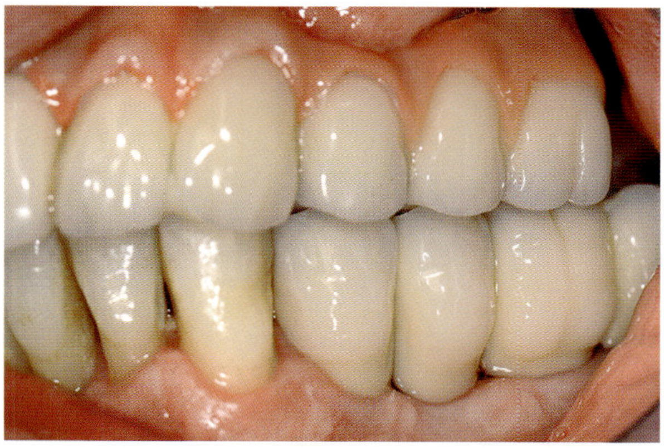

Fig 11.72

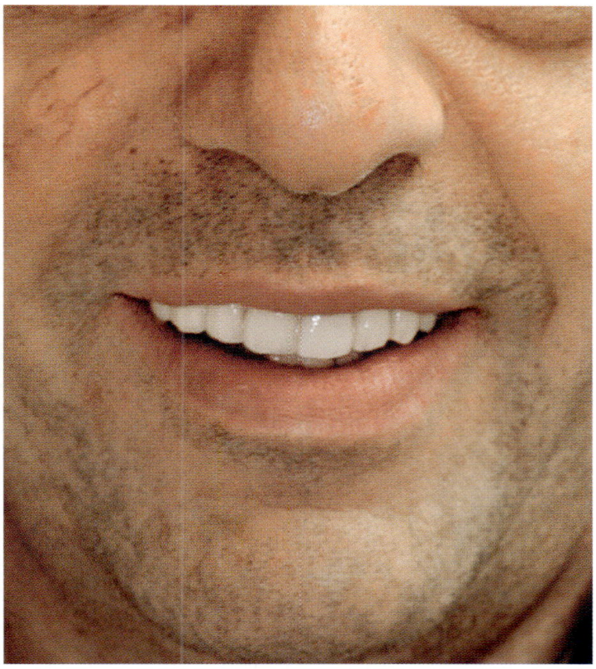

Fig 11.73

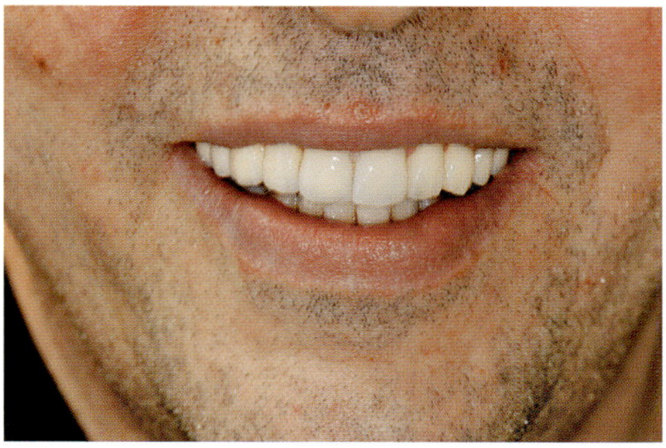

Fig 11.74

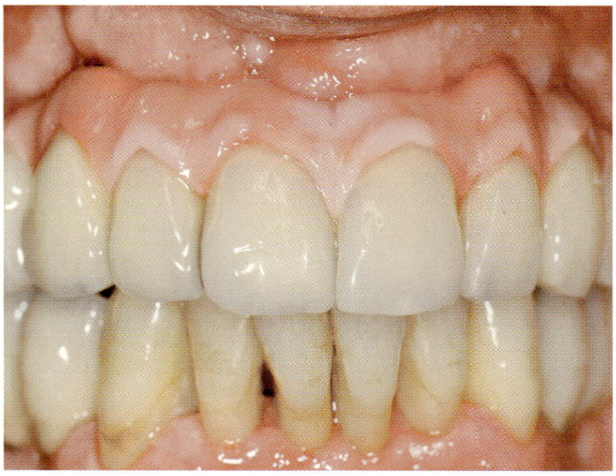

Fig 11.75

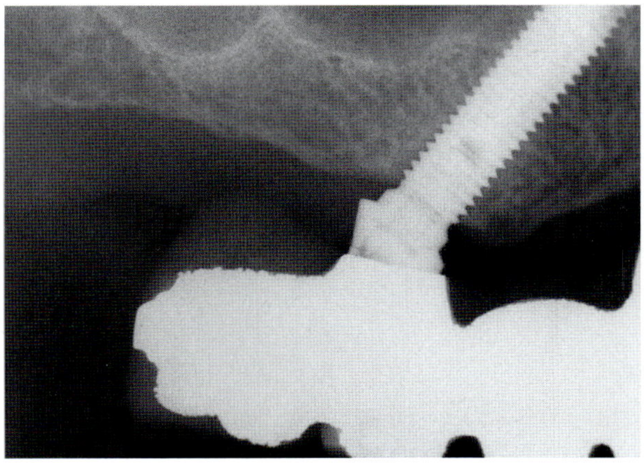

Fig 11.76

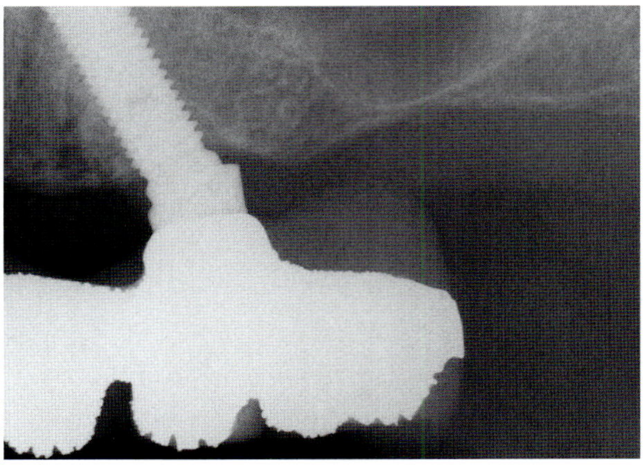

Fig 11.77

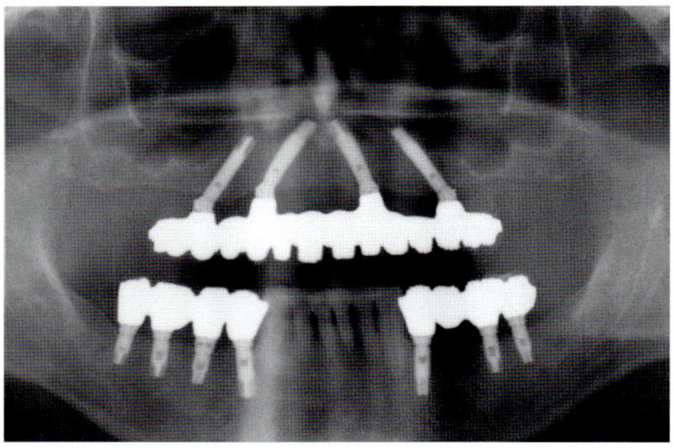

Fig 11.78

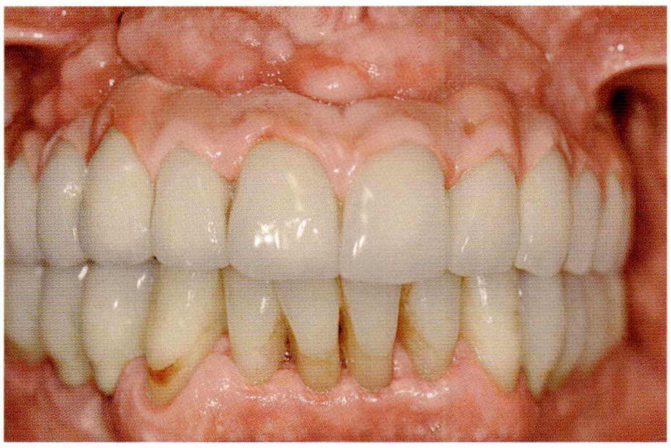

Fig 11.79

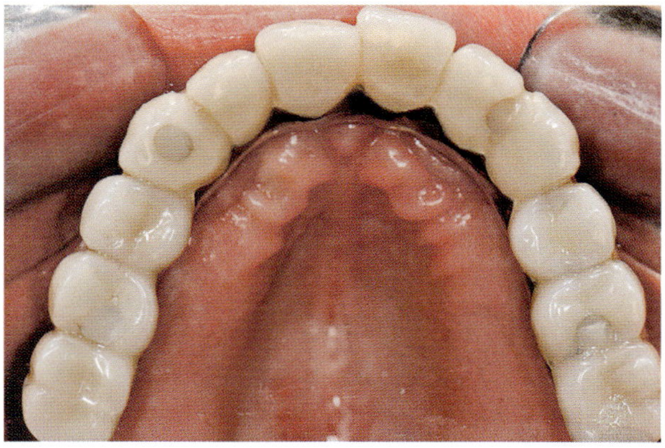

Fig 11.80

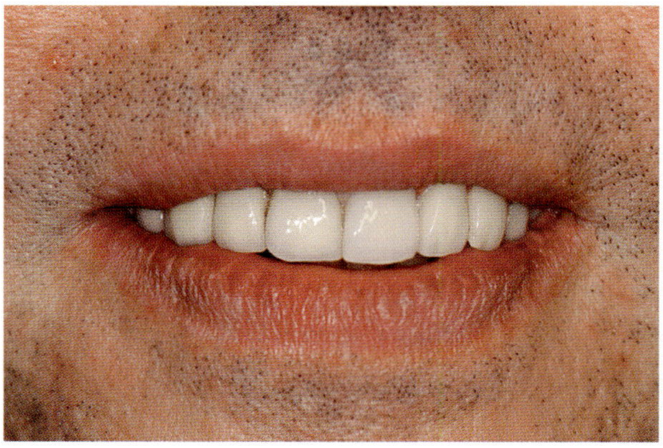

Fig 11.81

CHAPTER 12

FULL-ARCH FIXED PROSTHETIC TREATMENT WITHOUT RECONSTRUCTION OF SOFT TISSUES: THE NATURAL BRIDGE

This chapter illustrates the clinical (surgical and prosthetic) and laboratory procedures for a patient treated per the Columbus Bridge Protocol with a natural fixed bridge. The diagnostic work-up led the authors to recommend an immediate full-arch prosthesis without replacement of the supporting soft tissues since resorption was minimal. This treatment was distinctly different from the procedures described in chapter 11, where the missing hard and soft tissues were replaced with the prosthesis.

Background

The patient was a 51-year-old woman in good general health (American Society of Anesthesiologists Physical Status classification I [ASA PS I]) with a moderate smoking habit. She had been treated previously with combined fixed and removable prostheses in both jaws.

Physical and radiographic examinations

Thorough physical and radiographic examinations were conducted (Figs 12.1 to 12.10). Extraorally, the facial midline did not coincide with the maxillary dental midline. The esthetic analysis showed the presence of approximately 1 mm of maxillary anterior gingiva while smiling (see Figs 12.1 and 12.2), which the patient considered unattractive. She requested that this be changed so that no gingival tissues would show during speaking or smiling after prosthetic treatment was completed. The entire crowns of the maxillary anterior teeth were visible while smiling. The gingival margins of the central incisors teeth were uneven and asymmetric. The objective intraoral examination identified a defective preexisting fixed partial denture in the maxilla (see Figs 12.4 and 12.5). The margins of the preexisting restorations were supragingival and considered unsightly by the patient (see Fig 12.3), and the maxillary tissues demonstrated moderate inflammation secondary to coverage by the removable partial denture (see Fig 12.6).

The radiographic examination consisted of panoramic and periapical radiographs. Extensive bone loss was noted around all of the maxillary teeth (see Figs 12.7 to 12.9). The periodontal pockets were probed, and the values were recorded on the preoperative chart. The pocket measurements confirmed the loss of attachment and bone around the teeth; all of the teeth exhibited at least class I mobility (see Fig 12.10).

Diagnosis

The patient was diagnosed with advanced, generalized periodontal disease; a Class II jaw relationship; and a partially edentulous maxilla and mandible.

Treatment plan

The following treatment plan was developed and accepted by the patient. It addressed her chief complaints for improved esthetics and function:

1. Treatment of the maxillary dentition with extraction, immediate implant placement, and insertion of a fixed provisional prosthesis per the Columbus Bridge Protocol. This protocol was chosen because it eliminates dental disease, provides for immediate function and cross-arch stabilization, and permits placement of an immediate fixed prosthesis in the maxillary arch.
2. Treatment of the mandibular dentition with extraction, immediate implant placement, and insertion of a fixed provisional prosthesis per the Columbus Bridge Protocol.

Preliminary treatment: Diagnostic articulator mounting

The patient met with a hygienist for preliminary scaling and root planing of the remaining teeth to reduce inflammation by removing plaque and calculus. Preliminary alginate impressions were taken, and the first centric relation jaw record was made at the vertical dimension of occlusion (VDO). The jaw relation record was necessary to allow the casts to be mounted in the laboratory in preparation for making the surgical-prosthetic template as described in Chapter 3 (Figs 12.11 to 12.14). The facial midline was recorded on the wax interocclusal record so that the wax denture would be correctly centered on the articulator. The edentulous areas of the interocclusal record were relined with silicone to guarantee adequate stability of the casts during the articulator mounting.

Despite the presence of generalized periodontal pockets measuring 5 mm or more in depth, the proposed treatment plan called for the fabrication of a full-arch fixed denture without replacement of soft tissues associated with a Toronto Bridge–type prosthesis. This decision was based on several factors, including the preextraction clinical data and esthetic wax denture setup in the laboratory, the patient's request to eliminate any gingival tissues visible with smiling, the presence of a 3-mm overbite, and the relationship between lower lip position and the maxillary incisal edges while smiling.

Surgical treatment

Immediately prior to surgery, the VDO was determined by measuring the distance between two cutaneous points (pronasale and pogonion), one above and one below the mouth (Figs 12.15 and 12.16). Local anesthesia was administered, and the preexisting metal-ceramic fixed partial denture was sectioned and removed from the preparations (Figs 12.17 and 12.18). The extractions were performed one by one with utmost care to maintain the maxillary cortical plate of bone throughout the jaw. Generalized advanced bone loss was observed around the majority of the teeth, and periodontal probing confirmed significant bone loss on the distal surface of the maxillary right central incisor (Fig 12.20).

After the extractions were completed (Fig 12.19), extensive alveolar curettage was carried out in the extraction sockets, and then a bevelled incision for a full-thickness flap was made. The incisive papilla was avoided since it is an area of esthetic importance (Fig 12.21). The prosthetic design for this case was different than that used for the case illustrated in chapter 11. Because the emergence profiles of the artificial teeth in this treatment would be similar to the emergence profiles of the natural dentition, replacement of the gingival tissues was not needed. The flap was widened to fully expose the labial and buccal walls and the curvature of the palate (Fig 12.22). Before proceeding to implant placement, the surgical-prosthetic template was inserted, and the mandible was guided into centric relation. Since the surgical-prosthetic template was retained and stabilized by the occlusal surfaces of the mandibular teeth, it permitted the clinician to rapidly assess optimal positioning of the implants relative to the location of the teeth in the prosthesis (Fig 12.23). The facial-dental preoperative discrepancy was corrected in the wax denture, and the surgical-prosthetic template identified the locations of the emergence profiles of the artificial teeth.

After the flap was reflected on the lateral maxillary wall, the anterior wall of the right maxillary sinus was identified as described previously, the osteotomy was drilled parallel to the anterior wall of the sinus, and the distal implant was inserted (Fig 12.24; the asterisk indicates the bony window in the lateral wall of the sinus). When possible, extraction sites should be avoided by placing implants into residual bone for maximum primary stability (Fig 12.25). After the right distal implant was placed, the need for angle correction of the abutment was evaluated by reinserting the surgical-prosthetic template into the mouth. The location of the teeth was assessed relative to the location of the implant restorative platform, and the appropriate angulated abutment was placed (Fig 12.26).

The right anterior implant was placed next. The maxillary right central incisor site was avoided because it did not provide optimal support for the fixed provisional prosthesis. The anterior implant was placed in the interradicular bone between the sockets of the maxillary right incisors. The actual location was decided upon in conjunction with the location of the teeth in the surgical-prosthetic template (Fig 12.27). High levels of implant primary stability were obtained through the use of tapered implants and undersized osteotomy preparations. Insertion torque values ranged from 50 to 70 Ncm (Figs 12.28 to 12.30). With the use of two posterior tilted implants and two vertical implants, optimal cross-arch stabilization was obtained (Fig 12.31).

Prosthetic treatment

The prosthetic phase commenced with clinical abutment selection in conjunction with the position of teeth in the surgical-prosthetic template (Fig 12.32). The occlusal image demonstrates the emergence of the anterior implant relative to the position of the maxillary lateral incisor. This clinical step (Fig 12.33) enabled the clinician to identify the emergence of the abutment and screw access opening relative to the tooth in the surgical-prosthetic template.

After the conical abutments were placed, conical abutment pickup impression copings were screwed into the abutments (Figs 12.34 and 12.35). Holes were made in a stock plastic impression tray to permit access to the impression copings (Fig 12.36). The impression was taken with type III impression plaster (Fig 12.37). With the pickup impression protocol, the impression copings remain in the impression. The intaglio surface of the impression demonstrated the excellent anteroposterior spread and cross-arch stabilization obtained with the distal inclinations of the posterior implants.

Conical abutment healing caps were screwed into the conical abutments that remained in the implants, and the jaw relation records were made with the healing caps in place. The interocclusal wax record was made at the VDO that was determined preoperatively, prior to tooth extractions (Figs 12.38 and 12.39). The facial midline was recorded on the wax interocclusal record (Fig 12.40). Prior to sending the impression to the laboratory, the wax interocclusal record was carefully evaluated for accuracy (Figs 12.41 and 12.42). The treatment illustrated in this case demonstrated that with the appropriate diagnostic work-up and surgical-prosthetic treatment, optimal relationships were obtained relative to implant and abutment placement, and a screw-retained, fixed provisional prosthesis could be fabricated (Figs 12.43 and 12.44). The patient returned 24 hours after surgery with slight extraoral swelling but no bruising. She reported that she was comfortable and required only nonsteroidal anti-inflammatory medications for analgesia after the local anesthetic had worn off (Fig 12.45). Intraorally, minimal inflammation was observed (Fig 12.46).

The healing caps were removed from the conical abutments, and the provisional prosthesis was seated onto the conical abutments. The gold retaining screws were tightened progressively, cross-arch, to 10 Ncm. Provisional prostheses made per the Columbus Bridge Protocol are not made with cantilevered extensions (Fig 12.47).

To ensure high rates of osseointegration, it is important to use occlusal materials in the provisional prosthesis that provide sufficient shock absorption from the occlusal loads to the implants. Such a precaution helps to avoid overloading implants and prostheses with immediate occlusal function, as described in chapter 10. The intaglio surface of the provisional prosthesis resulted in discrete compression of the peri-implant soft tissues. This was done to create optimal gingival architecture prior to construction of the definitive prosthesis after osseointegration occurred (Figs 12.48 to 12.50). Further modifications in the gingival contours would be made as needed during follow-up visits over the next 4 months. By establishing the correct VDO and reestablishing harmony between the maxillary dental and facial midlines, optimal facial esthetics were obtained (Figs 12.51 and 12.52).

Ten days later, the patient returned for removal of the provisional prosthesis and sutures. The soft tissue contours were developing consistent with the contours of the intaglio surface of the provisional prosthesis (Figs 12.53 and 12.54). In this particular case, the peri-implant soft tissues resorbed significantly, resulting in excessive space between the provisional prosthesis and the edentulous ridge, especially in the area of the maxillary right incisor sites (Figs 12.55 and 12.56).

Autopolymerizing acrylic resin was added to the deficient areas of the prosthesis to reestablish optimal contours between the prosthesis and the peri-implant soft tissues (Figs 12.57 and 12.58).

Evaluation for fabrication of the definitive maxillary fixed prosthesis

The patient returned for further clinical follow-up approximately 4 months after the extractions, implant placement, and insertion of the provisional prosthesis per the Columbus Bridge Protocol. The following parameters were reevaluated:

- VDO
- Relationship between the smile line and the length of the teeth
- Relationship between the maxillary dental and facial midlines
- Lip support (increase, decrease, or maintain)
- Orientation and direction of angled abutments (Figs 12.59 and 12.60)
- Amount and location of occlusal wear (Fig 12.61)
- Adaptation of peri-implant soft tissues to the prosthesis and conical abutments (Figs 12.62 and 12.63)
- Phonetics

As far as the last point is concerned, the patient did report difficulties with the pronunciation of certain words. It was decided to reduce the palatofacial thickness of the definitive prosthesis relative to the original dimensions of the provisional prosthesis. Therefore, the two angulated conical abutments positioned on the mesial implants were scheduled to be removed prior to the definitive impression. The two anterior implant restorative platforms would be impressed directly, and new abutments would be selected in the laboratory on the master cast (Figs 12.64 and 12.65).

Fabrication of the definitive maxillary fixed prosthesis

The prosthetic protocol for the definitive prosthesis is similar to the protocol used for fabrication of the provisional prosthesis. The definitive impression was made with pickup implant impression copings for the two anterior implants and with conical abutment pickup impression copings for the two distal implants (Figs 12.65 and 12.66). Consistent with the Columbus Bridge Protocol, plaster impression material was used for the definitive impression (Figs 12.67 and 12.68).

In cases where patients present with high smile lines or other esthetic challenges related to the size of the artificial teeth, soft tissue recontouring can be accomplished as needed with rotary instruments prior to the bridge delivery (Figs 12.69 to 12.72). If soft tissues need to be surgically modified, the new soft tissue contours are generally impressed with regular body silicone impression material (Figs 12.73 to 12.76). A new cast is then poured in the laboratory to optimize the mucosal contact of the definitive prosthesis in this area. To maintain the contours of the soft tissues, it is important for the provisional prosthesis to be relined intraorally by rebasing the prosthesis with autopolymerizing acrylic resin (Figs 12.77 and 12.78).

In this case, it was observed that at the delivery appointment for the definitive prosthesis, the facial gingival contours established at the definitive impression appointment had matured and remained stable (Fig 12.79). Furthermore, the new surface gingival contours were confirmed after the provisional prosthesis was removed (Figs 12.80 to 12.82).

In the laboratory prosthetic phase, an angulated conical abutment was selected for use in the maxillary right lateral incisor implant site that decreased the thickness of the definitive prosthesis framework; a custom abutment was fabricated for use in the maxillary left lateral incisor implant site. The peri-implant soft tissues in this area were quite thin, and the custom abutment reduced the size of the abutment collar and optimized the esthetic results. This custom abutment was cast with a preformed retaining screw inside the occlusal surface of the abutment. This solution also continued the screw-retained philosophy inherent in the Columbus Bridge Protocol (Figs 12.83 to 12.88). Contrary to the design of the provisional prosthesis, the definitive prosthesis was designed with bilateral distal cantilevered supported by the cast metal framework and consisted of 12 masticatory units (Figs 12.89 and 12.90).

Clinically, the definitive prosthesis was screwed into the abutments with retaining screws torqued to 10 Ncm. During insertion of the prosthesis, soft tissues were slightly compressed to maintain the soft tissue contours established on the master cast (Figs 12.91 and 12.92). Postinsertion radiographs demonstrated *(1)* the absence of peri-implant radiolucencies, *(2)* crestal bone at the level of the first threads of the implants, and *(3)* optimal bone remodeling of the previous extraction sockets (Figs 12.93 to 12.95). The definitive prosthetic treatment reestablished optimal harmony of the inferior third of the face in both the frontal and sagittal planes and reestablished satisfactory masticatory function. The preoperative location of the smile line relative to the natural dentition and gingival margins was modified, and the amount of tooth display during speaking and smiling yielded an optimal esthetic result. Anatomical gingival contours were also developed within the framework of the prosthesis. The Columbus Bridge Protocol satisfied the patient's original expectations, avoided the use of a provisional removable prosthesis, and provided the patient with a fixed prosthesis within 24 hours of a single surgical appointment in which all of the procedures were accomplished (Figs 12.96 and 12.97).

Follow-up radiographs taken 3 years postoperatively demonstrated stable crestal bone levels relative to the radiographs taken at the insertion of the definitive prosthesis (Figs 12.98 to 12.102). The radiograph of the angled implant and prosthesis in the maxillary left posterior quadrant (see Fig 12.102) demonstrated that only one masticatory unit had to be added to the cantilevered framework to achieve occlusal function with the first molar. Clinical photographs taken at the same follow-up appointment show that occlusal, biologic, and esthetic stability were obtained with the definitive metal-ceramic prosthesis made according to the Columbus Bridge Protocol (Figs 12.103 to 12.107).

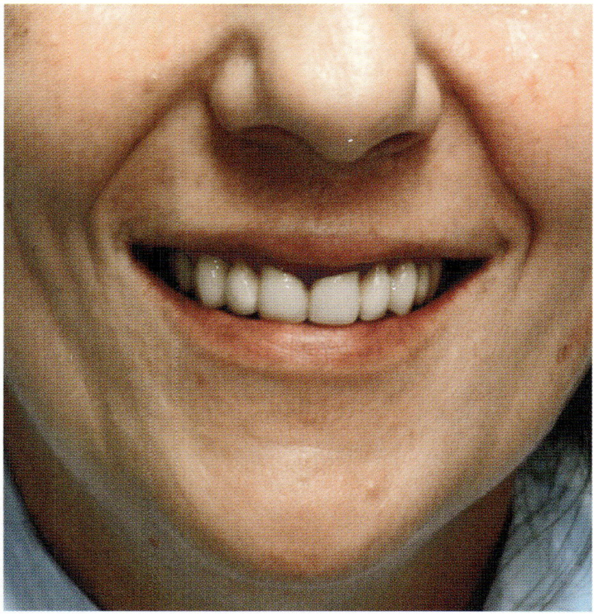

Fig 12.1

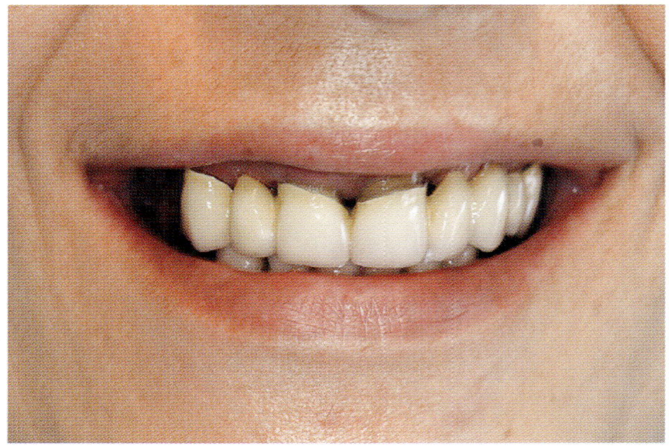

Fig 12.2

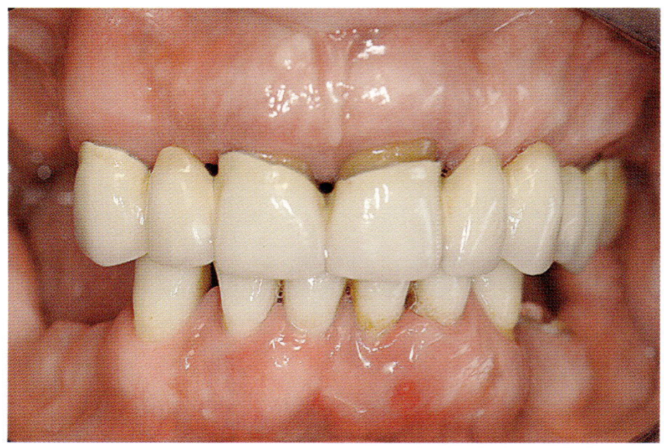

Fig 12.3

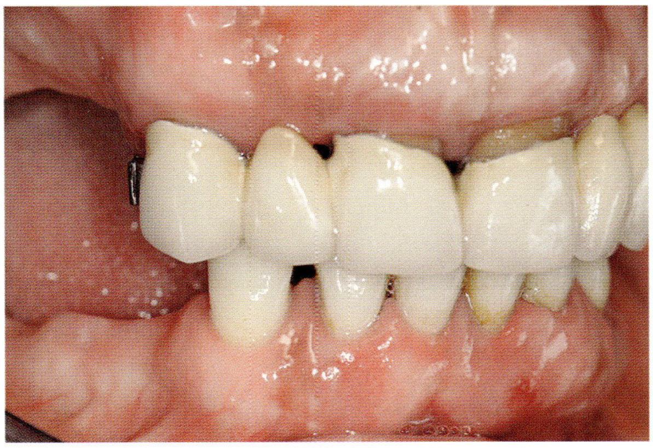

Fig 12.4

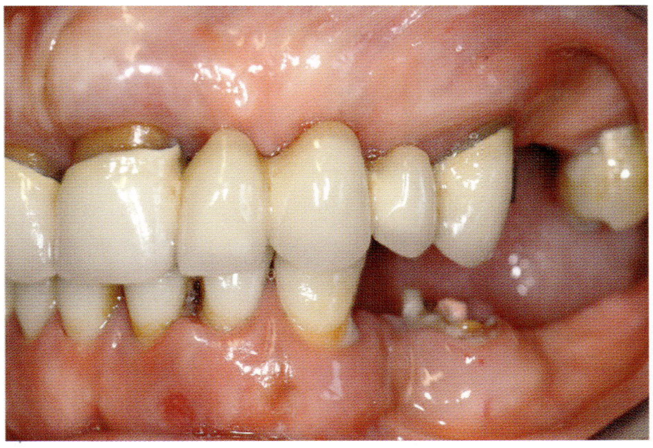

Fig 12.5

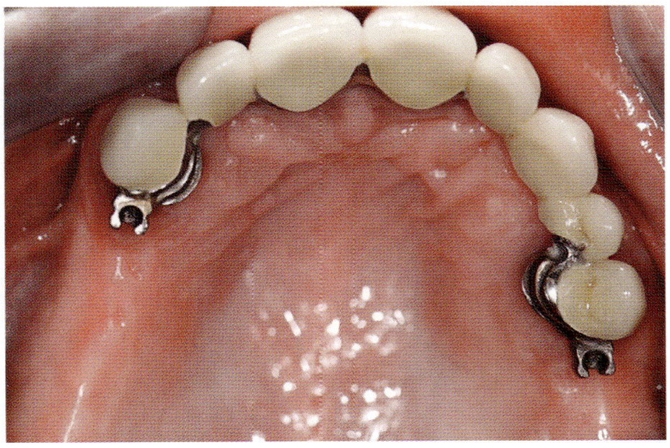

Fig 12.6

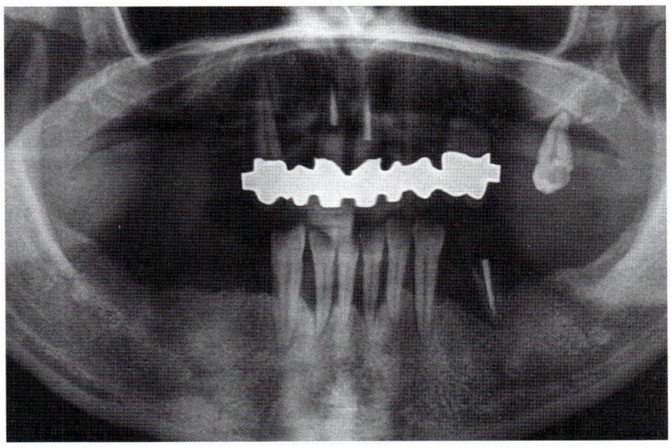

Fig 12.7

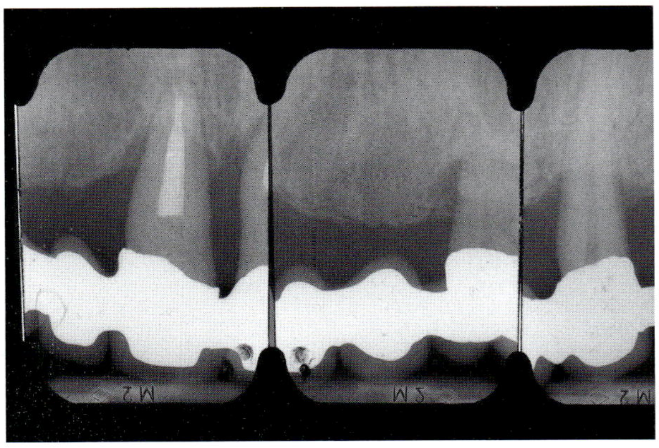

Fig 12.8

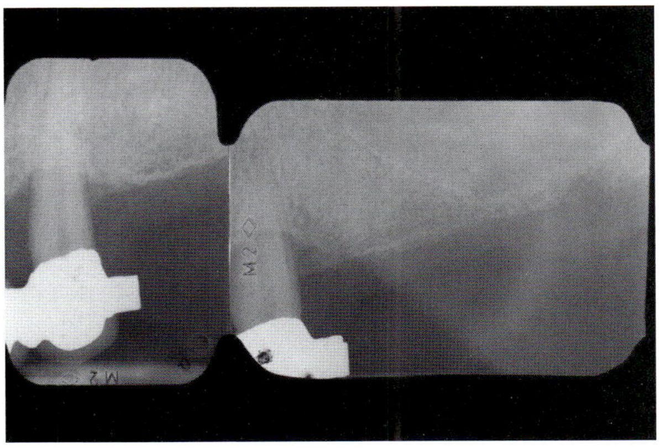

Fig 12.9

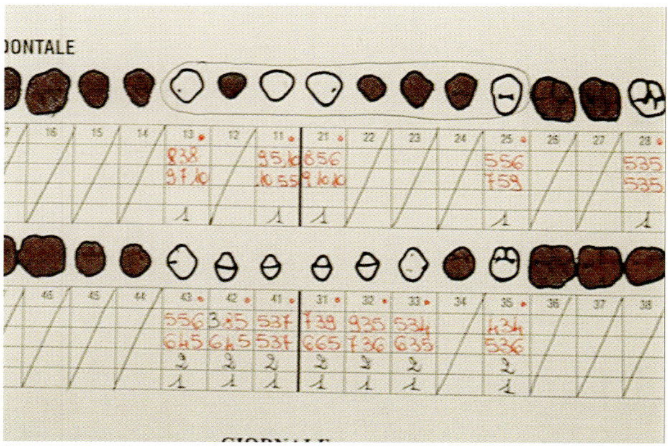

Fig 12.10

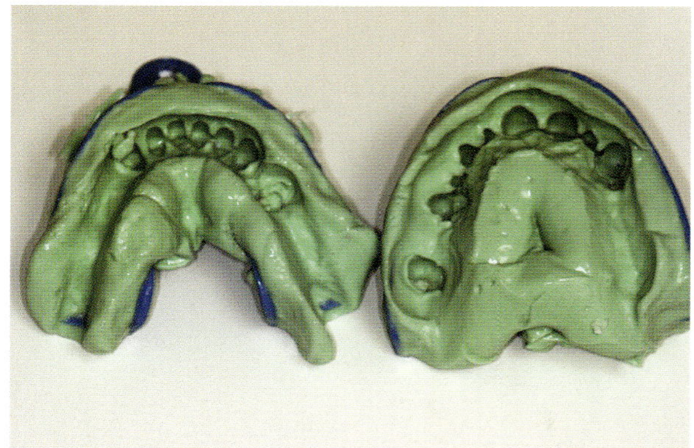

Fig 12.11

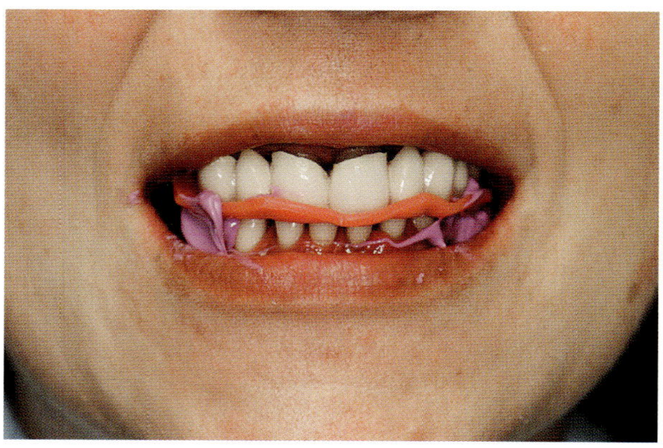

Fig 12.12

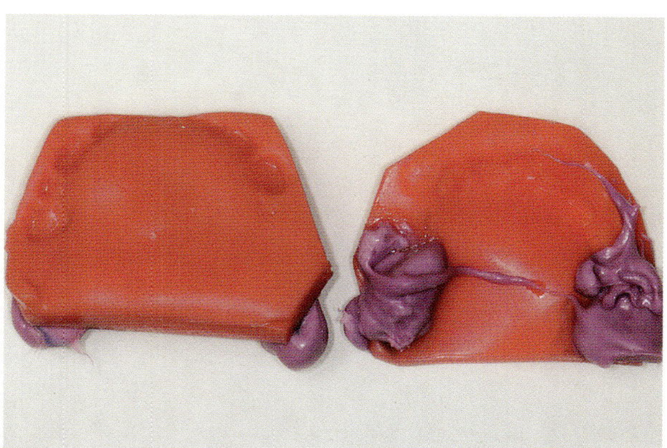

Fig 12.13

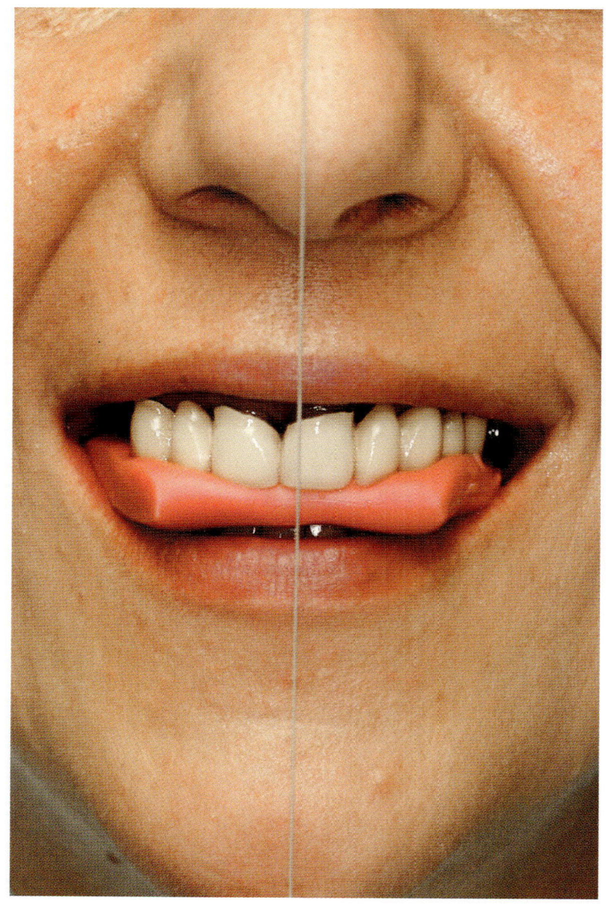

Fig 12.14

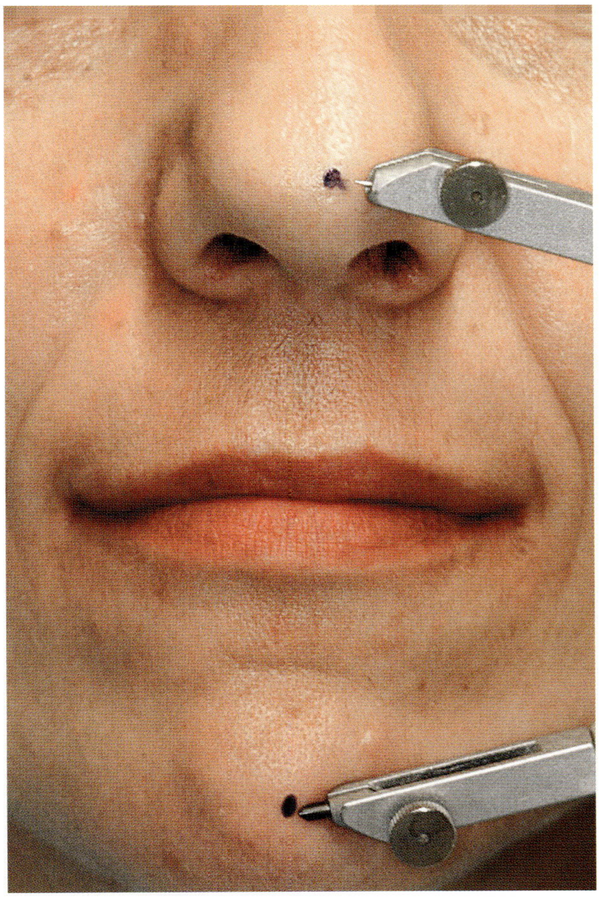

Fig 12.15

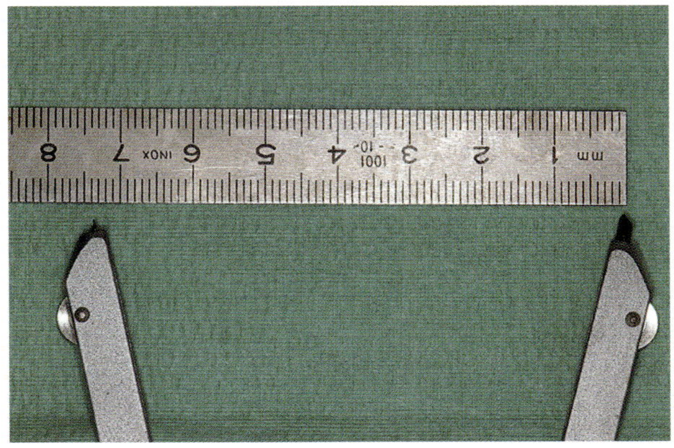

Fig 12.16

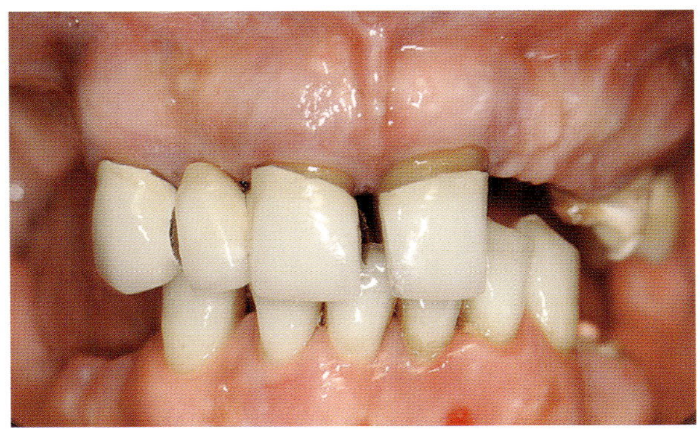

Fig 12.17

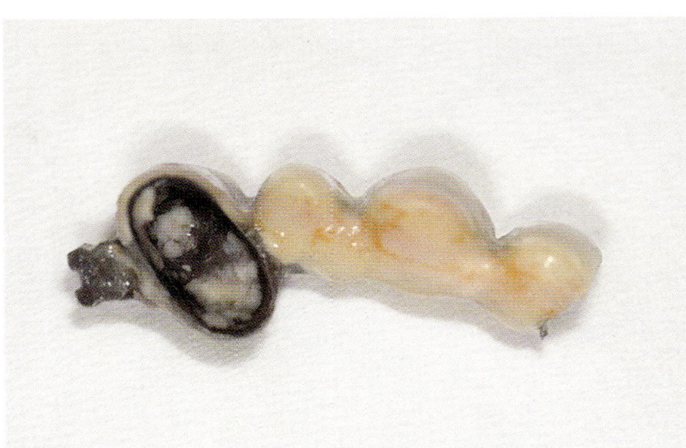

Fig 12.18

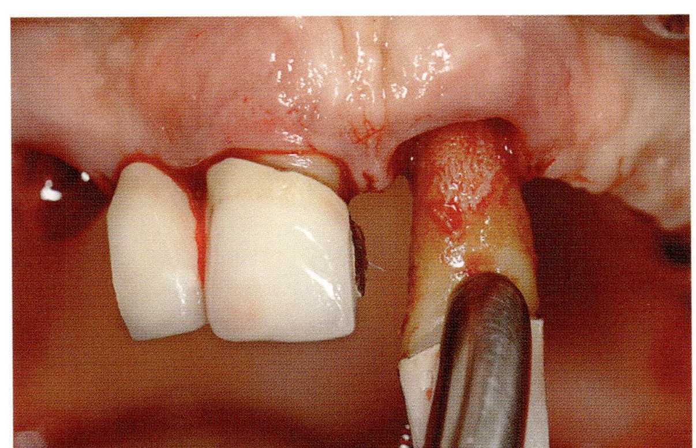

Fig 12.19

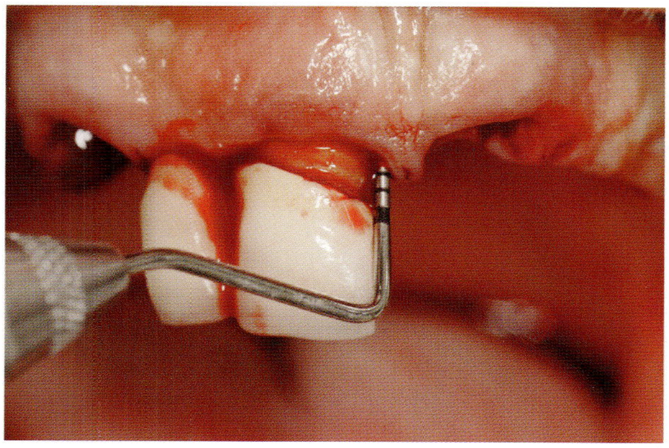

Fig 12.20

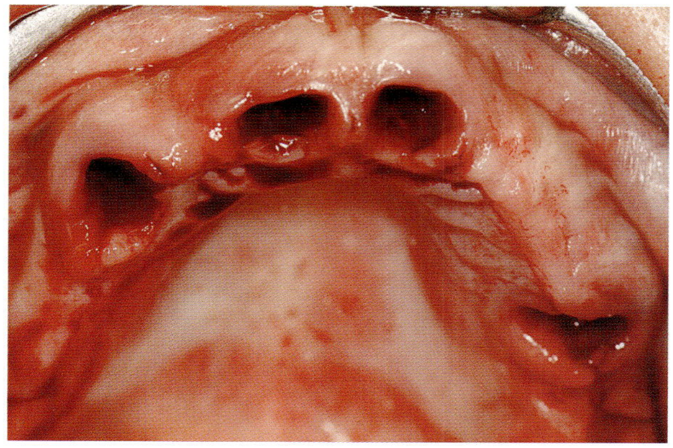

Fig 12.21

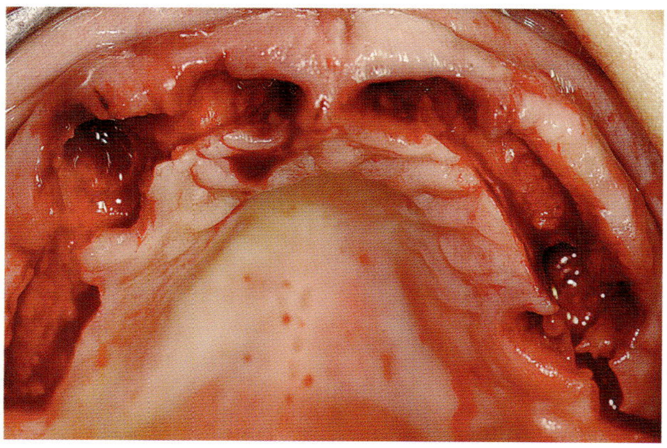

Fig 12.22

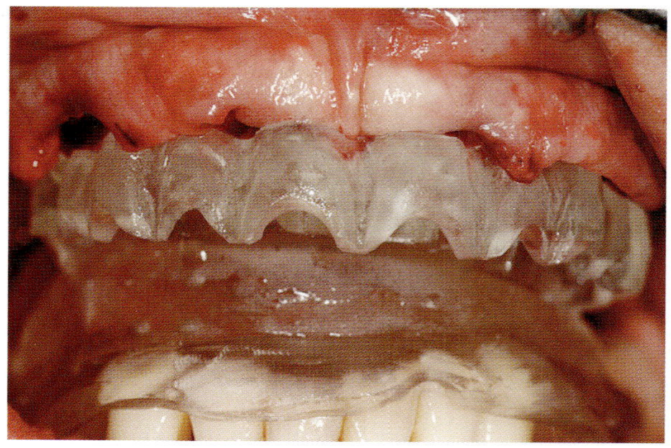

Fig 12.23

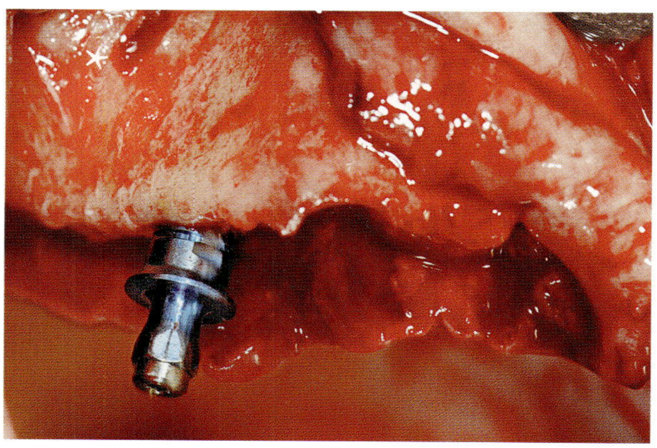

Fig 12.24

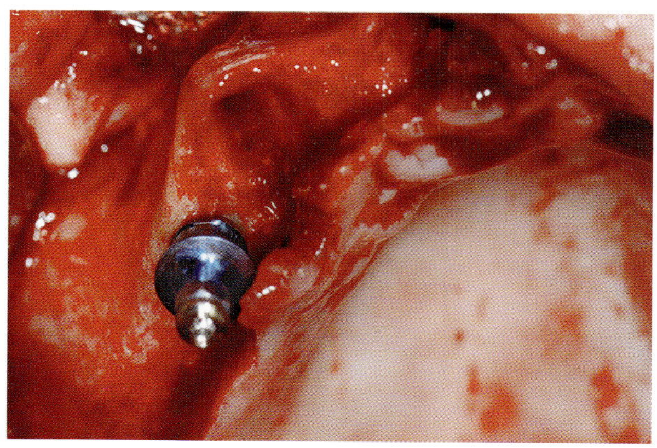

Fig 12.25

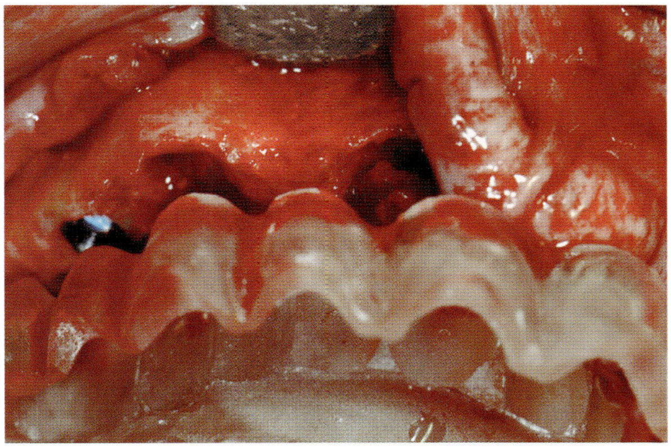

Fig 12.26

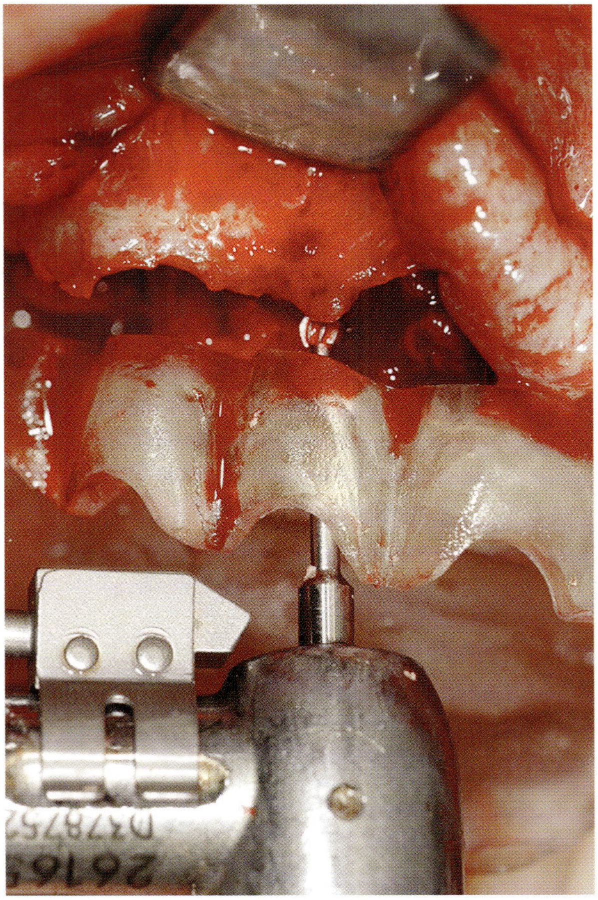

Fig 12.27

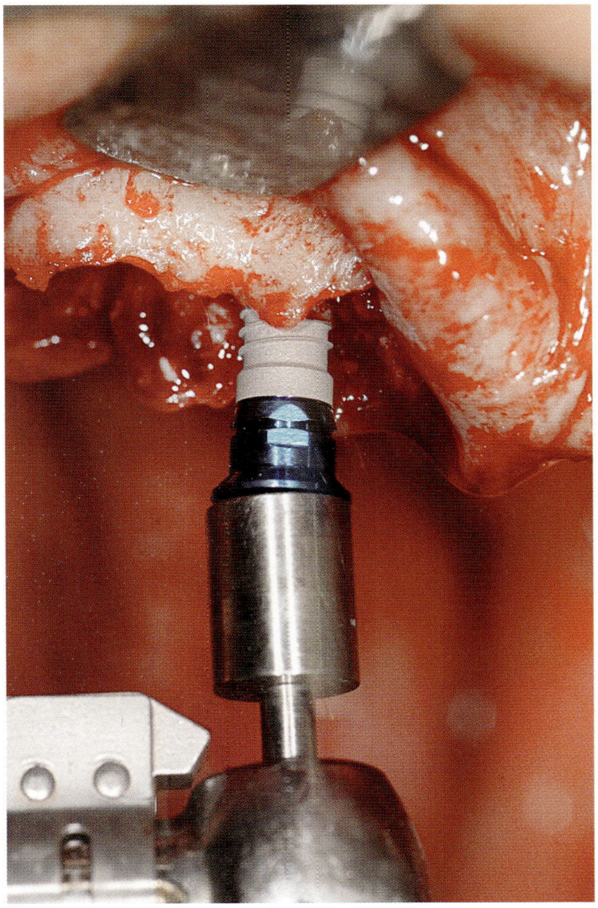

Fig 12.28

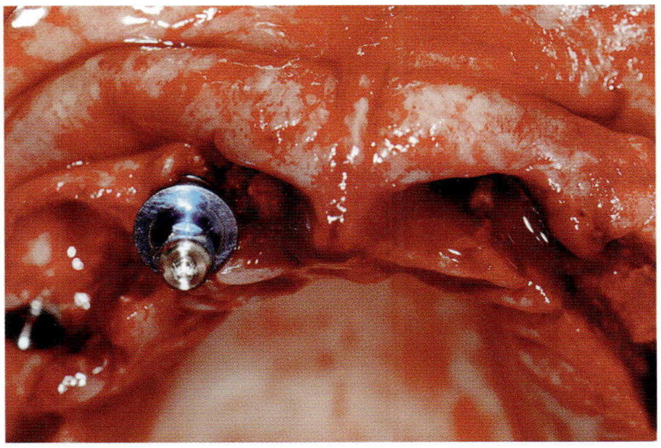

Fig 12.29

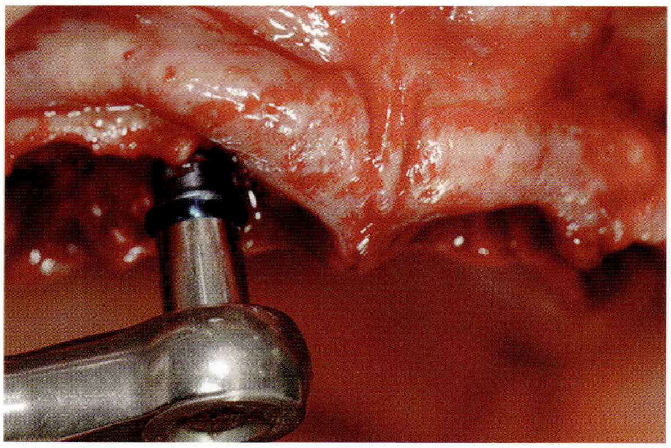

Fig 12.30

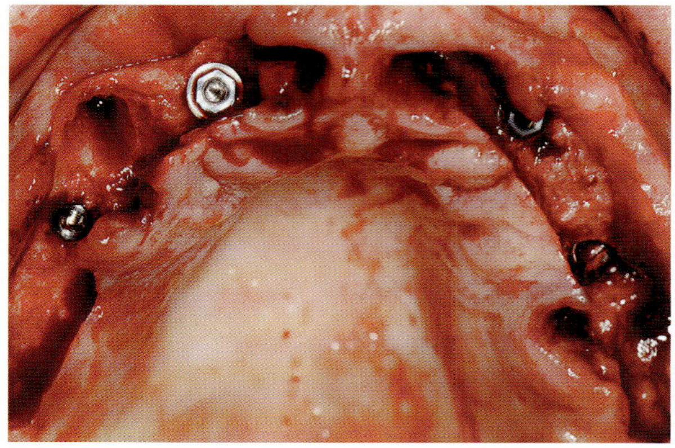

Fig 12.31

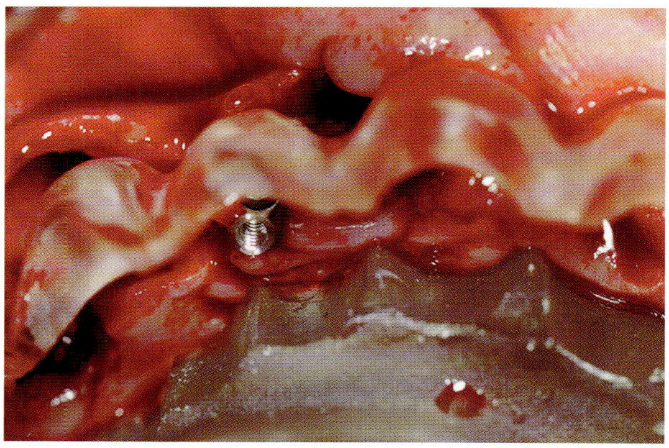

Fig 12.32

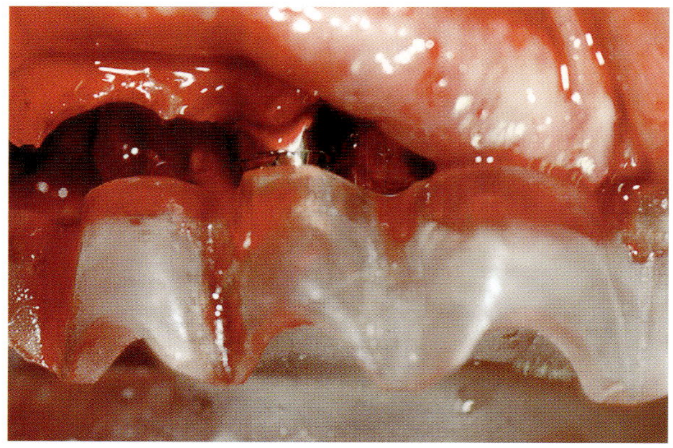

Fig 12.33

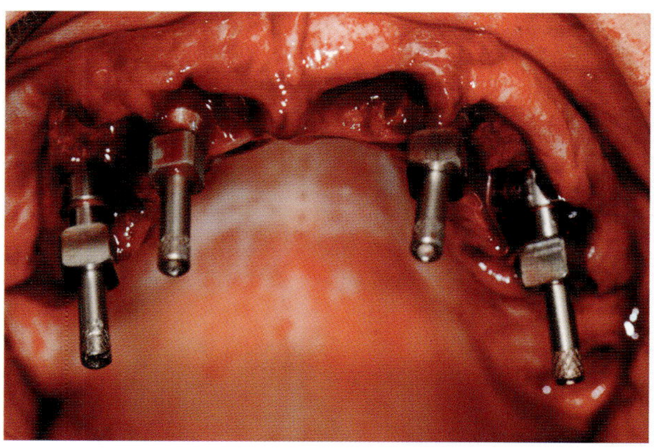

Fig 12.34

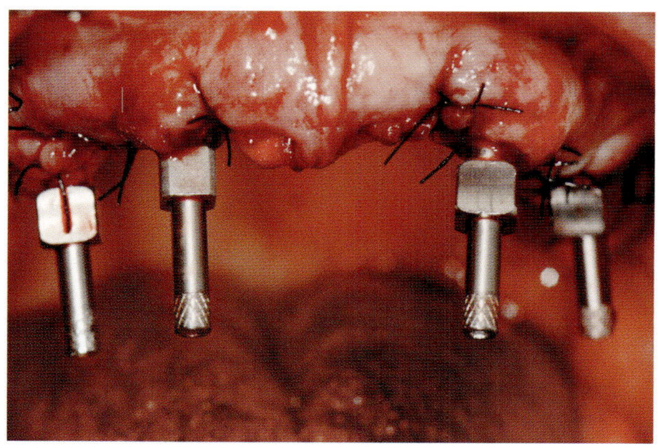

Fig 12.35

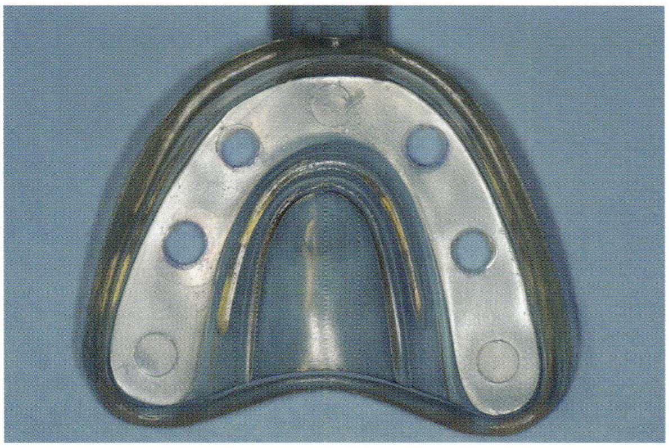

Fig 12.36

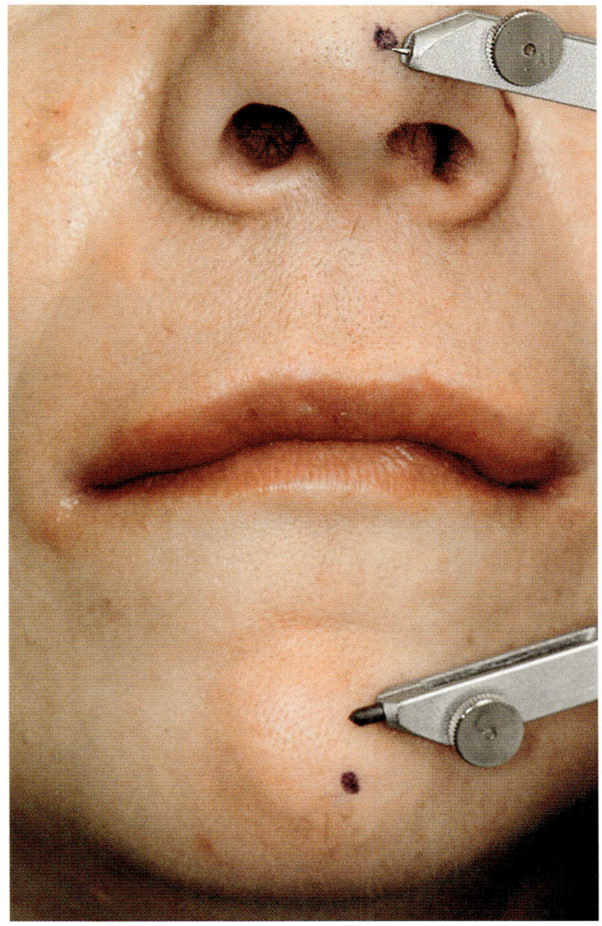

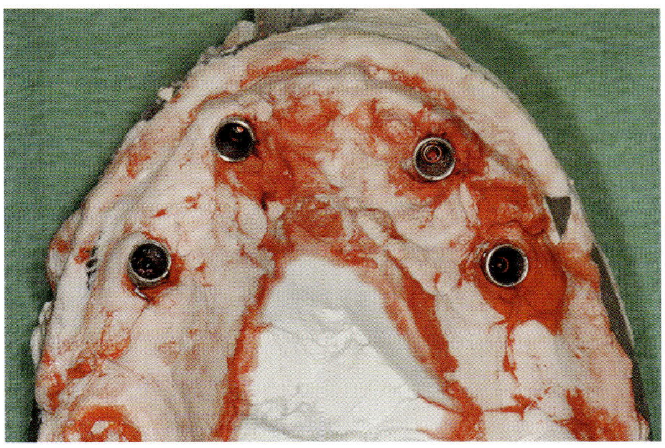

Fig 12.37

Fig 12.38

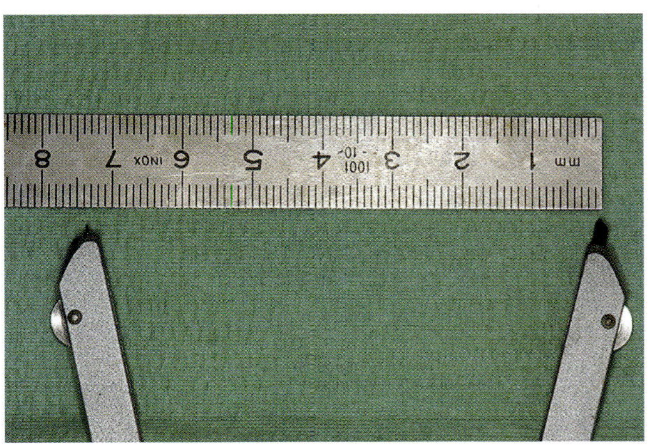

Fig 12.39

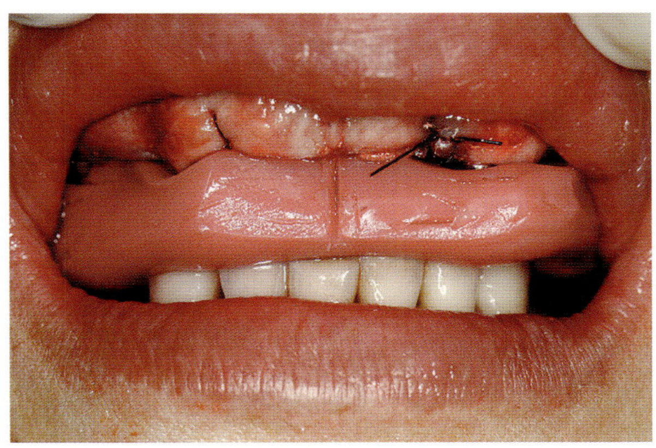

Fig 12.40

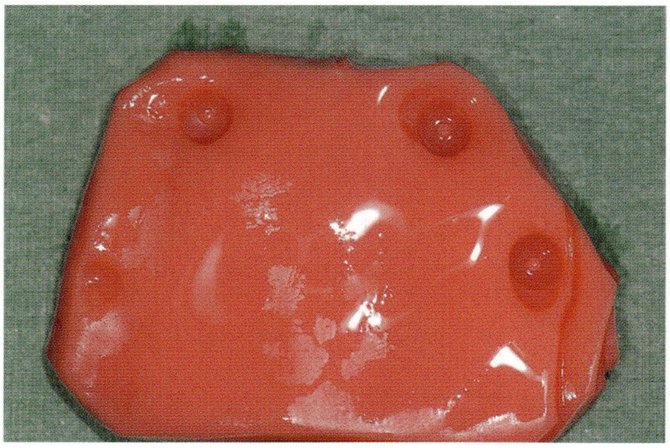

Fig 12.41

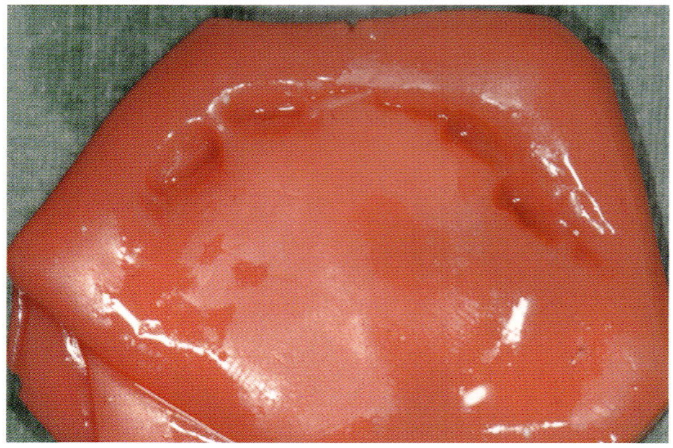

Fig 12.42

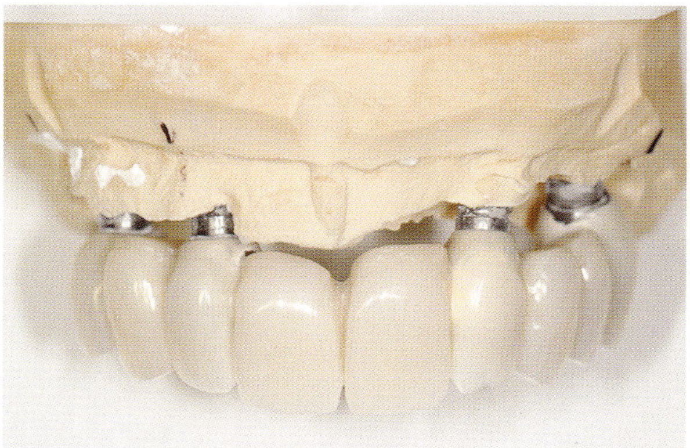

Fig 12.43

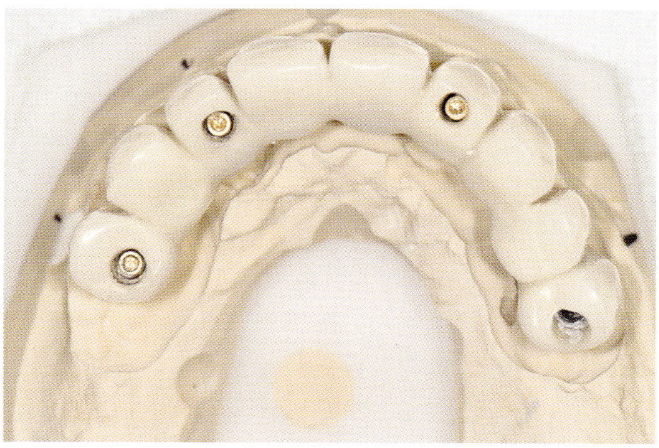

Fig 12.44

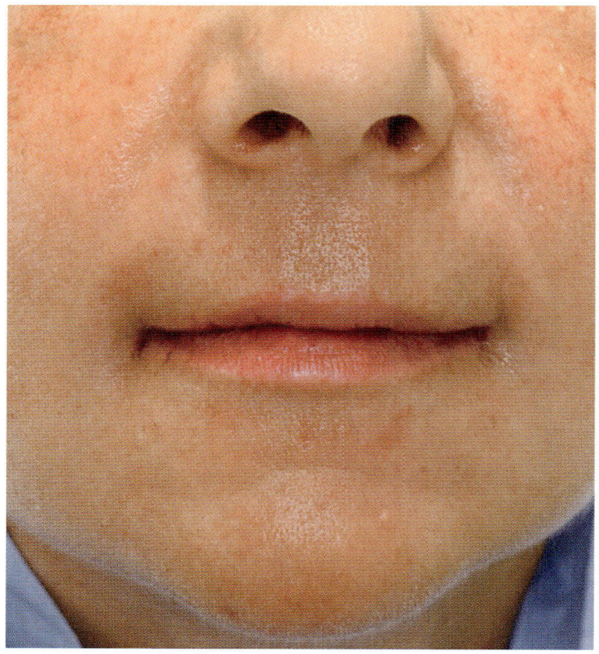

Fig 12.45

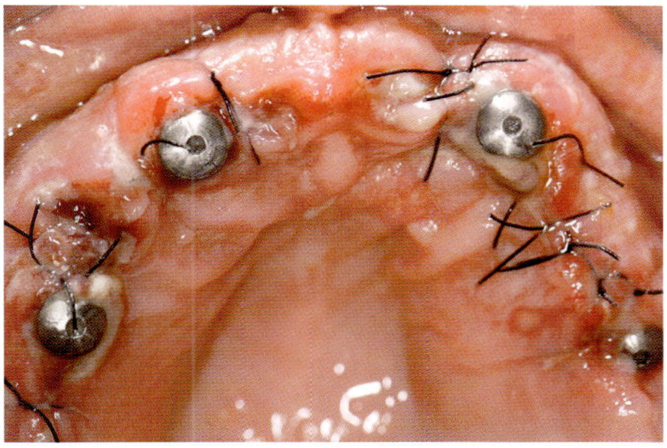

Fig 12.46

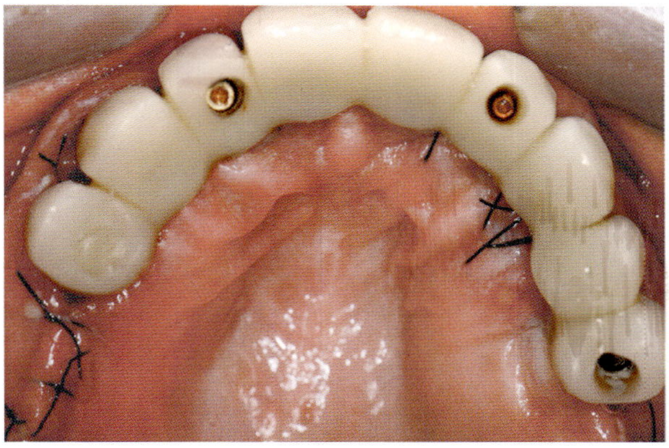

Fig 12.47

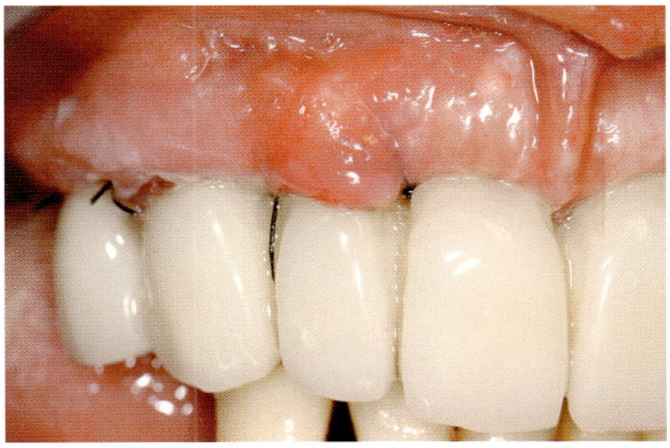

Fig 12.48

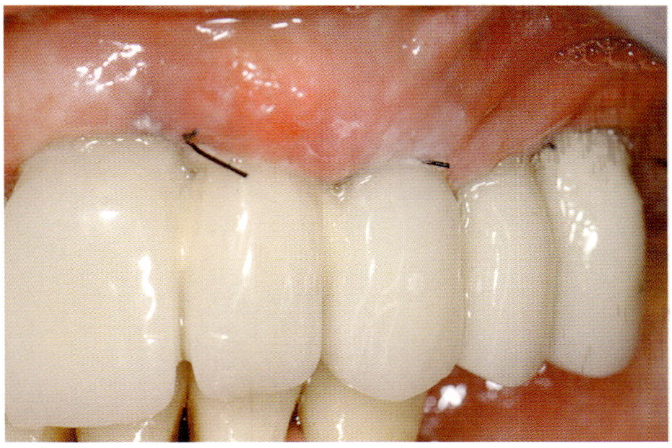

Fig 12.49

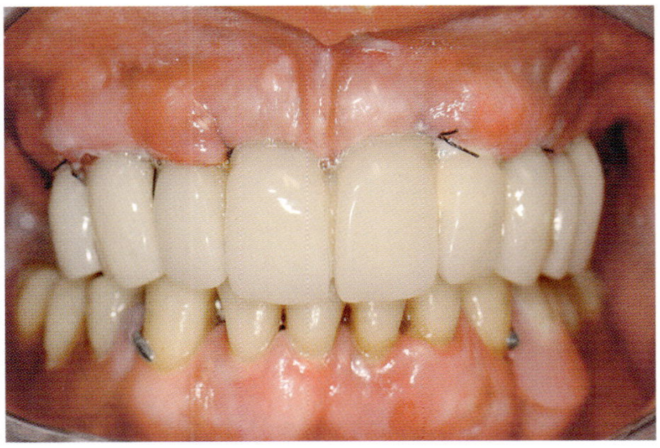

Fig 12.50

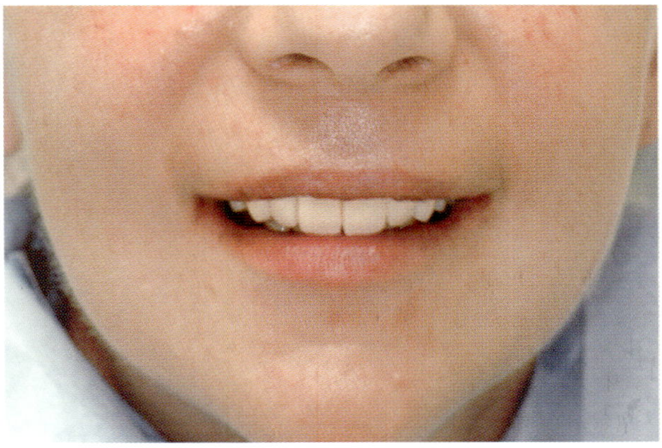

Fig 12.51

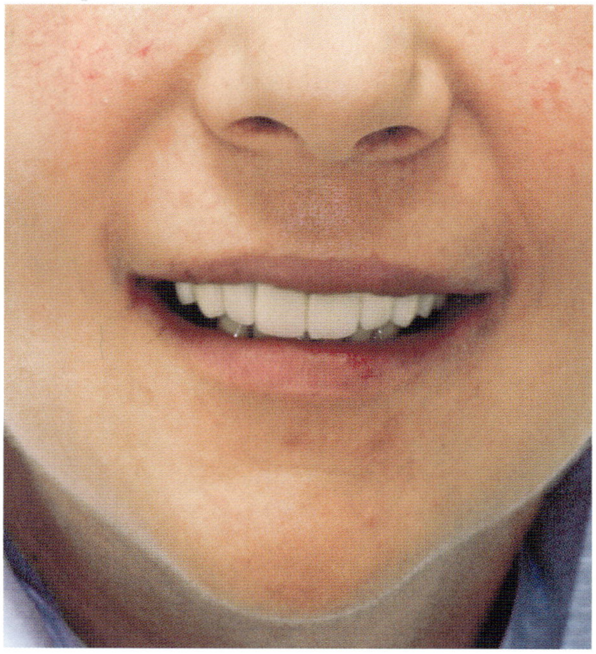

Fig 12.52

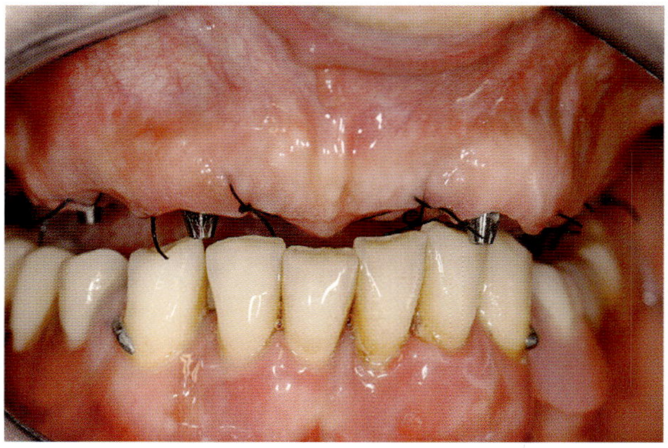

Fig 12.53

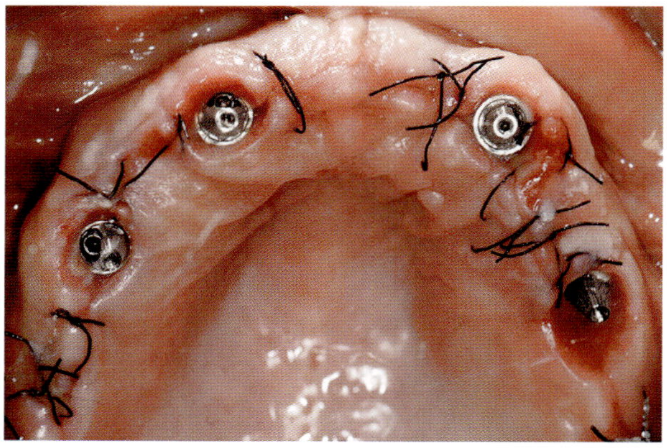

Fig 12.54

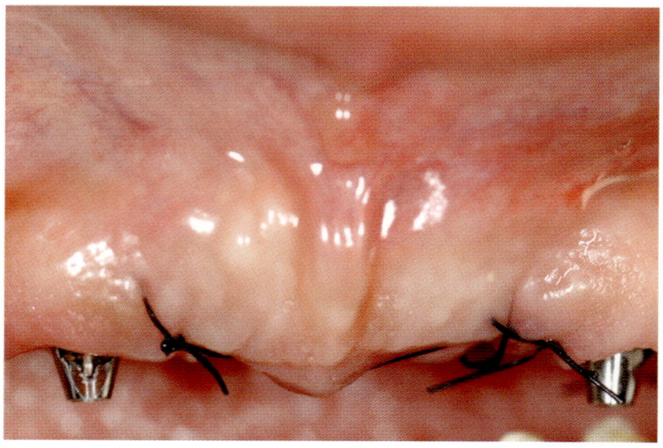

Fig 12.55

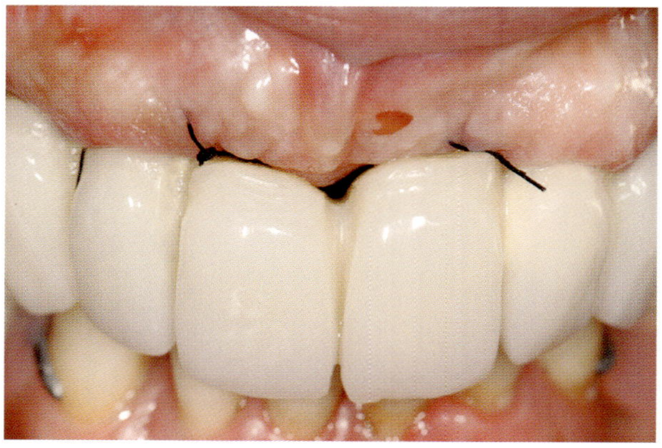

Fig 12.56

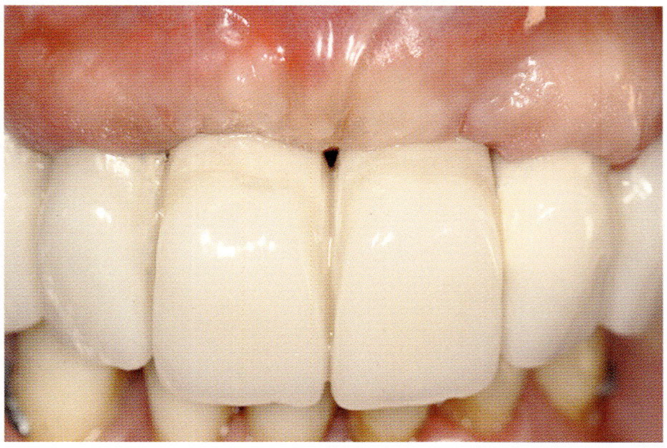

Fig 12.57

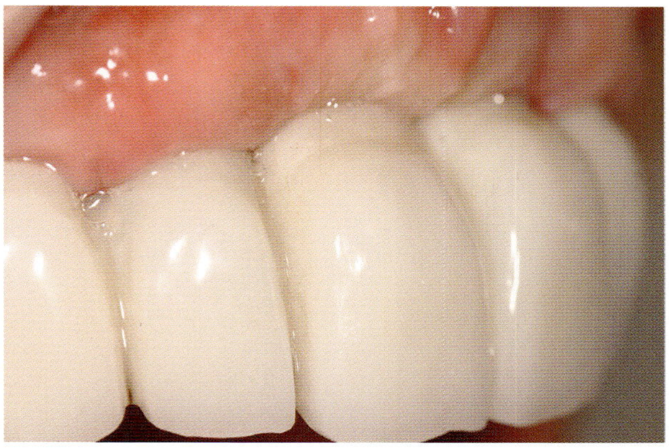

Fig 12.58

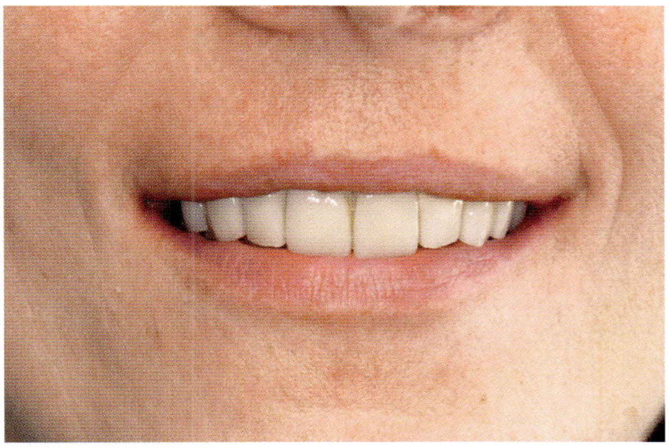

Fig 12.59

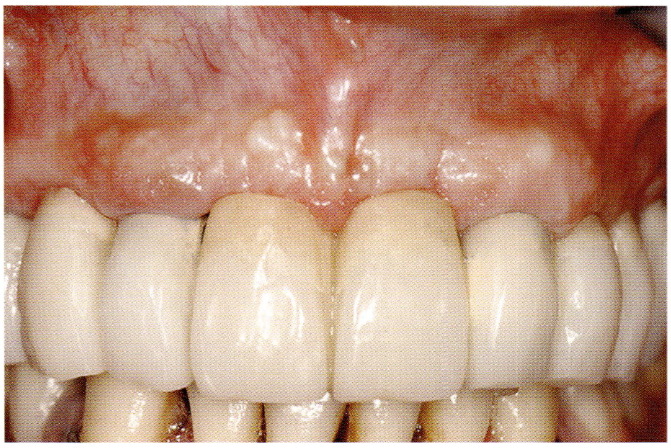

Fig 12.60

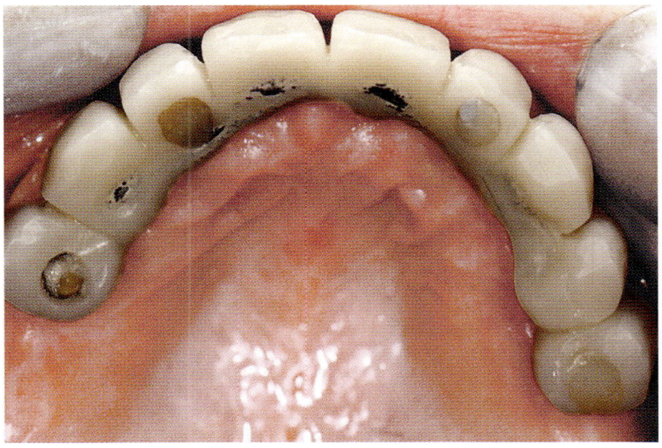

Fig 12.61

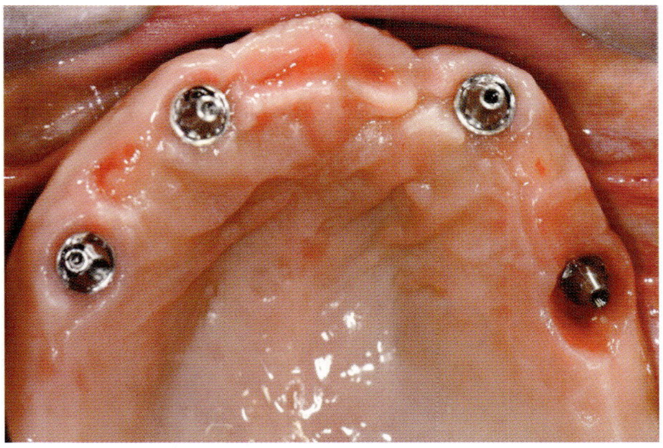

Fig 12.62

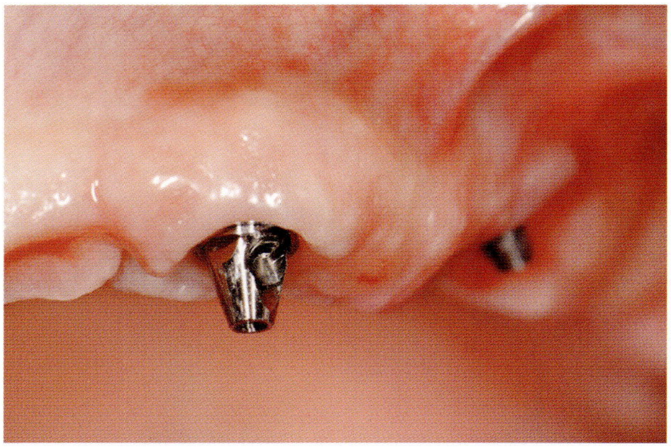

Fig 12.63

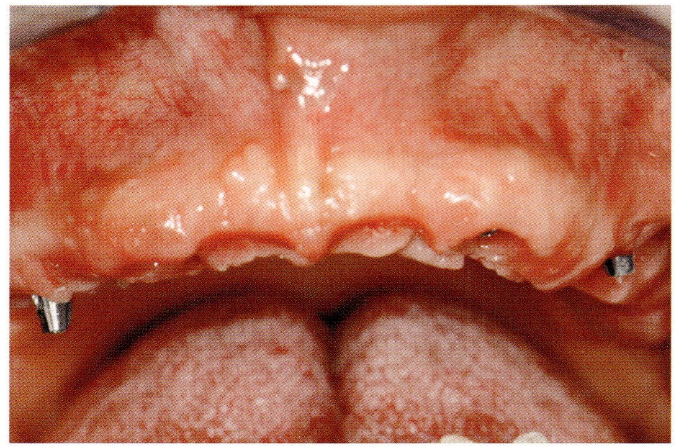

Fig 12.64

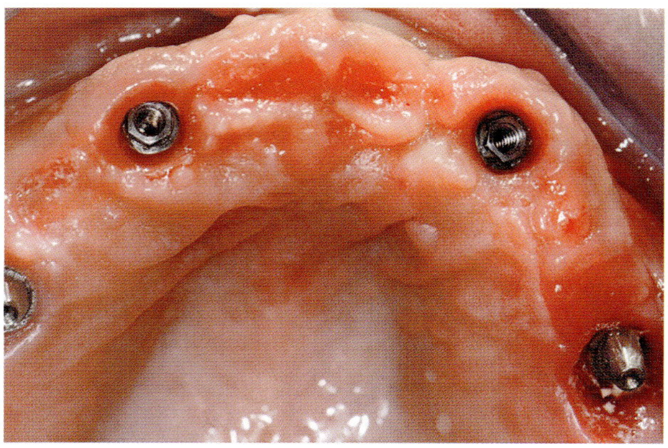

Fig 12.65

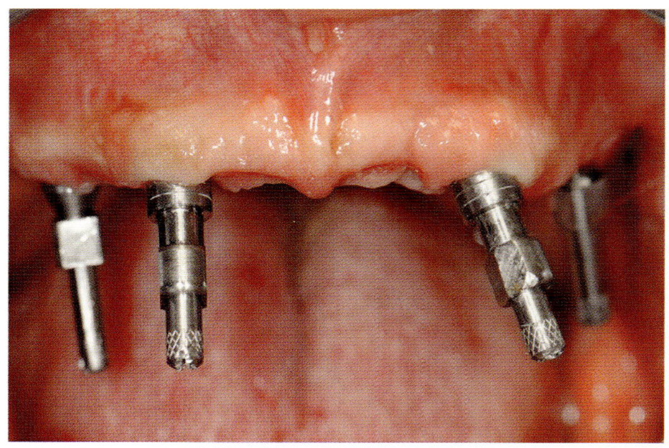

Fig 12.66

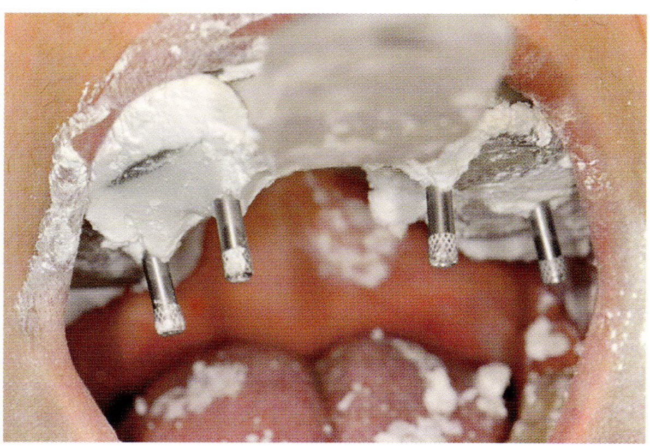

Fig 12.67

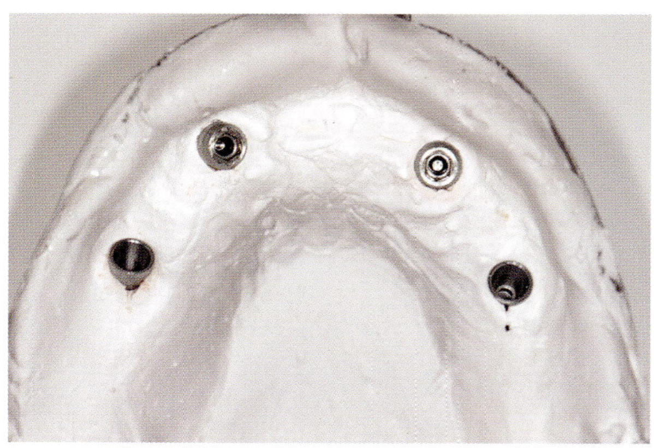

Fig 12.68

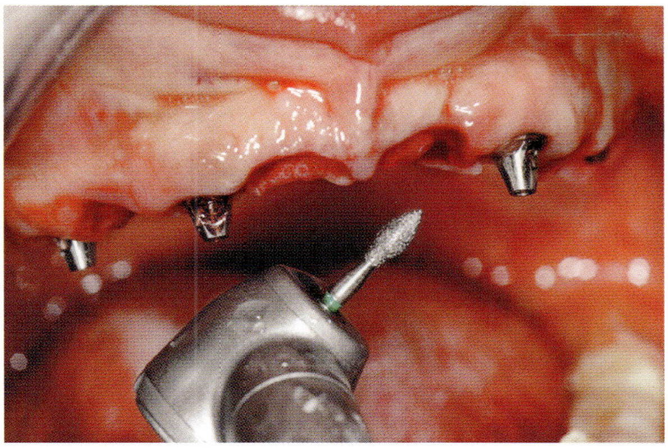

Fig 12.69

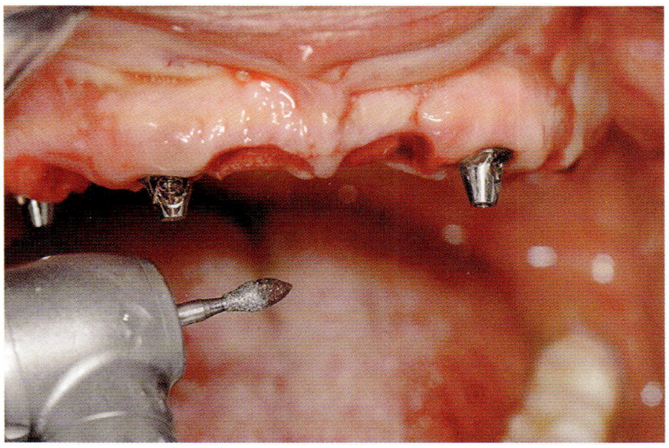

Fig 12.70

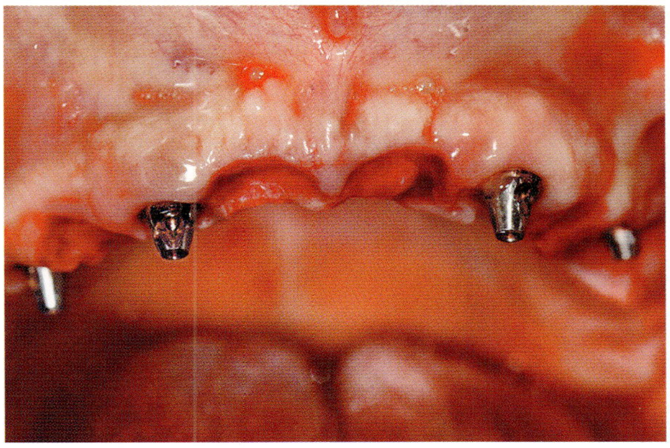

Fig 12.71

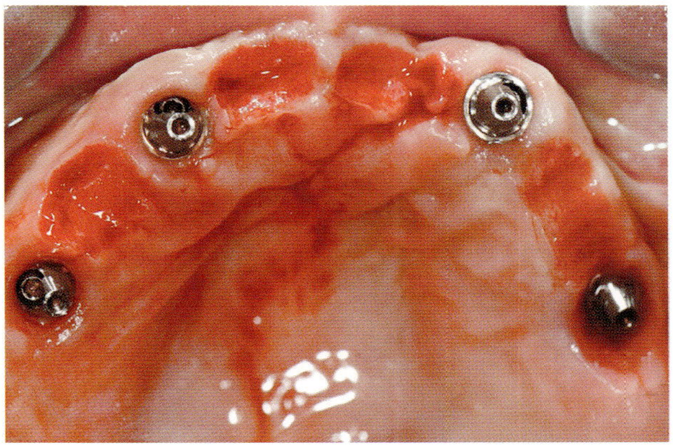

Fig 12.72

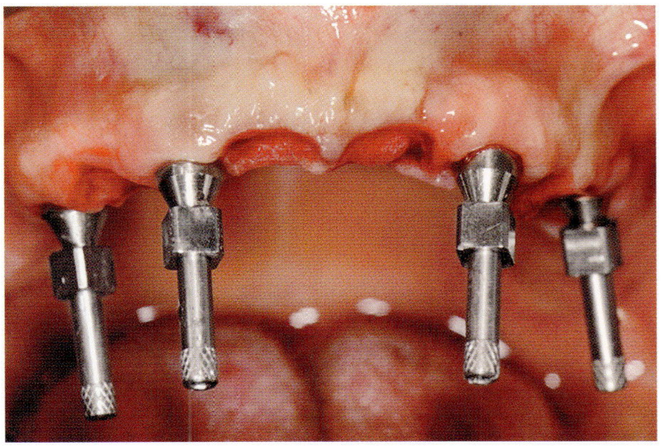

Fig 12.73

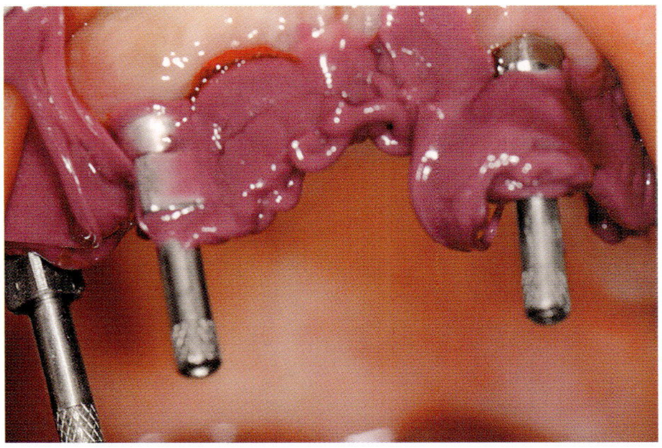

Fig 12.74

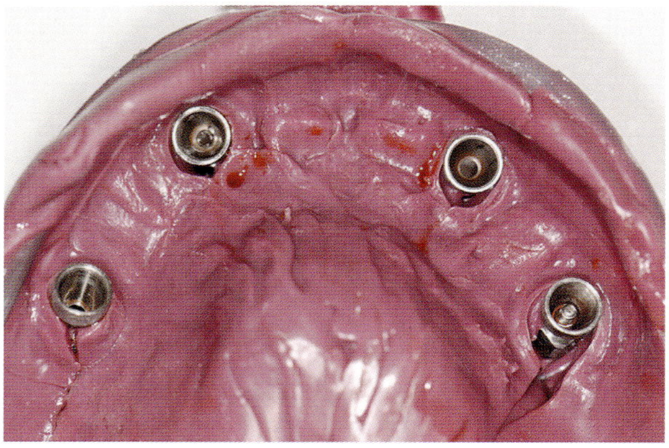

Fig 12.75

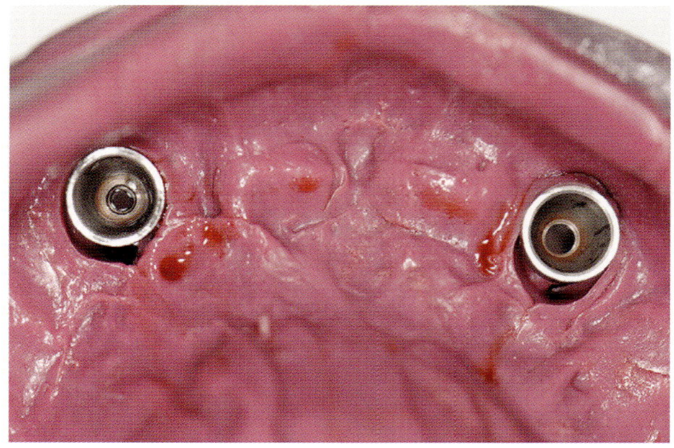

Fig 12.76

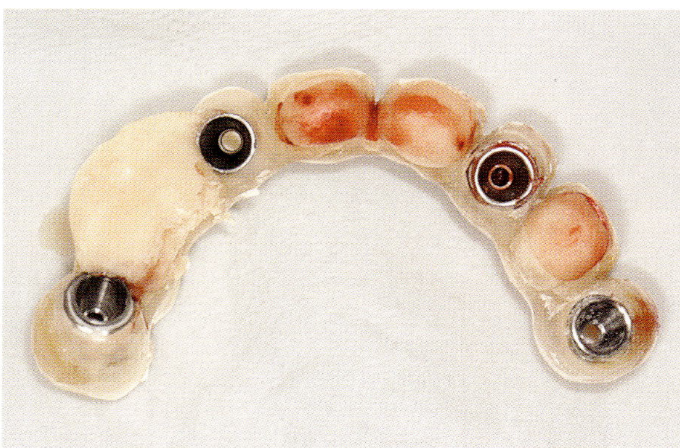

Fig 12.77

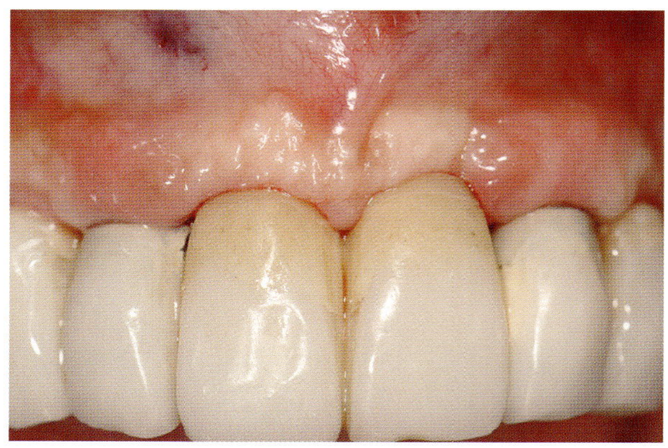

Fig 12.78

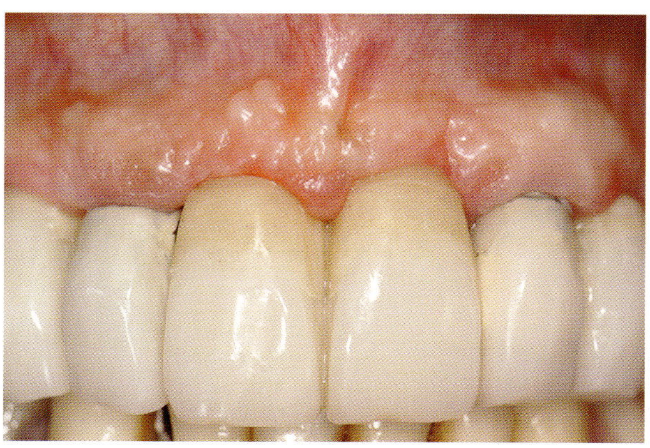

Fig 12.79

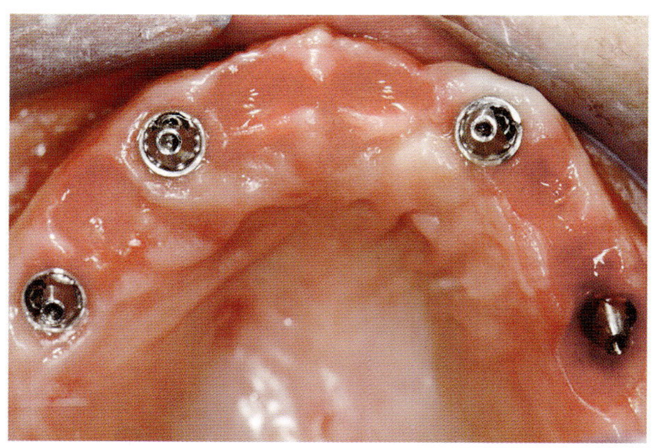

Fig 12.80

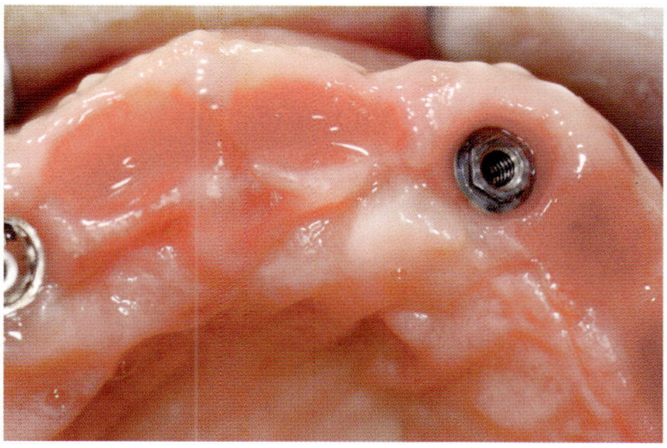

Fig 12.81

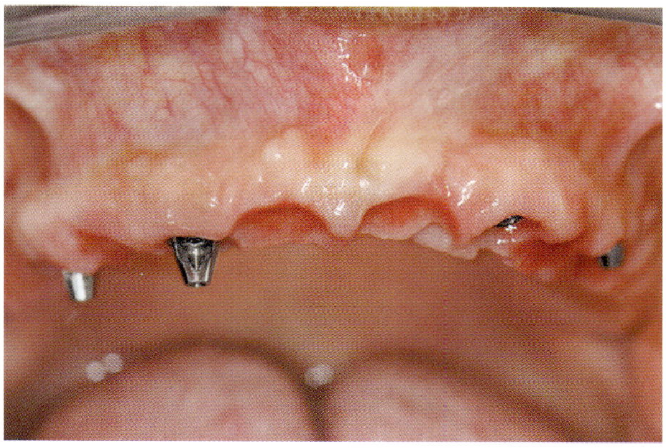

Fig 12.82

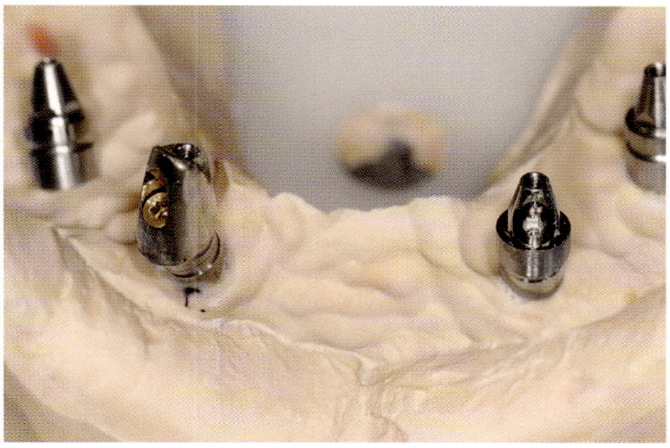

Fig 12.83

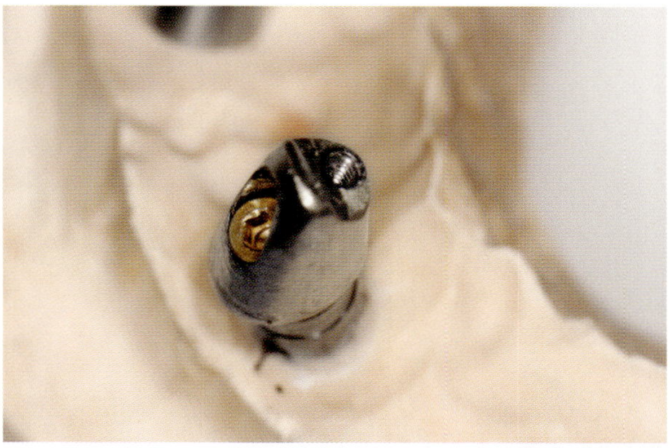

Fig 12.84

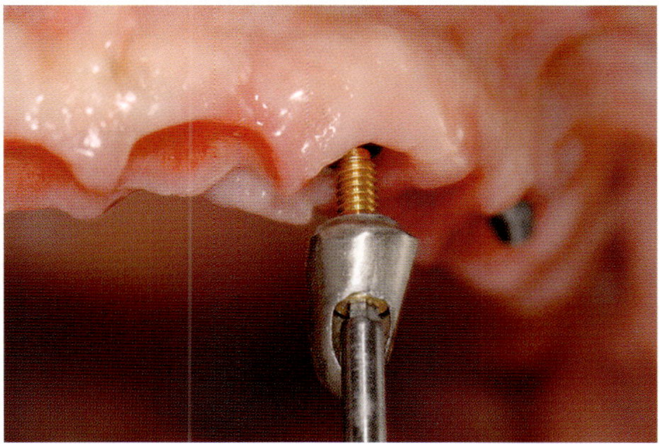

Fig 12.85

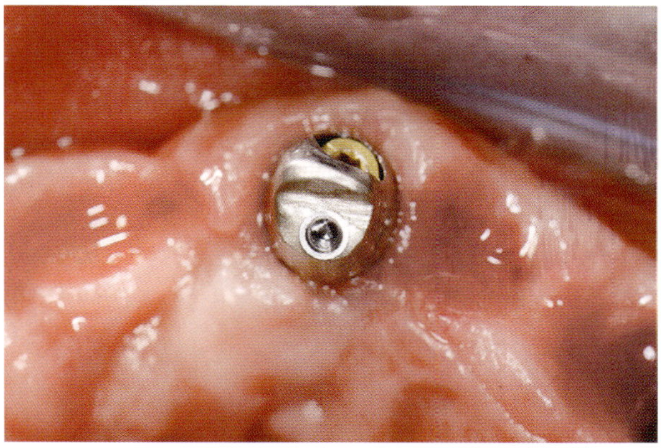

Fig 12.86

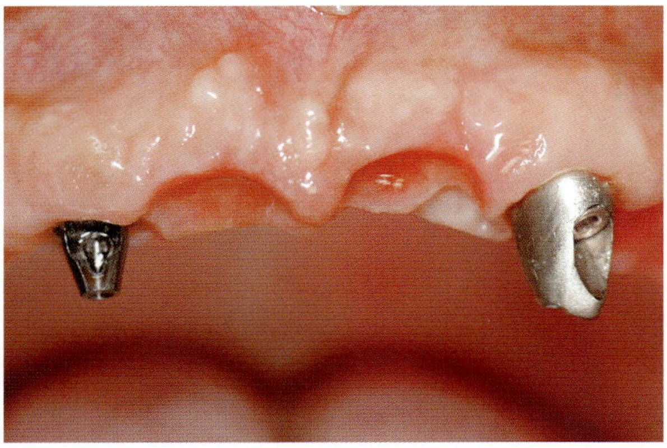

Fig 12.87

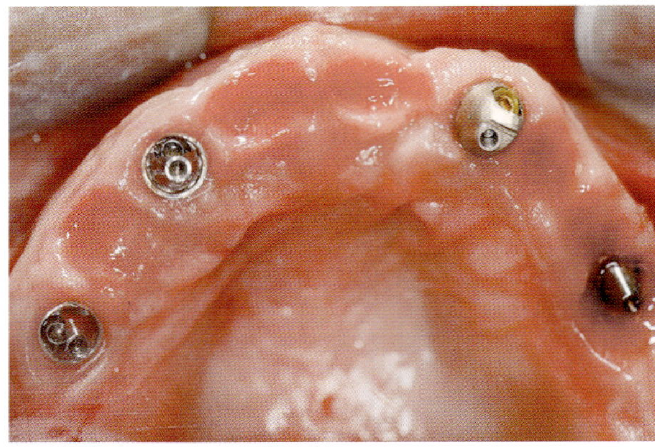

Fig 12.88

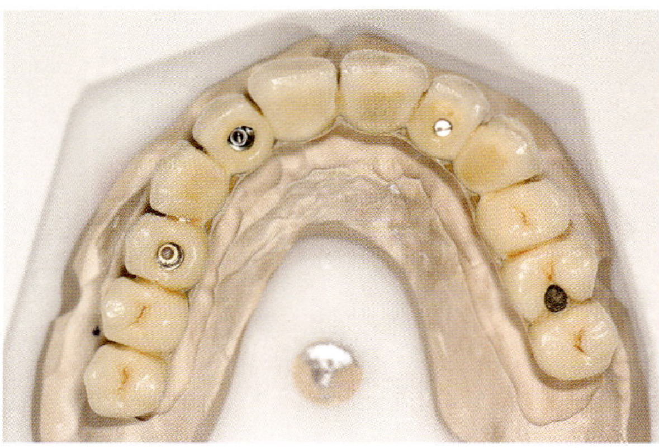

Fig 12.89

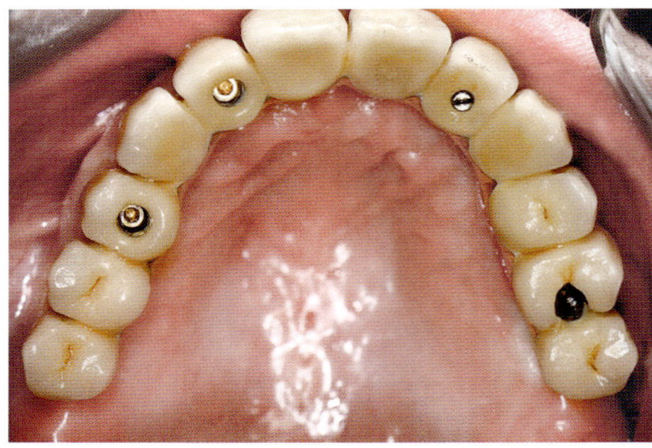

Fig 12.90

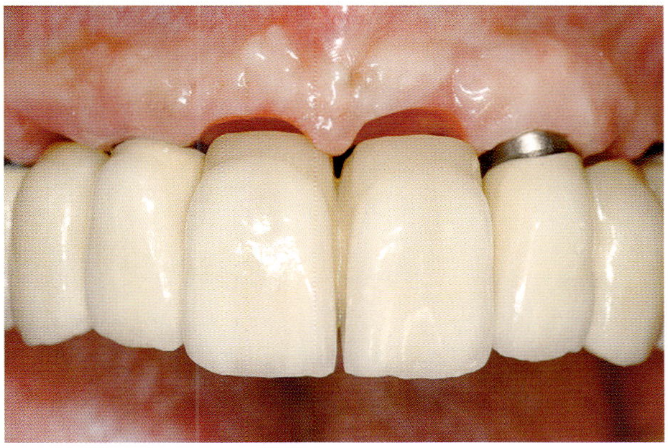

Fig 12.91

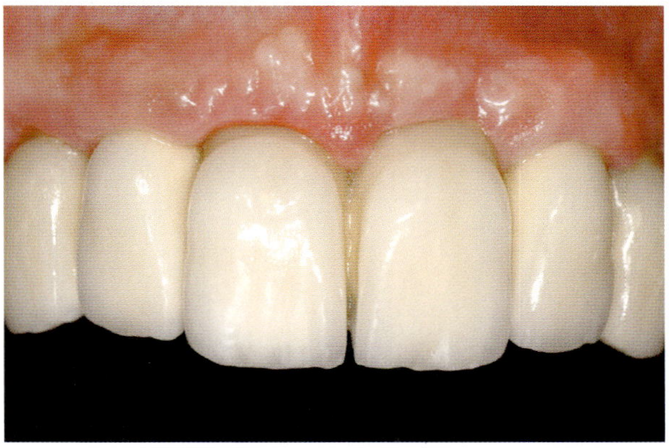

Fig 12.92

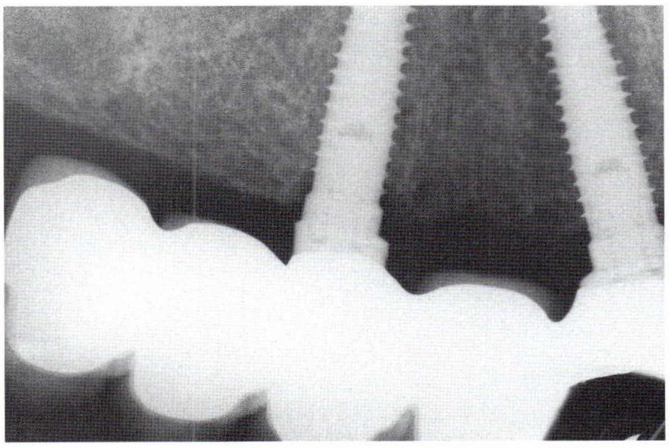

Fig 12.93

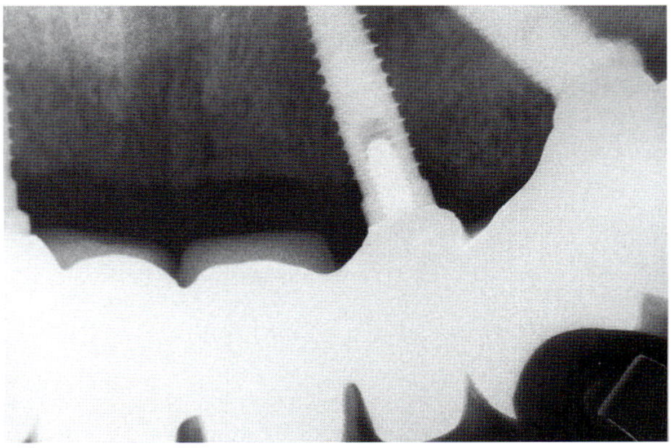

Fig 12.94

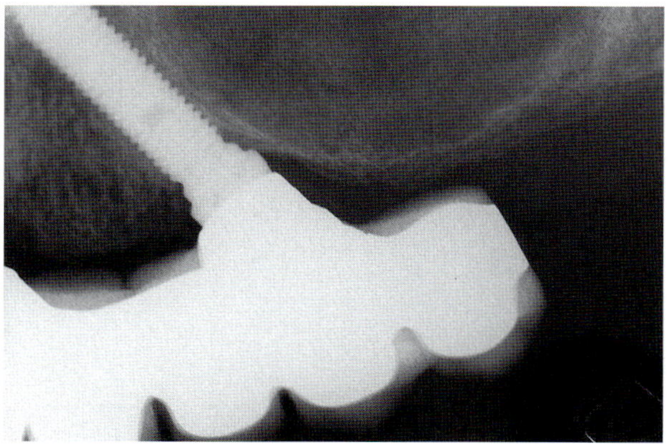

Fig 12.95

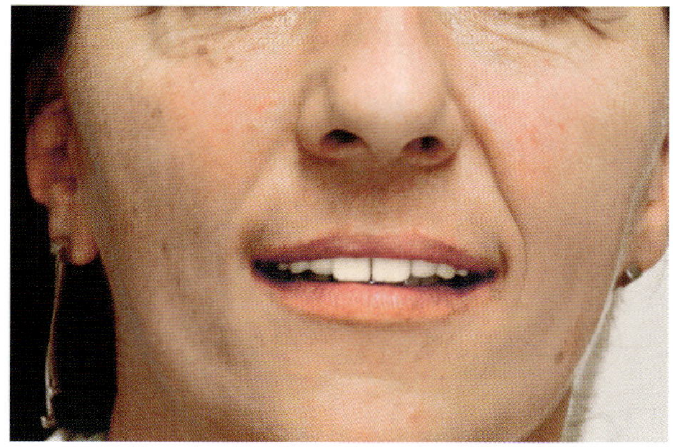

Fig 12.96

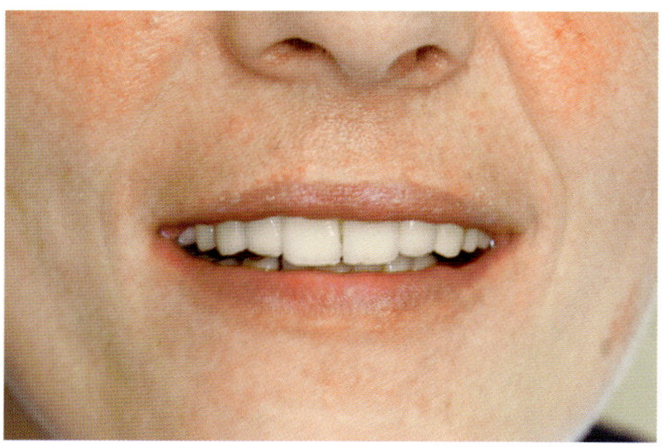

Fig 12.97

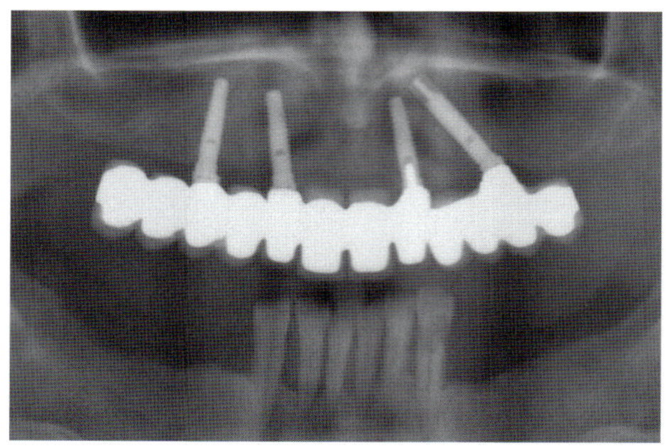

Fig 12.98

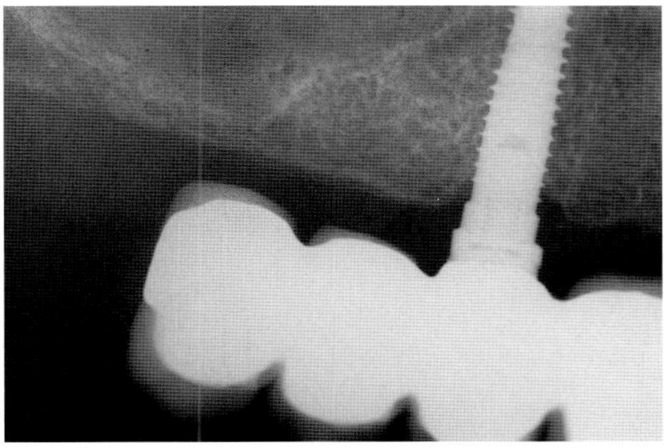

Fig 12.99

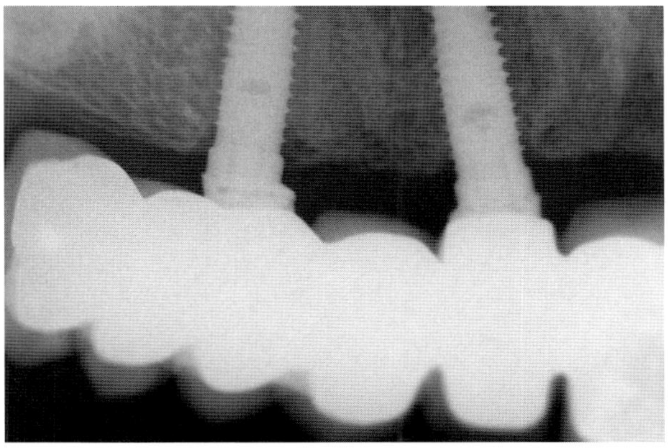

Fig 12.100

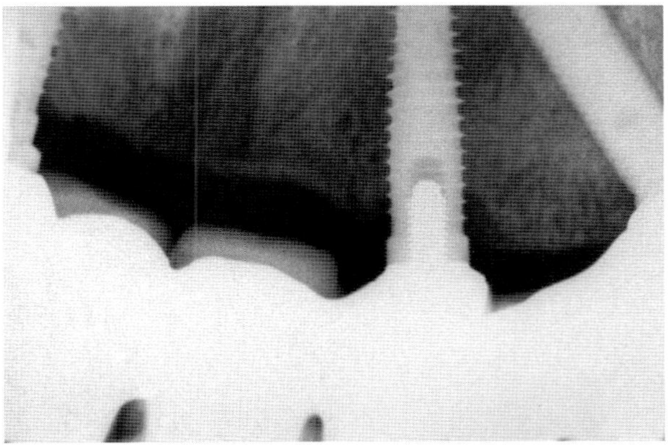

Fig 12.101

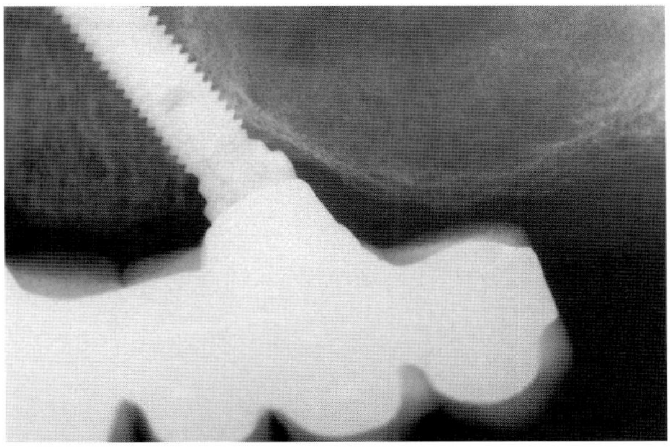

Fig 12.102

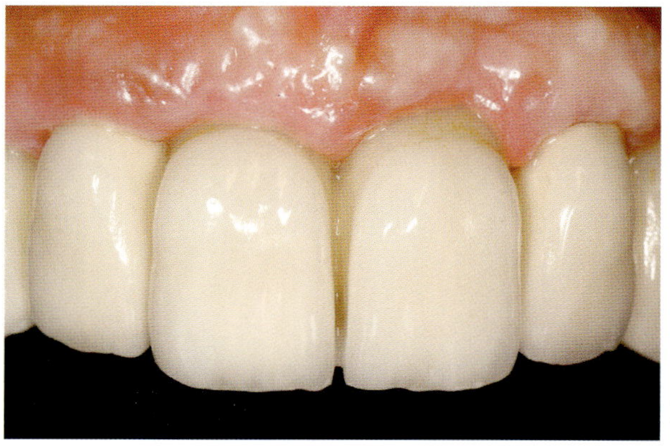

Fig 12.103

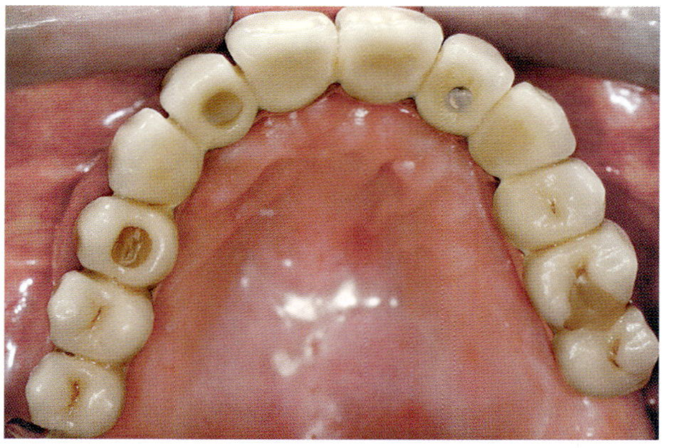

Fig 12.104

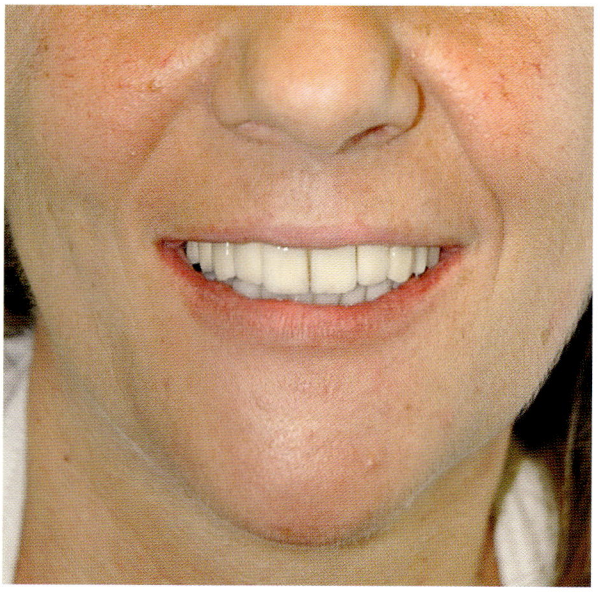

Fig 12.105

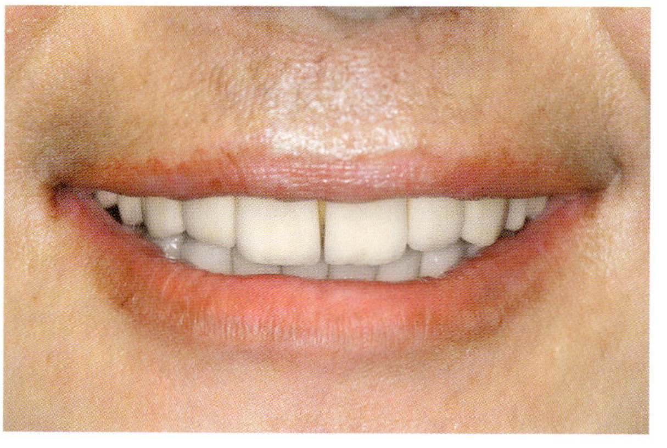

Fig 12.106

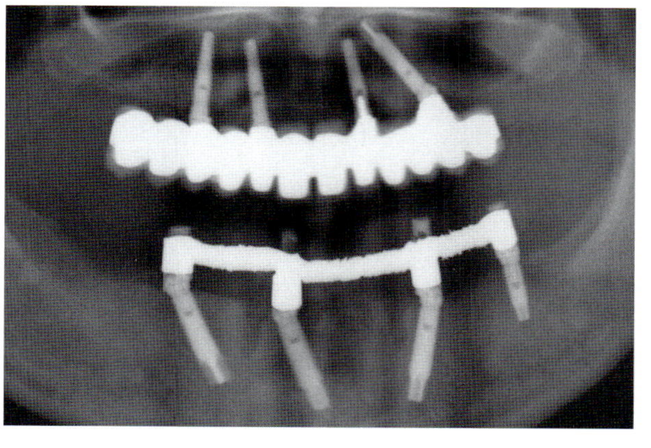

Fig 12.107

CHAPTER 13

CLINICAL AND RADIOGRAPHIC OUTCOMES OF PATIENTS TREATED WITH THE COLUMBUS BRIDGE PROTOCOL

Functional immediate loading of implants placed into edentulous mandibles is now recognized as a reliable and predictable procedure. The objective of an immediate loading protocol is a decrease in overall treatment time via single-stage surgery and immediate prosthesis function. The anterior zone of edentulous mandibles provides the most predictable results with both overdenture[1,2] and fixed prostheses.[3–8]

At the beginning of the 1980s, Schnitman et al[3] were among the first authors to propose an experimental technique that consisted of placing multiple implants (commercially pure titanium external hex Nobelpharma implants) splinted together into edentulous mandibles and loading them immediately with full functional occlusion. This protocol was developed to eliminate the postoperative discomfort patients experienced while wearing removable prostheses during osseointegration. Schnitman's group successfully treated seven patients by placing five or six interforaminal machined implants according to the classic protocol proposed by Brånemark for the treatment of edentulous mandibles. Unlike Brånemark's protocol, however, Schnitman loaded the implants within 24 hours of placement. He also placed additional rescue implants distal to the mental foramen in each posterior quadrant as a contingency if problems occurred with the loaded implants.

In 2000, Ericsson et al[4] published the clinical and radiographic results of a study that investigated the effects of reduced loading times compared with the classic two-stage protocol. Sixteen patients were treated with 88 machined implants. During the 18- to 60-month follow-up period, the research team reported no lost implants and an average bone resorption of 0.2 mm.

Using the Brånemark Novum concept–the first standardized surgical and prosthetic protocol for the treatment of mandibular edentulism with immediate loading–Engstrand et al[5] studied 95 patients treated with 285 interforaminal machined implants. The patients' progress was followed for 1 to 5 years (average, 2.5 years). Engstrand and his colleagues reported 18 failed implants in 13 patients and a cumulative survival rate (CSR) of 93.7%. The prosthetic survival rate was 99%. Average bone resorption was 0.73 mm after 1 year, 0.89 mm after 2 years, and 1.05 mm after 3 years.

Testori and coworkers[6] reported the results of a multicenter prospective study with 62 patients who each received five or six immediately loaded mandibular implants. All of the implants (N = 325) were manufactured with modified surfaces (Osseotite, Biomet 3i). Two implants were lost in the first 2 months of loading. The CSR was 99.4% after 12 to 60 months of follow-up (average, 28.6 ± 14.1 months). Similarly, Engquist and coworkers[7] followed the progress of 108 patients treated with early and delayed loading for 36 months and concluded that there were no differences in the CSRs between the two groups when early loading was applied to full-arch fixed prostheses in the anterior mandible.

The use of immediate loading protocols in edentulous maxillae, however, is not yet supported by comparable long follow-up periods as demonstrated in early research reports on osseointegration.[8–10]

In a 1997 study, Tarnow et al[11] followed four patients treated with immediate occlusal loading in edentulous maxillae and six patients treated with immediate occlusal loading in edentulous mandibles. All patients were treated with immediate fixed prostheses. Of the 69 implants placed with immediate occlusal loading, 67 integrated, resulting in a CSR of 98% after 1 to 5 years of follow-up.

Ibañez and coworkers[12] reported on the results of a clinical study where they treated 26 patients having edentulous maxillae with an immediate occlusal loading protocol. The patients' progress was followed for a period of 6 to 74 months. The reported CSR for 343 implants with modified surfaces was 99.42%. Average bone resorption was: 0.56 mm after 1 year; 0.76 mm after 2 years; 0.84 mm after 3 years; 0.82 mm after 4 years; 0.83 mm after 5 years, and 0.94 mm after 6 years.

Fischer et al[13] published a clinical report on maxillary implant treatment. The study included implants with modified surfaces and randomized controls; patients' progress was followed for 5 years. The implants were subjected to immediate functional and delayed loading, and the CSRs were 94.7% and 95.7%, respectively. Marginal bone resorption was slightly greater around immediately loaded implants (0.8 ± 1.2 mm) but not significantly different from that observed around the delayed loaded implants (0.3 ± 1.1 mm).

In a review of the literature on immediate and early loading, Attard and Zarb[14] developed a series of questions on this topic that needed further investigation. They affirmed that immediate functional loading protocols were predictable when applied to the anterior zone of the mandible and were independent of the type of implant used, its surface topography, and prosthetic design (success rates ranged from 90% to 100%). Attard and Zarb noted that little information was available regarding maxillary immediate occlusal loading. They also emphasized that the effect of the type of treatment on patients' quality of life still needs to be evaluated.

Most clinical studies in the literature have described the clinical success obtained in cases of immediate functional loading of splinted implants inserted into edentulous mandibles. The anterior edentulous mandibular bone is generally dense (type 1 or 2 according to Lekholm and Zarb) and has been considered favorable for the long-term survival of implants. Maxillary bone differs significantly from mandibular bone, and it presents unfavorable characteristics, from both macroscopic and microscopic viewpoints, for this type of treatment.

From the macroscopic point of view, the maxillary sinus and nasal cavities are important anatomical limitations to implant treatment (see chapter 6). In patients with atrophic maxillae (as in the case of edentulism following extraction of the maxillary teeth),[15] implants placed perpendicular to the occlusal plane are often of insufficient length to achieve adequate primary stability–an essential factor for osseointegration in immediate occlusal loading protocols.[16]

From the microscopic point of view, maxillary bone tends to be trabecular and, consequently, less dense than mandibular bone (type 3 or 4 according to Lekholm and Zarb). This characteristic negatively affects the potential to obtain implant primary stability in the maxilla.[17] Therefore, in cases with poor bone density, it is recommended that implant osteotomies be underprepared and that implants of the appropriate dimensions (length, width, and shape) be selected to facilitate obtaining implant primary stability.

Clinical reports have demonstrated that 40 Ncm of implant insertion torque is the minimum acceptable value for implants subjected to immediate occlusal loading.[18] It should be noted that there are significant differences and controversy in cases where single implants will be placed and restored with restorations that are out of occlusion and in cases where multiple, splinted implants will be subjected to immediate occlusal loading.

Maniatopoulos[19] reported that implant micromovements within the osteotomy site are likely to have deleterious effects on achieving predictable osseointegration. To ensure clinical success, clinicians must pay close attention to the details of their surgical and prosthetic protocols.[20] For instance, implants subjected to immediate loading with full-arch prostheses must be rigidly splinted together to avoid implant micromovements.[11]

In recent years, a number of articles have focused on the treatment of edentulous maxillae with prostheses that include implant support and immediate loading.[21–25] A literature review on immediate loading reported that a great variety of approaches have been described for this type of intervention.[26] These approaches have varied in both the surgical and prosthetic protocols applied and the number of implants placed, although the average number of implants placed for maxillary immediate occlusal loading is typically greater than eight.

This chapter presents an analysis of the clinical and radiographic outcomes for patients treated with the Columbus Bridge Protocol at the Department of Implant and Prosthetic Dentistry of Genoa University, Italy from 2004 to 2006.[27,28]

12-MONTH PILOT STUDY

Study Design

From March 2004 through December 2005, 21 edentulous maxillary patients (10 women, 11 men) with an average age of 58 years (women: 58.6 years; men: 57.4 years) were treated according to the Columbus Bridge Protocol.[27] All patients were in good general health and presented no contraindications to implant surgery. Maxillary tooth loss was classified according to three categories: periodontal disease (11 patients), dental caries (5 patients), and endodontic failures (5 patients).

The opposing mandibular jaws were restored with fixed prostheses supported by natural teeth or implants (n = 18) or with removable partial dentures (n = 3). Patients with mandibular complete dentures were excluded from this research project because of limitations to occlusal loading (decreased masticatory efficiency) associated with the dentures.

The Columbus Bridge Protocol requires the presence of sufficient bone volume for the placement of implants 4 mm in diameter and appropriate in length. The patients were treated in the maxilla with fixed prostheses supported by at least four implants (maximum of six implants per jaw). All of the implants (N = 111) were subjected to immediate occlusal loading with an average of 5.3 implants per patient (Table 13-1). The implant surfaces were roughened while maintaining machined cervical collars (Osseotite implants). Conical implants (Osseotite natural tapered [NT] implants) were used more frequently in immediate postextraction sites whereas cylindric shapes (Osseotite implants) were preferred in healed bone. If the implants reached insertion torque values of at least 40 Ncm, the implants were loaded immediately. All osteotomies were underprepared to increase

TABLE 13.1 - TYPE AND NUMBER OF IMPLANTS PLACED

	Implant length					
Implant type	**10 mm**	**11.5 mm**	**13 mm**	**15 mm**	**18 mm**	**TOTAL**
Cylindric implants, 4-mm diameter	1	2	20	30	20	73
Conical implants, 4-mm diameter	1	1	8	28	–	38

implant primary stability. To obtain bicortical stabilization, when possible, implant platforms were seated at the level of crestal bone. The use of longer implants in native bone was facilitated by angled implant placement. If necessary, the angles of the tilted implants were corrected with angulated conical abutments (17, 25, or 45 degrees).

The prostheses were fabricated according to the guidelines described in chapter 9. In review, the provisional prostheses were designed in accordance with the following parameters:

- Acrylic resin occlusal surfaces
- Metal frameworks for optimal rigidity
- Passively fitting frameworks fabricated through the luting technique
- Absence of distal cantilevered extensions
- Design permitting optimal hygienic maintenance

The screw-retained provisional prostheses were placed within 24 hours of the surgical appointments. Patients were instructed and motivated in home oral hygiene and adopted specific procedures depending upon healing. The definitive prostheses, also screw-retained, were delivered approximately 18 weeks after the initial surgical and prosthetic treatments were accomplished. The definitive prostheses were designed with distal extensions as needed to increase the number of masticatory units and, as a result, the masticatory efficiency. The occlusal surfaces of the definitive prostheses were fabricated with acrylic resin or ceramic.

The follow-up protocol included professional oral hygiene appointments. During the annual follow-up visits, the prostheses were removed, and the physical findings such as pain, mobility, and swelling around the implants were recorded. Retaining screws were evaluated for tightness. Centric occlusion and lateral excursions were also evaluated.

Follow-up radiographs were taken with customized Rinn holders. Radiographs were taken at the insertion of the provisional prosthesis (time 0) and at the 12-month follow-up visits. The radiographs were taken so that the implant threads on the mesial and distal surfaces were clear. The level of the crestal bone was calculated by measuring the distance between the implant-abutment interface and the most coronal bone-implant contact (Fig 13-1).[29] The measurements were made by a "blinded" radiologist not involved in the study, with the use of a diaphanoscope and a magnifying lens.

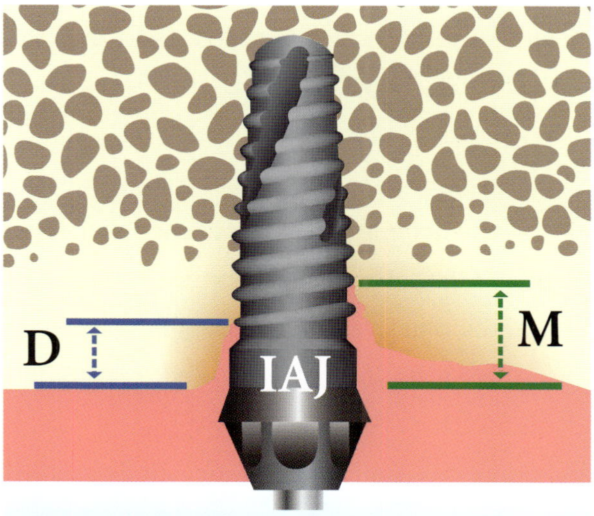

Fig. 13.1 - Illustration of how measurements were made in this study. Interproximal crestal bone levels were measured from the implant-abutment junction (IAJ) to the most coronal bone-implant levels on mesial (M) and distal (D) implant surfaces.

Statistical Analysis

The statistical analysis was made using SPSS 15.0 software (SPSS). The bone levels (mesial and distal) measured at time 0 and again at the 12-month follow-up visits were analyzed using the one-way analysis of variance (ANOVA). Various groups of implants were identified according to shape (cylindric or conical), inclination (straight or angled), and insertion site (healed or immediate postextraction site). Patients were identified as smokers or nonsmokers and as periodontal patients or nonperiodontal patients. Variables, such as bone quality (type 1, 2, or 3), angulations of prosthetic abutments (0, 17, 25, and 45 degrees), and type of opposing occlusion (fixed or removable partial), were also taken into consideration. Comparisons among these groups were performed with the two-way ANOVA corrected for the patient's effect. All tests were two-tailed and the alpha was set to .05.

Results

All 21 patients appeared at the scheduled recall visits, and their progress was followed for at least 12 months. The average follow-up for the study was 20 months. The implant CSR was 92.8% (Table 13-2).

Eight implants (four conical, four cylindric) failed within the first 3 months (Table 13-3). Two patients lost two implants each, and four patients lost one implant each. Five of the eight lost implants were in distal areas; 40% of the short implants (< 13 mm) failed. Five of the eight failed implants were replaced with new implants that were attached to the preexisting provisional prostheses. After 12 months of follow-up, the CSR for the definitive prostheses was 100%. All patients maintained the full-arch fixed prostheses for the entire follow-up period.

The average crestal bone levels at time 0 were 0.65 mm from the implant-abutment connection on the mesial surfaces and 0.41 mm on the distal surfaces. At the 12-month follow-up visits, crestal bone levels were 1.39 mm from the implant-abutment connection on the mesial surfaces and 1.35 mm on the distal surfaces. No statistically significant differences were observed in crestal bone loss between straight and angled implants, nor did bone resorption appear to be dependent upon prosthetic abutment angulations (0, 17, 25, or 45 degrees).

No statistically significant differences were observed in crestal bone loss adjacent to conical implants versus cylindric implants or adjacent to implants placed immediately into postextraction sites when compared with implants placed into healed bone. Bone quality had no statistically significant effect on bone resorption. Although greater levels of interproximal crestal bone loss were recorded in patients who became edentulous secondary to periodontal disease, these results were not significant when compared with interproximal crestal bone loss in patients who did not lose their teeth secondary to periodontal disease. Patients who smoke did demonstrate significantly greater crestal bone loss compared with patients who do not smoke ($P < .03$).

Finally, patients with a fixed prosthesis in the opposing dentition showed significantly increased bone resorption compared with patients having a partially removable prosthesis in the opposing arch ($P < .05$). The results among the groups examined are displayed in Table 13-4.

Discussion

This analysis of patients treated per the Columbus Bridge Protocol at the University of Genoa demonstrated an overall CSR of 92.8% for maxillary implants subjected to immediate functional loading with at least 12 months of follow-up. This CSR is similar to CSRs reported in the literature for similar clinical treatments with maxillary implants placed into immediate occlusal function (Fischer et al[13]: 94.7%; Maló et al[30]: 97.6%, and Bergkvist et al[31]: 98.2%).

The results of this research suggest that for patients treated per the Columbus Bridge Protocol, four implants (up to maximum of six in some clinical situations; see chapter 7) appear to be sufficient to support full-arch prostheses subjected to immediate occlusal loading.

It is important to note that careful treatment planning is necessary. Clinicians must take the necessary steps to obtain high implant primary stability, which is critical for achieving the success noted in this study on immediate occlusal loading of maxillary implants. In the Columbus Bridge Protocol, implant primary stability is obtained by *(1)* underpreparation of the implant osteotomies; *(2)* insertion torque values ≥ 40 Ncm; and *(3)* use of implants with a length mostly greater than 11.5 mm that are placed into native bone. The protocol also requires that patients be treated with scaling and root planing procedures around their remaining teeth and return for regularly scheduled recall appointments.

The average bone loss recorded around all implants at the 12-month follow-up visits (ie, difference between T12 and T0 values) was 0.84 mm (Cl 95%; 0.68–0.99 mm). The bone loss was also comparable with values published by the following authors for fixed implant treatment with maxillary, full-arch, immediate occlusal loading: Ibañez et al,[12] 0.76 mm; Fischer et al,[13] 0.80 mm; and Maló et al,[30] 0.90 mm.

No differences in bone resorption were noted between straight and angled implants subjected to immediate occlusal loading, which is consistent with the results reported in the literature:

- Calandriello and Tomatis[32] reported that after 12 months of occlusal loading, 0.82 mm of crestal bone loss was noted adjacent to straight implants and 0.34 mm adjacent to angled implants.
- Testori et al[33] reported that after 12 months of occlusal loading 0.90 mm of crestal bone loss was noted adjacent to straight implants and 0.80 mm adjacent to angled implants.

These results appear to validate the use of long, angled implants placed into native bone in distal segments of edentulous maxillae since the vertical placement of implants is not possible secondary to maxillary atrophy. In posterior atrophic maxillae, angled implants may actually be preferred to straight implants because

TABLE 13.2 - CUMULATIVE SURVIVAL RATE (CSR) 12 MONTHS AFTER IMPLANT PLACEMENT

Follow-up (months)	Implants placed	Failed implants	CSR (%)
0	111	0	100
6	103	8	92.8
12	103	8	92.8

TABLE 13.3 - TYPE AND NUMBER OF FAILED IMPLANTS

Implant type	Implant length					TOTAL
	10 mm	11.5 mm	13 mm	15 mm	18 mm	
Cylindric implants, 4-mm diameter	–	1	–	1	2	4
Conical implants, 4-mm diameter	1	–	2	1	–	4
Percentage compared to inserted implants	50%	33.3%	7.1%	3.4%	10%	7.2%

the angled implants *(1)* improve anteroposterior spread and cross-arch stabilization and *(2)* reduce posterior cantilevered prostheses and the potential of occlusal overload. Angled implants significantly decrease the need to graft maxillary sinuses and, therefore, the surgical morbidity associated with grafting procedures. Per the Columbus Bridge Protocol, bone grafts are generally not necessary to increase bone volume in posterior maxillae because distal implants can be placed into native bone, parallel to the anterior wall of the maxillary sinus.

Another advantage of this protocol is that successful prosthetic treatment can be accomplished with a limited number of implants (four to six) without compromising the CSRs of implants and/or prostheses. In fact, optimal biomechanical support for prostheses can be obtained with angled distal implants. During the course of this study, there were no implant fractures and no mechanical failures in the abutments. No statistical difference in screw loosening between angled and straight abutments was observed in this study.

This biomechanical aspect seems to match the laboratory results of a recent study on the influence of abutment angulation on screw loosening.[34] The authors reported angled abutments showed significantly higher removal torque values than straight abutments. The divergent angles of the conical abutments did not affect crestal bone loss adjacent to any of the implants. These findings are particularly encouraging if one considers that some of the patients were treated with 45-degree angulated conical abutments. Further studies are required to validate the use of these custom-made components in long-term, multicenter clinical studies.

The two patient risk factors regarded as most likely to be responsible for middle- to long-term implant failure are smoking and periodontal disease.[35] In this study, significantly higher levels of bone resorption were observed in smokers than in nonsmokers ($P < .03$). Patients with periodontal disease also demonstrated higher degrees of bone resorption, but the differences were not statistically significant when compared with patients who did not have periodontal disease. A larger difference among the various patient groups may have been masked by improved oral hygiene practices and rigid follow-up protocols for the patients who maintained their teeth. For instance, smoking is known to affect the health of peri-implant tissues only marginally when oral hygiene is optimal, but its noxious side effects are exacerbated in patients with poor hygiene, especially postsurgery.[36]

In this study, several procedures were carried out to increase the potential for osseointegration to occur. Both the provisional and definitive prostheses were fabricated with metal frameworks. Metal frameworks are more rigid than all–acrylic resin fixed dentures, so they increase prosthesis rigidity for splinting implants. The fit of the metal framework was enhanced through the specific luting technique associated with the Columbus Bridge Protocol (see chapter 9), thereby decreasing the potential for micromotion. None of the 21 patients treated in this study demonstrated prosthesis fracture. Certainly, the accurate and precise methods used to fabricate the prostheses played an essential role in reaching the optimal prosthetic CSR value recorded (100%) with the Columbus Bridge Protocol. In a pilot study, Grunder[37] treated five edentulous maxillary patients with immediately loaded full-arch prostheses and reported that five of the seven implant failures occurred in patients whose prostheses were made of acrylic resin without metal substructures. However, other researchers have reported high levels of clinical success with all-acrylic resin provisional prostheses.[23,30,38] All of the provisional prostheses and some of the definitive prostheses were fabricated with acrylic resin occlusal surfaces. There are contrasting opinions on this topic,[39–41] but many authors assert that the occlusal surfaces of implant prostheses should be made from materials that have a shock absorption capacity similar to acrylic resin to reduce the stresses transmitted to the bone-implant interface[20,42–45] and, consequently, to reduce the risk of overload.

TABLE 13.4 - MEAN DIFFERENCE IN BONE RESORPTION (T12–T0) AMONG SITES, IMPLANT SHAPES, IMPLANT INCLINATIONS, AND TYPES OF SOCKET				
	Number of Implants	**Mean Difference (T12–T0) (mm)**	**Lower 95%**	**Upper 95%**
Mesial site (tapered)	34	0.97	0.48	1.46
Mesial site (cylindric)	69	0.63	0.38	0.88
Distal site (tapered)	34	1.03	0.53	1.53
Distal site (cylindric)	69	0.88	0.68	1.09
Mesial site (upright)	61	0.62	0.32	0.93
Mesial site (angled)	42	0.92	0.56	1.27
Distal site (upright)	61	0.86	0.60	1.12
Distal site (angled)	42	1.04	0.67	1.41
Mesial site (healed bone)	56	0.98	0.64	1.33
Mesial site (extraction sockets)	47	0.46	0.18	0.73
Distal site (healed bone)	56	1.14	0.84	1.45
Distal site (extraction sockets)	47	0.68	0.40	0.96

36-MONTH PROSPECTIVE STUDY

Study Design

Between September 2005 and January 2006, the Department of Implant and Prosthetic Dentistry of Genoa developed a prospective clinical study to evaluate the clinical and radiographic outcomes of immediate versus delayed loading in a convenience sample of patients with edentulous maxillae.

A sample of 49 patients (25 women, 24 men) with edentulous maxillae or significant unfavorable prognoses for their maxillary dentitions was identified for this study. Patients presented with a mean age of 58.2 years and were treated with fixed screw-retained prostheses supported by implants (N = 260).

Patients were divided into two groups: the patients in the test group were selected for treatment with the immediate loading protocol on the basis of both their expectations and demand for immediate, fixed implant prostheses; they sought to avoid the use of a transitional complete denture. On the other hand, the patients in the control group were willing to accept wearing a complete denture for a short time interval, and this cohort was composed of older patients relative to the test group.

The test group comprised 34 patients (19 women, 15 men) with bad prognoses for their maxillary teeth. These subjects underwent postextraction implant placement with immediate loading according to the Columbus Bridge Protocol. Provisional fixed screw-retained prostheses were placed within 24 hours of implant placement. The definitive prostheses were placed after a mean healing period of 4.5 months.

The control group comprised 15 patients (6 women, 9 men) with hopeless maxillary teeth who were made edentulous 3 months prior to implant surgery and treated with transitional complete dentures. These subjects underwent the standard two-stage ad modum Brånemark implant protocol with delayed loading. Definitive fixed screw-retained prostheses were placed after a mean healing period of 8.75 months.

Except for the time sequence for extraction, implant loading, and the number of implants, the control and test group did not differ in surgical-prosthetic protocols or maintenance programs.

A total of 163 4-mm-diameter implants (Osseotite and Osseotite natural tapered [NT] implants) were placed in the test group; implant numbers ranged from 4 to 6 per subject (mean: 4.8 implants per patient). Ninety-seven implants (Osseotite) were placed in the control group. These patients received 6 to 9 implants each (mean: 6.5 implants per patient). In the control group, cover screws were placed onto the implants before the surgical sites were closed. Mean healing time in the control group was 6.8 months. During this period, patients wore complete dentures relined with a soft material at 14 days and every month thereafter. During the first 2 weeks, patients were asked not to wear their dentures to allow the peri-implant soft tissues to heal without pressure from the dentures. Later, implants were exposed during a second surgical procedure; prosthetic abutments were then placed onto the implants prior to fabrication of the definitive prostheses.

Radiographic examinations were accomplished to assess interproximal bone levels at baseline (provisional prosthesis placement for the test group; implant placement for the control group) and at the 12-, 24-, and 36-month follow-up appointments. The implant-abutment interface was used as the reference point for the bone level measurements. Interproximal bone levels were assessed from these reference points to the most coronal bone levels at the mesial and distal surfaces of each implant.[29]

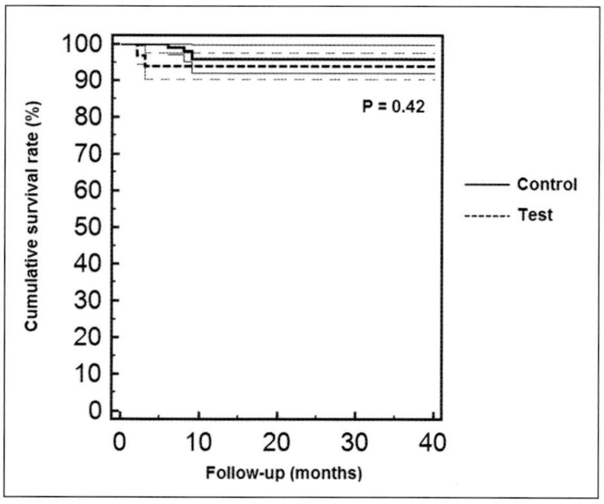

Fig. 13.2 - Life table analysis for implants in the test and control groups.

Statistical Analysis

The Shapiro-Wilk test was used to evaluate normality of the dependent variables used, and the data were rank transformed if normality was rejected. Differences between test and control groups with respect to time-dependent bone loss (mesial and distal) were analyzed with repeated measures analysis of variance, and contrasts among baseline and successive measures were assessed. Survival analysis was per- formed by means of a marginal Cox model to evaluate the effect of group on survival and compute a survival curve.

Clinical Outcomes

No patients were lost to recall, and they were all followed for at least 36 months, with the average follow-up period being 40.5 months (range: 36 to 47 months). Ten implants (6.1%) failed in the test group, which occurred during the first 3 months after implant placement and occlusal loading. Of the 10 implants that failed in the test group, 6 new implants were placed into the distal areas to increase molar support in the prostheses and were immediately loaded. These implants were not considered in the survival calculations or for peri-implant bone level evaluations. The cumulative implant survival rate at the 36-month follow-up visit (after implant placement) was 93.9% (95% confidence interval [CI]: 90% to 97.8%) for the test group (Fig 13.2).

In the control group, four implants (4.1%) failed during the first 12 months after implant placement. One implant failed before it was uncovered, and three implants were lost 2 months postloading, approximately 8 months after implant placement. No patient had more than one implant failure, and no additional implants were placed after implant failure. The CSR at the 36-month follow-up visit (after implant placement) was 95.9% (95% CI: 90 to 99.8%) for the control group (see Fig 13-2). The difference in CSRs between test and control groups was not statistically significant ($P = .42$). At the 36-month follow-up appointments, no prosthetic failures were found in either group.

Radiographic Outcomes

Average bone level at baseline was 0.5 mm from the implant-abutment connection both in the test and control groups. After 12 months, it was 1.3 ± 0.8 mm in the test group and 1.9 ± 0.8 mm in the control group. At the 24-month recall, it was at 1.5 ± 0.9 mm in the test group and 2.2 ± 0.9 mm in the control group.

Finally, after 36 months, it was 1.6 ± 0.9 mm in the test group and 2.3 ± 1.1 mm in the control group. Bone loss revealed moderate peri-implant bone resorption during the first 12 months, and a steady-state condition during all other intervals (Fig 13.3).

Discussion

It has been noted by the authors that immediate full-arch treatment (test group) yields instant significant improvement in patient satisfaction and perceptions related to comfort and function. In contrast, patients submitted to the standard two-stage protocol with delayed loading (control group) did not initially show particular interest in a management protocol that automatically included treatment time reduction. However, they were concerned when they were instructed to avoid wearing the complete dentures for the first 2 weeks after implant placement and experienced increased intraoral discomfort during the first month of treatment. Discomfort associated with the second surgical procedure to uncover the implants was less, but some patients required additional analgesics to manage the discomfort. Increased chairtime was noted relative to the two-stage protocol and was regarded as an unfavorable occurrence by some patients.

The clinical observations reported that more implants failed in the test group (CSR: 93.9%) than in the control group (CSR: 95.9%), but this difference was not statistically significant ($P = .42$). The apparent context of the observed implant failures seemed to be different for the two groups. For the test group (immediate loading), osseointegration failed to occur earlier in the process, during the first 3 months after immediate occlusal loading. No implants in the test group were lost after definitive prostheses were placed (4.5 months after implant placement). In the control group, three patients had implants that failed after fixed prosthesis delivery, and they needed their

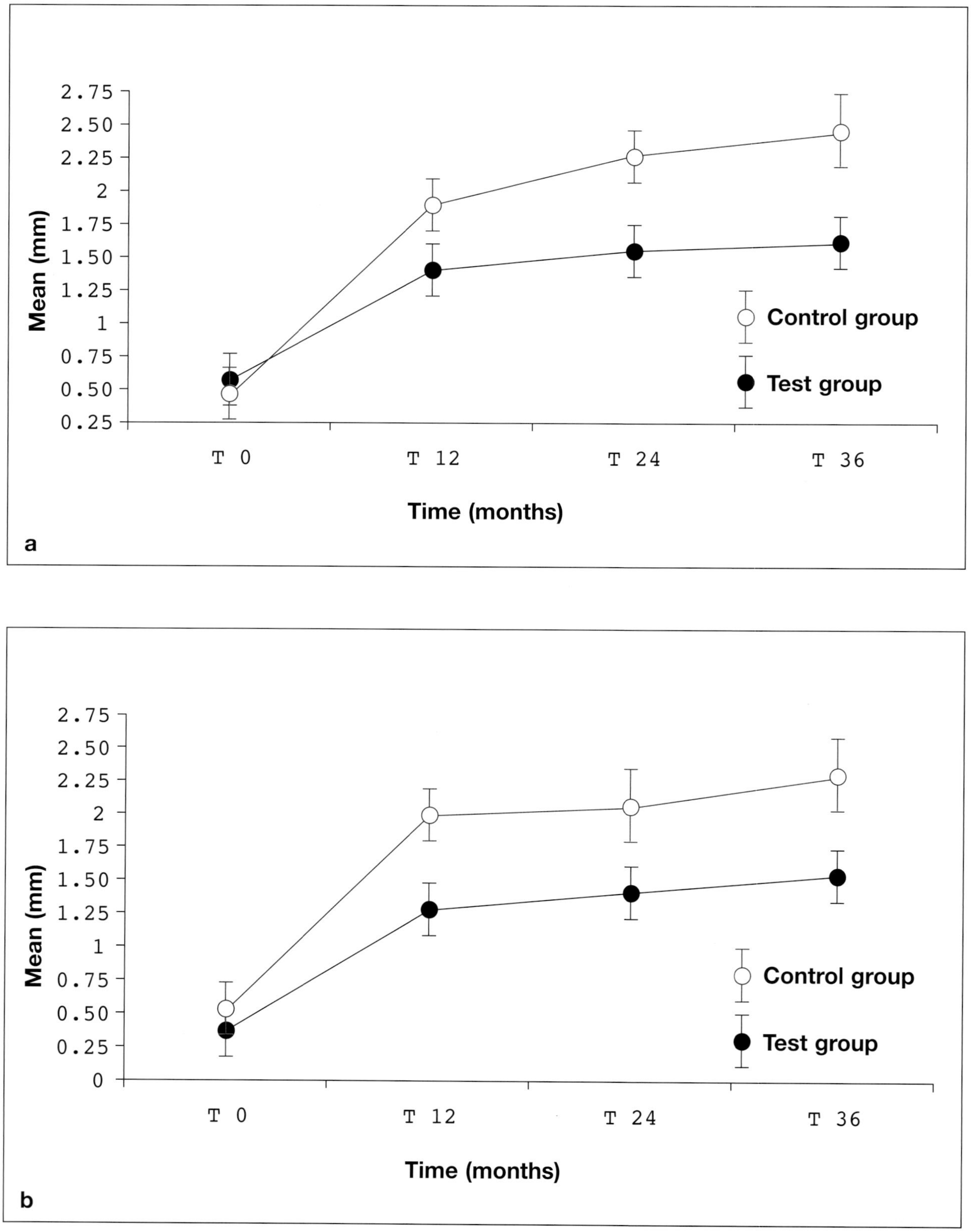

Fig 13.3 - Bone level comparisons between baseline (T0) and 3-year follow-up appointments (T36) for mesial *(a)* and distal *(b)* implant surfaces.

definitive prostheses modified secondary to implant failures.

While recognizing the inherent limits of the radiographic monitoring technique used, a statistically significant difference was nonetheless observed in peri-implant bone resorption at 12 months as well as at all following intervals (higher values in the control group).

Conclusion

In the mid-term follow-up, the application of the Columbus Bridge Protocol for immediate rehabilitation of edentulous maxillae led to similar clinical and radiologic results (implant cumulative survival rate and peri-implant bone resorption) with the traditional two-stage protocol. The advantages of the proposed protocol for a fixed implant-retained prosthesis in edentulous maxillae are the possibility to maintain the high predictability of the two-stage surgical procedures even with moderate to severe maxillary bone atrophy, multiple extraction sockets, and a reduced number of implants. The delivery of the provisional fixed denture in 24 hours, and the possibility to avoid the use of a provisional complete removable denture, make the Columbus Bridge Protocol an elective option in the treatment of the maxillary full-arch. The significance of a learning curve to better manage surgical and prosthodontic application and possible complications of this novel approach demands consideration.

The following pages present a series of clinical cases treated from 2004 to 2007 per the Columbus Bridge Protocol. The case presentations include tables with basic patient and treatment information (Fédération Dentaire International [FDI] tooth-numbering system used for all implant sites) as well as intraoral radiographs (taken at implant placement and at the 12- and 24-month follow-ups), panoramic radiographs, and clinical images.

Patient I

Age	49 years
General health	Good
Smoking habit	No
Cause of tooth loss	Endodontic failures
Bone quality	Type 2
Type of implants	Cylindric 4 × 15–mm
	Full Osseotite (sites 16, 15, 25)
	Conical 4 × 15–mm
	Full Osseotite NT (site 23)
Type of conical abutments	17 degrees (sites 12, 23)
	25 degrees (sites 15, 25)

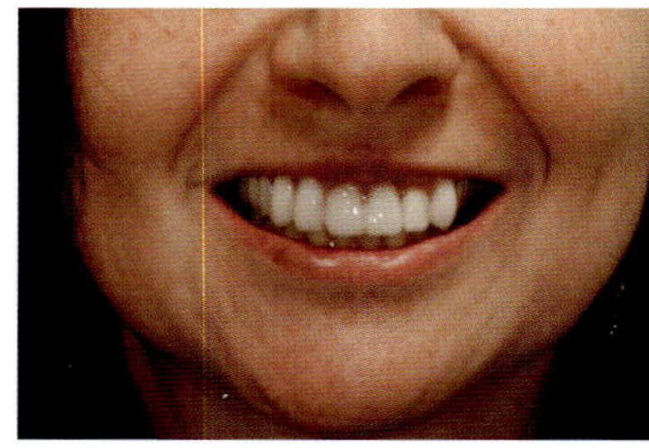

Preoperative smile

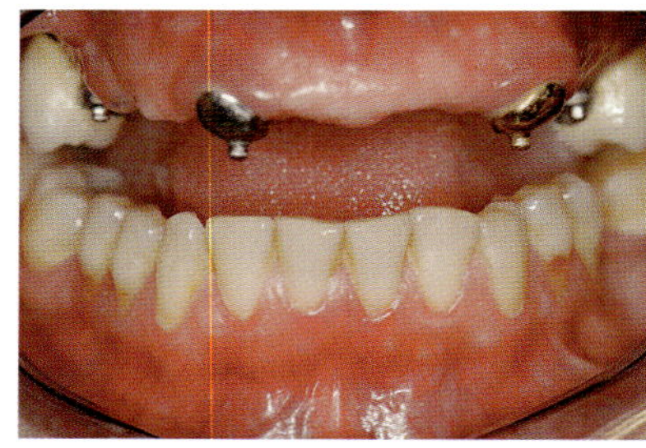

Preoperative frontal view with patient in centric occlusion

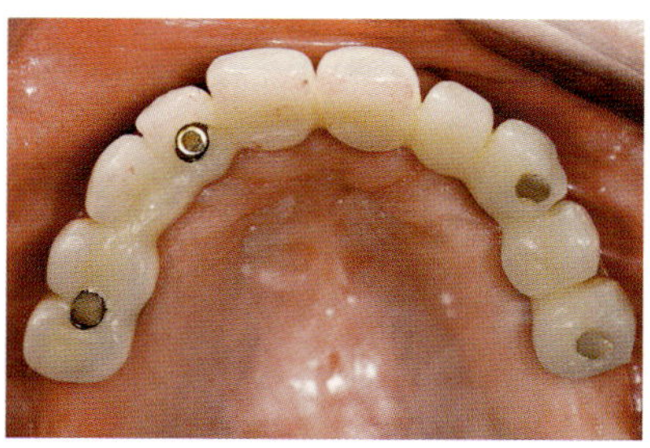

Occlusal view of provisional full fixed prosthesis (FFP)

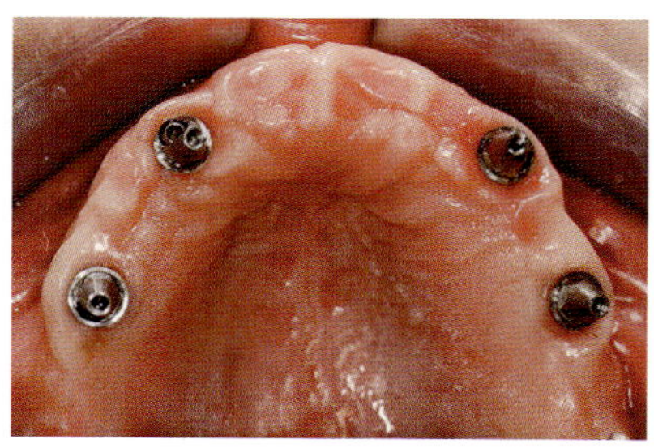

Maxillary occlusal view of soft tissue healing

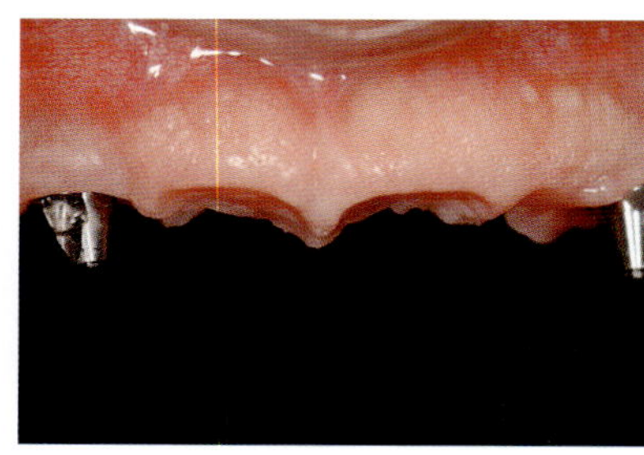

Frontal maxillary view, 4 months postsurgery

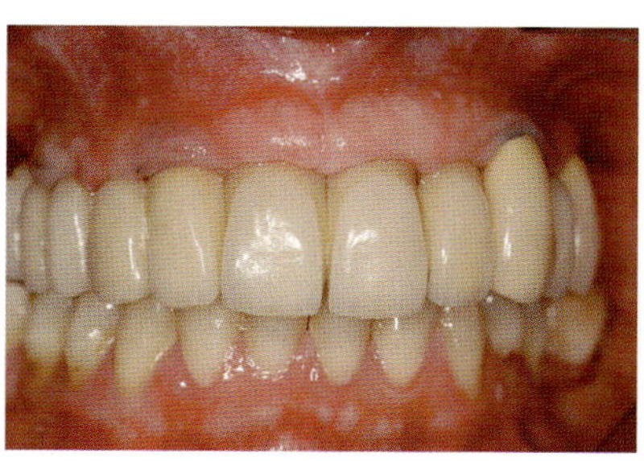

Frontal view of definitive FFP with patient in centric occlusion

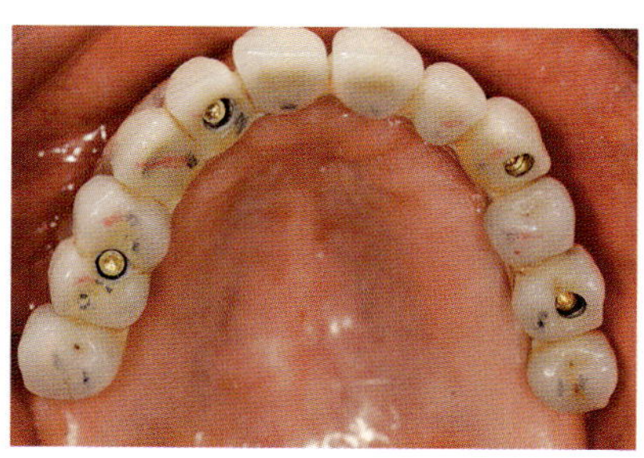

Occlusal view of definitive FFP

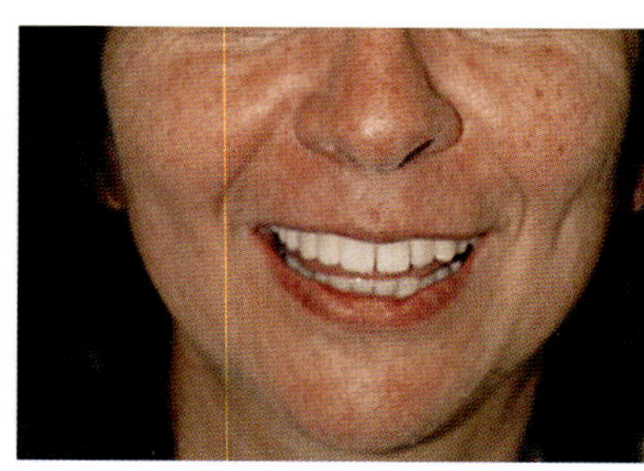

Smile with definitive FFP in place

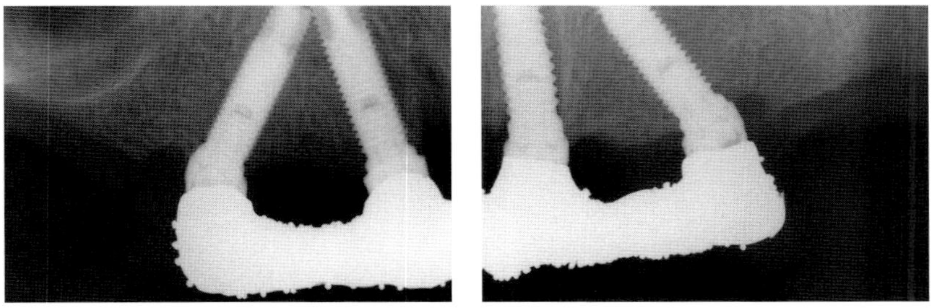

Intraoral radiographs at time 0

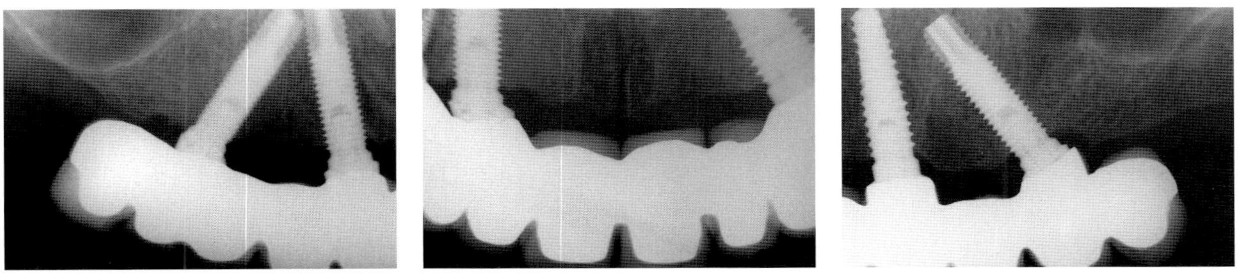

Postoperative intraoral radiographs at 12 months

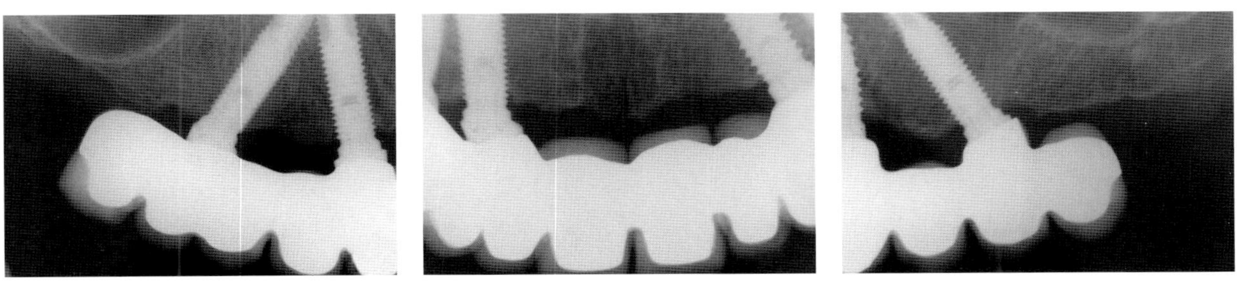

Postoperative intraoral radiographs at 24 months

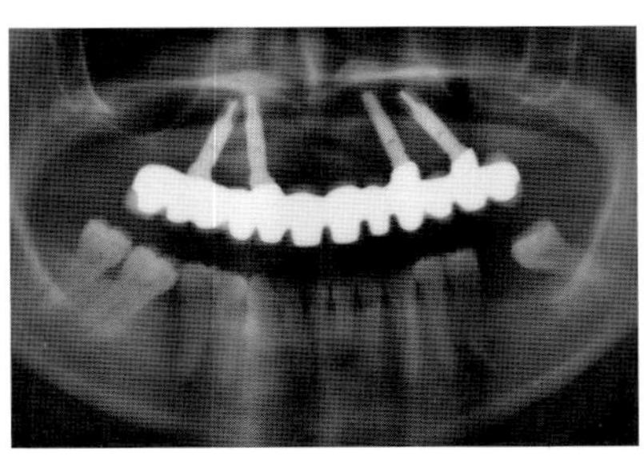

Postoperative panoramic radiograph at 24 months

Patient II

Age	48 years
General health	Good
Smoking habit	Yes
Cause of tooth loss	Endodontic failures
Bone quality	Type 3
Type of implants	Conical 4 × 15–mm Full Osseotite NT (sites 11, 15, 22, 25)
Type of conical abutments	17 degrees (sites 11, 22, 25) 25 degrees (site 15)

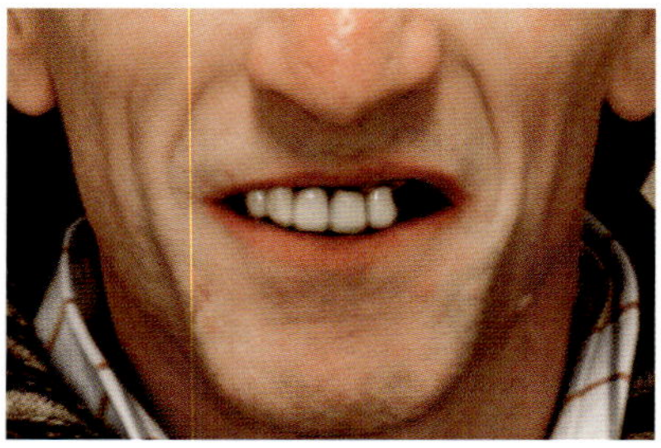

Preoperative smile

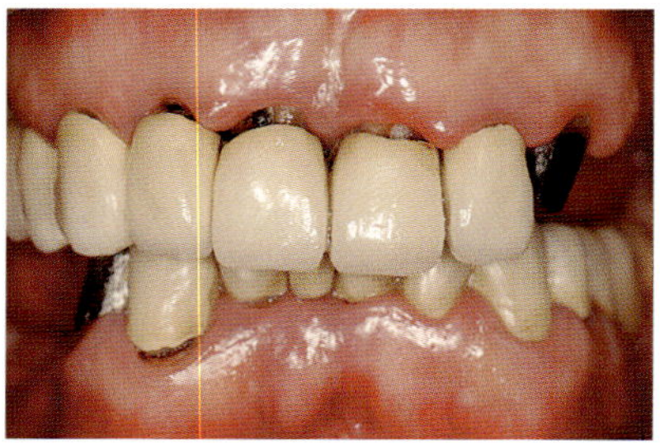

Preoperative frontal view with patient in centric occlusion

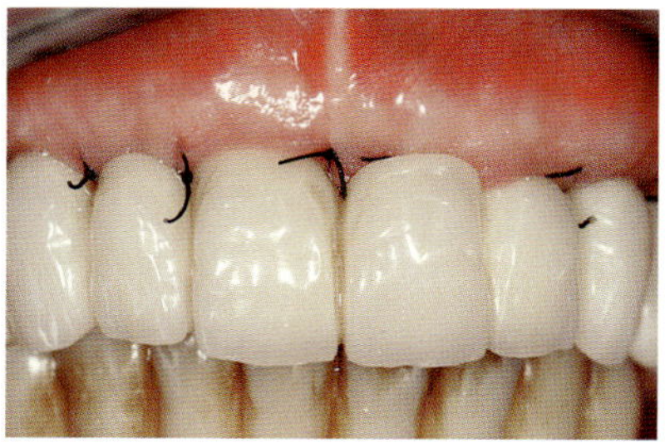

Frontal view at suture removal appointment with provisional FFP in place

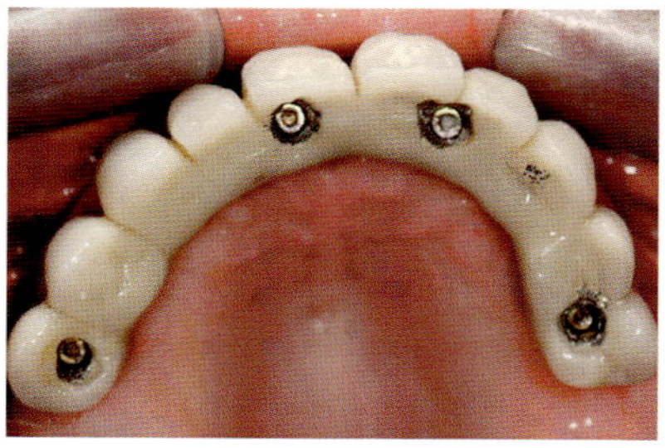

Maxillary occlusal view of provisional FFP

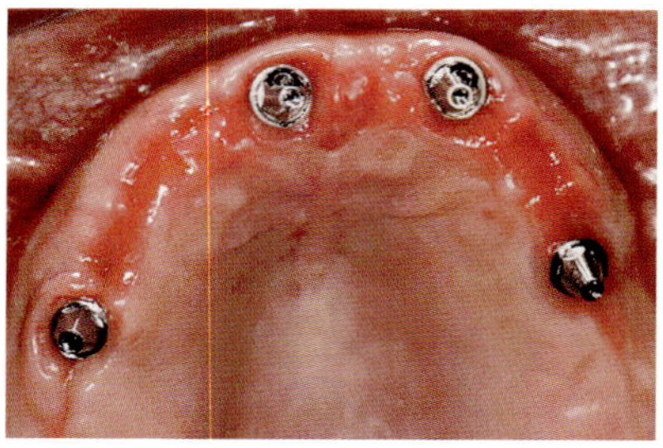

Occlusal view of soft tissue healing, 4 months postsurgery

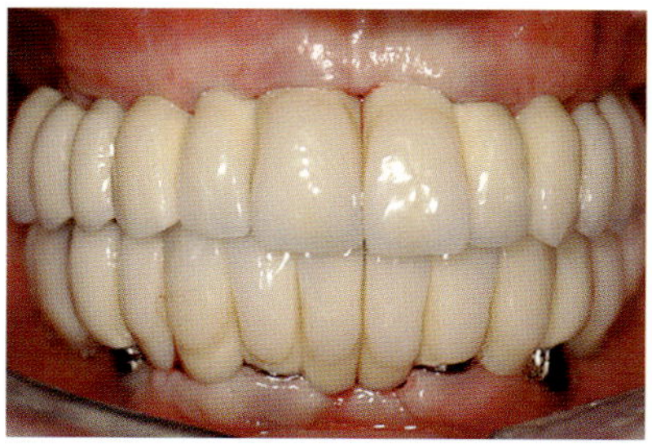

Frontal view of definitive FFPs with patient in centric occlusion

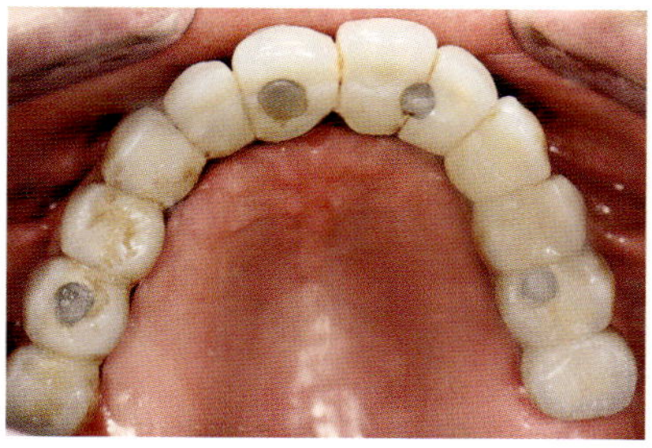

Occlusal view of definitive FFPs

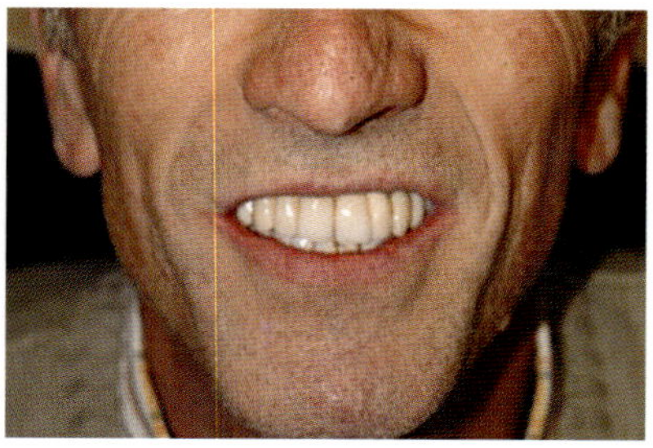

Smile with definitive FFPs in place

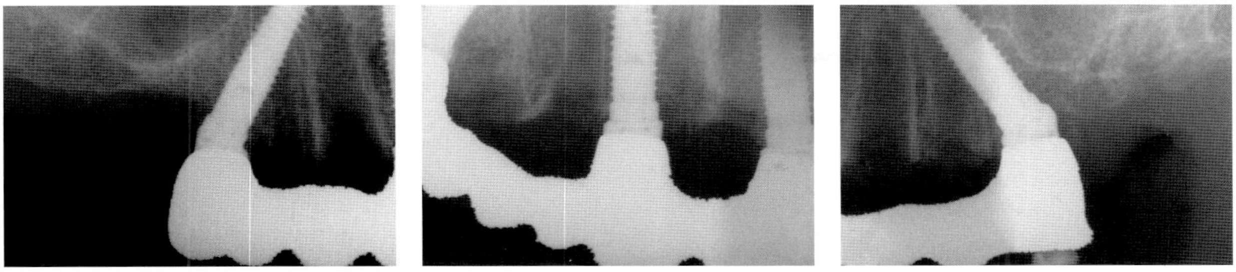

Intraoral radiographs at time 0

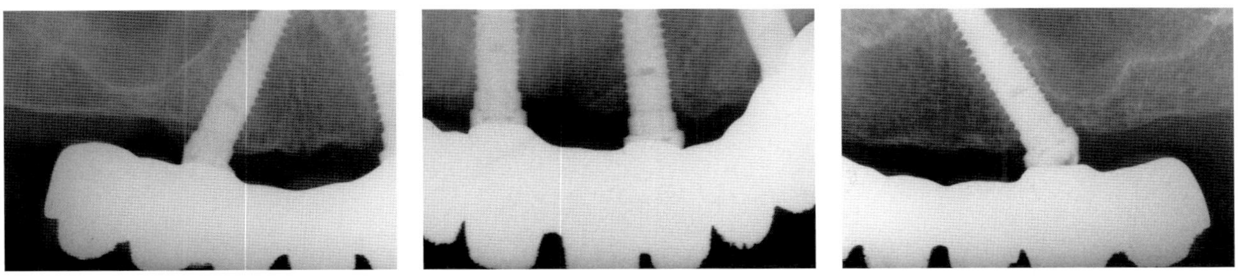

Postoperative intraoral radiographs at 12 months

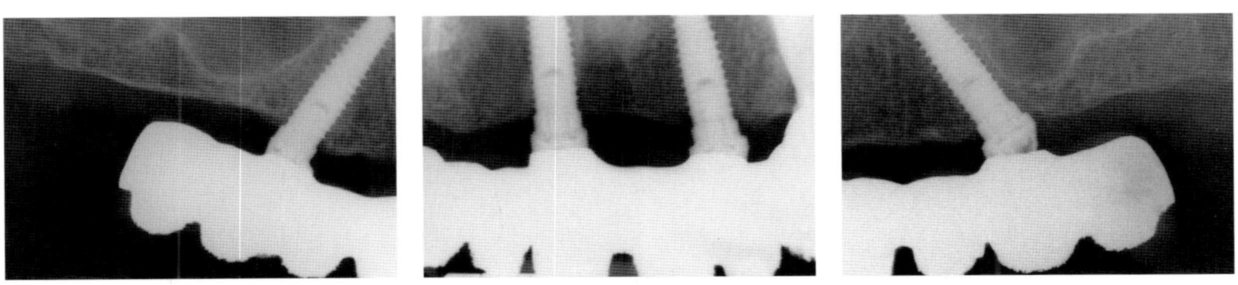

Postoperative intraoral radiographs at 24 months

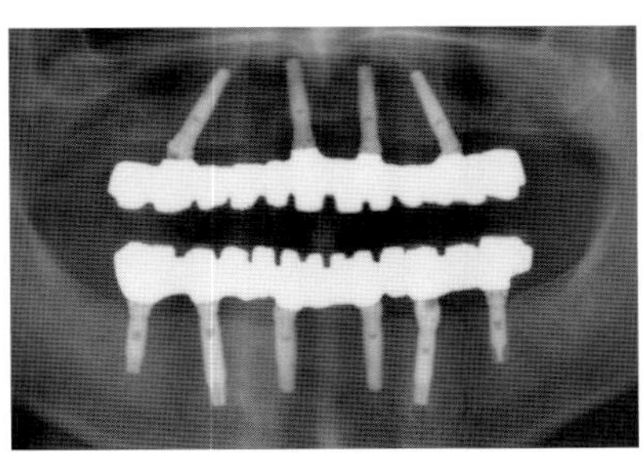

Postoperative panoramic radiograph at 36 months

Patient III

Age	50 years
General health	Hypertension
Smoking habit	No
Cause of tooth loss	Generalized severe periodontitis
Bone quality	Type 2
Type of implants	Conical 4 × 11.5–mm
	Full Osseotite NT
	(sites 12, 14, 22, 24)
Type of conical abutments	17 degrees (site 12)
	25 degrees (sites 22, 24)
	45 degrees (site 14)

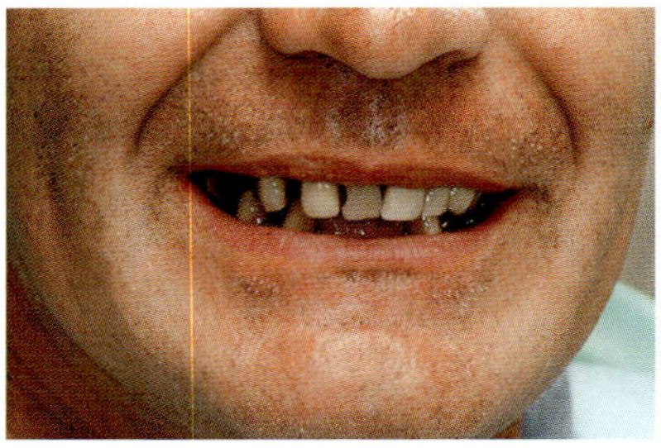

Preoperative smile

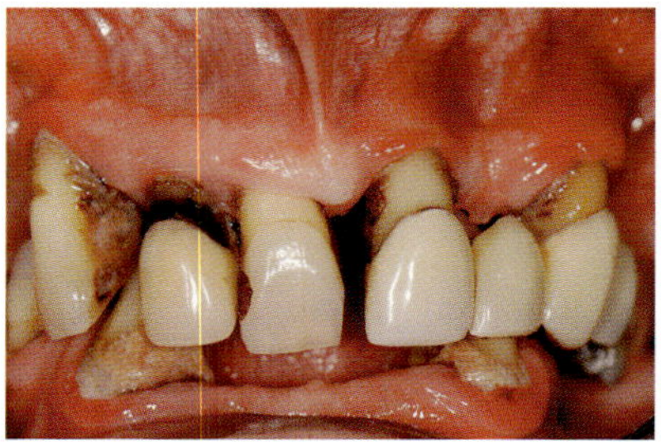

Preoperative frontal view with patient in centric occlusion

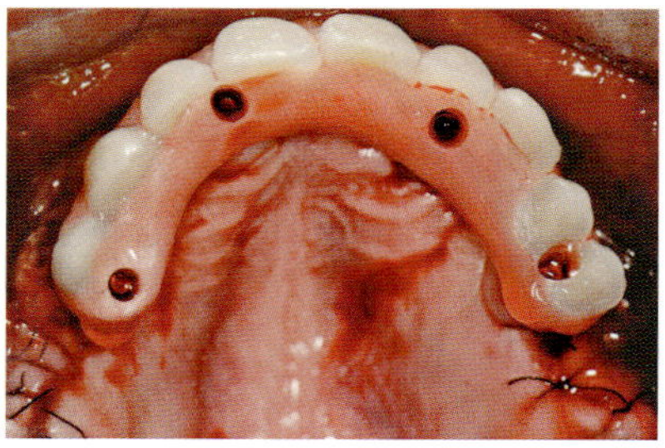

Occlusal view of provisional FFP

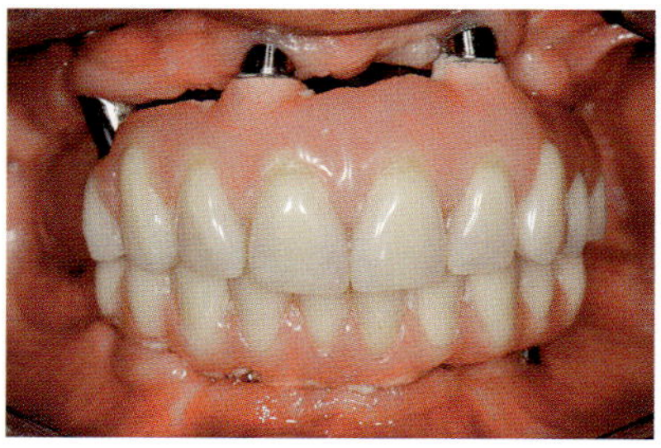

Frontal view at insertion appointment with provisional FFPs in place

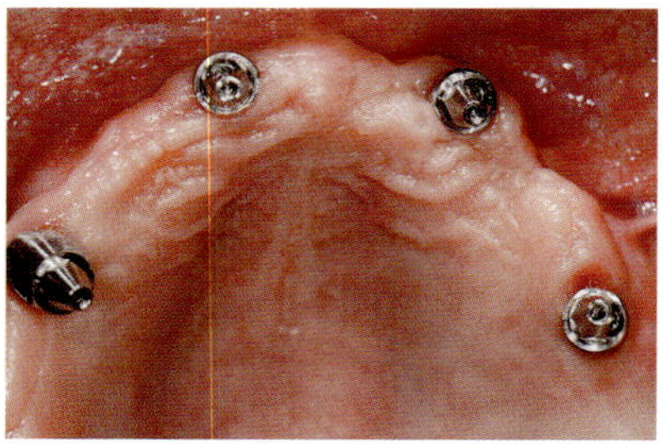

Occlusal view of soft tissue healing, 4 months postsurgery

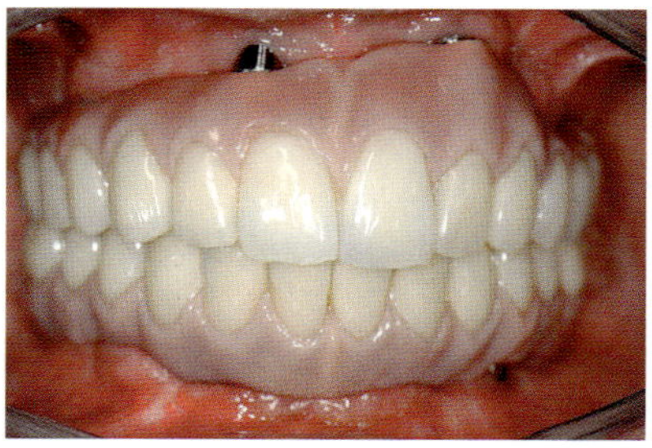

Frontal view of definitive FFPs with patient in centric occlusion

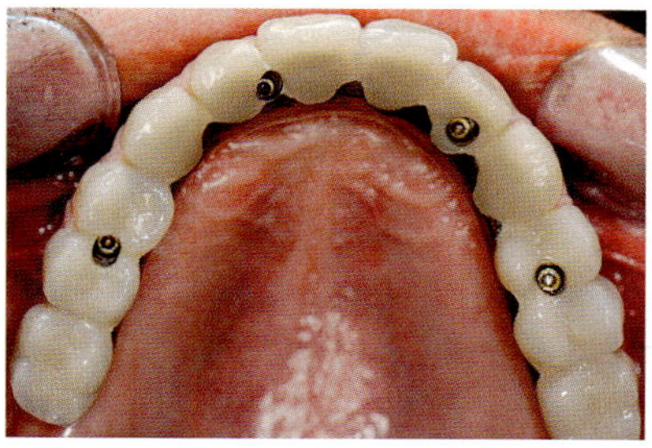

Occlusal view of definitive FFP

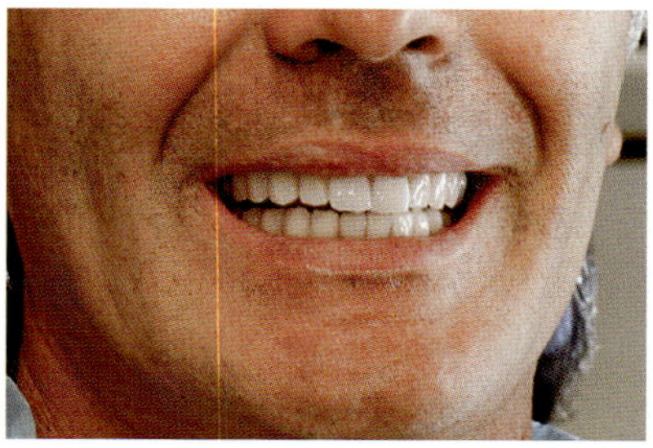

Smile with definitive FFPs in place

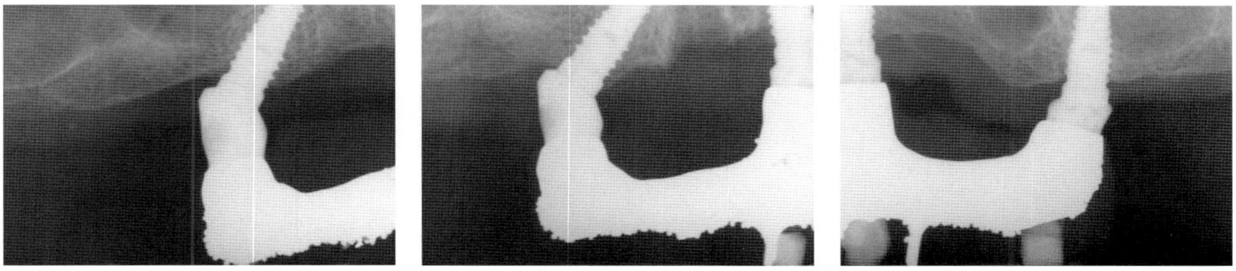

Intraoral radiographs at time 0

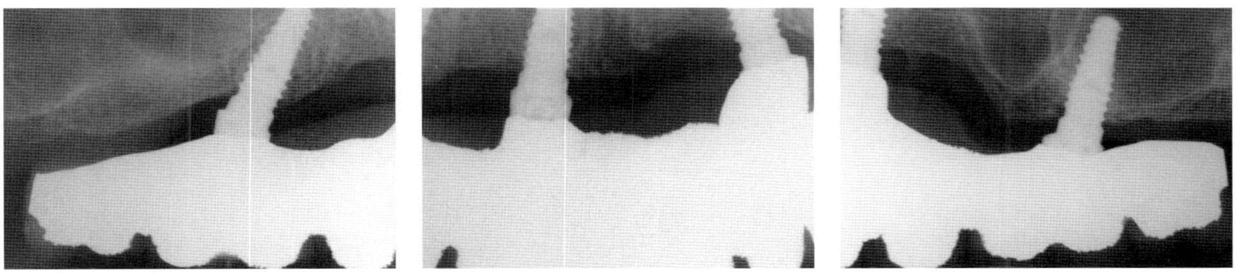

Postoperative intraoral radiographs at 12 months

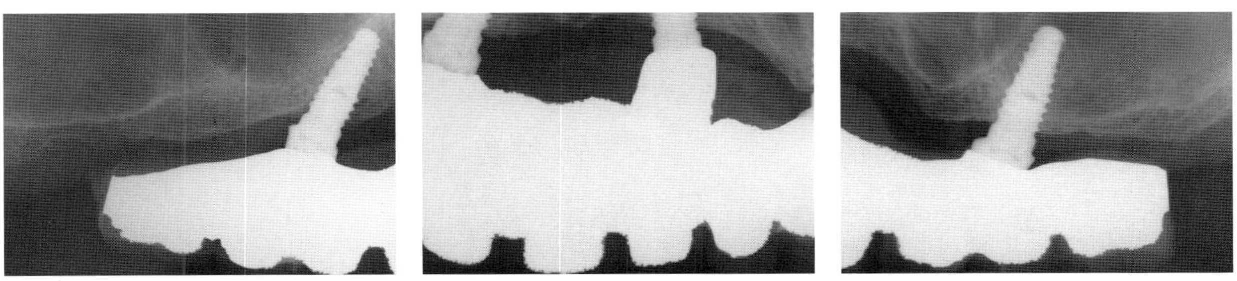

Postoperative intraoral radiographs at 24 months

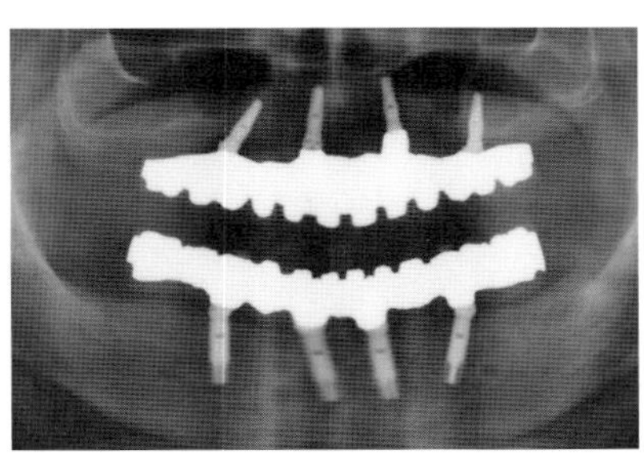

Postoperative panoramic radiograph at 36 months

Patient IV

Age	67 years
General health	Good; hyperthyroidism
Smoking habit	No
Cause of tooth loss	Endodontic failures
Bone quality	Type 3
Type of implants	Cylindric 4 × 15–mm Full Osseotite NT (sites 11, 15, 22, 25)
Type of conical abutments	25 degrees (sites 15, 25)
	45 degrees (sites 11, 22)

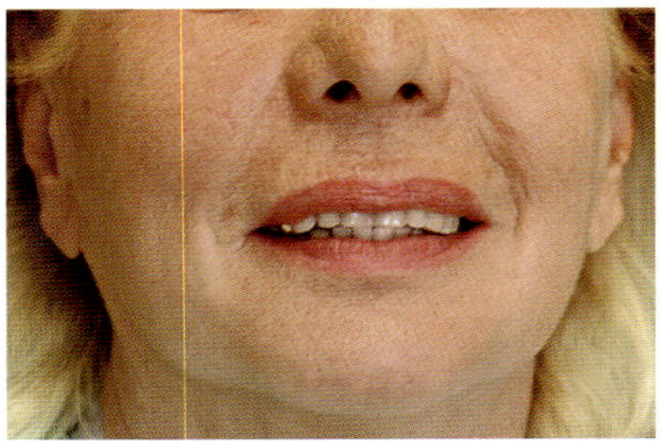

Preoperative smile

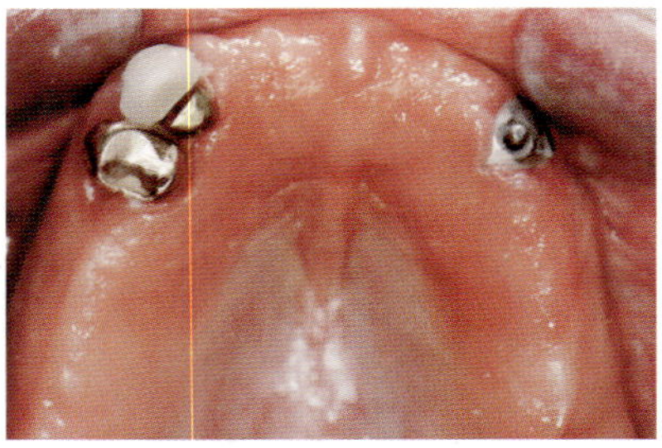

Preoperative occlusal view

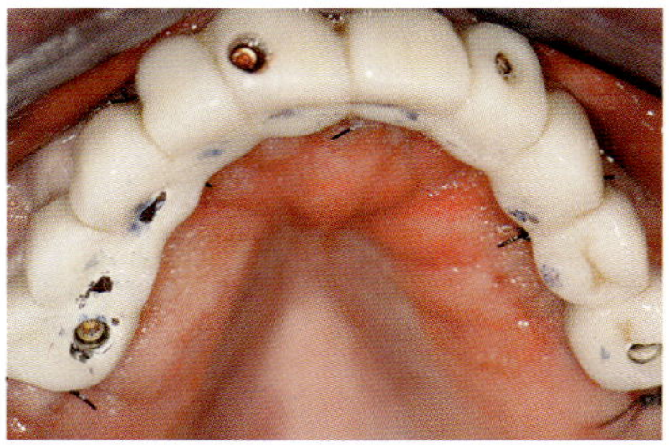

Occlusal image at insertion appointment with provisional FFP in place

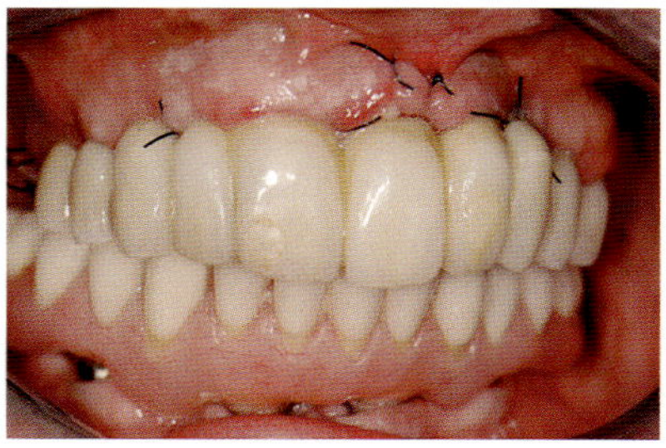

Frontal view at suture removal appointment

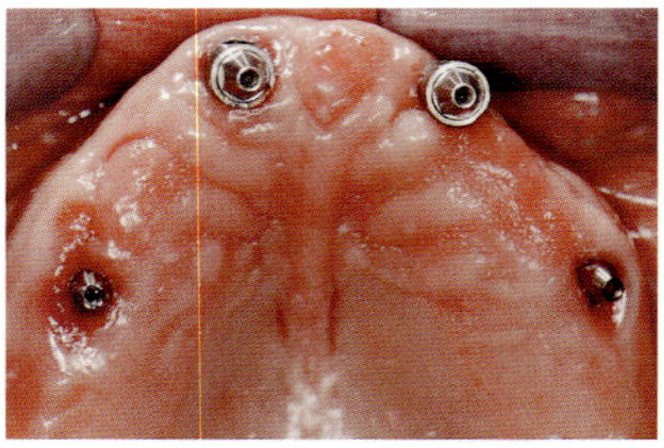

Occlusal view of soft tissue healing, 4 months postsurgery

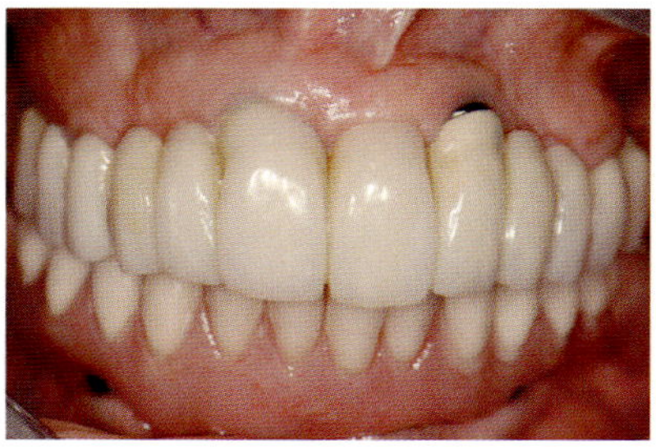

Frontal view of definitive FFPs with patient in centric occlusion

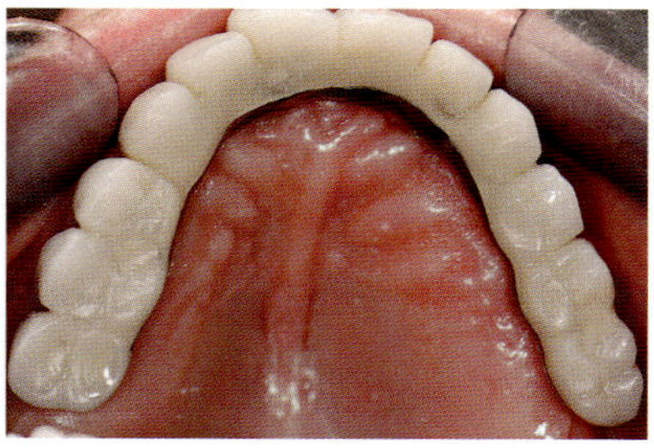

Occlusal view of definitive FFP

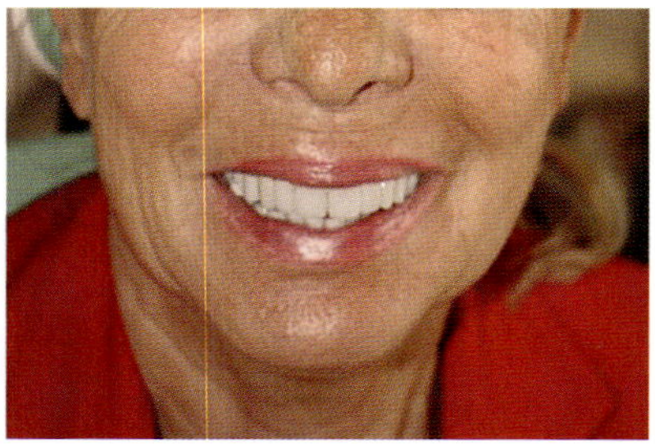

Smile with definitive FFPs in place

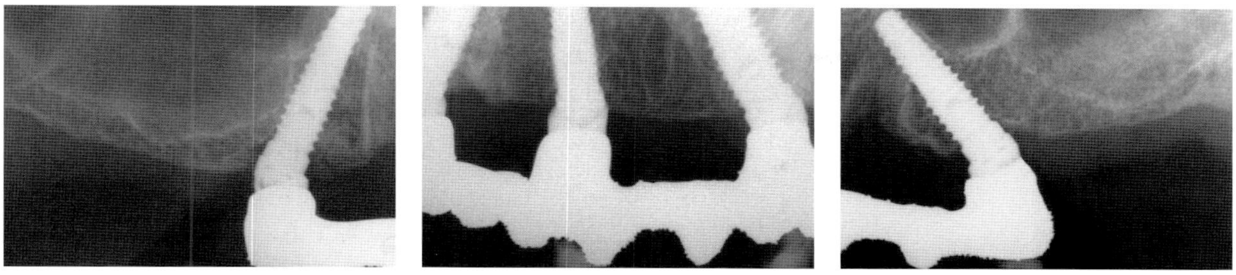

Intraoral radiographs at time 0

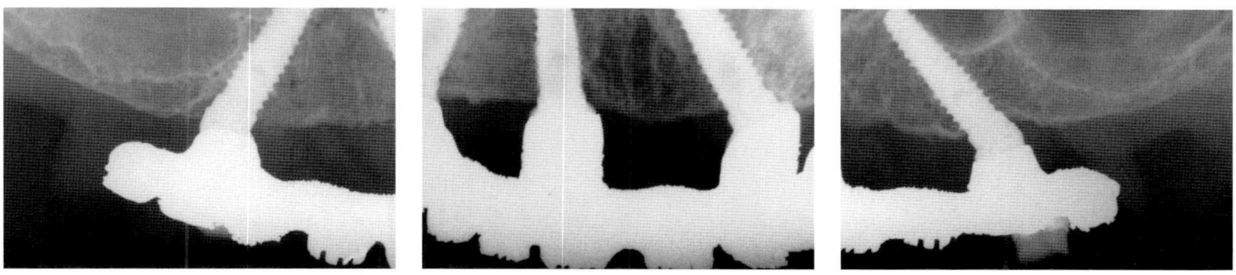

Postoperative intraoral radiographs at 12 months

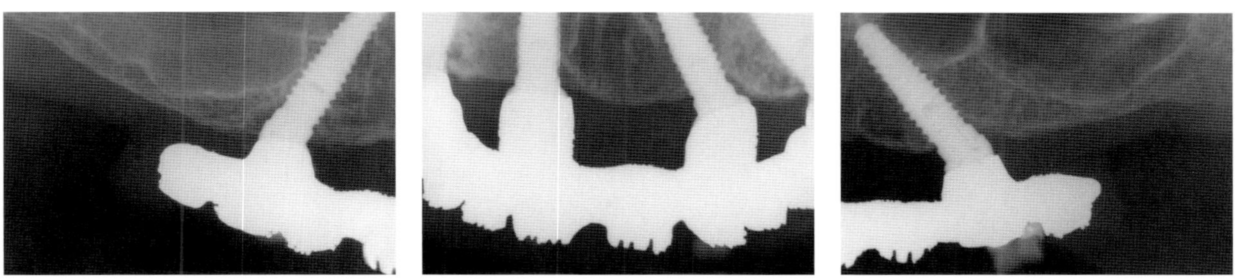

Postoperative intraoral radiographs at 24 months

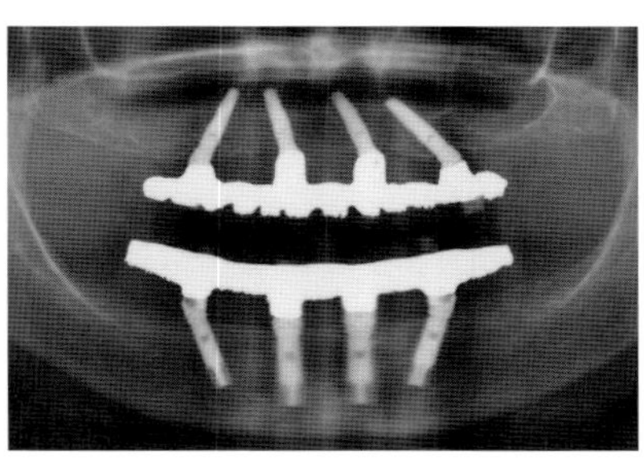

Postoperative panoramic radiograph at 36 months

Patient V

Age	77 years
General health	Hypertension
Smoking habit	No
Cause of tooth loss	Generalized severe periodontitis
Bone quality	Type 2
Type of implants	Cylindric 4 × 18–mm NanoTite (sites 13, 16, 26)
	Conical 4 × 15–mm NanoTite (site 24)
Type of conical abutments	25 degrees (sites 16, 24, 26)
	45 degrees (site 13)

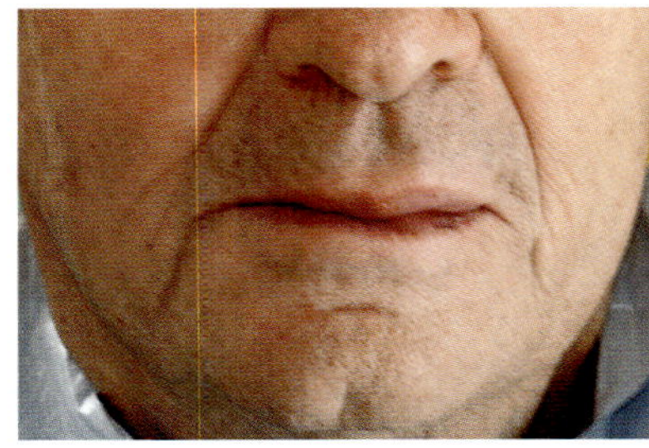

Preoperative frontal view

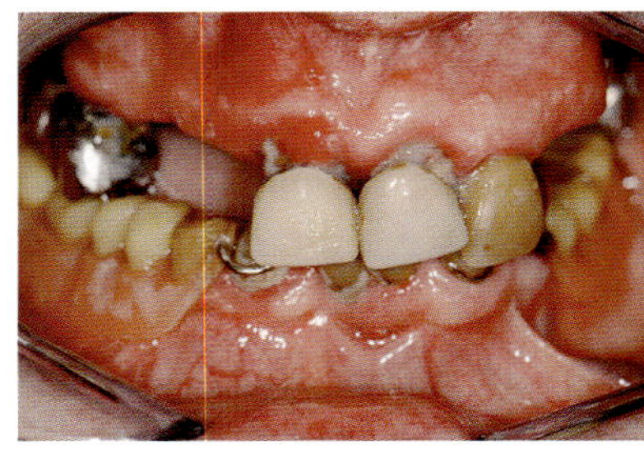

Preoperative frontal view with patient in centric occlusion

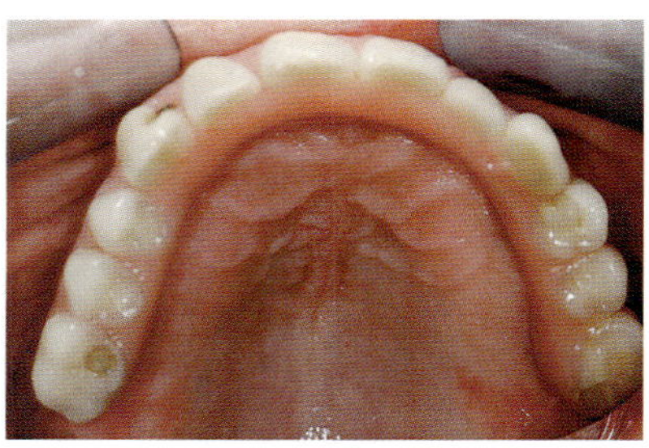

Occlusal image with provisional FFP in place

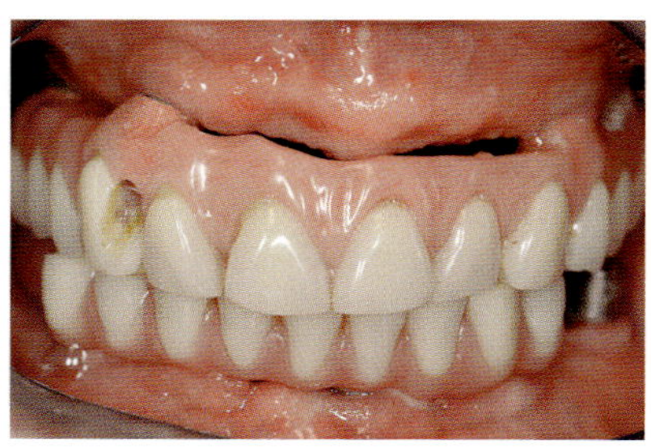

Frontal view of provisional FFPs

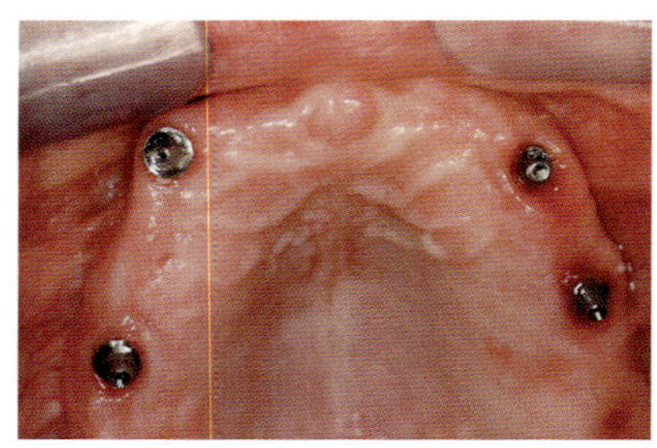

Occlusal view of soft tissue healing, 4 months postsurgery

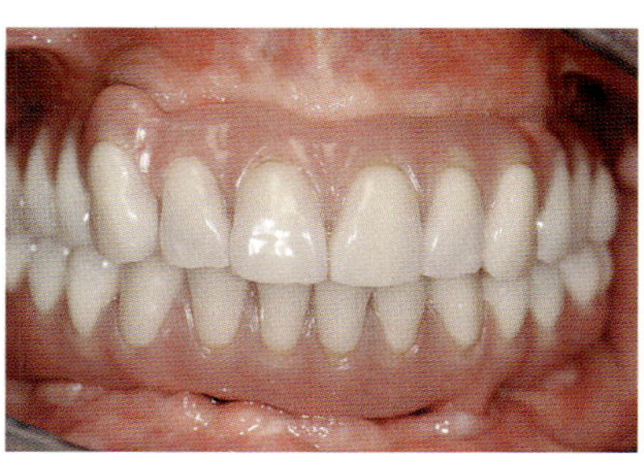

Frontal view of definitive FFPs with patient in centric occlusion

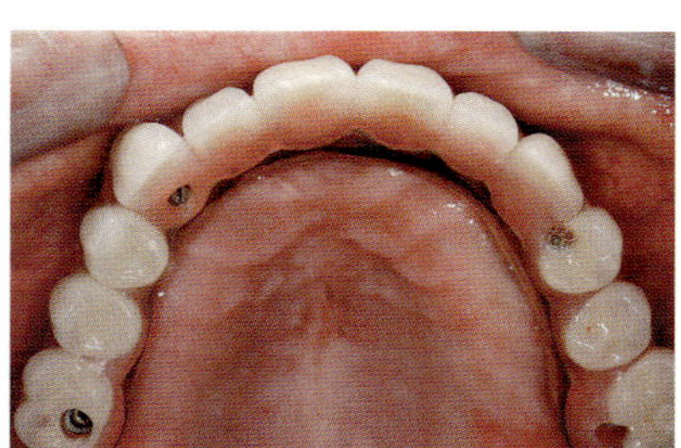

Occlusal view of definitive FFP

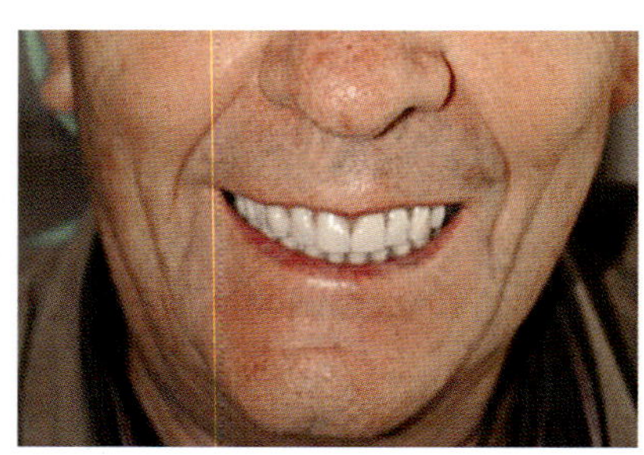

Smile with definitive FFPs in place

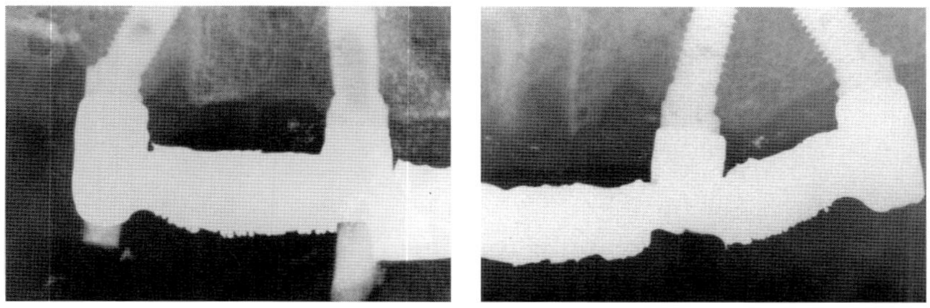

Intraoral radiographs at time 0

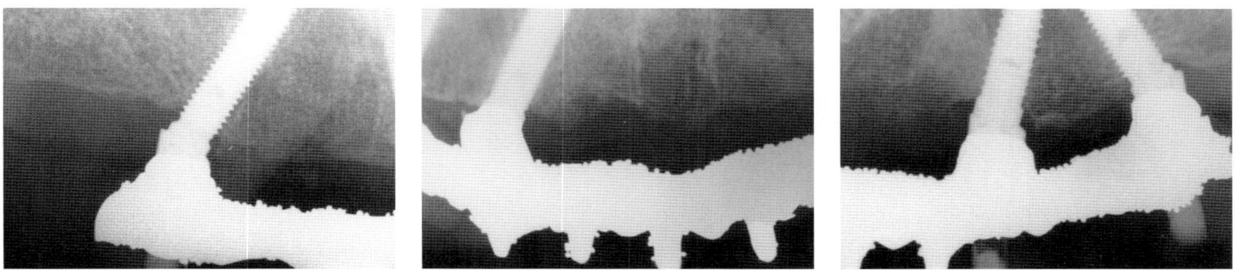

Postoperative intraoral radiographs at 12 months

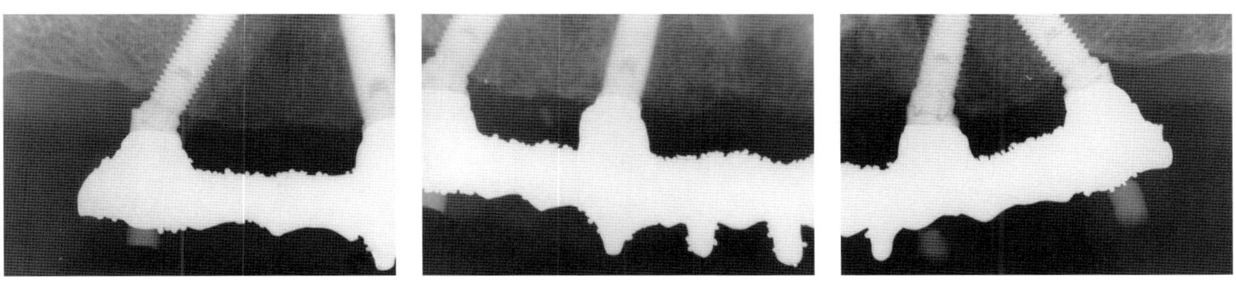

Postoperative intraoral radiographs at 24 months

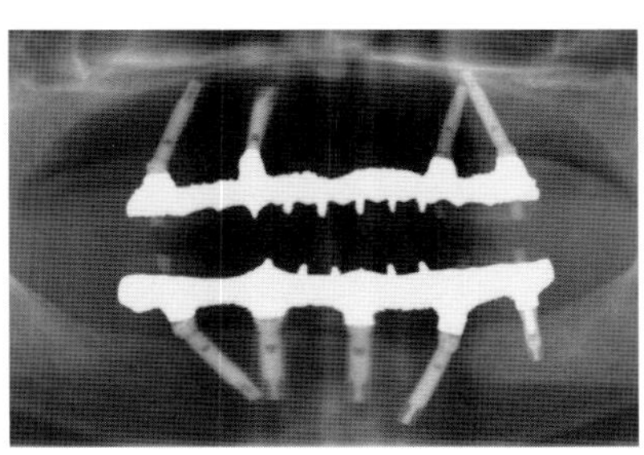

Postoperative panoramic radiograph at 24 months

Patient VI

Age	74 years
General health	Good
Smoking habit	No
Cause of tooth loss	Dental caries
Bone quality	Type 3
Type of implants	Cylindric 4 × 18–mm Osseotite (sites 15, 22, 25)
	Cylindric 4 × 15–mm Osseotite (site 12)
Type of conical abutments	17 degrees (site 22)
	25 degrees (sites 12, 15, 25)

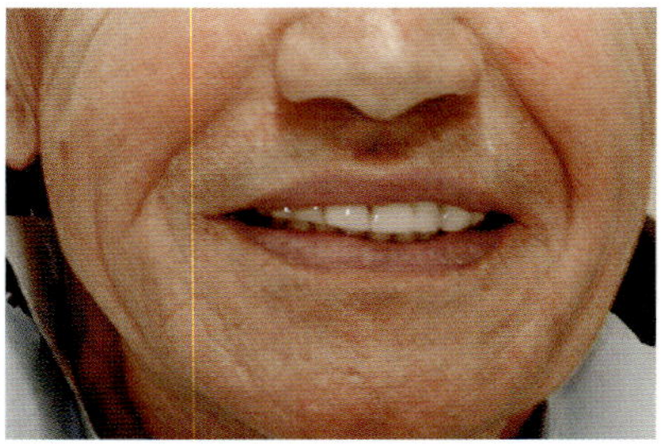
Preoperative smile

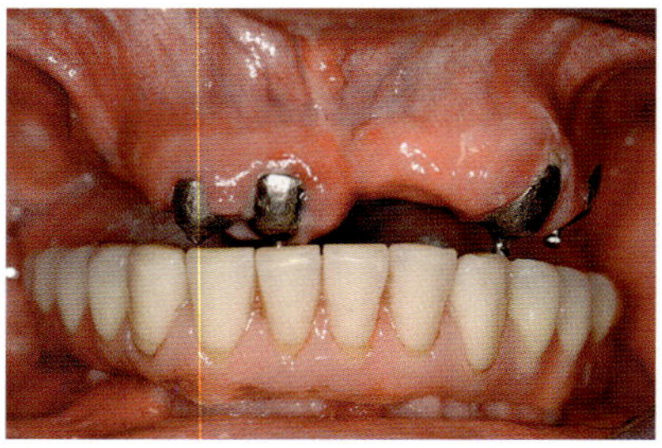
Preoperative frontal view

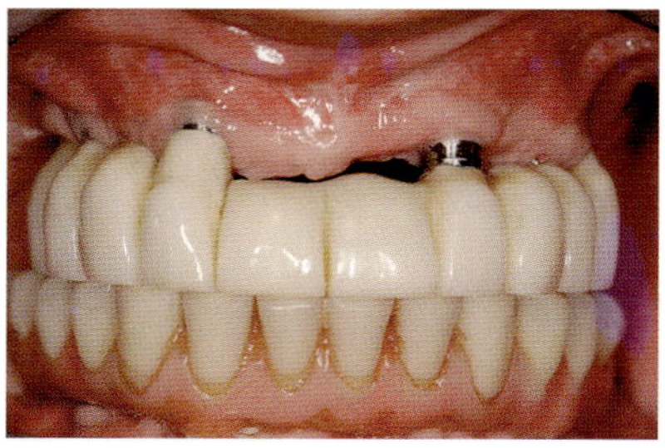
Frontal view with provisional FFP in place

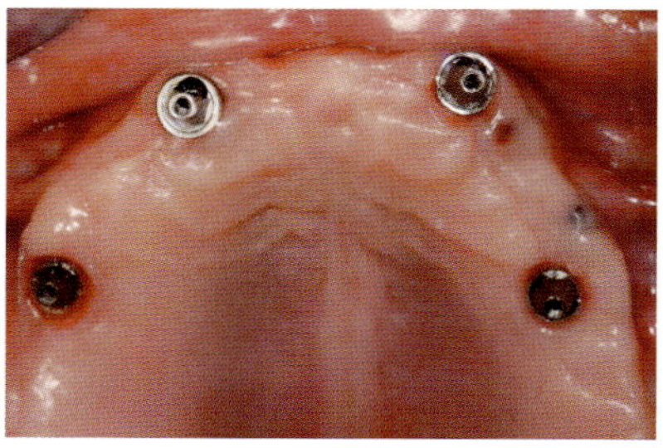
Occlusal view of soft tissue healing

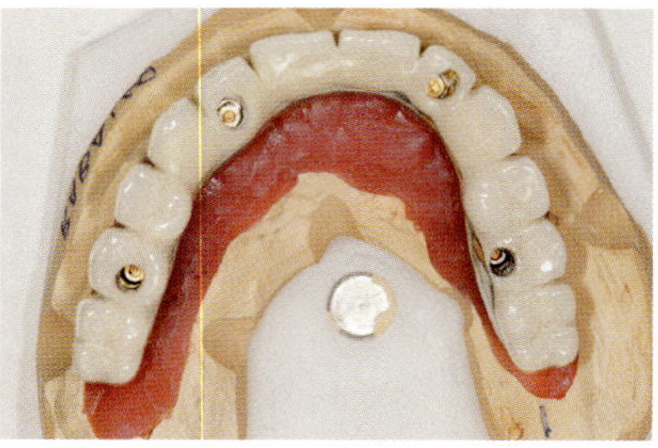
Laboratory maxillary occlusal view

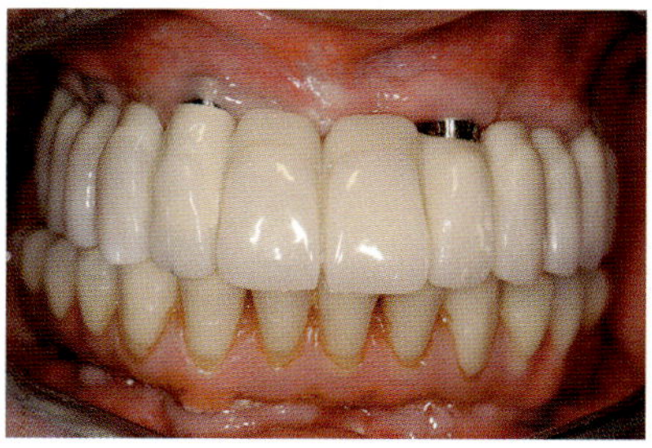
Frontal view of definitive FFPs with patient in centric occlusion

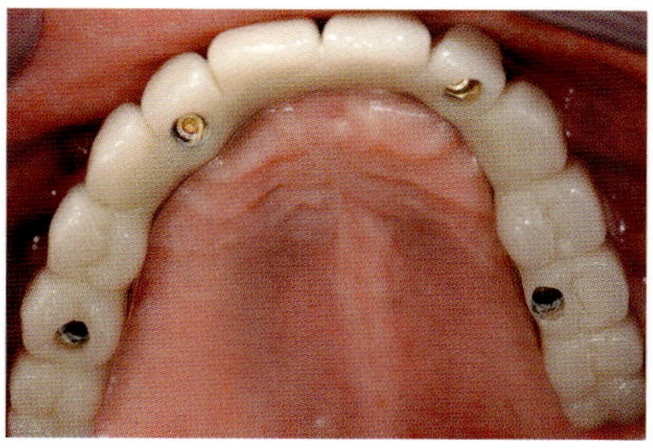
Occlusal view of definitive FFP

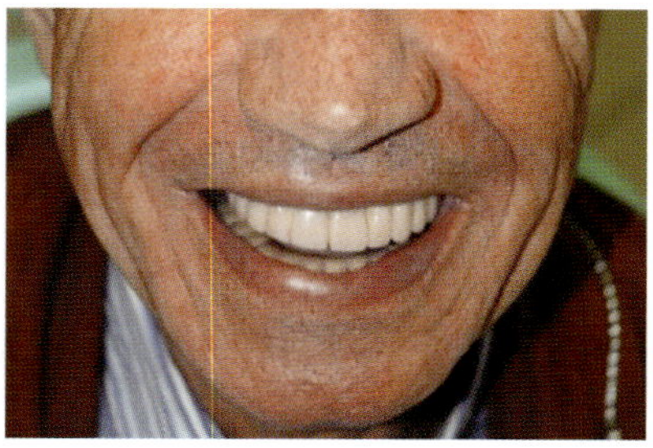
Smile with definitive FFPs in place

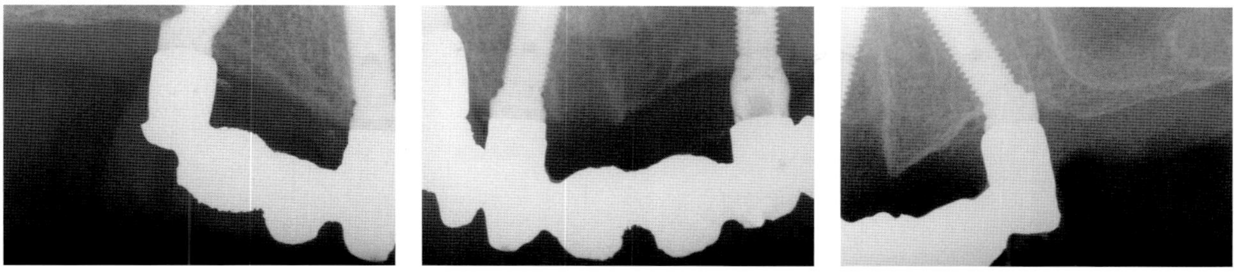

Intraoral radiographs at time 0

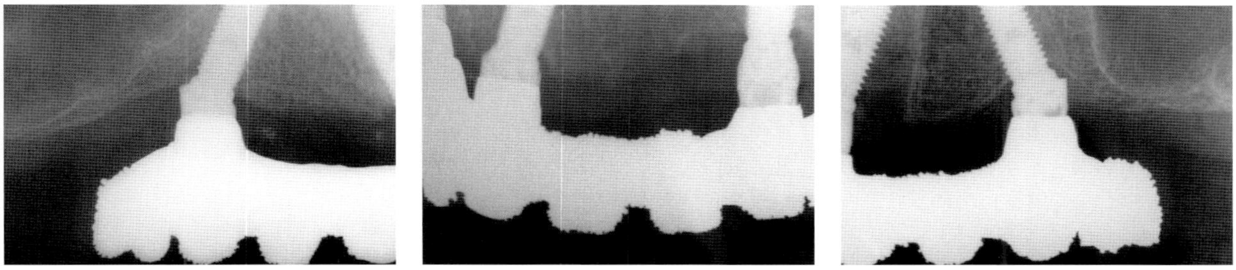

Postoperative intraoral radiographs at 12 months

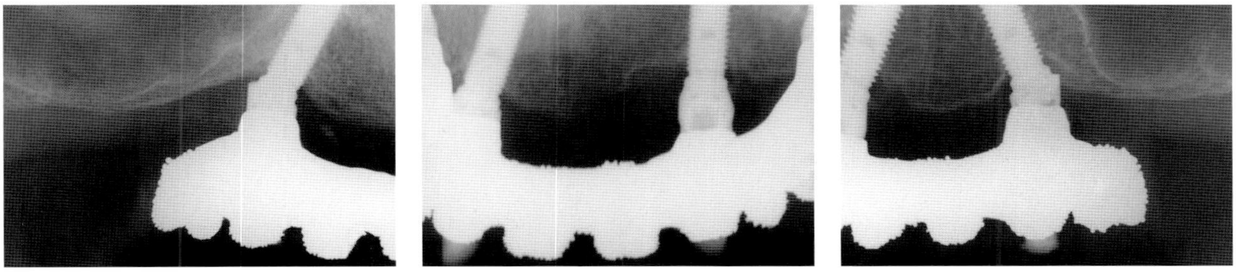

Postoperative intraoral radiographs at 24 months

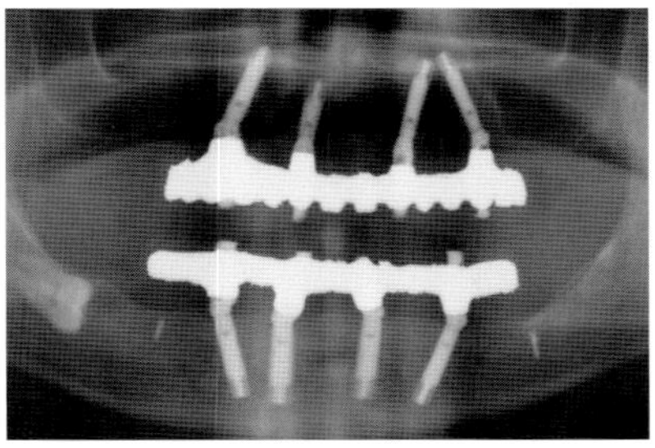

Postoperative panoramic radiograph at 36 months

Patient VII

Age	56 years
General health	Good
Smoking habit	Yes
Cause of tooth loss	Generalized severe periodontitis
Bone quality	Type 1
Type of implants	Cylindric 4 × 15–mm Full Osseotite (sites 11, 14, 21, 25)
Type of conical abutments	0 degrees (site 11)
	17 degrees (site 21)
	25 degrees (sites 14, 25)

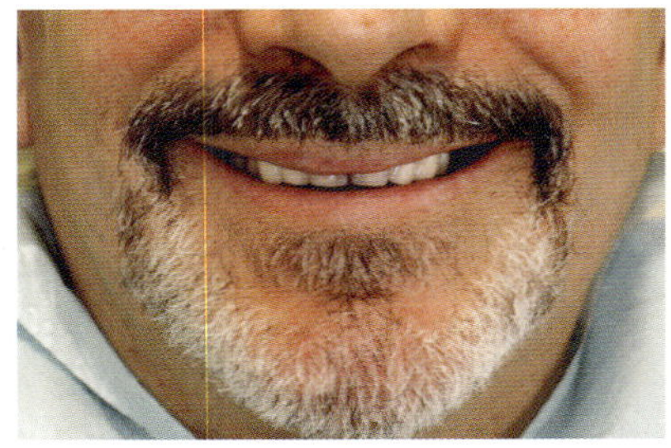

Preoperative smile

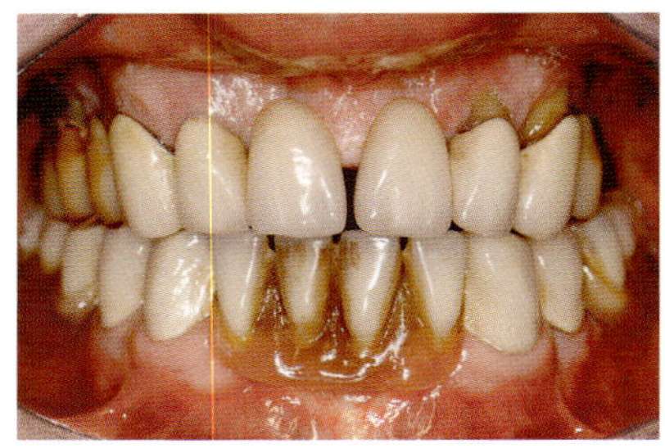

Preoperative frontal view with patient in centric occlusion

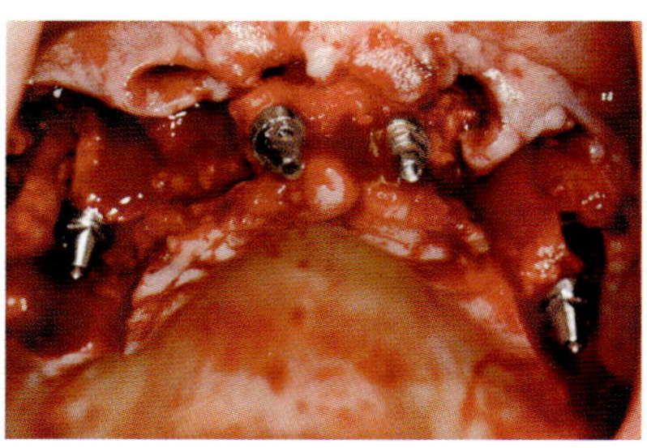

Occlusal view following extractions and implant and abutment placement

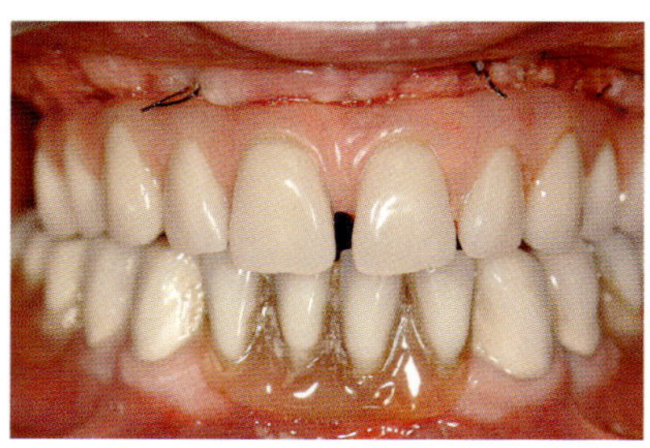

Frontal view with immediate provisional FFP in place

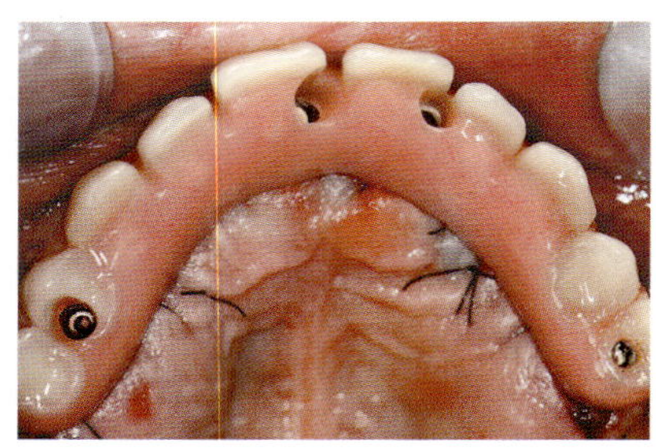

Occlusal view with immediate provisional FFP in place

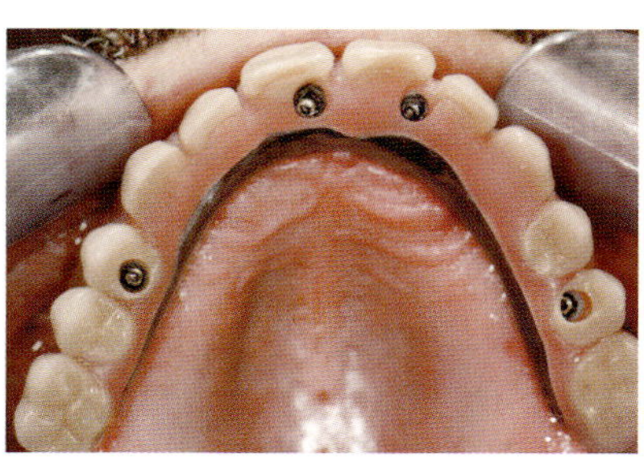

Occlusal view of definitive FFP

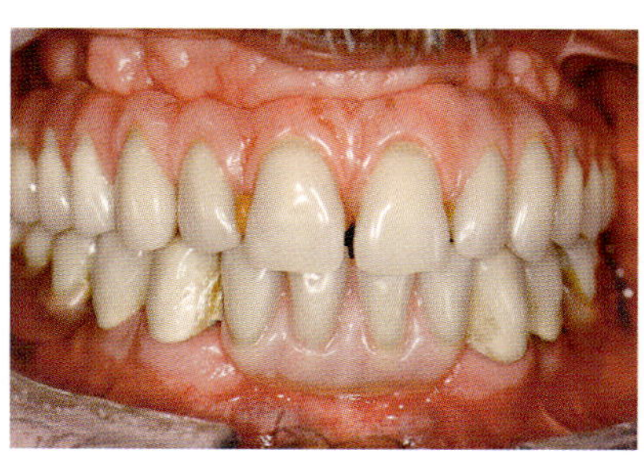

Frontal view of definitive FFP with patient in centric occlusion

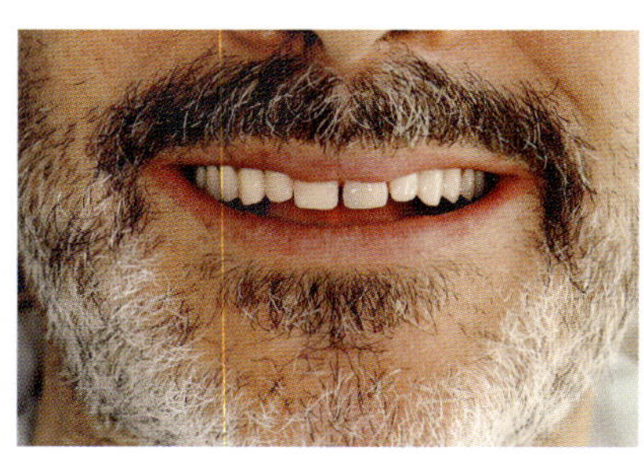

Smile with definitive FFP in place

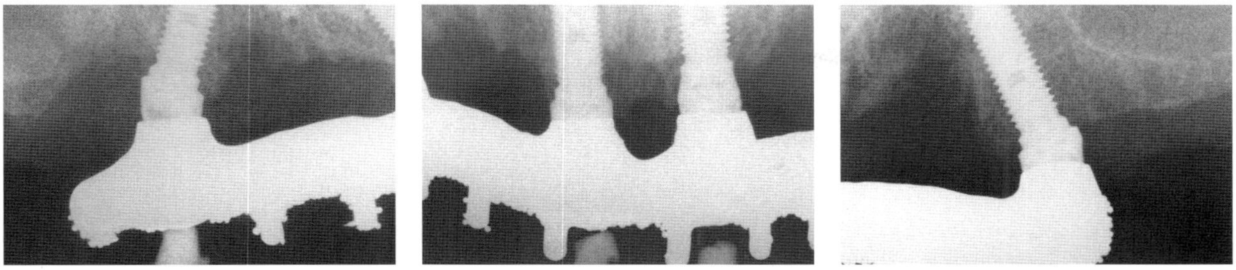

Intraoral radiographs at time 0

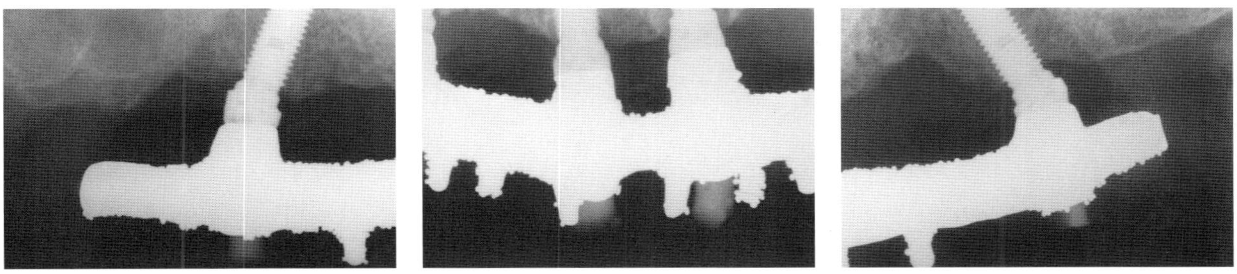

Postoperative intraoral radiographs at 12 months

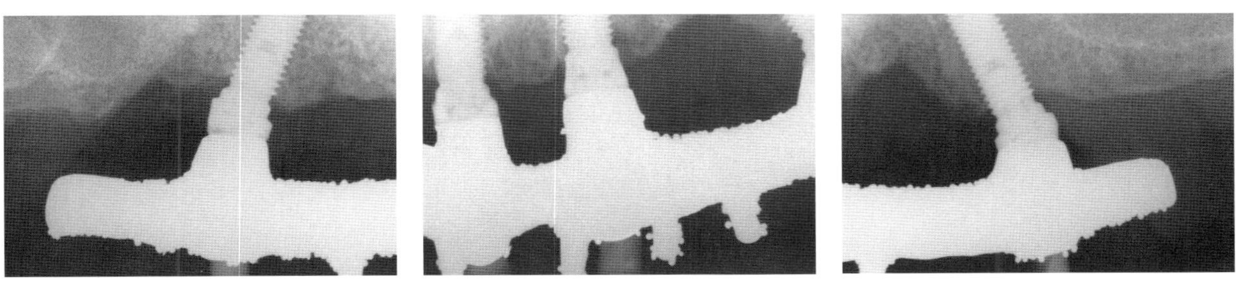

Postoperative intraoral radiographs at 24 months

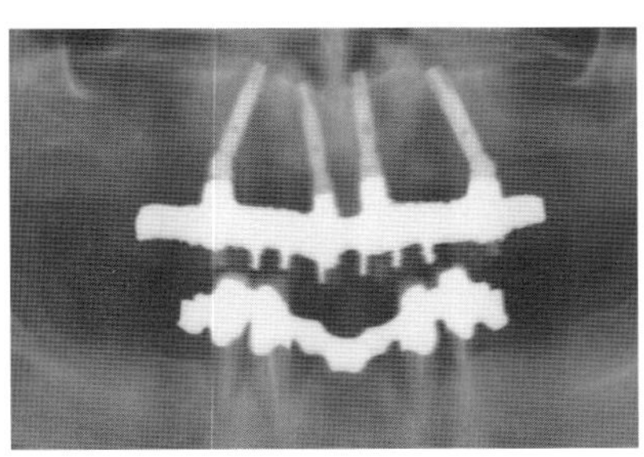

Postoperative panoramic radiograph at 36 months

Patient VIII

Age	77 years
General health	Diabetes mellitus type 1
Smoking habit	No
Cause of tooth loss	Generalized severe periodontitis
Bone quality	Type 2
Type of implants	Conical 4 × 15–mm NanoTite (sites 15, 23, 26)
	Cylindric 4 × 15–mm NanoTite (site 13)
Type of conical abutments	17 degrees (sites 13, 23)
	25 degrees (sites 16, 26)

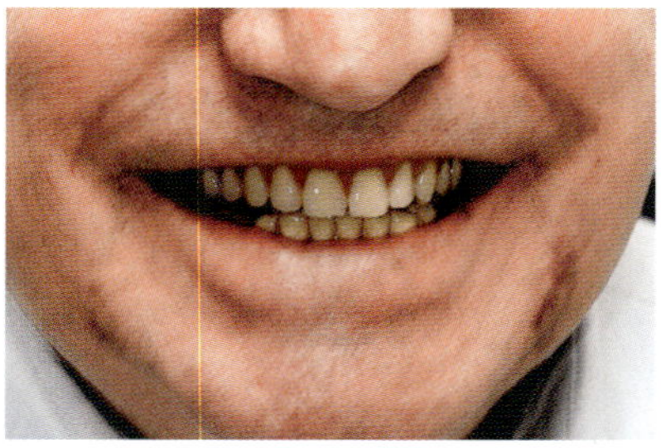

Frontal view with maxillary full denture

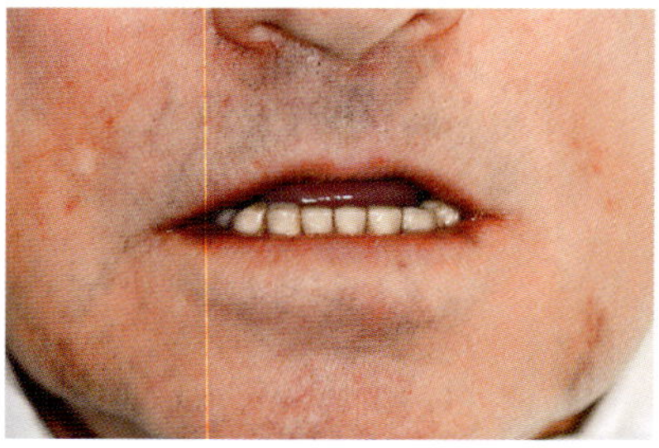

Frontal view 24 hours postsurgery

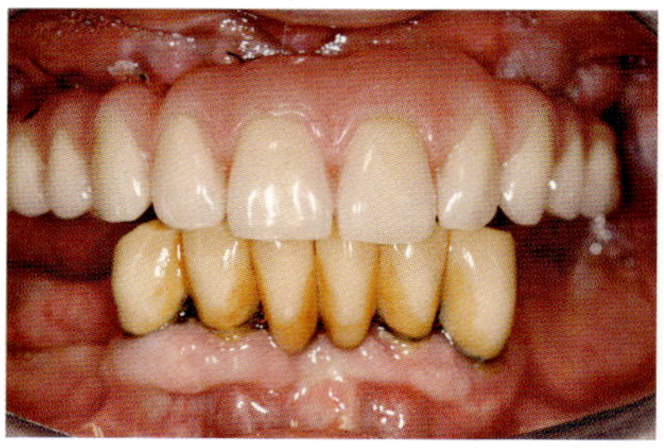

Frontal view with immediate provisional FFP in place and patient in centric occlusion

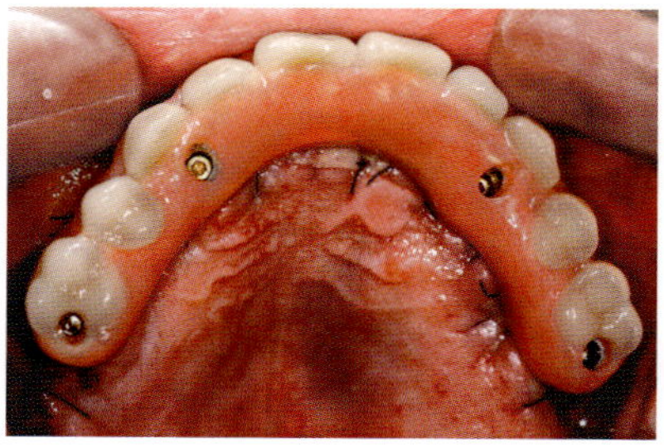

Occlusal view with immediate provisional FFP in place

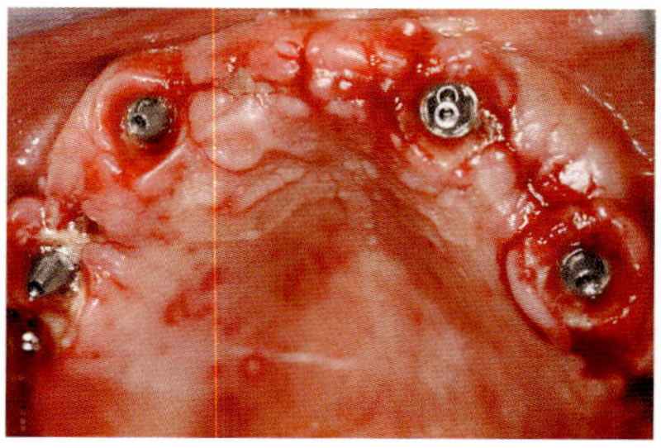

Occlusal view of edentulous maxilla and abutments at the suture removal appointment

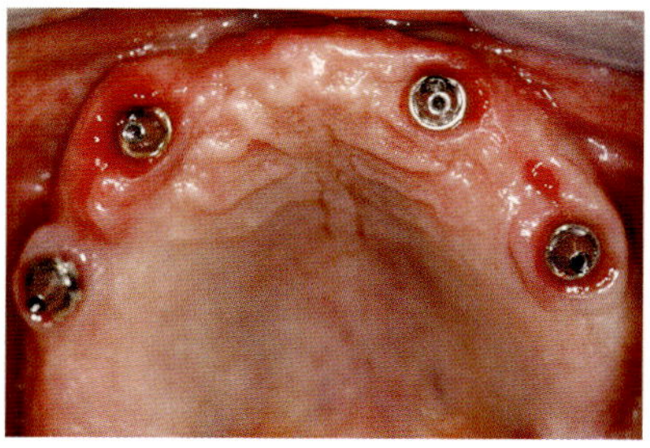

Occlusal view of edentulous maxilla and abutments prior to insertion of the definitive FFP

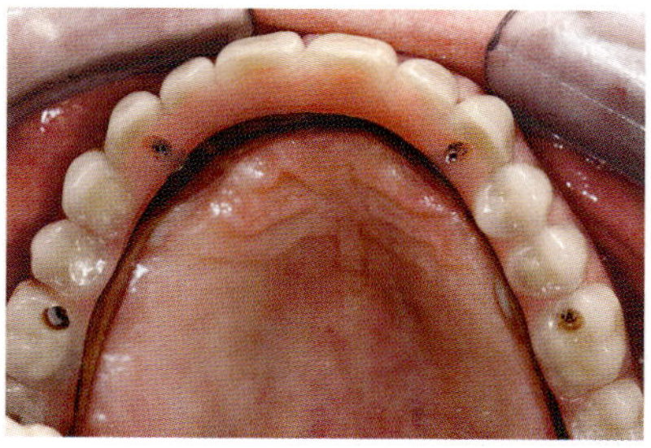

Occlusal view of definitive FFP in place

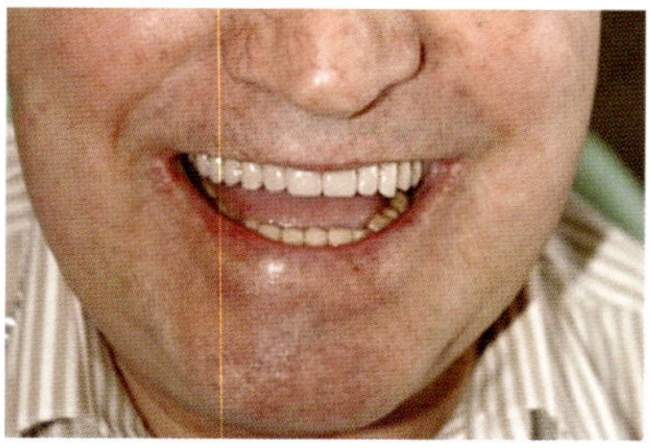

Smile with definitive FFP in place

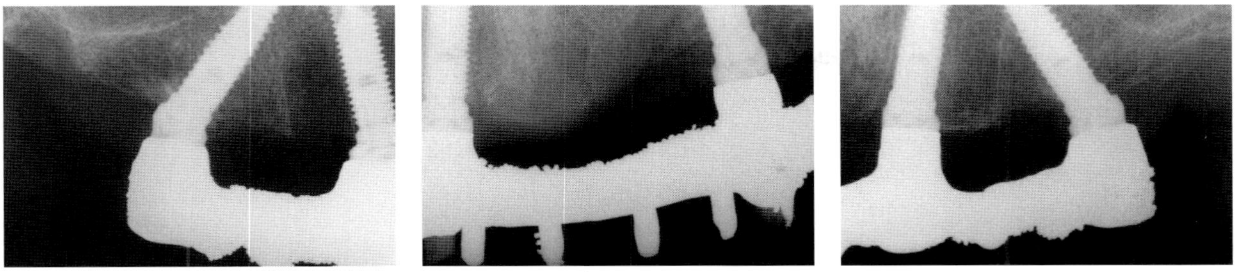

Intraoral radiographs at time 0

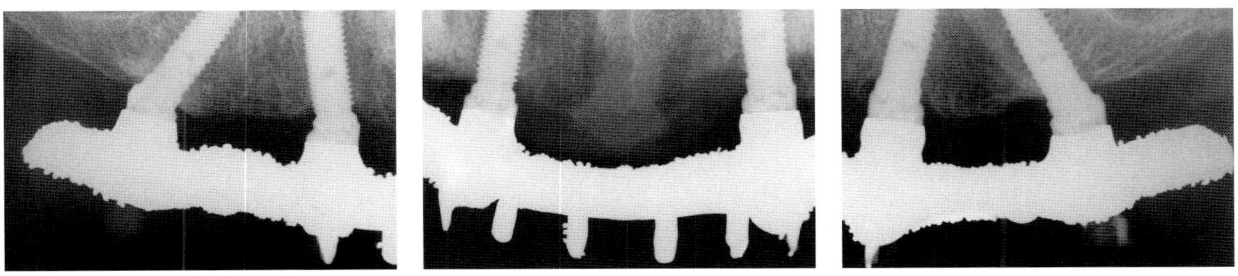

Postoperative intraoral radiographs at 12 months

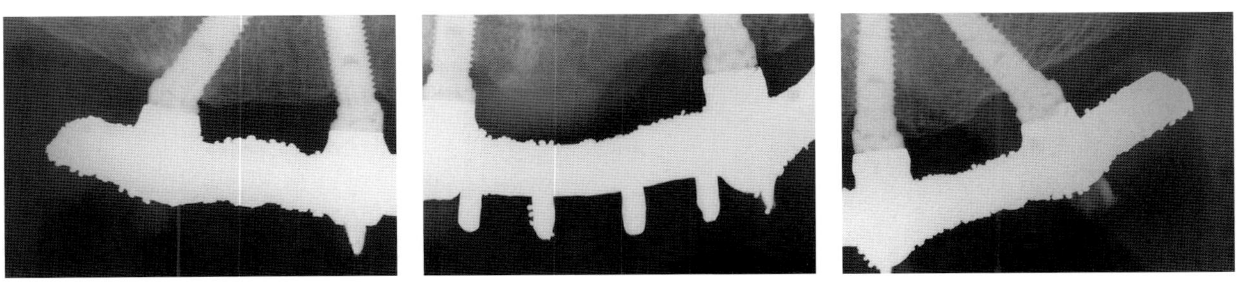

Postoperative intraoral radiographs at 24 months

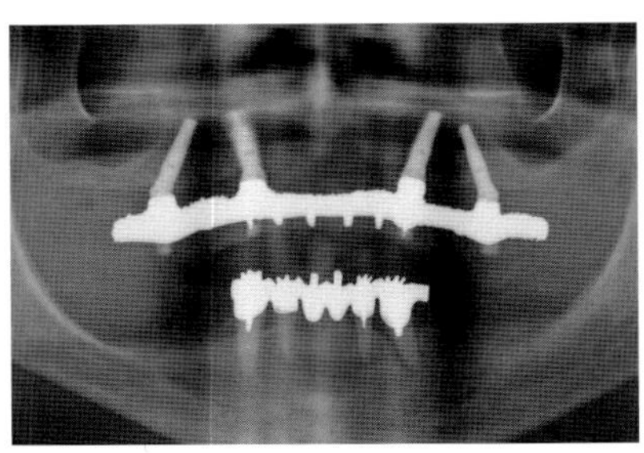

Postoperative panoramic radiograph at 24 months

Patient IX

Age	42 years
General health	Good
Smoking habit	No
Cause of tooth loss	Dental caries
Bone quality	Type 1
Type of implants	Cylindric 4 × 15–mm Full Osseotite (sites 12, 15, 22, 25)
Type of conical abutments	25 degrees (sites 12, 15, 22, 25)

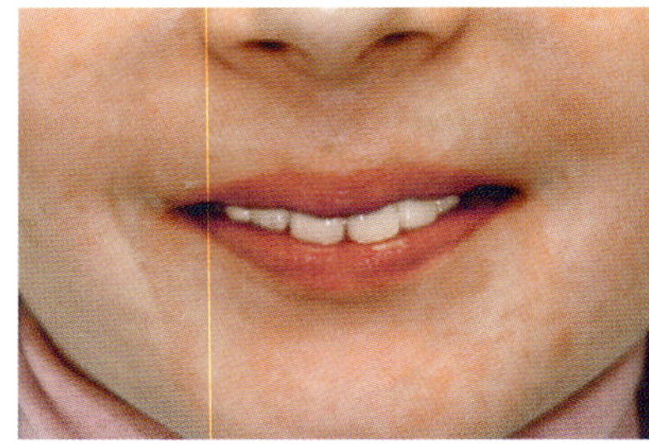

Preoperative smile

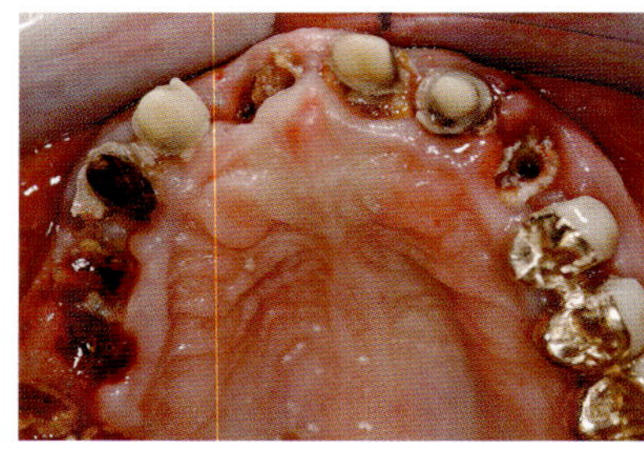

Preoperative occlusal view after removal of defective fixed partial dentures

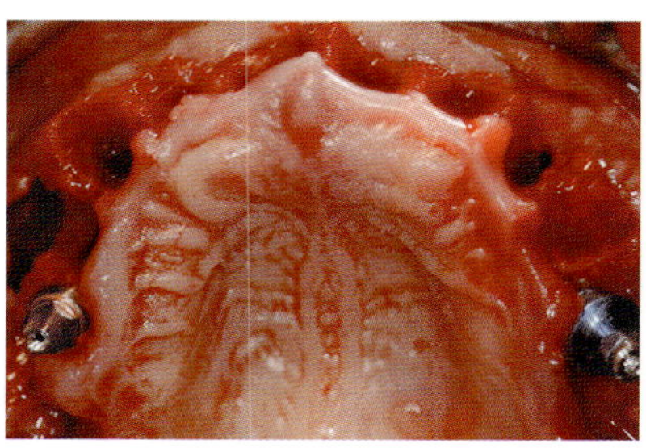

Occlusal view after tooth extractions with posterior implants in place

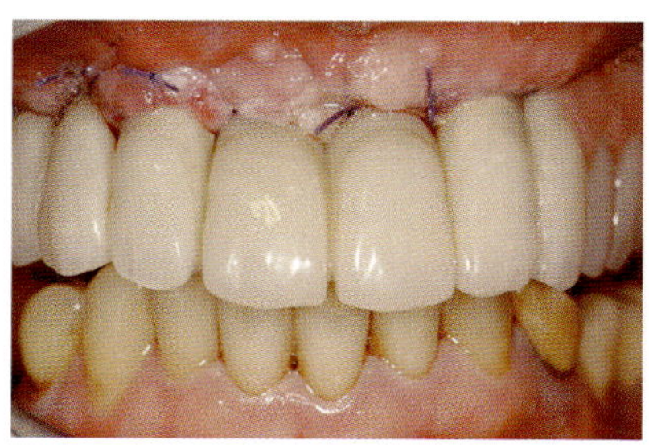

Frontal view with immediate provisional FFP in place

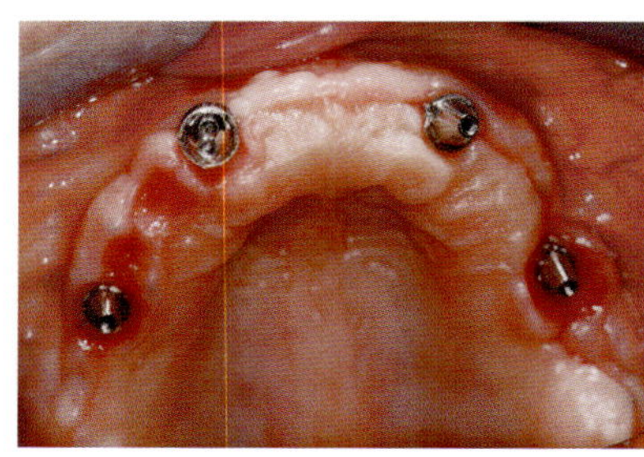

Occlusal view of edentulous maxilla and abutments

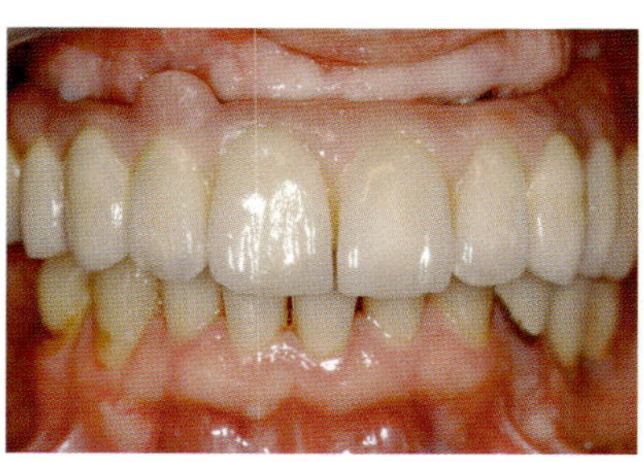

Frontal view of definitive FFP in place

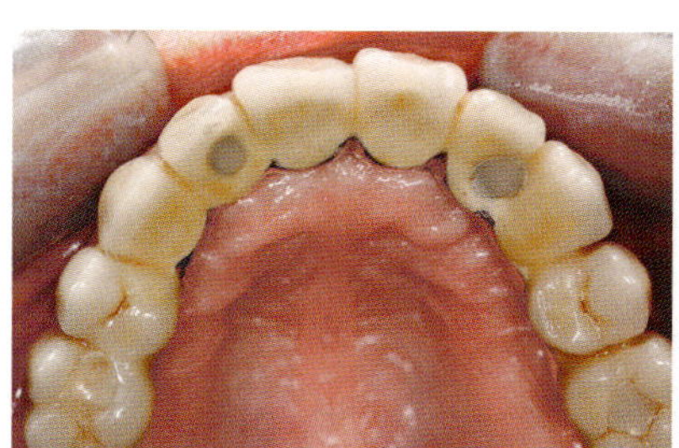

Occlusal view of definitive FFP in place

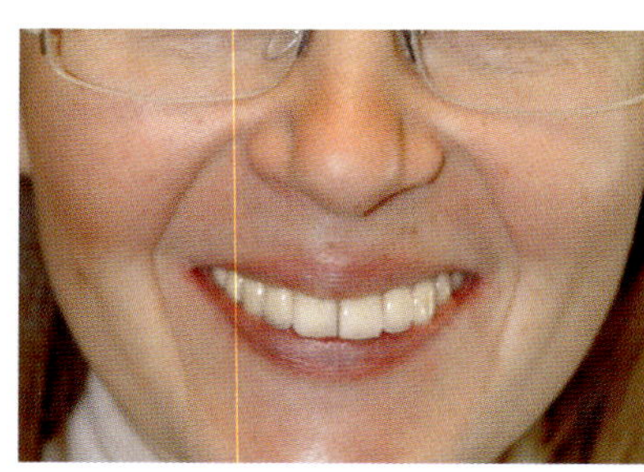

Smile with definitive FFP in place

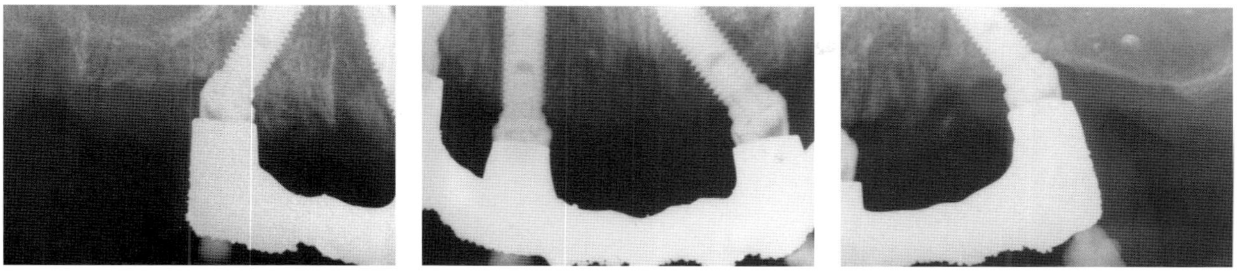

Intraoral radiographs at time 0

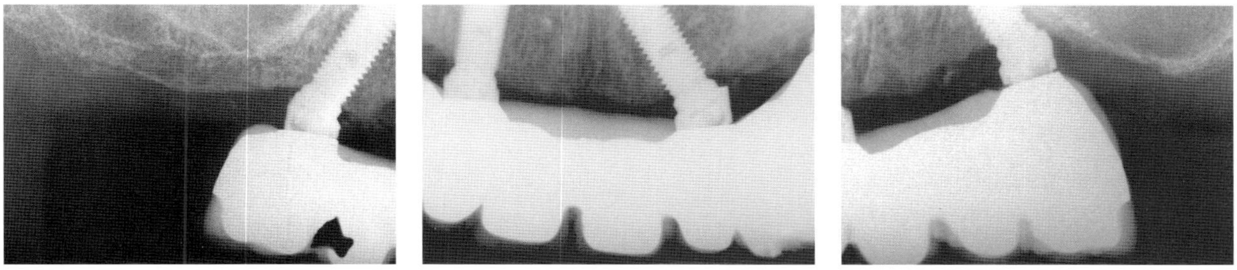

Postoperative intraoral radiographs at 12 months

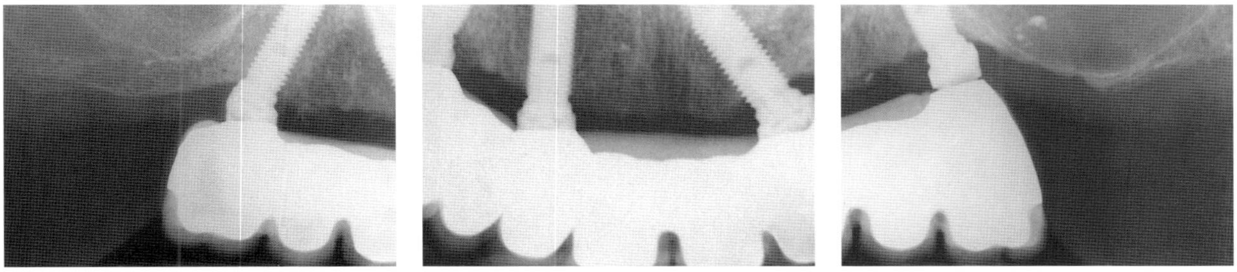

Postoperative intraoral radiographs at 24 months

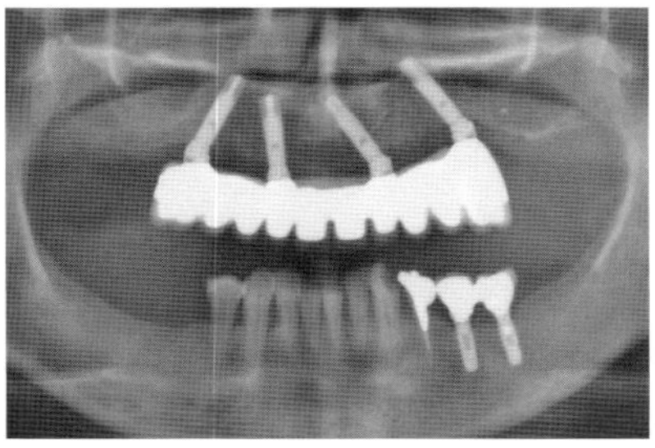

Postoperative panoramic radiograph at 36 months

Patient X

Age	56 years
General health	Good
Smoking habit	Yes
Cause of tooth loss	Endodontic failures
Bone quality	Type 3
Type of implants	Cylindric 4 × 19–mm Osseotite (sites 13, 23)
	Conical 4 × 15–mm Full Osseotite NT (sites 15, 25)
Type of conical abutments	17 degrees (sites 13, 23)
	25 degrees (sites 15, 25)

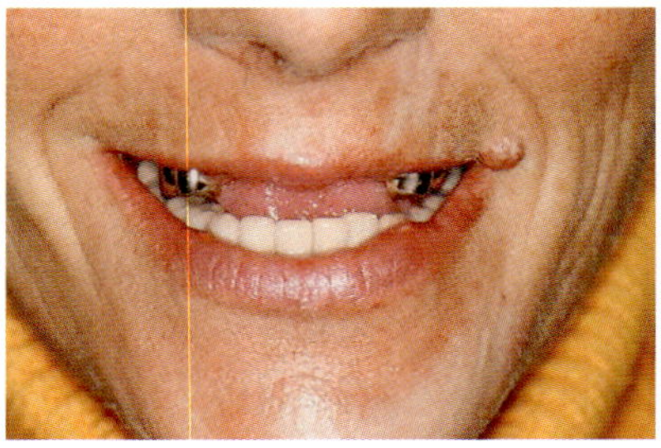

Preoperative smile

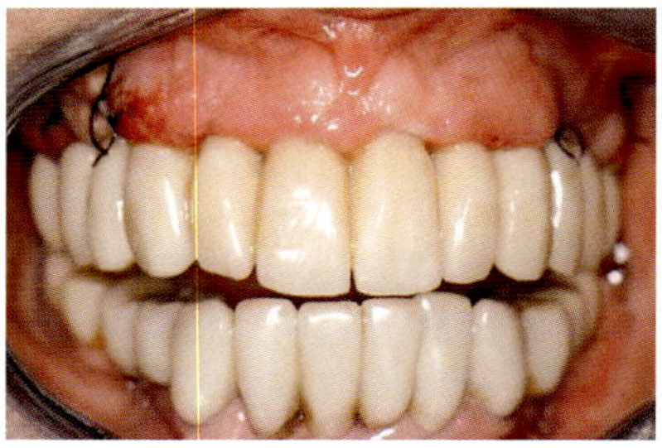

Frontal view with immediate provisional FFP in place

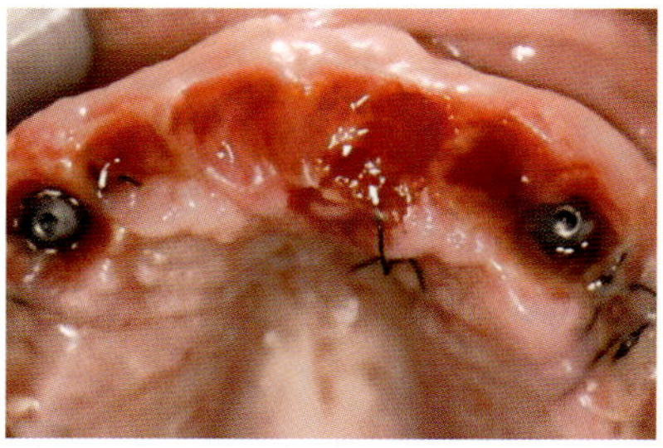

Occlusal view at the suture removal appointment

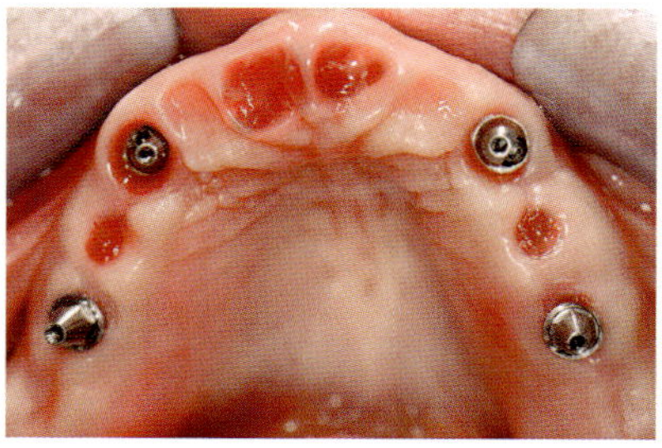

Occlusal view of soft tissue healing

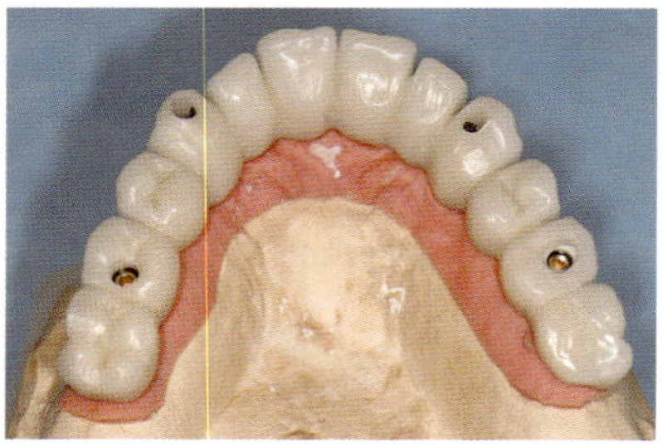

Occlusal view of definitive FFP on the master cast

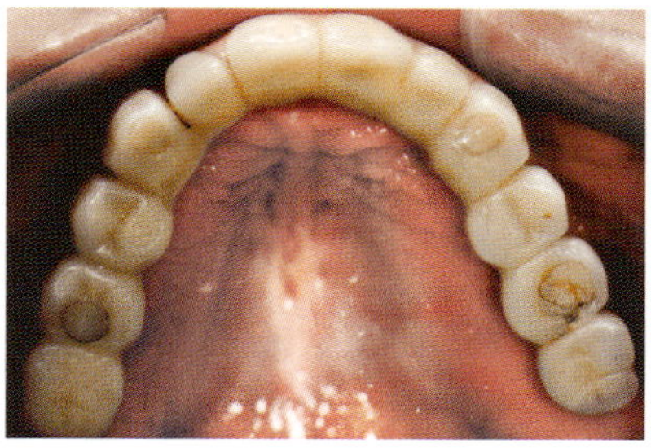

Occlusal image of definitive FFP in place

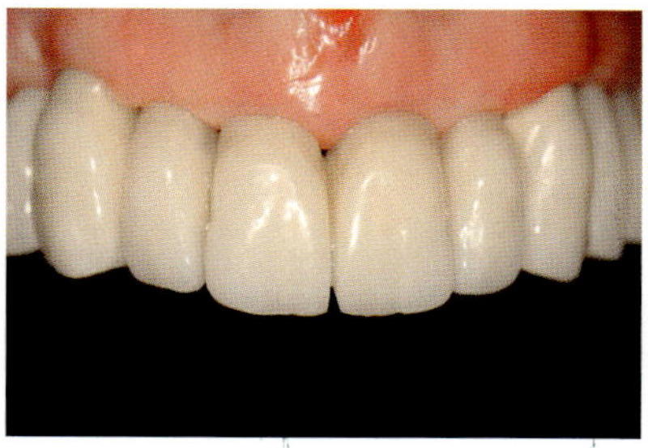

Frontal view of definitive FFP in place

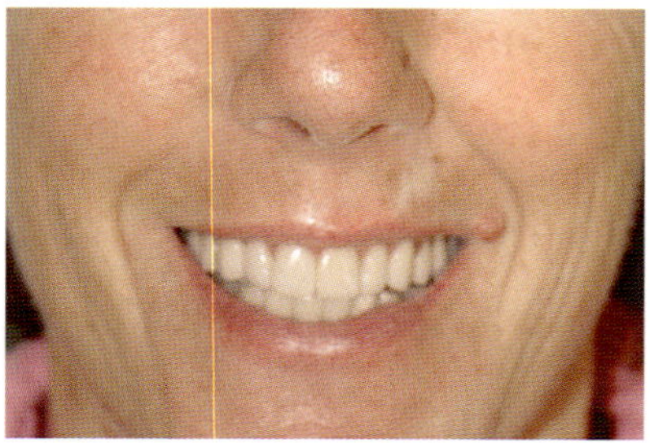

Smile with definitive FFP in place

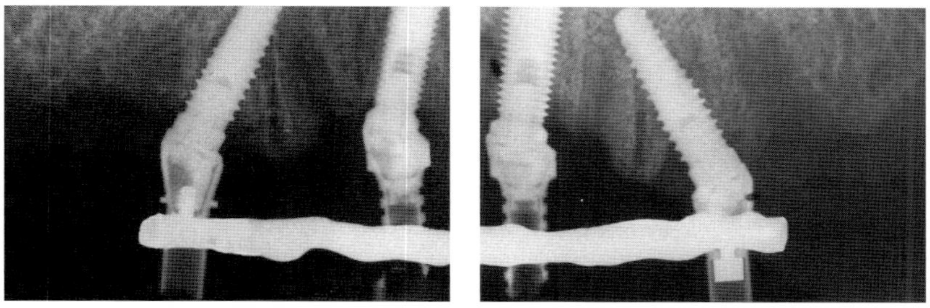

Intraoral radiographs at time 0

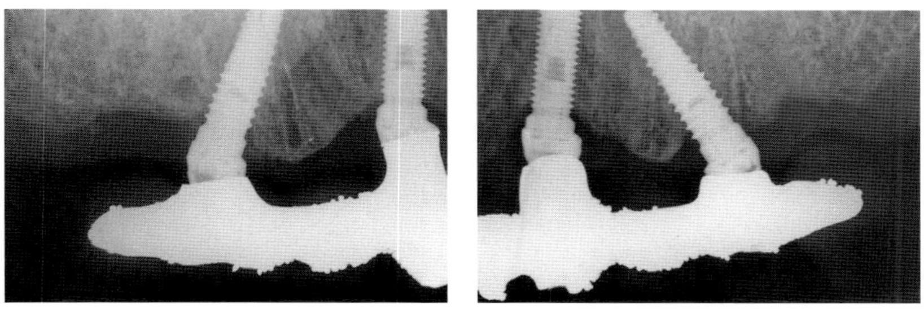

Postoperative intraoral radiographs at 12 months

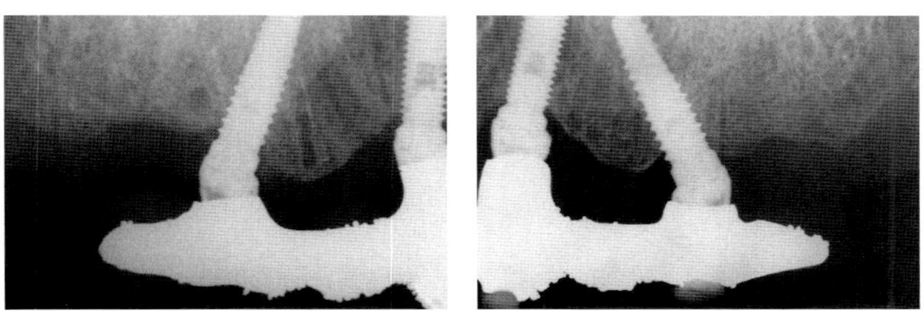

Postoperative intraoral radiographs at 24 months

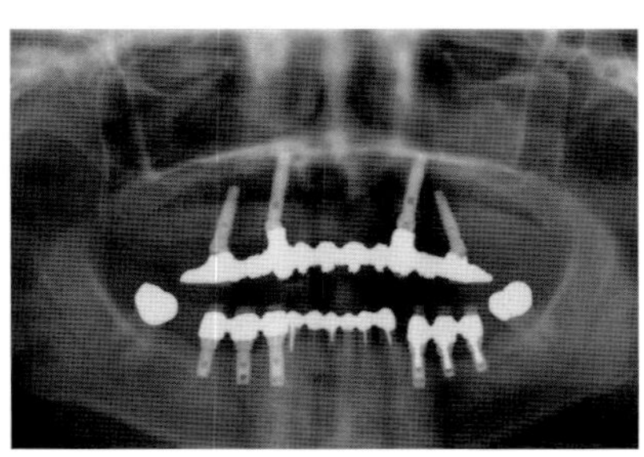

Postoperative panoramic radiograph at 36 months

Patient XI

Age	56 years
General health	Good
Smoking habit	Yes
Cause of tooth loss	Dental caries
Bone quality	Type 2
Type of implants	Cylindric 4 × 18–mm NanoTite (sites 14, 25)
	Cylindric 4 × 15–mm NanoTite (sites 11, 22)
Type of conical abutments	17 degrees (sites 11, 22)
	25 degrees (sites 14, 25)

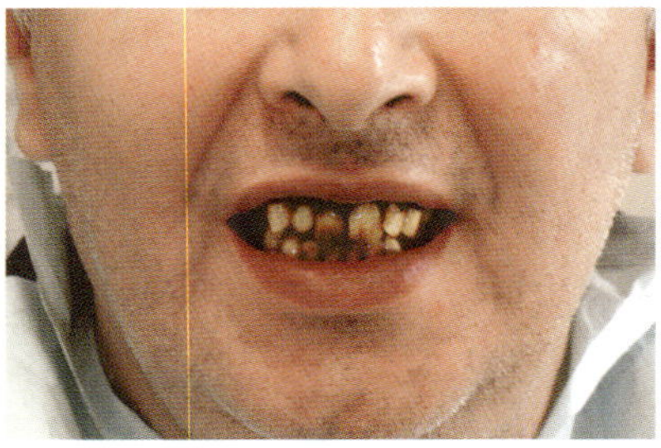

Preoperative smile

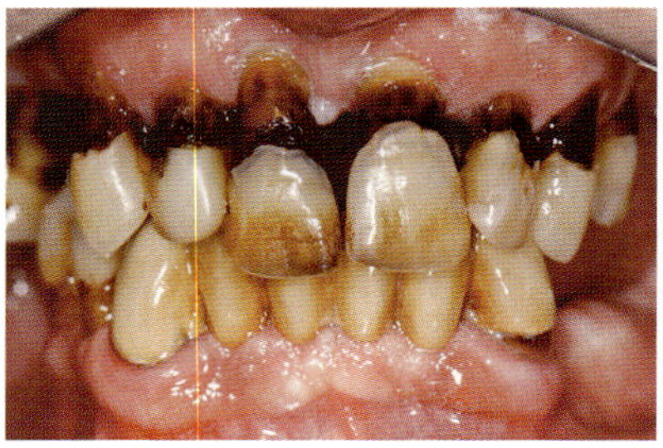

Preoperative view
with the patient in centric occlusion

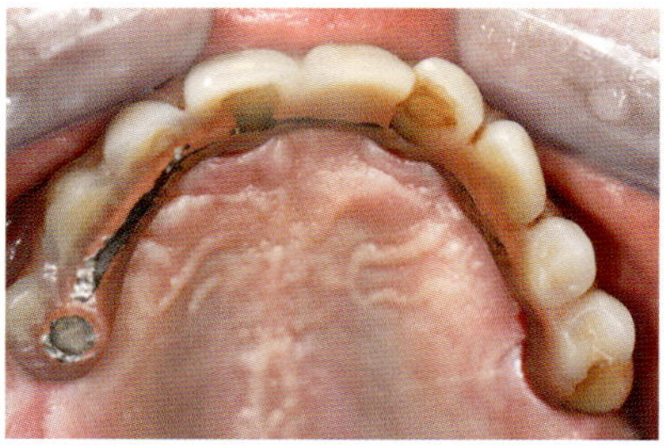

Occlusal view of immediate provisional FFP in place

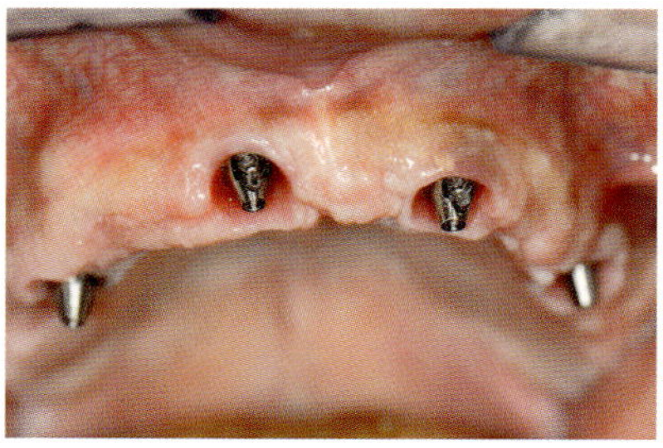

Frontal view of edentulous maxilla and abutments

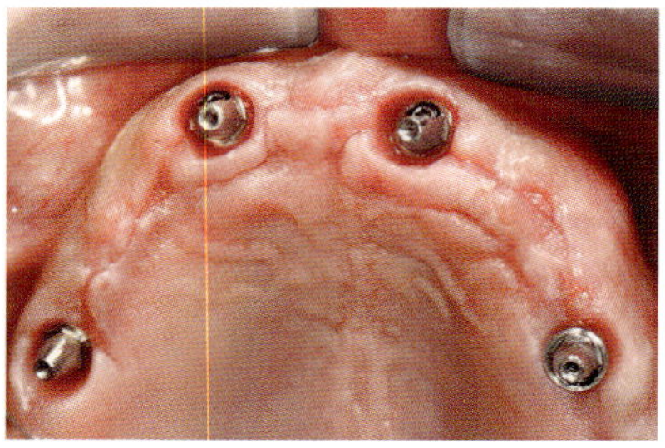

Occlusal view of edentulous maxilla and abutments

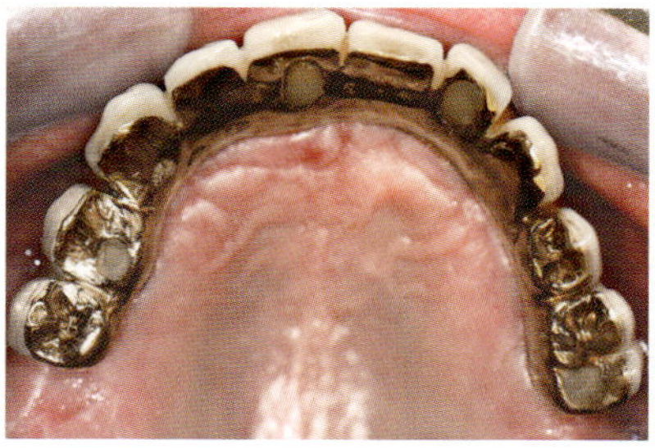

Occlusal view of definitive FFP in place

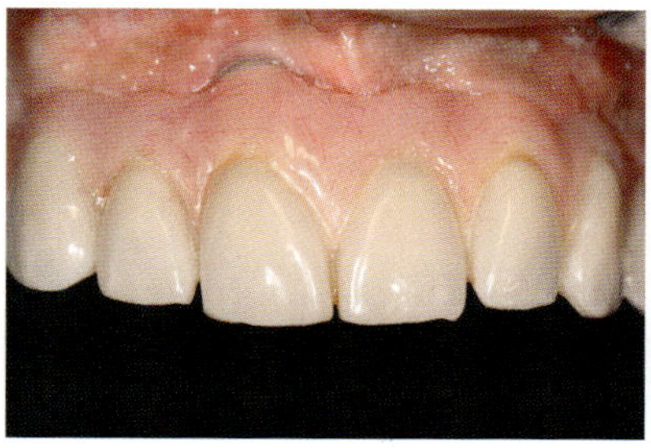

Frontal view of definitive FFP in place

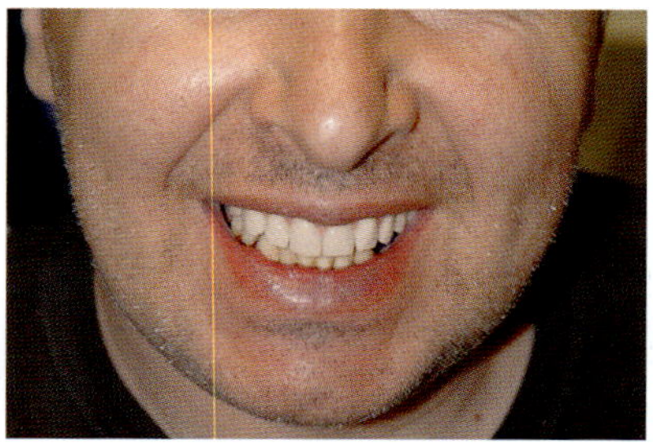

Smile with definitive FFP in place

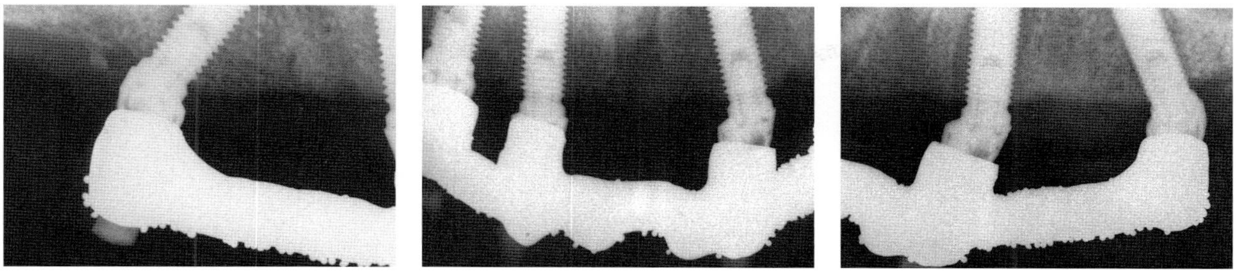

Intraoral radiographs at time 0

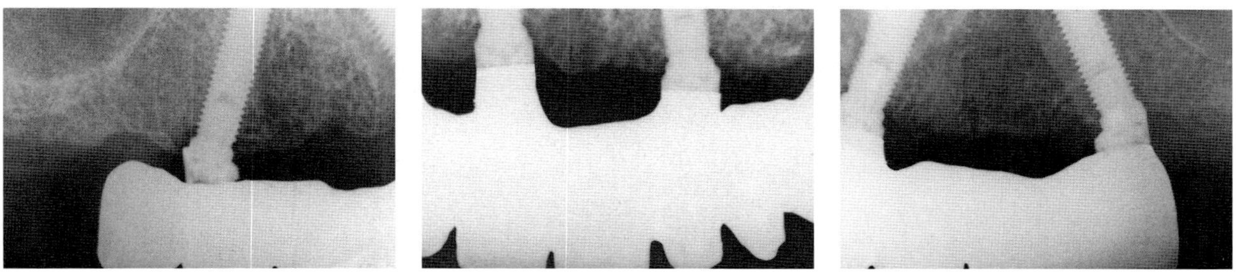

Postoperative intraoral radiographs at 12 months

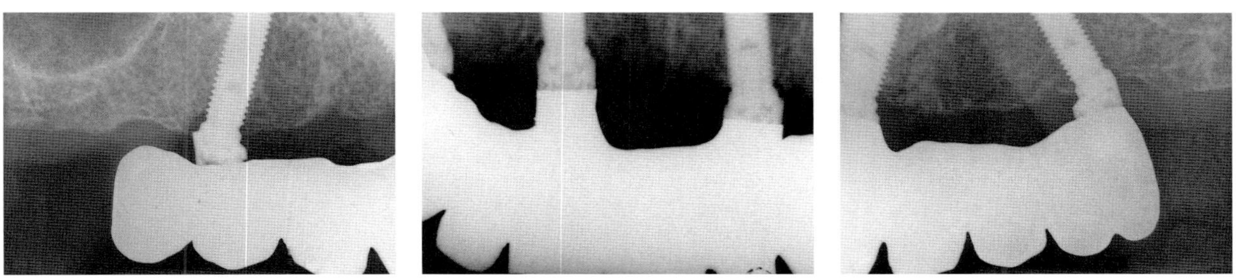

Postoperative intraoral radiographs at 24 months

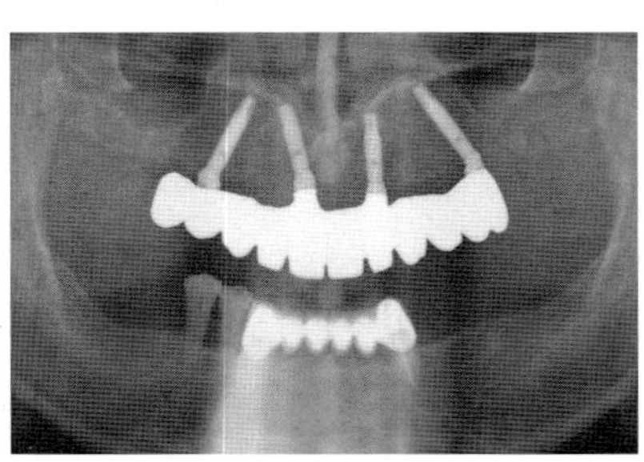

Postoperative panoramic radiograph at 24 months

Patient XII

Age	51 years
General health	Depression
Smoking habit	No
Cause of tooth loss	Dental caries
Bone quality	Type 2
Type of implants	Conical 4 × 15–mm NanoTite (sites 11, 21)
	Cylindric 4 × 18–mm NanoTite (sites 14, 25)
Type of conical abutments	25 degrees (sites 11, 14, 21, 25)

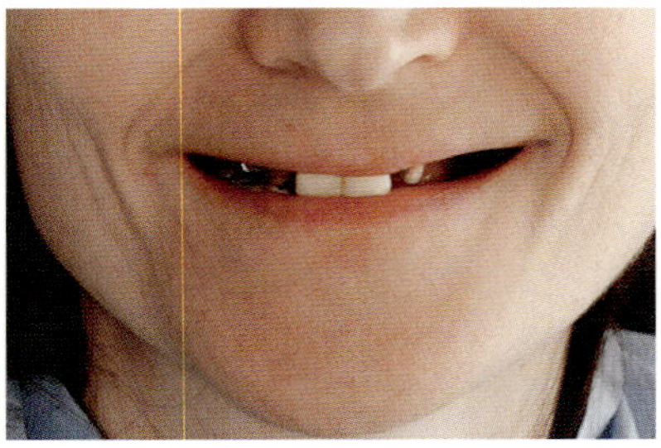

Preoperative smile

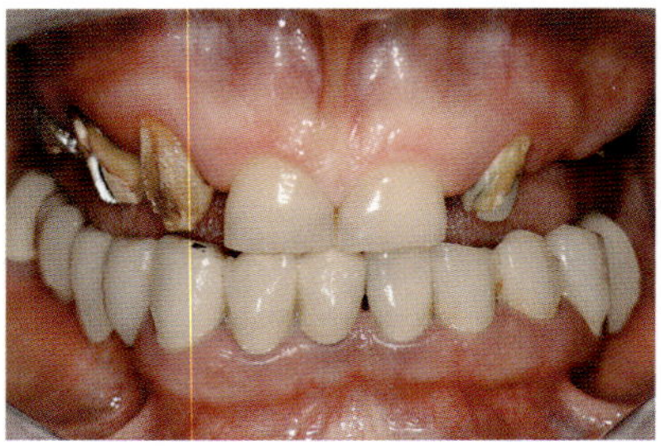

Preoperative frontal view with the patient in centric occlusion

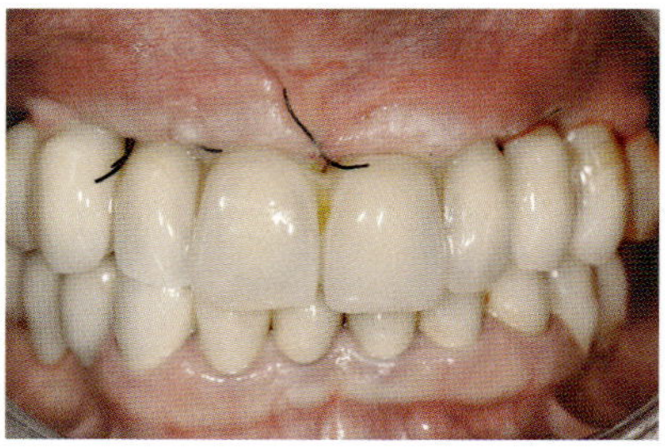

Frontal view with immediate provisional FFP in place

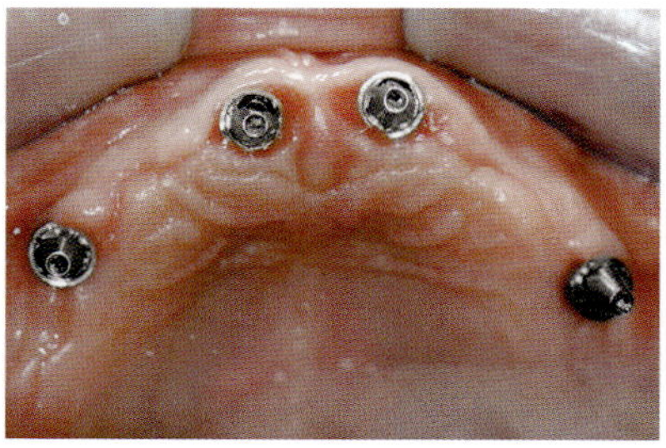

Occlusal view of edentulous maxilla and abutments, 4 months postsurgery

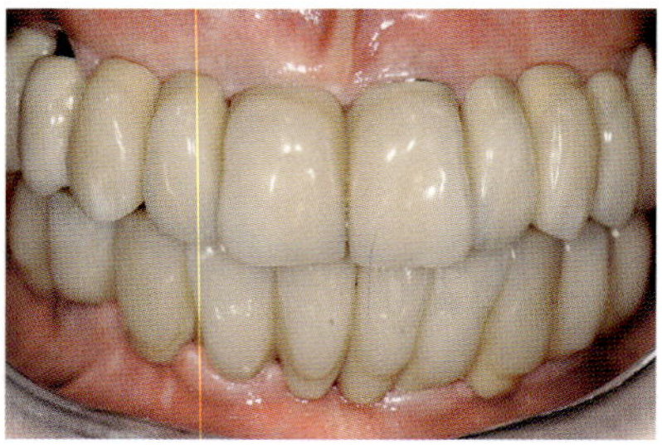

Frontal view with definitive FFPs in place and patient in centric occlusion

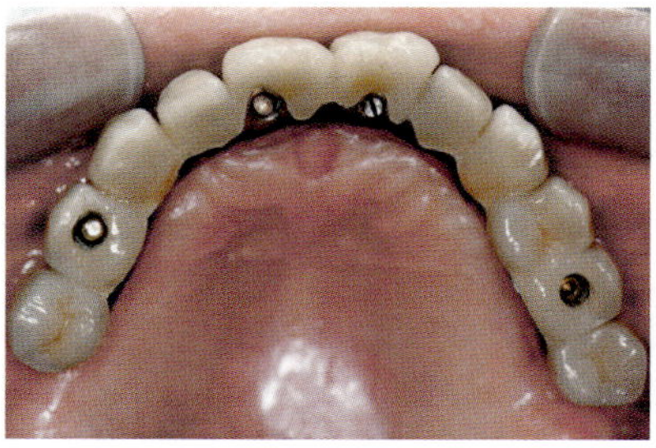

Occlusal view with definitive FFP in place

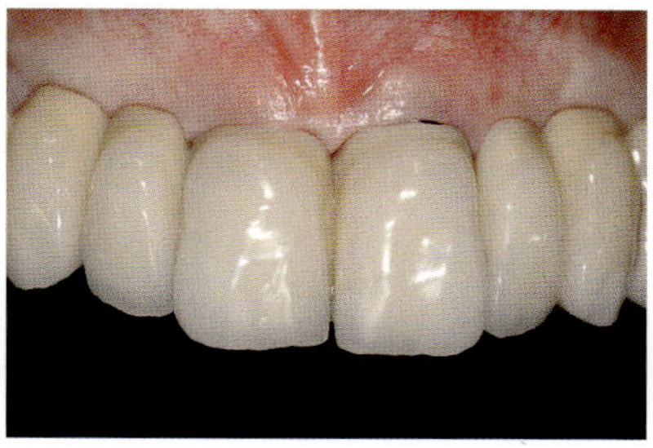

Frontal view with definitive FFP in place

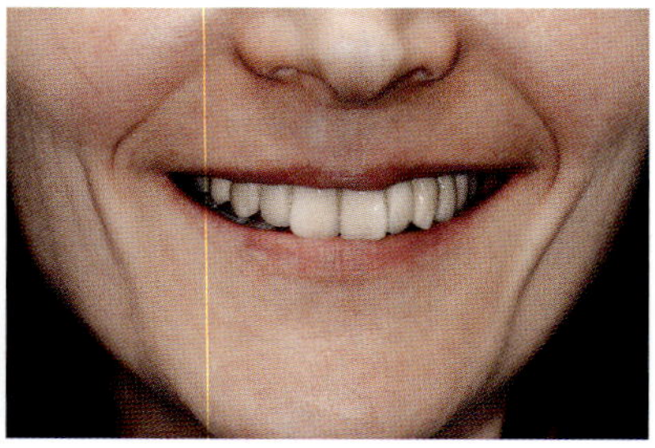

Smile with definitive FFPs in place

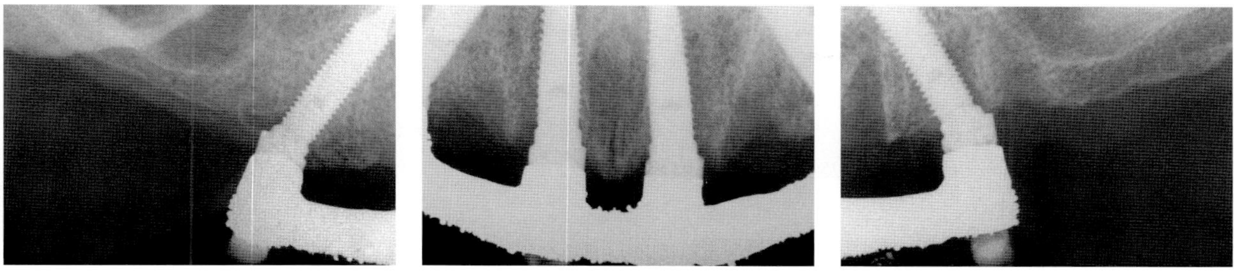

Intraoral radiographs at time 0

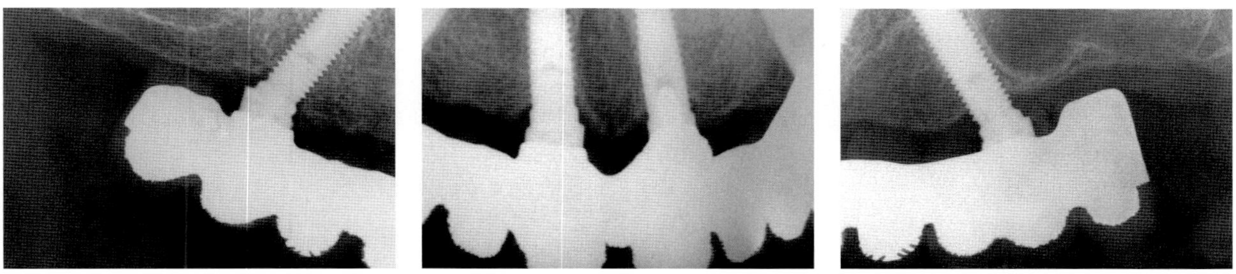

Postoperative intraoral radiographs at 12 months

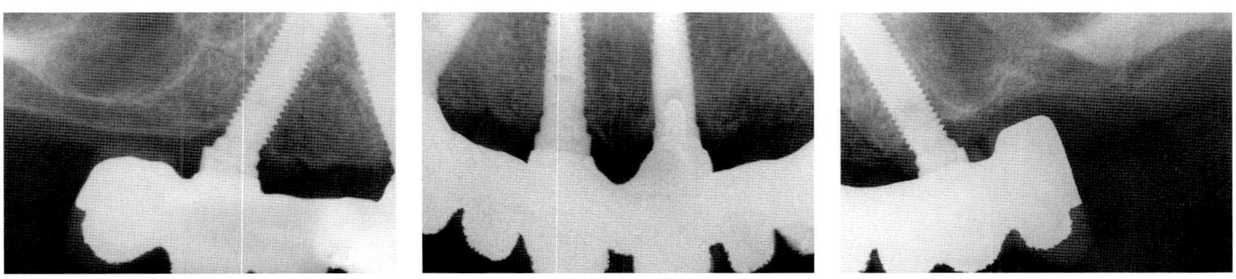

Postoperative intraoral radiographs at 24 months

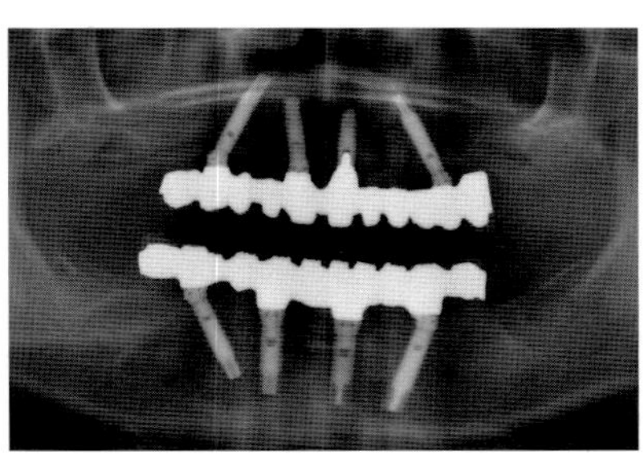

Postoperative panoramic radiograph at 24 months

REFERENCES

1. Chiapasco M, Gatti C. Implant-retained mandibular overdentures with immediate loading: A 3- to 8-year prospective study on 328 implants. Clin Implant Dent Relat Res 2003;5:29–38.
2. Alfadda SA, Attard NJ, David LA. Five-year clinical results of immediately loaded dental implants using mandibular overdentures. Int J Prosthodont 2009;22:368–373.
3. Schnitman PA, Wohrle PS, Rubenstein JE. Immediate fixed interim prostheses supported by two-stage threaded implants: Methodology and results. J Oral Implantol 1990;16:96–105.
4. Ericsson I, Randow K, Nilner K, Peterson A. Early functional loading of Brånemark dental implants: 5-year clinical follow-up study. Clin Implant Dent Relat Res 2000;2:70–77.
5. Engstrand P, Gröndahl K, Ohrnell LO, Nilsson P, Nannmark U, Brånemark PI. Prospective follow-up study of 95 patients with edentulous mandibles treated according to the Brånemark Novum concept. Clin Implant Dent Relat Res 2003;5:3–10.
6. Testori T, Meltzer A, Del Fabbro M, et al. Immediate occlusal loading of Osseotite implants in the lower edentulous jaw. A multicenter prospective study. Clin Oral Implants Res 2004;15:278–284.
7. Engquist B, Astrand P, Anzén B, et al. Simplified methods of implant treatment in the edentulous lower jaw: A 3-year follow-up report of a controlled prospective study of one-stage versus two-stage surgery and early loading. Clin Implant Dent Relat Res 2005;7:95–104.
8. Brånemark PI, Hansson BO, Adell R, et al. Osseointegrated implants in the treatment of the edentulous jaw. Experience from a 10-year period. Scand J Plast Reconstr Surg Suppl 1977;16:1–132.
9. Adell R, Lekholm U, Rockler B, Brånemark PI. A 15-year study of osseointegrated implants in the treatment of the edentulous jaw. Int J Oral Surg 1981;10:387–416.
10. Brånemark PI, Svensson B, van Steenberghe D. Ten-year survival rates of fixed prostheses on four or six implants ad modum Brånemark in full edentulism. Clin Oral Implants Res 1995;6:227–231.
11. Tarnow DP, Emtiaz S, Classi A. Immediate loading of threaded implants at stage 1 surgery in edentulous arches: Ten consecutive case reports with 1- to 5-year data. Int J Oral Maxillofac Implants 1997;12:319–324.
12. Ibañez JC, Tahhan MJ, Zamar JA, et al. Immediate occlusal loading of double acid-etched surface titanium implants in 41 consecutive full-arch cases in the mandible and maxilla: 6- to 74-month results. J Periodontol 2005;76:1972–1981.
13. Fischer K, Stenberg T, Hedin M, Sennerby L. Five-year results from a randomized, controlled trial on early and delayed loading of implants supporting full-arch prosthesis in the edentulous maxilla. Clin Oral Implants Res 2008;19:433–441.
14. Attard NJ, Zarb GA. Immediate and early implant loading protocols: A literature review of clinical studies. J Prosthet Dent 2005;94:242–258.
15. Sharan A, Madjar D. Maxillary sinus pneumatization following extractions: A radiographic study. Int J Oral Maxillofac Implants 2008;23:48–56.
16. Lioubavina-Hack N, Lang NP, Karring T. Significance of primary stability for osseointegration of dental implants. Clin Oral Implants Res 2006; 17:244–250.
17. Friberg B, Jemt T, Lekholm U. Early failures in 4641 consecutively placed Brånemark dental implants. A study from stage I surgery to the connection of completed prostheses. Int J Oral Maxillofac Implants 1991;6:142–146.
18. Adriaenssens P, Hermans M. Immediate implant function in the anterior maxilla: A surgical technique to enhance primary stability for Brånemark MKIII and MKIV implants. A randomized, prospective clinical study at the 1-year follow-up. Appl Osseointegration Res 2001;2:17–21.

19. Maniatopoulos C, Pilliar RM, Smith DC. Threaded versus porous-surfaced designs for implant stabilization in bone-endodontic implant model. J Biomed Mater Res 1986;20:1309–1333.
20. Skalak R. Biomechanical considerations in osseointegrated prostheses. J Prosthet Dent 1983;49: 843–848.
21. Balshi SF, Wolfinger GJ, Balshi TJ. A prospective study of immediate functional loading, following the Teeth in a Day protocol: A case series of 55 consecutive edentulous maxillas. Clin Implant Dent Relat Res 2005;7:24–31.
22. van Steenberghe D, Glauser R, Blombäck U, et al. A computed tomographic scan-derived customized surgical template and fixed prosthesis for flapless surgery and immediate loading of implants in fully edentulous maxillae: A prospective multicenter study. Clin Implant Dent Relat Res 2005;7(suppl 1):111S–120S.
23. Maló P, Nobre Mde A, Petersson U, Wigren S. A pilot study of complete edentulous rehabilitation with immediate function using a new implant design: Case series. Clin Implant Dent Relat Res 2006;8:223–232.
24. Duarte LR, Filho HN, Francischone CE, Peredo LG, Brånemark PI. The establishment of a protocol for the total rehabilitation of atrophic maxillae employing four zygomatic fixtures in an immediate loading system: A 30-month clinical and radiographic follow-up. Clin Implant Dent Relat Res 2007;9:186–196.
25. Ostman PO, Hellman M, Sennerby L,Wennerberg A. Temporary implant-supported prosthesis for immediate loading according to a chair-side concept: Technical note and results from 37 consecutive cases. Clin Implant Dent Relat Res 2008; 10:71–77.
26. Del Fabbro M, Testori T, Francetti L, Taschieri S, Weinstein R. Systematic review of survival rates for immediately loaded dental implants. Int J Periodontics Restorative Dent 2006;26:249–263.
27. Tealdo T, Bevilacqua M, Pera F, et al. Immediate function with fixed implant-supported maxillary dentures: A 12-month pilot study. J Prosthet Dent 2008;99:351–360.
28. Tealdo T, Bevilacqua M, Menini M, et al. Immediate versus delayed loading of dental implants in edentulous maxillae: A 36-month prospective study. Int J Prosthodont 2011;24:294–302.
29. Bergkvist G, Sahlholm S, Nilner K, Lindh C. Implant-supported fixed prostheses in the edentulous maxilla. A 2-year clinical and radiological follow-up of treatment with non-submerged ITI implants. Clin Oral Implants Res 2004;15:351–359.
30. Maló P, Rangert B, Nobre M. All-on-4 immediate-function concept with Brånemark System implants for completely edentulous maxillae: A 1-year retrospective clinical study. Clin Implant Dent Relat Res 2005;7(suppl 1):88S–94S.
31. Bergkvist G, Nilner K, Sahlholm S, Karlsson U, Lindh C. Immediate loading of implants in the edentulous maxilla: Use of an interim fixed prosthesis followed by a permanent fixed prosthesis: A 32-month prospective radiological and clinical study. Clin Implant Dent Relat Res 2009;11:1–10.
32. Calandriello R, Tomatis M. Simplified treatment of the atrophic posterior maxilla via immediate/early function and tilted implants: A prospective 1-year clinical study. Clin Implant Dent Relat Res 2005;7(suppl 1):1S–12S.
33. Testori T, Del Fabbro M, Capelli M, Zuffetti F, Francetti L, Weinstein RL. Immediate occlusal loading and tilted implants for the rehabilitation of the atrophic edentulous maxilla: 1-year interim results of a multicenter prospective study. Clin Oral Implants Res 2008;19:227–232.
34. Ha CY, Lim YJ, Kim MJ, Choi JH. The influence of abutment angulation on screw loosening of implants in the anterior maxilla. Int J Oral Maxillofac Implants 2011;26:45–55.

35. Klokkevold PR, Han TJ. How do smoking, diabetes, and periodontitis affect outcomes of implant treatment? Int J Oral Maxillofac Implants 2007; 22(suppl):173–202.
36. Horning GM, Cohen ME. Necrotizing ulcerative gingivitis, periodontitis, and stomatitis: Clinical staging and predisposing factors. J Periodontol 1995;66:990–998.
37. Grunder U. Immediate functional loading of immediate implants in edentulous arches: Two-year results. Int J Periodontics Restorative Dent 2001;21:545–551.
38. Maló P, Rangert B, Nobre M. "All-on-Four" immediate-function concept with Brånemark System implants for completely edentulous mandibles: A retrospective clinical study. Clin Implant Dent Relat Res 2003;5(suppl 1):2–9.
39. Wood MR, Vermilyea SG, Committee on Research in Fixed Prosthodontics of the Academy of Fixed Prosthodontics. A review of selected dental literature on evidence-based treatment planning for dental implants: Report of the Committee on Research in Fixed Prosthodontics of the Academy of Fixed Prosthodontics. J Prosthet Dent 2004;92:447–462.
40. Sahin S, Cehreli MC, Yalçin E. The influence of functional forces on the biomechanics of implant-supported prostheses–A review. J Dent 2002;30: 271–282.
41. Taylor TD, Wiens J, Carr A. Evidence-based considerations for removable prosthodontic and dental implant occlusion: A literature review. J Prosthet Dent 2005;94:555–560.
42. Ciftçi Y, Canay S. Stress distribution on the metal framework of the implant-supported fixed prosthesis using different veneering materials. Int J Prosthodont 2001;14:406–411.
43. Juodzbalys G, Kubilius R, Eidukynas V, Raustia AM. Stress distribution in bone: Single-unit implant prostheses veneered with porcelain or a new composite material. Implant Dent 2005; 14:166–175.
44. Conserva E, Menini M, Tealdo T, et al. Robotic chewing simulator for dental materials testing on a sensor-equipped implant setup. Int J Prosthodont 2008;21:501–508.
45. Conserva E, Menini M, Tealdo T, et al. The use of a masticatory robot to analyze the shock absorption capacity of different restorative materials for prosthetic implants: A preliminary report. Int J Prosthodont 2009;22:53–55.

CHAPTER 14
COMPLICATIONS AND THEIR MANAGEMENT

This chapter identifies complications that could arise between the surgical phase and delivery of the definitive fixed prosthesis. Clinical problems associated with the traditional delayed loading implant surgical protocol are not discussed since they have been identified previously by numerous authors.[1–5] Implant prosthetic treatment per the Columbus Bridge Protocol provides clinicians with guidelines for fabricating provisional full-arch prostheses within 24 to 48 hours of implant placement and provides solutions for complications that may arise during treatment. A benefit of the Columbus Bridge Protocol is that it enables patients to function with fixed prostheses even in the event that one implant fails to integrate.

Complications can be divided into two groups based on the time that they occur (Table 14.1): Immediate complications[6] occur during the immediate surgical-prosthetic appointments. Late complications occur between insertion of the provisional prosthesis and insertion of the definitive prosthesis approximately 4 months later.

Complications that arise after insertion of the definitive full-arch prosthesis are not described in this chapter. The authors believe that these complications, better classified as middle- or long-term complications, are similar to those associated with traditional delayed-loading protocols, which have already been amply covered in the literature.

Immediate and late complications can be further subdivided into biologic and mechanical complications.[7–10] Biologic complications are associated with problems in the soft and hard tissues. Management of complications as described in this chapter is the result of the clinical evaluation discussed in chapter 13.

TABLE 14.1		
	1 - IMMEDIATE COMPLICATIONS	**2 - LATE COMPLICATIONS**
BIOLOGIC COMPLICATIONS OF THE PERI-IMPLANT SOFT TISSUES	1.1 Excessive pressure between soft tissues (mucosa) and the full-arch prosthesis	2.1 Exposure of the abutment collar secondary to peri-implant soft tissue recession
BIOLOGIC COMPLICATIONS OF HARD TISSUES	1.2 Failure to obtain sufficient primary implant stability 1.3 Fracture of vestibular cortical bone during implant placement 1.4 Excessive subcrestal implant placement	2.2 Failure to obtain osseointegration
MECHANICAL COMPLICATIONS	1.5 Stripping of external hexagon implant restorative platform 1.6 Incorrect abutment positioning 1.7 Incorrect impression coping positioning 1.8 Mobility of pick up impression coping in the impression 1.9 Difficult provisional full-arch prosthesis insertion due to nonparallel abutments 1.10 Difficult to mask access openings to retaining screws	2.3 Stripping of abutment screws or retaining screws 2.4 Fracture of abutment screws or retaining screws 2.5 Fracture or displacement of artificial teeth 2.6 Fracture of the full-arch provisional prosthesis 2.7 Changing orientation or angle of conical abutments 2.8 Changing the palatal contours of the prosthesis for phonetics

Table 14.1 - Complications classification associated with the Columbus Bridge Protocol. Complications associated with conventional implant and prosthodontic treatments have been excluded.

1. IMMEDIATE COMPLICATIONS

1.1 Excessive Pressure Between Soft Tissues (Mucosa) and the Full-Arch Prosthesis

At the time of delivery of the fixed provisional prosthesis, 24–48 hours after surgery, swelling and inflammation may be significant enough to make it difficult or even impossible to seat the provisional prosthesis. The swollen tissues also may prevent the retaining screws from being tightened into the conical abutments for optimal seating (Fig 14.1). In addition, incomplete seating of the prosthesis onto the abutments may occur secondary to excessive relief on the stone of the master cast during the fabrication of the provisional prosthesis. In these cases, the patient will generally show signs of moderate to significant discomfort. When unable to tighten the screws, the clinician may have to relieve the pontic area of the prosthesis until such time that the prosthesis can be seated completely onto the abutments (Fig 14.2).

Management

It is critical to find the areas of the provisional prosthesis responsible for incomplete seating onto the abutments. The authors recommend the use of Pressure Indicator Paste (Mizzy) to highlight the areas of greatest pressure. The prosthesis is then adjusted accordingly, polished, and reinserted onto the abutments. The tissues will tolerate some pressure, and blanching of the tissues may be visualized. Once the prosthesis is completely seated, the retaining screws may be tightened across the arch to 10 Ncm (Figs 14.3 and 14.4). After placement of the prosthesis onto the abutments, periapical radiographs should be taken to confirm that the cylinders of the prosthesis are completely seated onto the abutments. In cases where the clinician suspects that significant swelling will occur between the surgical and prosthetis insertion appointments, a customized postsurgical silicone dressing can help control the swelling between appointments to ensure that the conical abutment healing caps remain supragingival. The patient wears the post-surgical dressing overnight to control the swelling, and the clinician removes it the next morning. The postsurgical dressing may be fabricated directly in the mouth, or it can be made in the laboratory on the master cast. It is made by injecting silicone impression material (Fresh Clear, Dreve) around impression copings placed onto the conical abutments or around tissue conditioning cylinders specifically designed to work with the silicone dressing (see chapter 16).The postsurgical dressing remains in place intraorally until the patient returns for insertion of the provisional prosthesis the next day. Periodontal gel may be used in and around the flaps prior to insertion of the silicone dressing (Figs 14.5 to 14.20).

1.2 Failure to Obtain Sufficient Implant Primary Stability

High levels of implant primary stability may not be achieved in cases with inadequate osteotomy preparation associated with poor bone quality (type 3 or 4). Inadequate implant primary stability also may be caused by the use of an implant site that is not conducive to osteotomy preparation, such as a postextraction site (Fig 14.21).[2]

Management

An implant with insufficient primary stability (insertion torque < 20 Ncm) should not be used in the Columbus Bridge Protocol. Rather, it should be replaced with an implant that has a larger diameter, a longer length, or a different angulation compared with the original implant–steps that are likely to increase the insertion torque values. In the worst-case scenario, the portion of the prosthesis directly over the unstable implant may be fabricated out of occlusion.
If an implant with less-than-optimal insertion torque is placed in an anterior position, the failure to reach the default torque value can be tolerated if the provisional prosthesis is not removed until osseointegration has occurred. In this case, the sutures must be resorbable.

1.3 Fracture of Vestibular Cortical Bone During Implant Placement

The vestibular cortical bone can fracture in the case of erroneous implant placement. In implant sites with significant quantities of cortical bone (type 1 or 2), underpreparation of the osteotomy may generate insertion torque values that exceed the strength of the bone and cause the facial cortical plate to fracture. If the bone segment involved in the fracture site shows significant mobility, long-term consequences often include loss of the implant and, potentially, a significant alveolar defect in the labiopalatal dimension (Figs 14.22 to 14.24).

Management

When the fractured cortical plate has not completely separated from the alveolar process, and the implant has primary stability, a solution may be to allow patients to heal on their own. However, it is advisable to substitute this implant as soon as possible by changing its position and removing the fractured bone fragment.

1.4 Excessive Subcrestal Implant Placement

Excessive subcrestal implant placement is often the direct result of continued vertical placement of an implant in an attempt to achieve the appropriate level of insertion torque and implant primary stability. This generally results in prosthetic complications associated with the inability to accurately seat the conical abutments (Fig 14.25). In a clinical case where a natural fixed bridge has been treatment planned, the anterior implants should all be positioned at the same level (coronoapically). An excessive subcrestal implant placement will cause the peri-implant bone to resorb to the level of the first implant thread according to the biologic width.[11]

Management

To ensure an accurate abutment-implant connection, some areas of the supraimplant bone may need to be removed with a bone profiler (Fig 14.26).

1.5 Stripping of External Hexagon Implant Restorative Platform

An external hexagon implant restorative platform may be stripped when the insertion torque at implant placement exceeds the tolerance values of implants[12] because of improper use of a hand wrench. Stripping the external hexagon may necessitate implant removal and replacement.

Management

If the external hex was stripped at the last stage of implant placement, the surgeon may accept the implant position but must be careful to remove any metal filings that remain on the implant platform. Stripping the external hexagon may compromise the accuracy and long-term survival of the implant-abutment connection since the implant restorative platform has lost its anti-rotation component. If this is the case, it is advisable for the definitive prosthesis to be made from an implant level impression or to use a straight conical abutment since an accurate hex is required to properly orient angled abutments. If, on the contrary, stripping the external hex occurs before the implant has been correctly seated in the coronoapical direction, the implant should be removed by turning it counterclockwise with an appropriate instrument. Removal should be done very carefully to avoid fracturing the alveolus (Figs 14.27 and 14.28). The implant site must be reprepared with larger drills for the insertion of a new implant.

1.6 Incorrect Abutment Positioning

Incorrect abutment positioning primarily occurs when angled implants are used (Fig 14.29). The correction of an angled implant axis with an angled abutment demands that the surgeon prepare a countersink into the coronal aspect of the peri-implant bone so the shoulder of the angled abutment can be optimally seated onto the implant restorative platform (Fig 14.30). If complete seating between an angled abutment and an implant is not obtained, the implant-abutment connection may not be stable and could lead to screw loosening with occlusal function (Figs 14.31 and 14.32).

Management

If the clinician suspects that an abutment is not correctly seated onto its corresponding implant during surgery, an intraoral radiograph must be taken and evaluated before proceeding with screw tightening. If incorrect seating is observed after a provisional prosthesis has been delivered but before insertion of the definitive prosthesis, it is necessary to remove the prosthesis, reposition the abutment correctly, take another intraoral radiograph, and then tighten the abutment screw. If the abutment cannot be seated, it may be necessary to use a bone profiler to remove the peri-implant bone interfering with abutment seating (Fig 14.33). This operation should be performed after osseointegration has occurred and requires that the provisional prosthesis be modified.

1.7 Incorrect Impression Coping Positioning

The impression coping may be incorrectly positioned when bone or soft tissue interferes with complete seating of a conical abutment impression coping onto a conical abutment. This complication usually arises when the protocol was not followed. It may occur if impression copings were placed onto abutments after flap closure and the impression coping-abutment interface was not visualized (Fig 14.34).

Management

If a clinician can feel that an impression coping is not completely seated onto its corresponding abutment, an intraoral periapical radiograph should be taken and evaluated for complete seating (Fig 14.35). If the misfit is not detected during the surgical or the provisional prosthetic phase, then the provisional prosthesis will not fit correctly (Fig 14.36). If the misfit is so pronounced that the prosthesis cannot be seated, a new impression must be made so that a new master cast can be fabricated and the provisional prosthesis can be modified. If it is discovered that one titanium cylinder of the prosthesis is causing the interference, the cylinder can be removed from the prosthesis and correctly repositioned directly in the mouth (Figs 14.37 to 14.42).

1.8 Mobility of Pick up Impression Coping in the Impression

Loose impression copings within the plaster impression are caused by insufficient retention of the most coronal portions of impression copings inside the plaster (Figs 14.43 and 14.44). Instability will lead to errors when laboratory analogs are attached and tightened to the impression copings within the impression, and the analogs will not be correctly positioned within the master casts when compared with the clinical intraoral abutment positions.

Management

If the thickness of peri-implant soft tissues obscures the retentive portions of the impression copings, it is recommended to use modified pickup abutment impression copings with longer impression coping bodies (see Fig 8.8 and chapter 16). The impression coping within the impression must be examined visually or with a probe. If a loose impression coping is detected within the plaster impression, the impression must be remade.

1.9 Difficult Provisional Full-Arch Prosthesis Insertion Due to Nonparallel Abutments

Angulated abutments are often used to generate a common path of insertion for nonparallel implants. In some clinical cases, divergent paths of insertion may remain between anterior and posterior abutments. Usually, a nonparallel implant can be managed with a back-and-forth movement during placement of the provisional prosthesis.

Management

In some cases where it is impossible to connect a provisional prosthesis to abutments, the internal aspects of the prefabricated titanium cylinders used in the luting technique may be adjusted clinically (Fig 14.45). During reevaluation of the definitive prosthesis design, a decision can be made to change the angle of one or more of the abutments prior to fabricating the definitive prosthesis.

1.10 Difficult to Mask Access Openings to Retaining Screws

If implant treatment planning, abutment selection, and positioning were not performed optimally, the access openings to the retaining screws may be positioned in the esthetic zone (Fig 14.46).

Management

This complication in the provisional prosthesis can be easily solved by using composite resin restorative materials to disguise the inappropriately placed screw access openings.[7] Once this is done, the treatment plan for the definitive prosthesis will be changed such that an implant level impression will be made at the appropriate time. The master cast fabricated from this type of impression will allow the dental laboratory technician to place the correct angulated abutment on the cast in its correct position relative to the contours of the definitive prosthesis. In some cases, a custom abutment may be need to be fabricated (Fig 14.47).

In some patients with limited restorative volume available for the definitive prosthesis, the access openings for the retaining screws may be so short that a hex retaining screw access restoration may be interfering intraorally. In rare cases, the heads of retaining screws may need to be altered to place them inside the prosthesis. It is also possible to use slotted retaining screws since the heads of slotted screws are shorter than the heads of hexed retaining screws (Figs 14.48 to 14.50).

2. LATE COMPLICATIONS

2.1 Exposure of the Abutment Collar Secondary to Peri-Implant Soft Tissue Recession

Exposure of abutment collars occurs more frequently around angled conical abutments than straight conical abutments because angled conical abutments generally have longer collar heights (≥ 2 mm).

Management

When this complication occurs, the exposed collars must be concealed by fabricating the definitive prosthesis with a framework and esthetic veneer that covers the exposed collars (Figs 14.51 to 14.54). In patients who are restored with the natural fixed bridge (no soft tissue replacement), clinicians are advised not to place implants in the intercanine zone to avoid this complication.

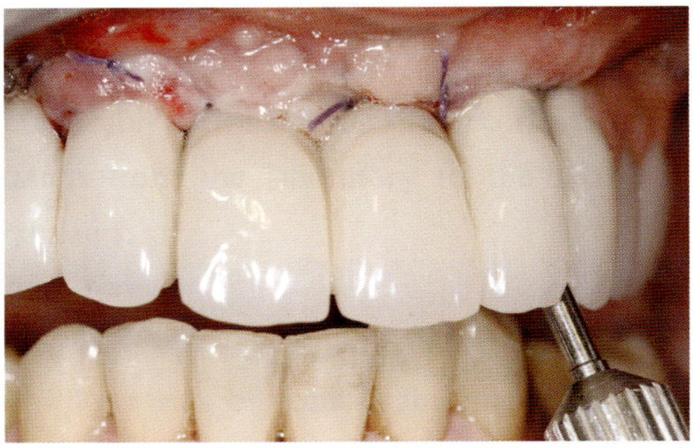

Fig 14.1 - Insertion of the provisional prosthesis 24 hours postsurgery may be compromised in the presence of soft tissue swelling that prevents the prosthesis from going into place.

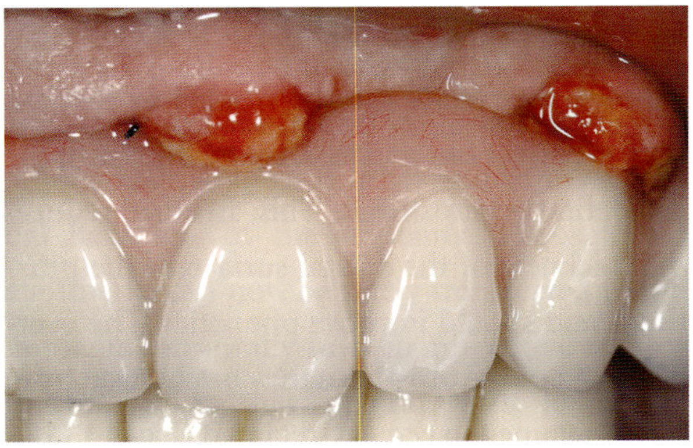

Fig 14.2 - A patient with a maxillary fixed prosthesis in place 10 days postsurgery. An excessive soft tissue contact with the intaglio surface of the prosthesis is present.

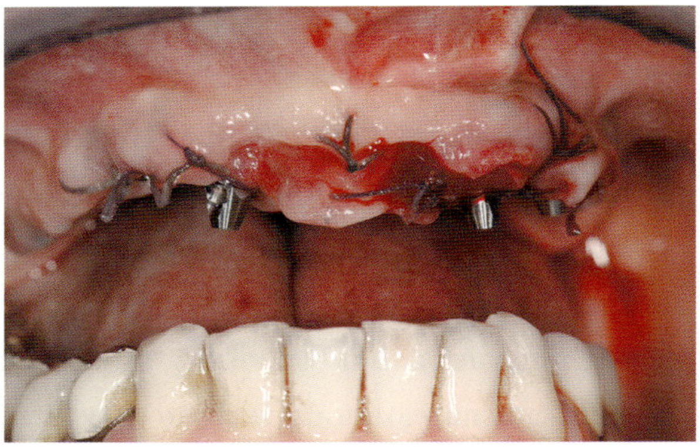

Fig 14.3 - Labial intraoral image of the patient in Fig 14.2 after the provisional prosthesis was removed, prior to suture removal.

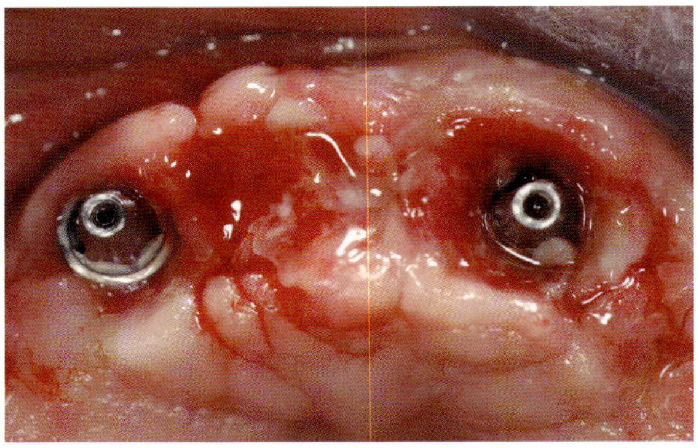

Fig 14.4 - Maxillary occlusal image of the patient in Figs 14.2 and 14.3 after suture removal. Soft tissue swelling and hemorrhage are seen secondary to removal of the prosthesis.

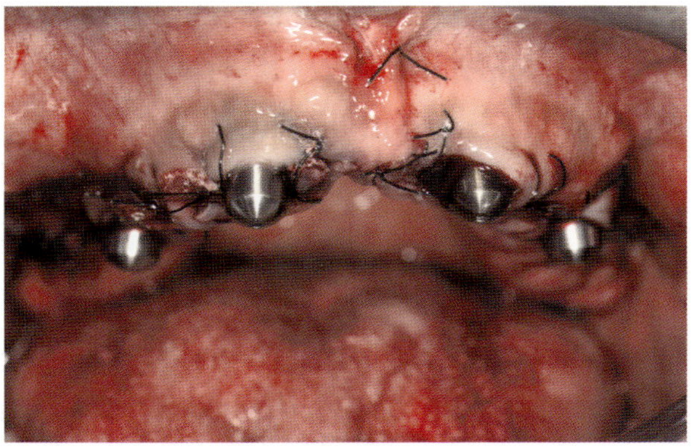

Fig 14.5 - Image of a patient taken after the plaster pickup impression was made. Healing caps were placed onto the conical abutments.

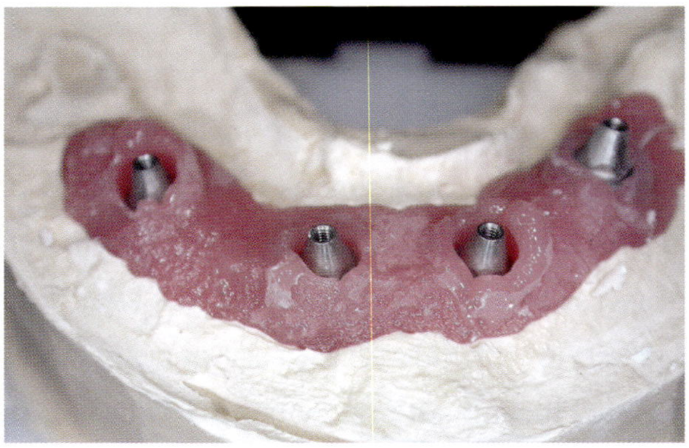

Fig 14.6 - Master cast of the patient in Fig 14.5 with the conical abutment analogs in place.

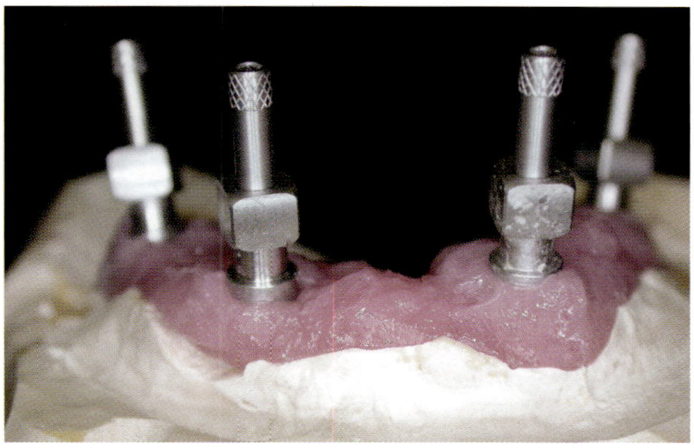

Fig 14.7 - Master cast with four pickup impression copings in place in the master cast.

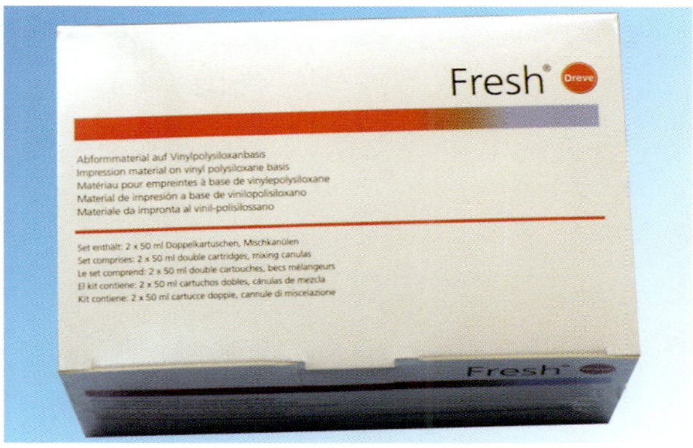

Fig 14.8 - Silicone material was used to make the postsurgical dressing that the patient was to wear to control soft tissue swelling between the surgical appointment and the prosthesis insertion appointment.

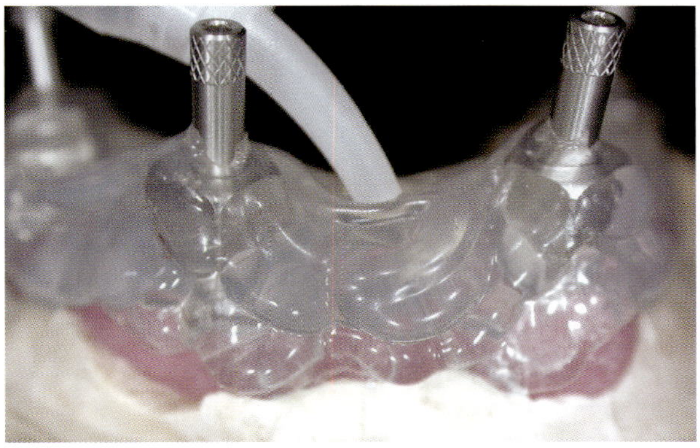

Fig 14.9 - Silicone was injected around the pickup impression copings on the master cast.

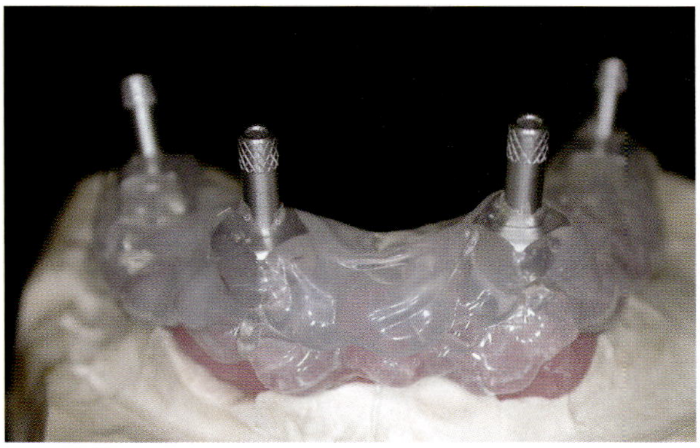

Fig 14.10 - Before the postsurgical dressing is delivered to the patient, the long impression coping screws will be replaced with shorter retaining screws.

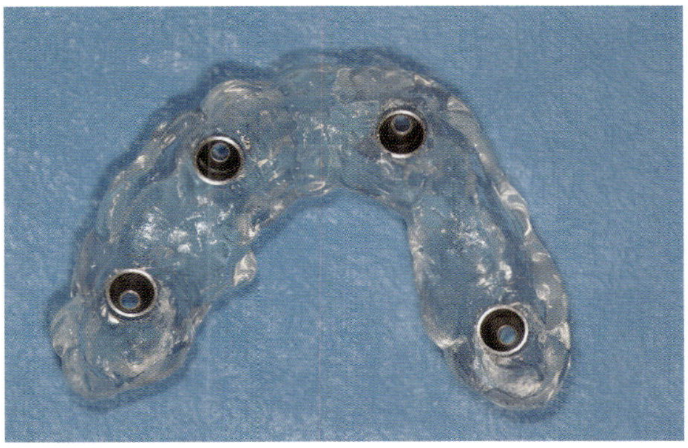

Fig 14.11 - Intaglio surface of the postsurgical dressing made with transparent silicone.

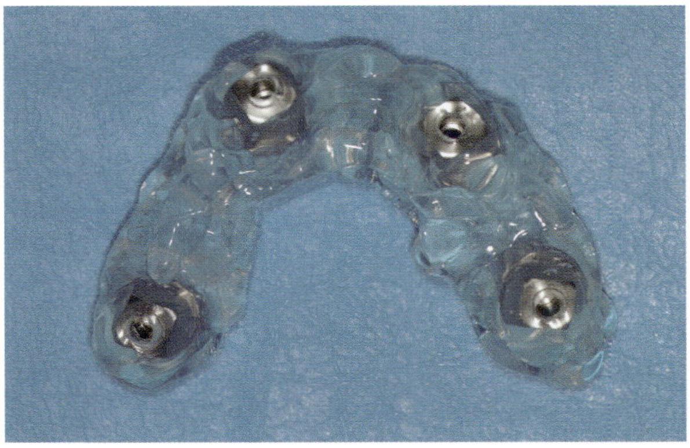

Fig 14.12 - Occlusal surface of the postsurgical dressing made with transparent silicone.

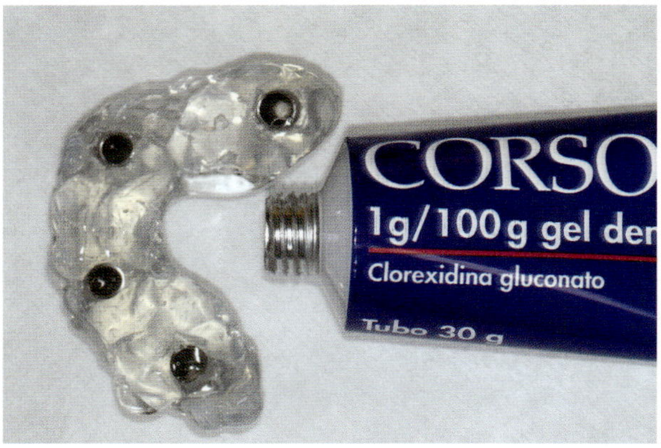

Fig 14.13 - Chlorhexidine gel (Corsodyl dental gel, GlaxoSmithKline) is placed in the intaglio surface of the postsurgical dressing prior to insertion onto the abutments.

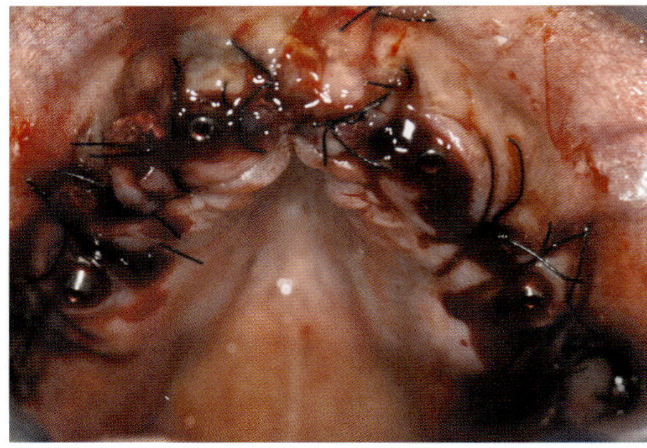

Fig 14.14 - Prior to insertion of the postsurgical dressing, the conical abutment healing caps were removed. Note that the conical abutments have been obscured by the soft tissues.

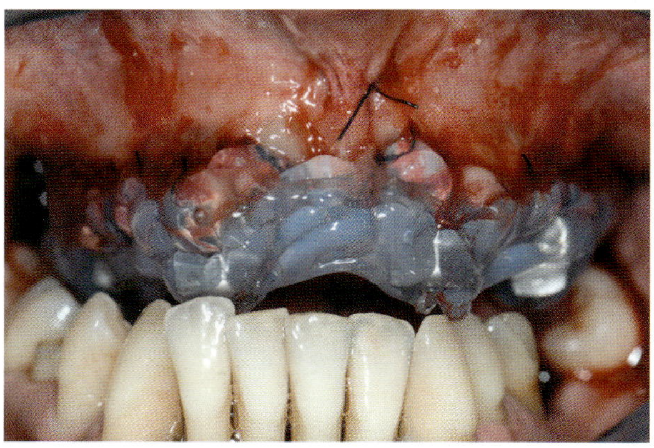

Fig 14.15 - The patient was discharged with the postsurgical dressing in place.

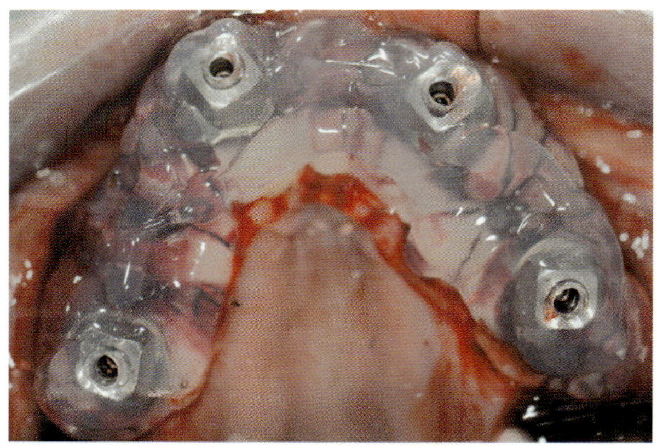

Fig 14.16 - Occlusal surface of the postsurgical dressing in place.

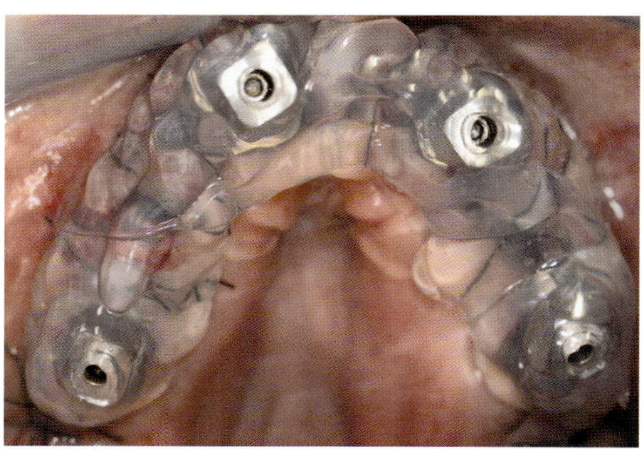

Fig 14.17 - Occlusal surface of the postsurgical dressing in place 24 hours after surgery. The soft tissue contours have been stabilized; no bleeding was noted.

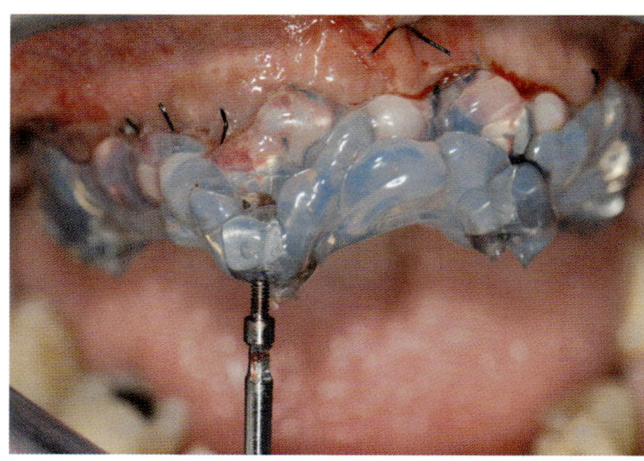

Fig 14.18 - The postsurgical dressing was removed the day after the implants and abutments were placed.

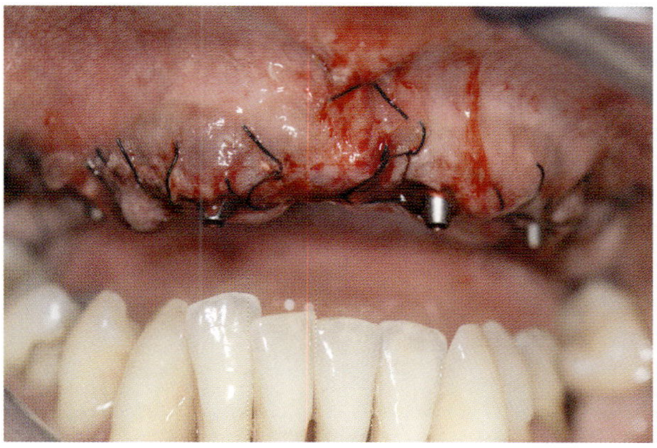

Fig 14.19 - Twenty-four hours after surgery, the peri-implant soft tissues were significantly less swollen than they were prior to insertion of the postsurgical dressing.

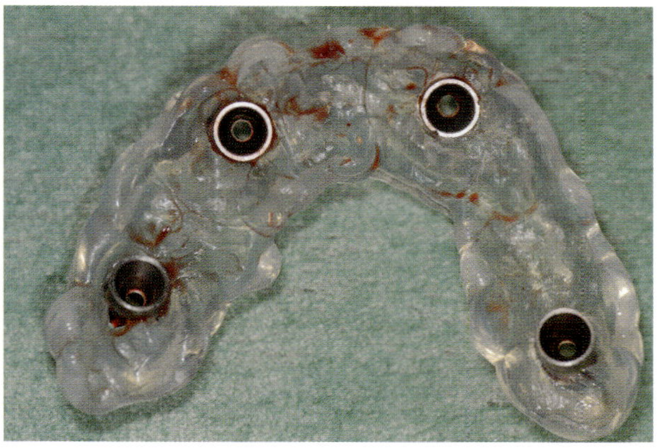

Fig 14.20 - Intaglio surface of the postsurgical dressing made with transparent silicone after it was removed from the intraoral abutments.

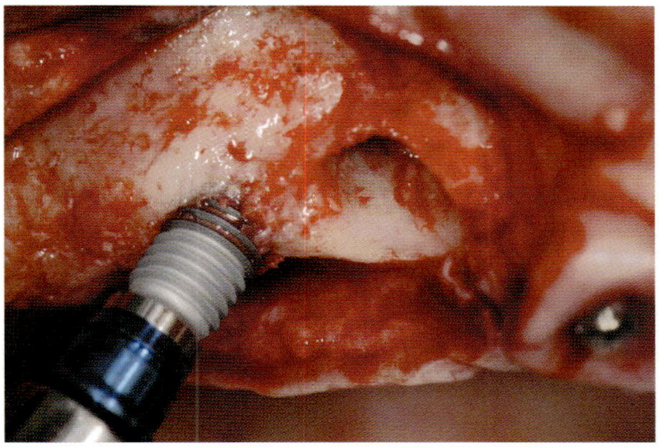

Fig 14.21- During implant placement, the extraction site was partially avoided to optimize implant primary stability.

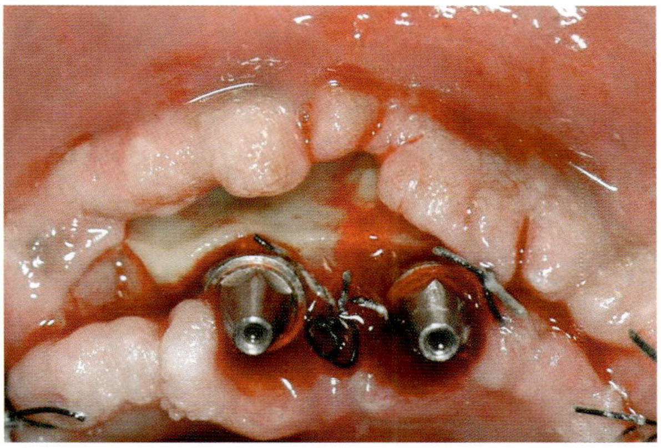

Fig 14.22 - Photograph taken 7 days after insertion of the provisional prosthesis. A labial dehiscence with exposure of the labial cortical plate was evident.

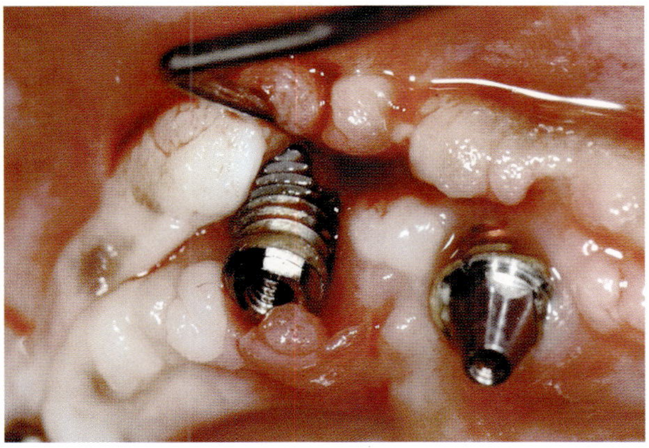

Fig 14.23 - The labial cortical plate was fractured and removed. The implant no longer had primary stability, displayed mobility, and was also removed.

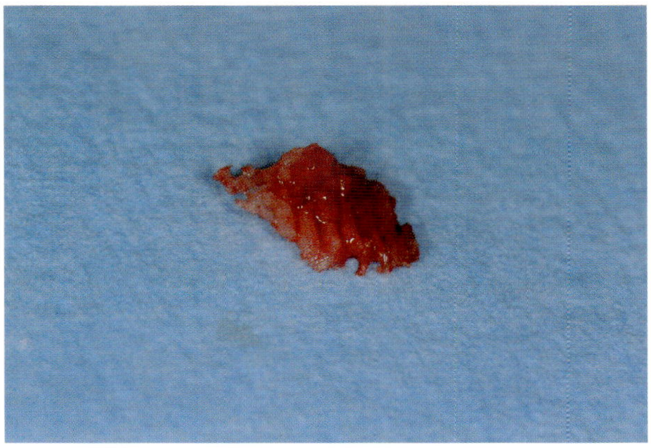

Fig 14.24 - Labial cortical plate that was removed from the patient in Figs 14.22 and 14.23. The internal aspect of the segment revealed the presence of threads that corresponded to the implant threads of the mobile implant.

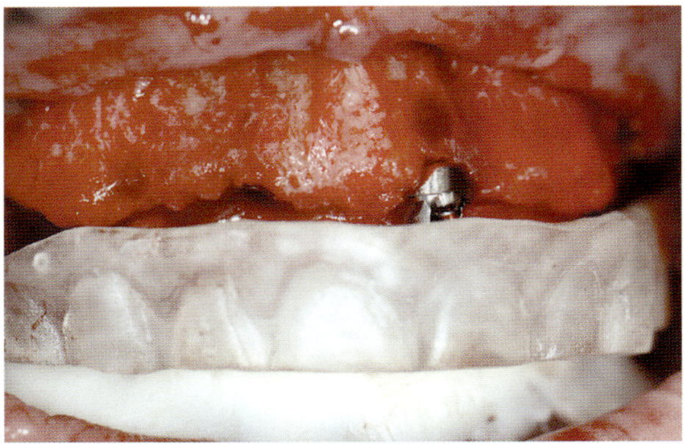

Fig 14.25 - Deep implant placement, relative to the location of the alveolar crest, creates clinical challenges regarding optimal, correct seating of angled abutments.

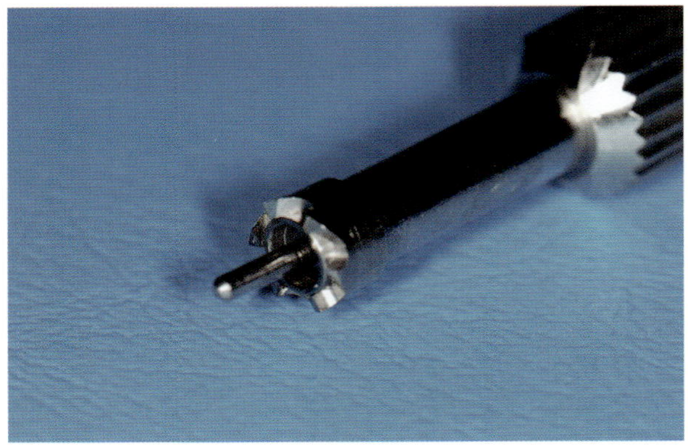

Fig 14.26 - A bone profiler may be used for removing crestal bone interferences.

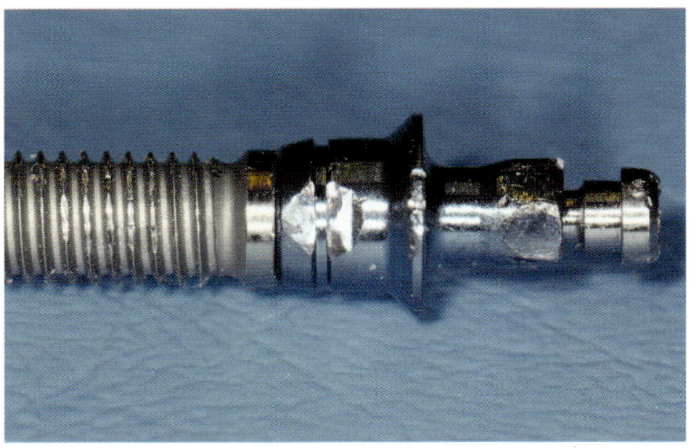

Fig 14.27 - The external hexagon implant restorative platform was damaged during implant placement.

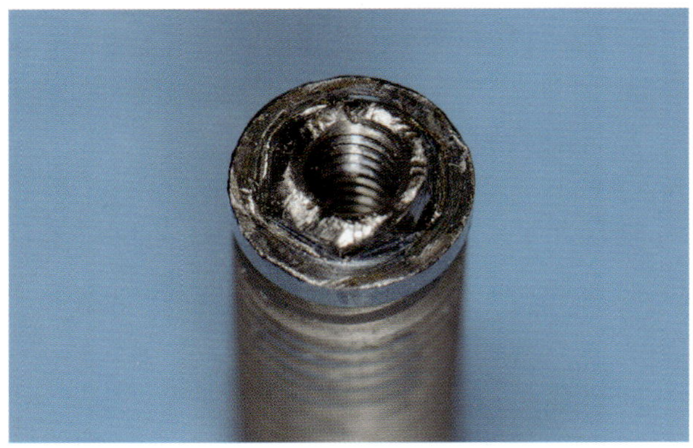

Fig 14.28 - Close-up image of the damaged implant platform in Fig 14.27. This was noted after the implant mount was removed. The implant was not usable and had to be removed.

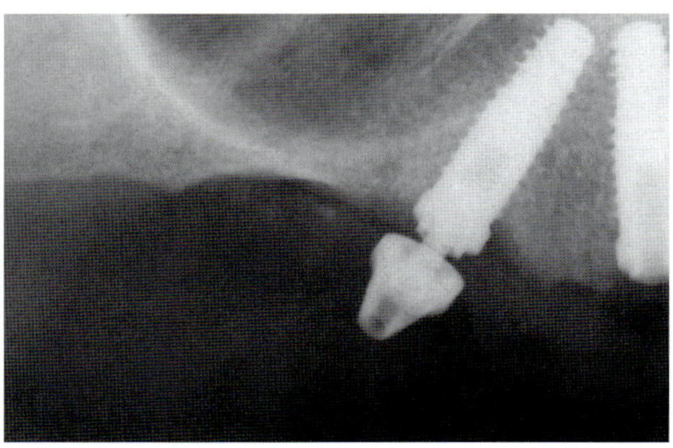

Fig 14.29 - This radiograph demonstrates an angled conical abutment that was not correctly seated onto the external hexagon of an implant.

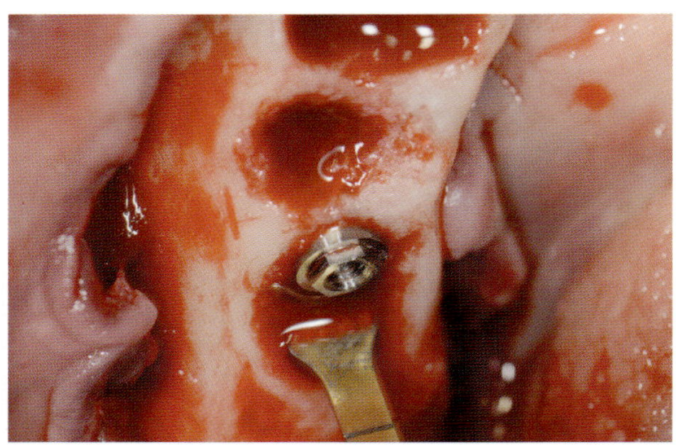

Fig 14.30 - Peri-implant bone being recontoured with an ultrasonic instrument (Piezosurgery, Mectron).

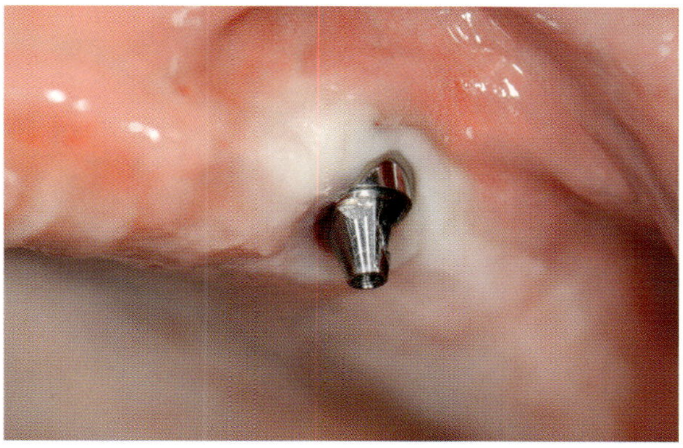

Fig 14.31 - A fistulous tract associated with an incompletely seated abutment.

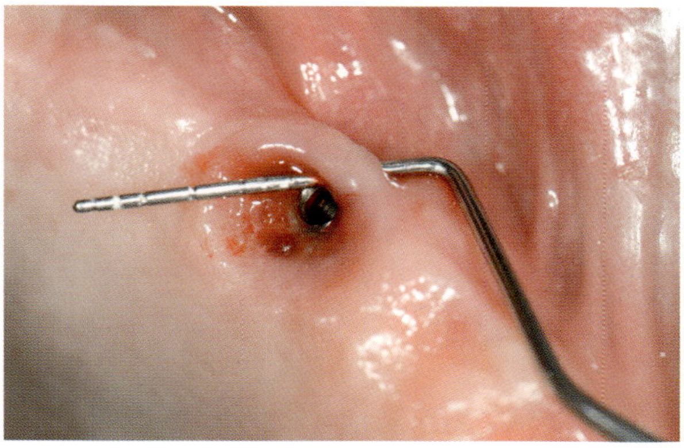

Fig 14.32 - A periodontal probe clearly demonstrated the fistulous tract identified in Fig 14.31.

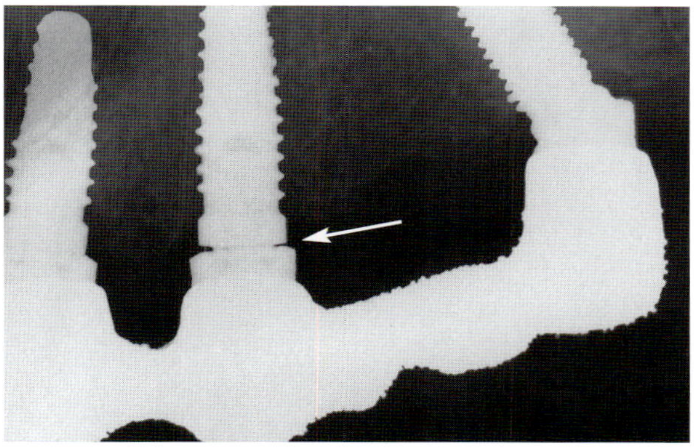

Fig 14.33 - This radiograph clearly demonstrated an inaccurate fit between an abutment and an implant (*arrow*) after the provisional prosthesis was inserted.

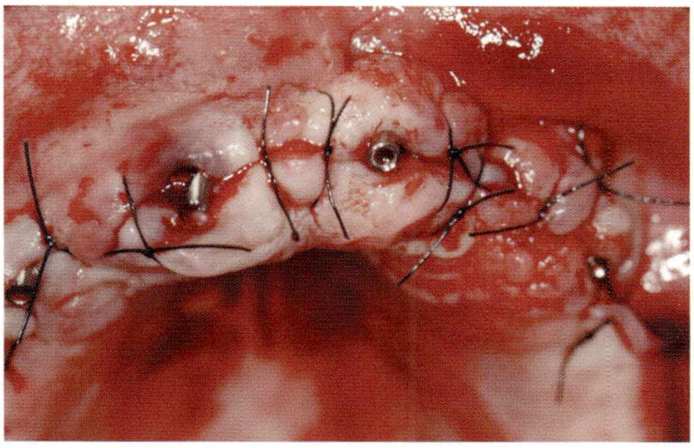

Fig 14.34 - In this case, the flaps were closed prior to placement of the pickup impression copings. It is more difficult to seat impression copings after flap closure; the authors prefer to seat the impression copings onto the abutments and then close the flaps with sutures.

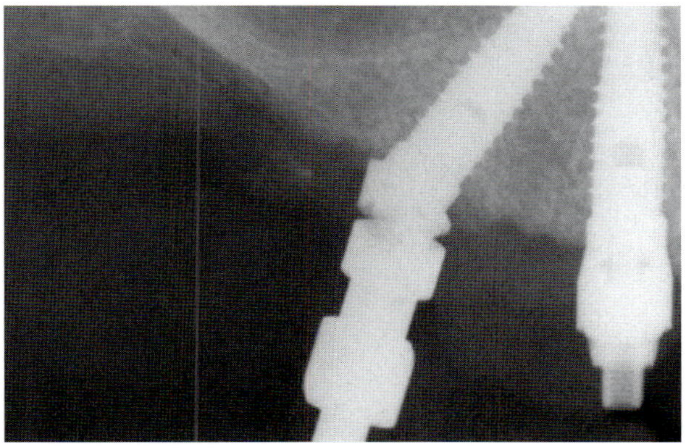

Fig 14.35 - This radiograph clearly demonstrated an inaccurate fit between a pickup impression coping and a conical abutment prior to making the impression. The coping was tightened in its proper position prior to making the impression.

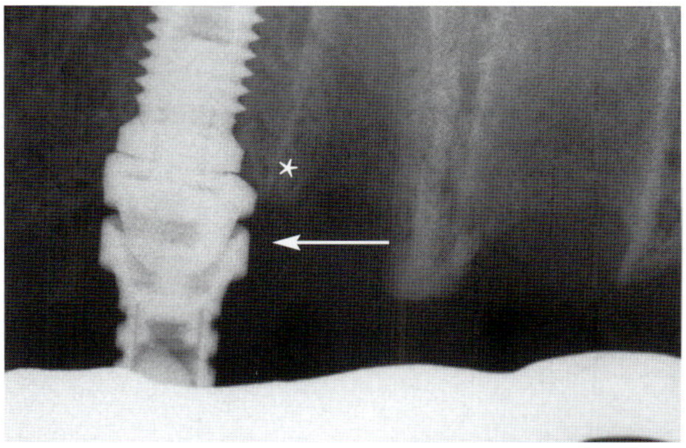

Fig 14.36 - This radiograph clearly demonstrated an inaccurate fit between a titanium cylinder and an abutment after the patient functioned for several months. The prosthesis no longer fit the abutment correctly (*arrow*). The authors believe that the abutment screw loosened secondary to an ill-fitting prosthesis (*).

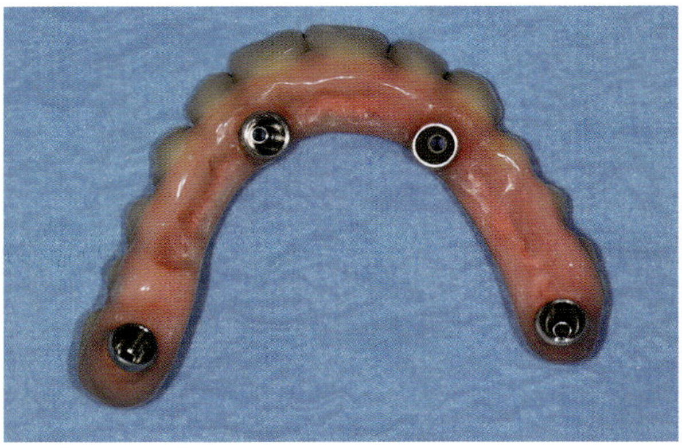

Fig 14.37 - Intaglio surface of a misfitting fixed provisional prosthesis fabricated with a metal framework.

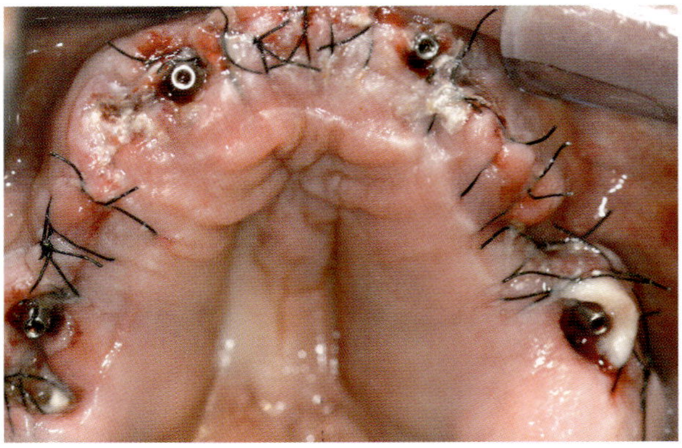

Fig 14.38 - Maxillary occlusal image of a patient 24 hours after implant placement. The provisional prosthesis in Fig 14.37 did not go into place at the maxillary left lateral incisor implant site.

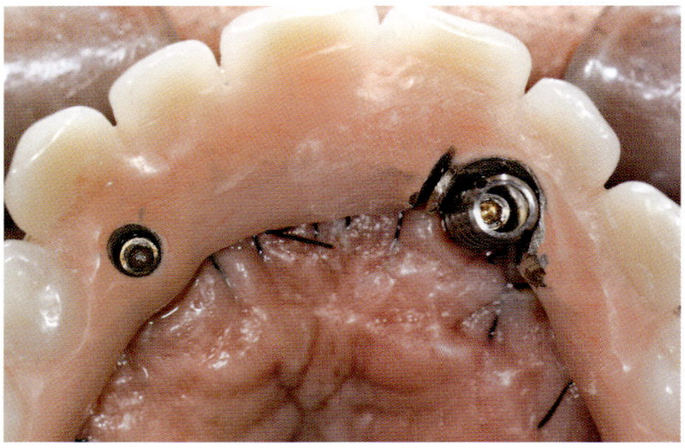

Fig 14.39 - The titanium cylinder that corresponded to the maxillary left lateral incisor implant site was removed from the prosthesis. A new titanium cylinder was placed onto the abutment such that it did not touch the prosthesis, and the prosthesis was correctly seated on the remaining abutments.

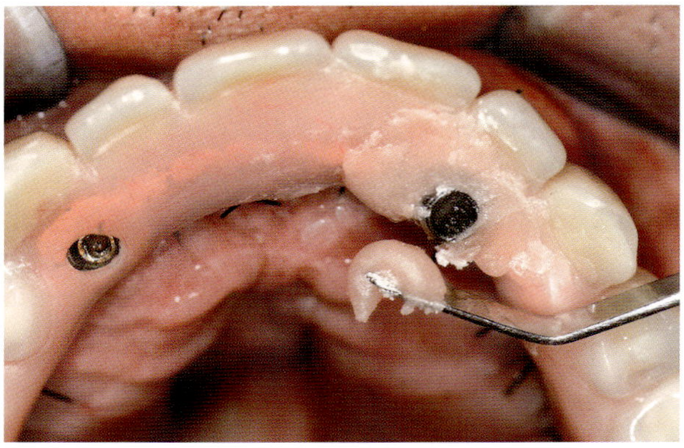

Fig 14.40 - The titanium cylinder was splinted to the provisional prosthesis with autopolymerizing acrylic resin.

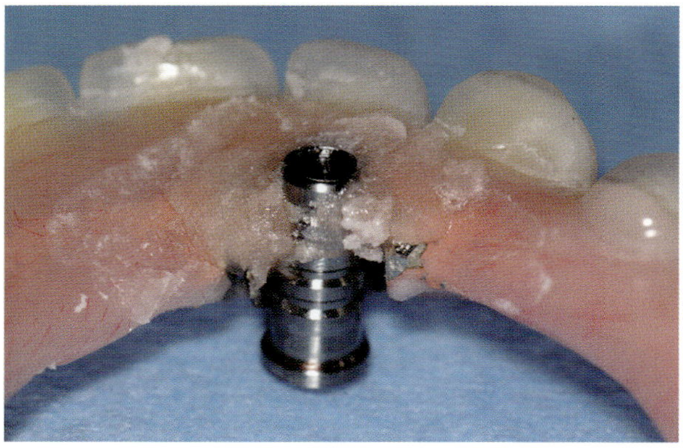

Fig 14.41 - After the acrylic resin polymerized, the provisional prosthesis was removed from the implants. The titanium cylinder remained attached to the prosthesis.

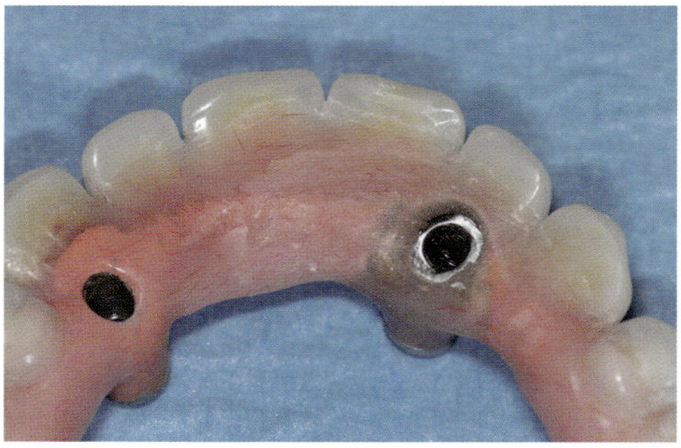

Fig 14.42 - Additional autopolymerizing acrylic resin was placed around the titanium cylinder, consistent with the preexisting contours of the provisional prosthesis. The prosthesis was finished, polished, and reinserted onto the abutments.

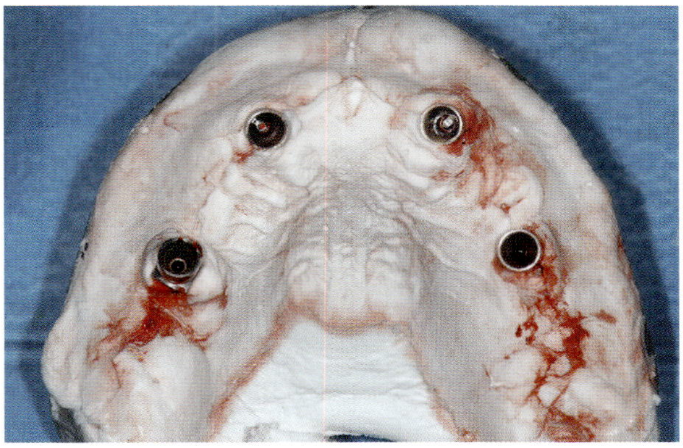

Fig 14.43 - The accuracy of the pickup impression depends on the physical retention generated by the coronal portions of the impression copings.

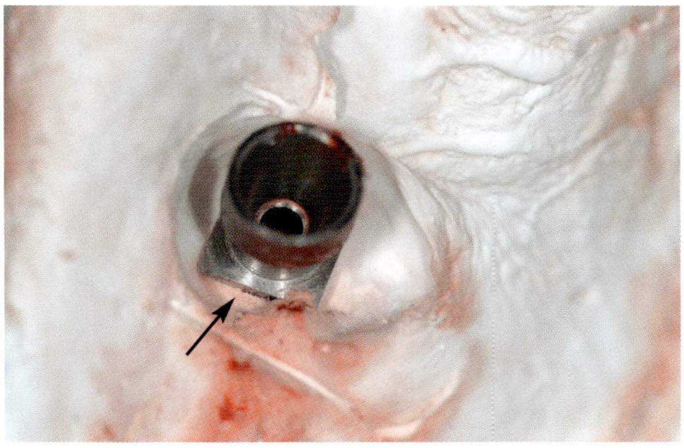

Fig 14.44 - Close-up image of one of the pickup impression copings from Fig 14.43. The distal impression coping was mobile within the plaster impression (*arrow*). The impression had to be redone.

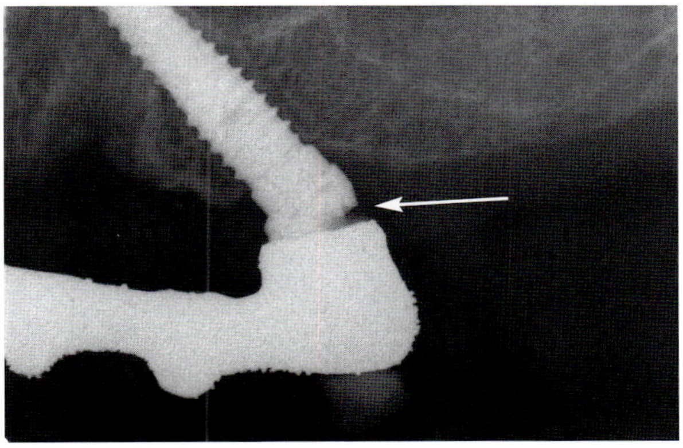

Fig 14.45 - The internal surface of the titanium cylinder on the distal implant was adjusted (*arrow*) to connect the provisional prosthesis.

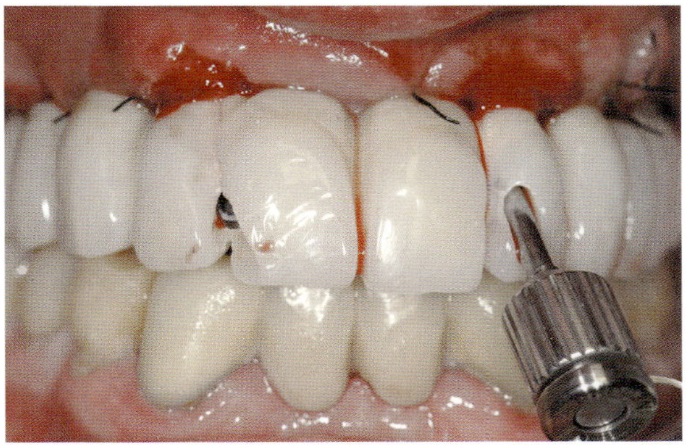

Fig 14.46 - In this case, the anterior screw access openings exited the prosthesis through the facial surfaces of the artificial teeth.

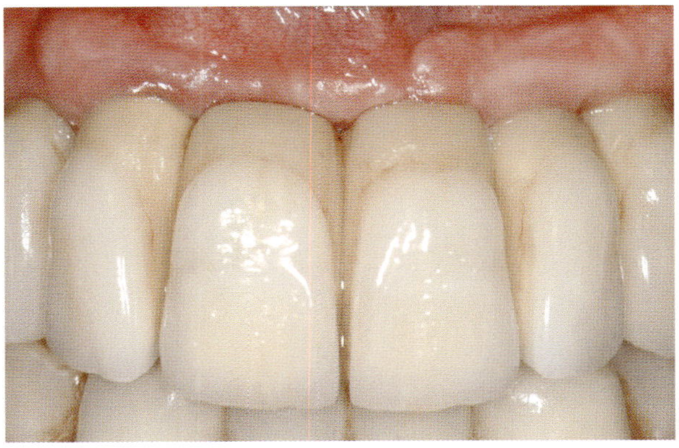

Fig 14.47 - The locations of the screw access openings, noted in Fig 14.46, were changed in the definitive prosthesis by changing the anterior abutments from straight (0 degrees) to angulated (25 degrees).

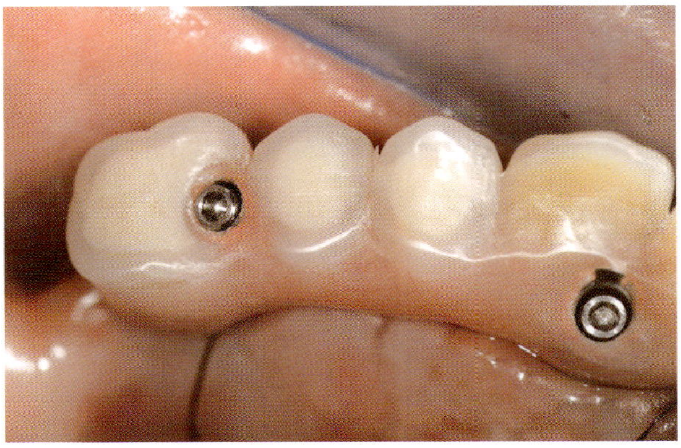

Fig 14.48 - In this case, there was minimal interocclusal clearance around the distal implant. A hex retaining screw could not be used because it was higher than the occlusal surface of the artificial tooth.

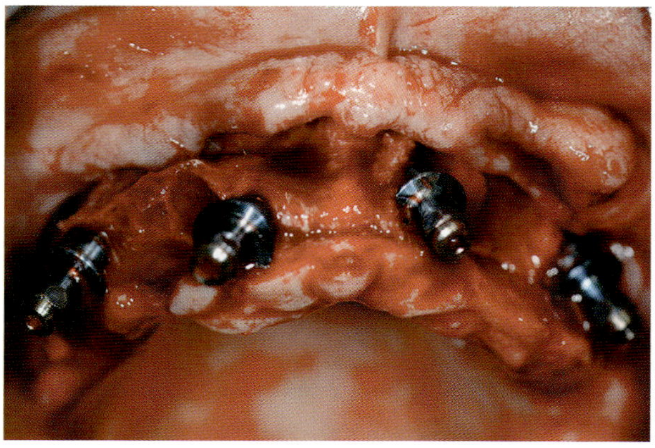

Fig 14.61 - Maxillary occlusal image of the patient in Figs 14.55 to 14.60. The implants were placed with a minimal anteroposterior spread.

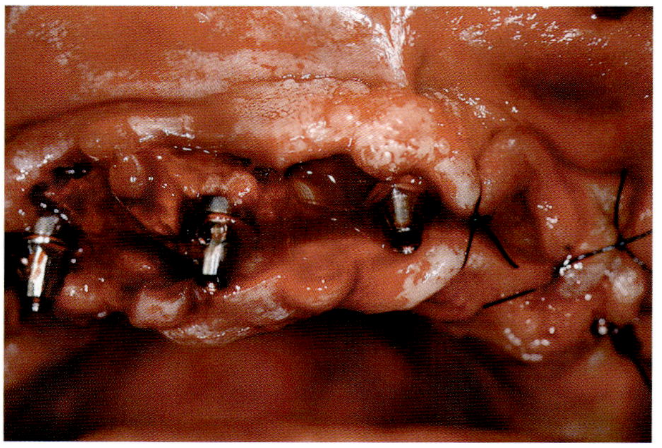

Fig 14.62 - The nonparallel implant angulations were corrected with four 25-degree angled conical abutments.

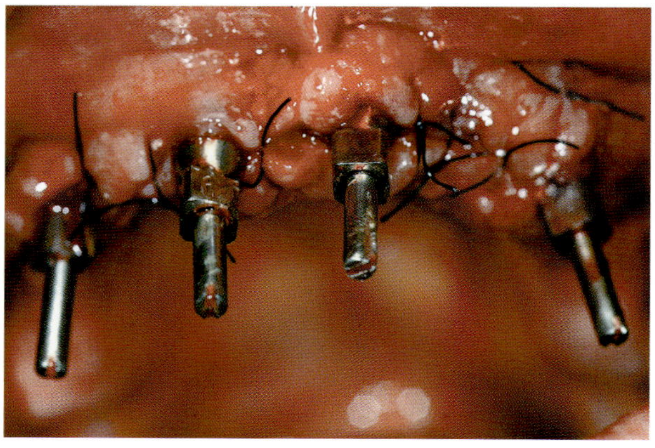

Fig 14.63 - Pickup conical abutment impression copings were screwed into the conical abutments consistent with the pickup impression protocol.

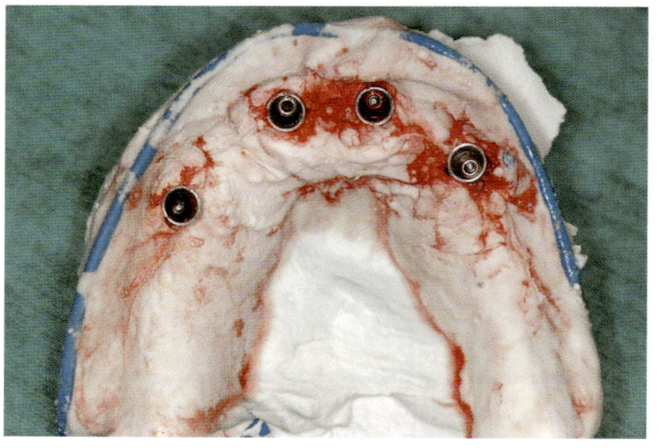

Fig 14.64 - The intaglio surface of the pickup plaster impression.

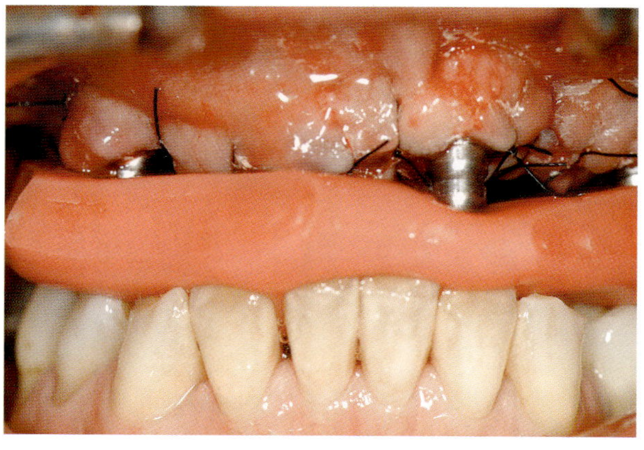

Fig 14.65 - Anterior image of the centric relation wax record in place. The record was made at the predetermined vertical dimension of occlusion.

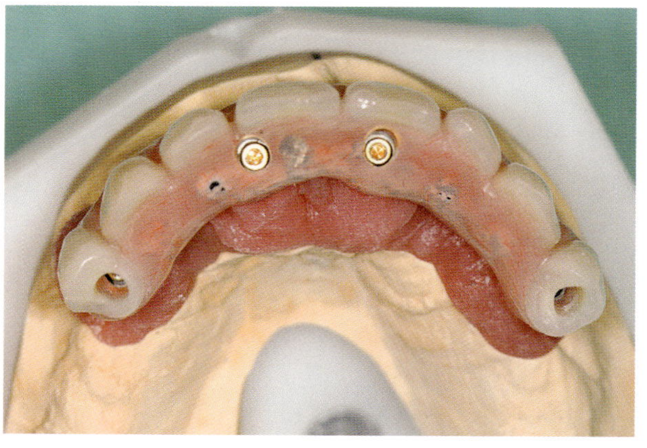

Fig 14.66 - Occlusal image of the provisional prosthesis fabricated per the Columbus Bridge Protocol. The anteroposterior spread is not pronounced.

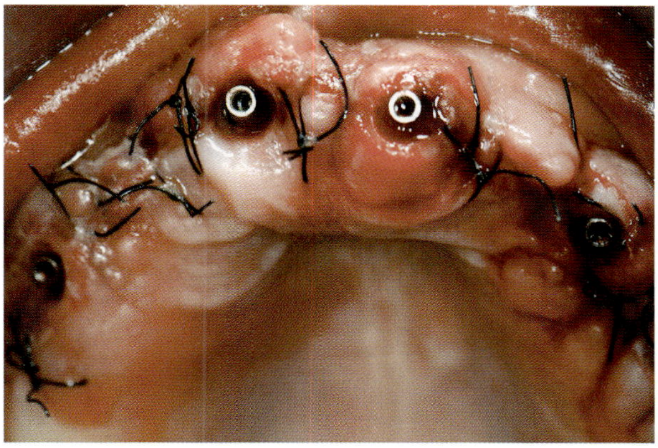

Fig 14.67 - Maxillary occlusal image of the patient 24 hours postsurgery.

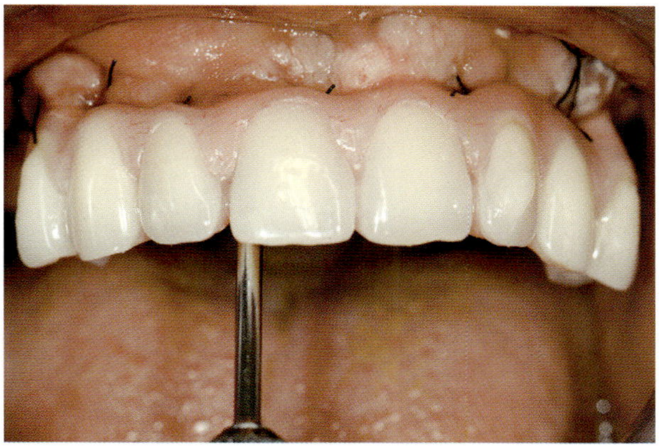

Fig 14.68 - The immediate fixed prosthesis being placed 24 hours postsurgery. The prosthesis was screw-retained per the Columbus Bridge Protocol.

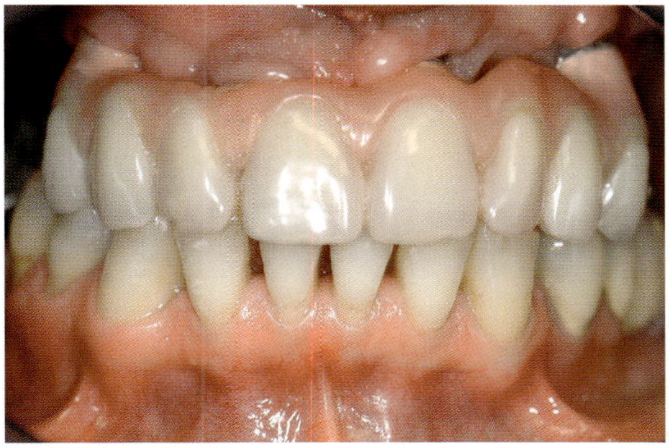

Fig 14.69 - The patient treated in Figs 14.55 to 14.68 1 month postsurgery. The patient reported mild discomfort around the left distal implant with chewing.

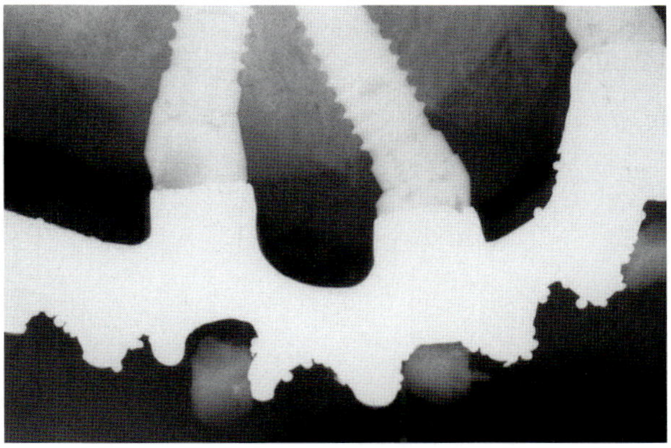

Fig 14.70 - Intraoral radiograph of the anterior implants.

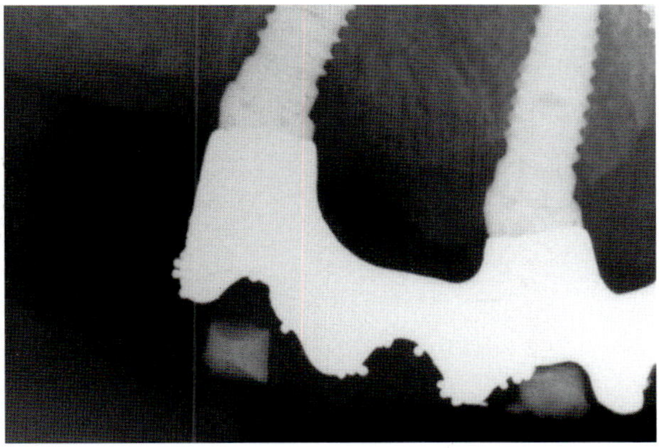

Fig 14.71 - Implants in the maxillary right quadrant.

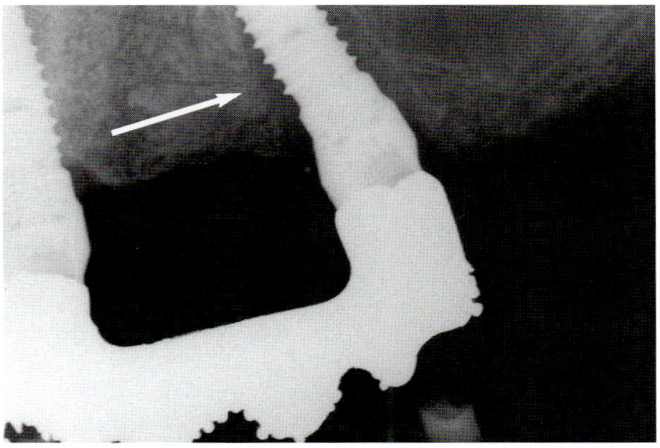

Fig 14.72 - Implants in the maxillary left quadrant. A peri-implant radiolucency was evident around the coronal portion of the left distal implant (*arrow*).

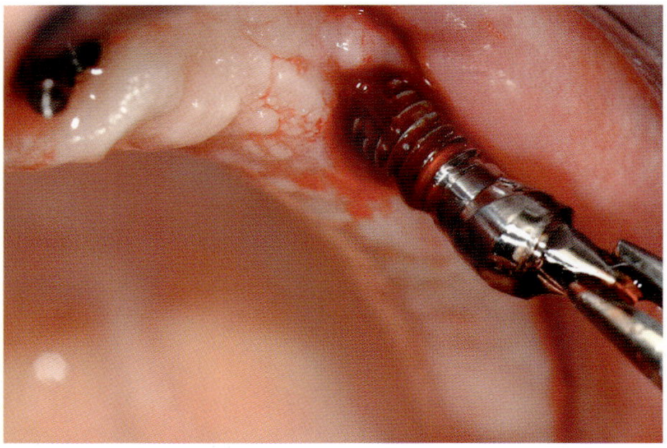

Fig 14.73 - Removing the fibrointegrated (mobile) implant depicted in Fig 14.72.

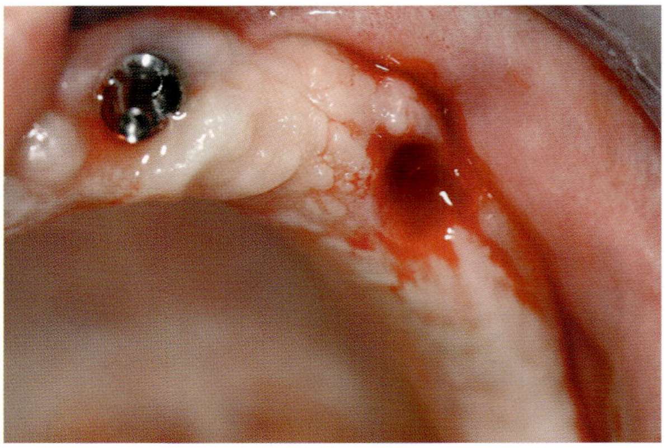

Fig 14.74 - Maxillary left first premolar implant site immediately after removal of the mobile implant.

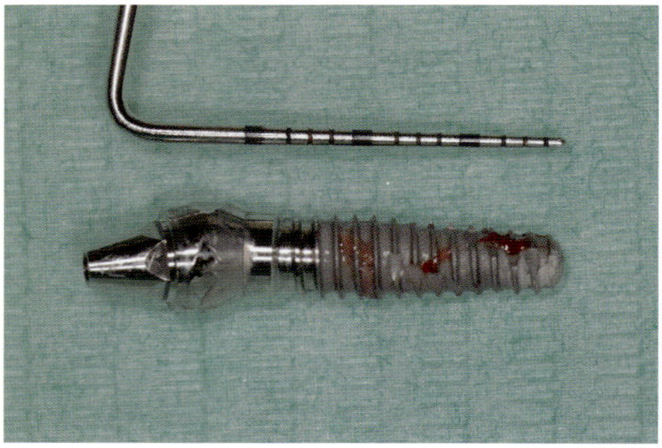

Fig 14.75 - The failed, tapered implant: 4 mm in diameter, 15 mm in length, with a machined collar.

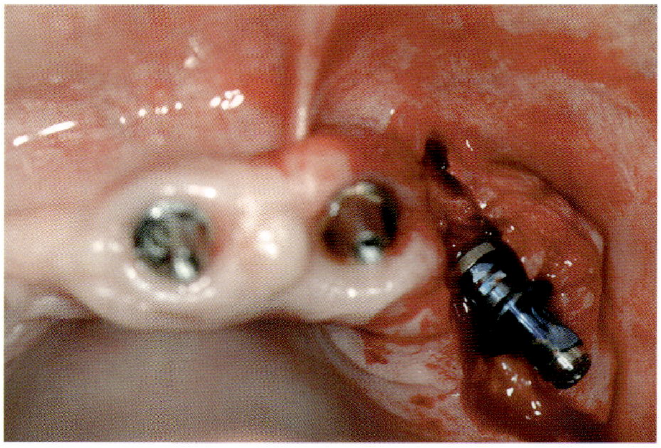

Fig 14.76 - A small full-thickness mucoperiosteal flap was reflected and a new 4 × 15–mm implant was placed.

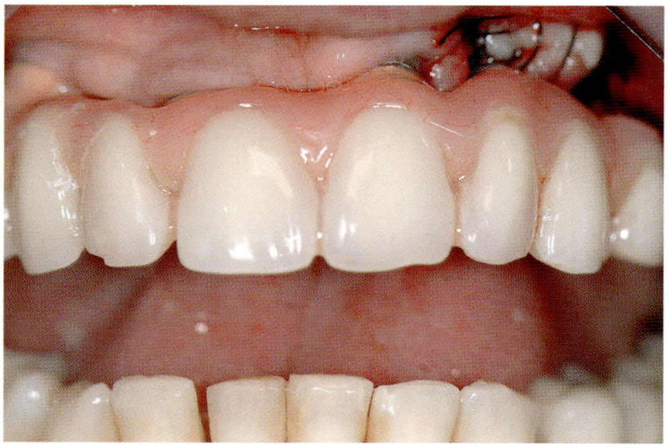

Fig 14.77 - The provisional prosthesis was adjusted in the area of the failed implant. A new angled conical abutment was placed onto the implant. A new titanium cylinder was placed on the new abutment, and the cylinder was attached to the provisional prosthesis.

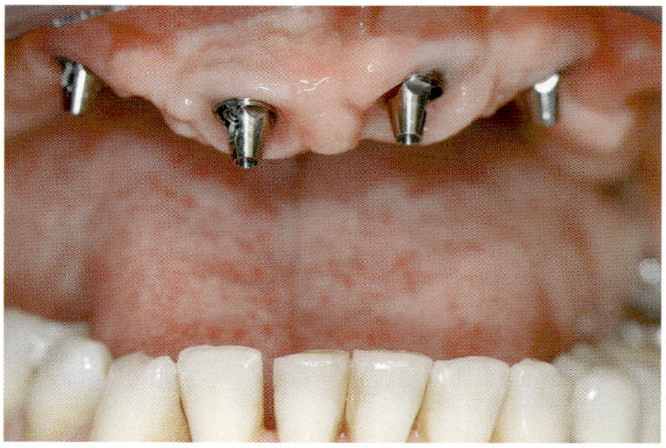

Fig 14.78 - Four months after the procedures were accomplished (Figs 14.73 - 14.77), the provisional prosthesis was removed, and the implants were evaluated for osseointegration.

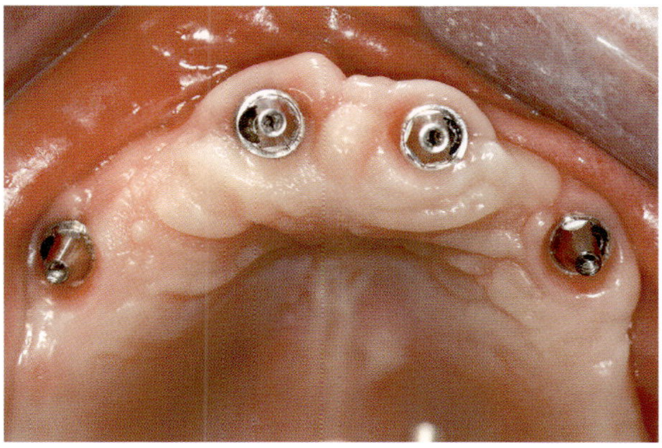

Fig 14.79 - Maxillary occlusal view of the implants after the provisional prosthesis was removed. All of the implants were stable and appeared to be osseointegrated. Arrangements were made to begin fabrication of the definitive prosthesis.

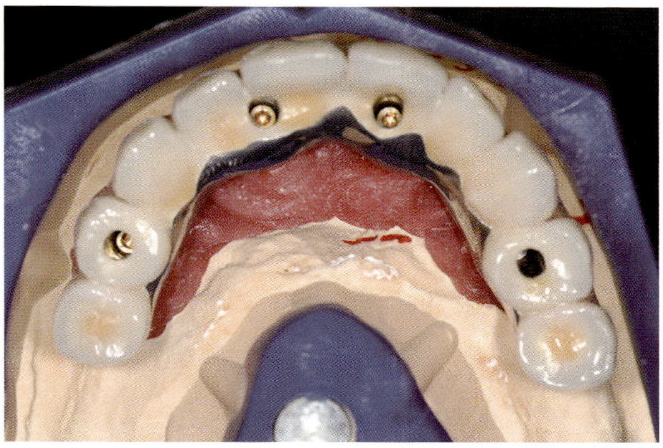

Fig 14.80 - Occlusal image of the definitive prosthesis. Note the cantilevered extensions of both distal segments. The prosthesis now consists of 10 masticatory units.

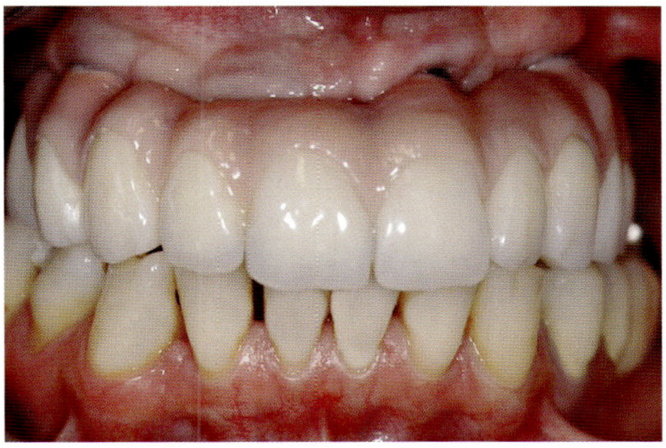

Fig 14.81 - Facial view of the definitive prosthesis.

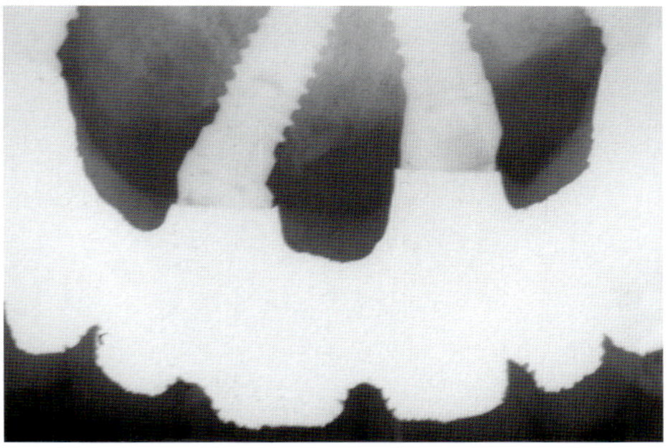

Fig 14.82 - Periapical radiograph of the anterior implants with the definitive prosthesis in place.

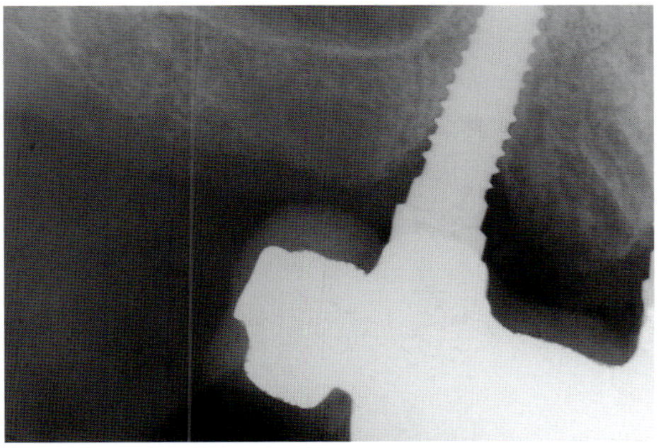

Fig 14.83 - The implant with the definitive prosthesis in place (maxillary right quadrant).

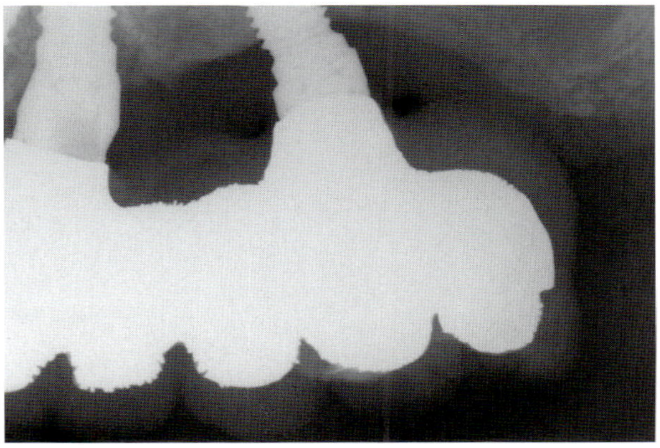

Fig 14.84 - The implant with the definitive prosthesis in place (maxillary left quadrant).

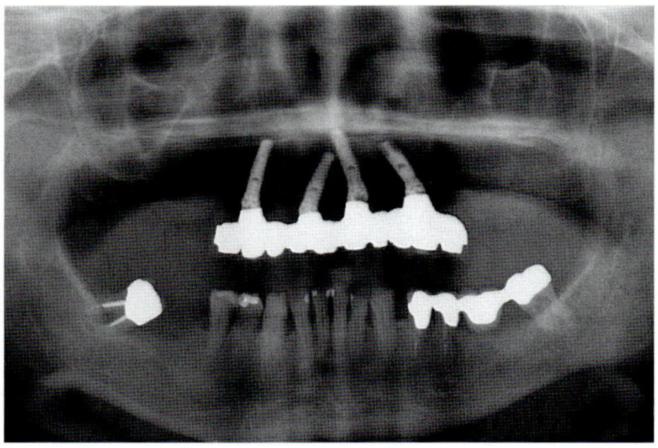

Fig 14.85 - Three-year postinsertion panoramic radiograph of the implants with the definitive prosthesis in place.

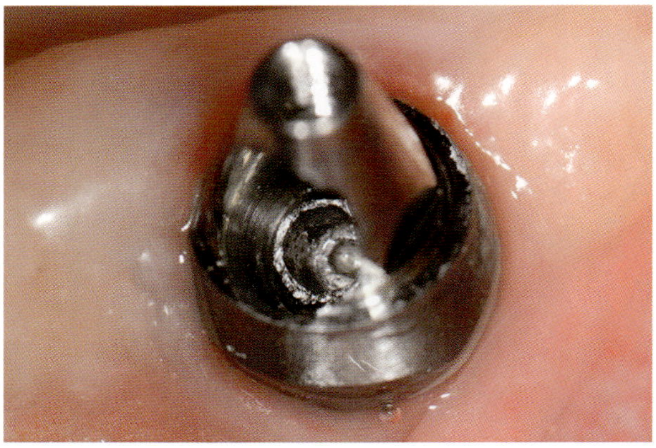

Fig 14.86 - A stripped hex abutment screw.

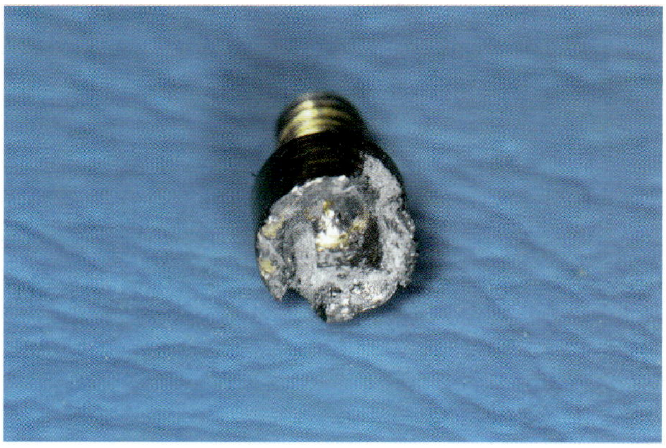

Fig 14.87 - A stripped hex retaining screw. To remove this screw, it must be converted into a slotted screw head.

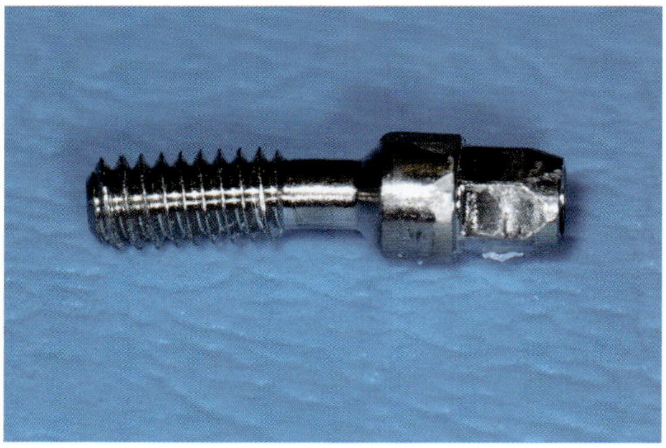

Fig 14.88 - A deformed abutment screw.

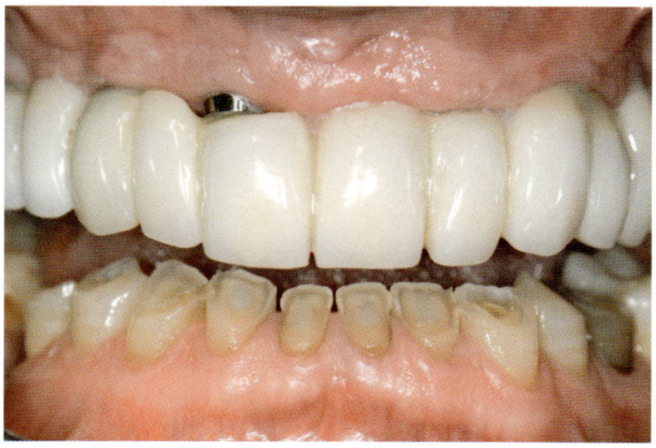

Fig 14.89 - This patient fractured a retaining screw secondary to heavy occlusal forces associated with parafunctional activity.

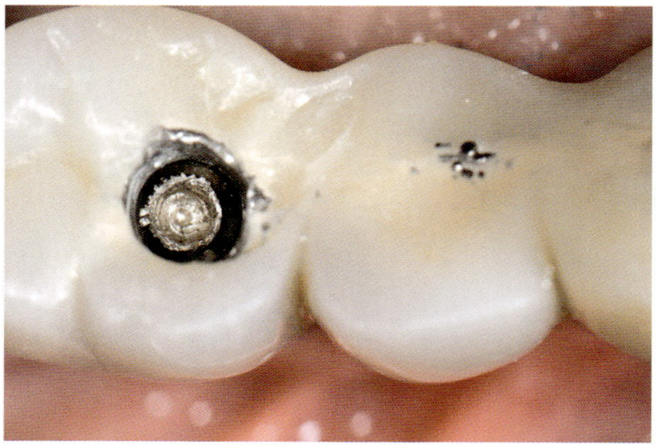

Fig 14.90 - The posterior occlusal surface of the prosthesis in Fig 14.89 that demonstrated wear associated with heavy occlusal abrasion.

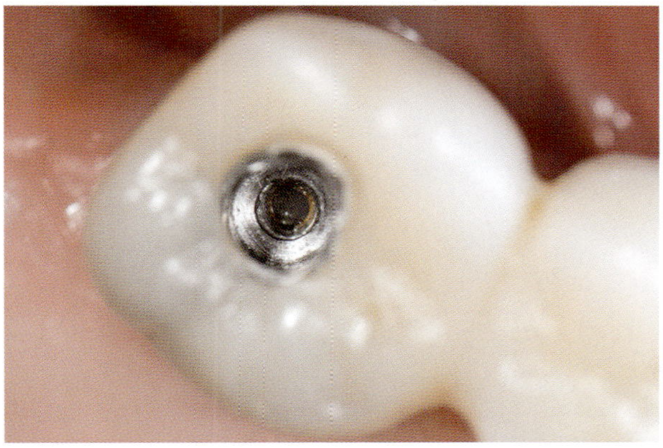

Fig 14.91 - A molar portion of a provisional prosthesis. The fractured hex screw head has been removed.

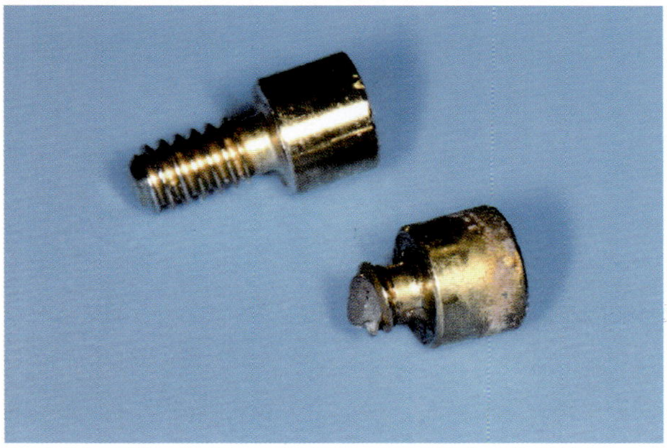

Fig 14.92 - An intact retaining screw (*left*) and the fractured retaining screw in Fig 14.91 (*right*). The fracture occurred beneath the screw head.

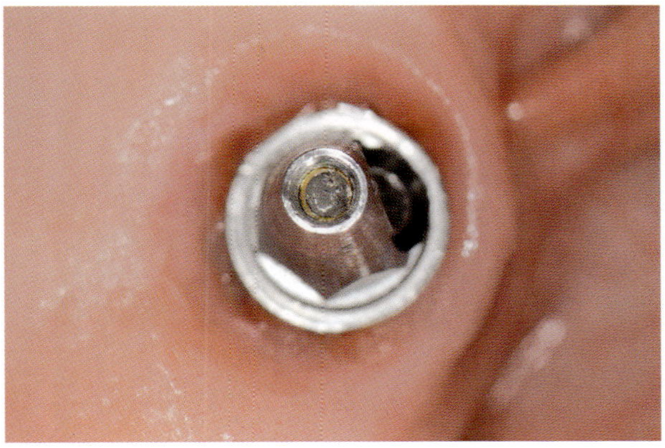

Fig 14.93 - The portion of a fractured retaining screw that remained inside the angled conical abutment.

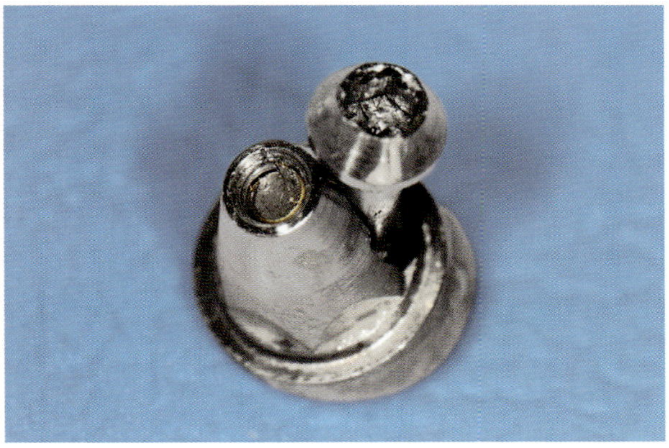

Fig 14.94 - The angulated conical abutment (in Fig 14.93) was removed by unscrewing the abutment screw. The fractured retaining screw remained inside the angled conical abutment.

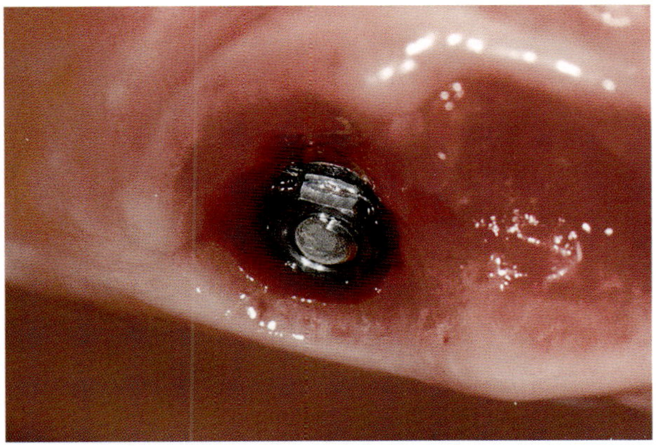

Fig 14.95 - A fractured abutment screw.

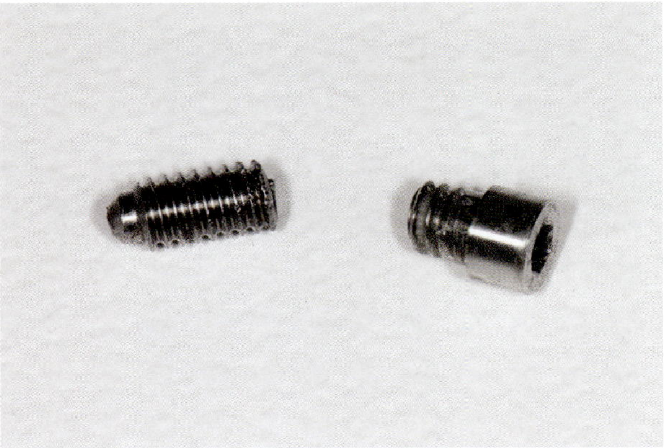

Fig 14.96 - The portions of the fractured abutment screw in Fig 14.95.

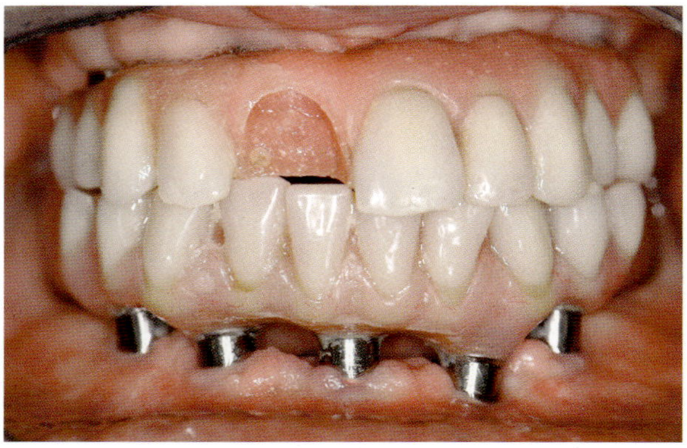

Fig 14.97 - A prosthesis where an acrylic resin denture tooth fractured completely from the prosthesis in a cohesive type of fracture.

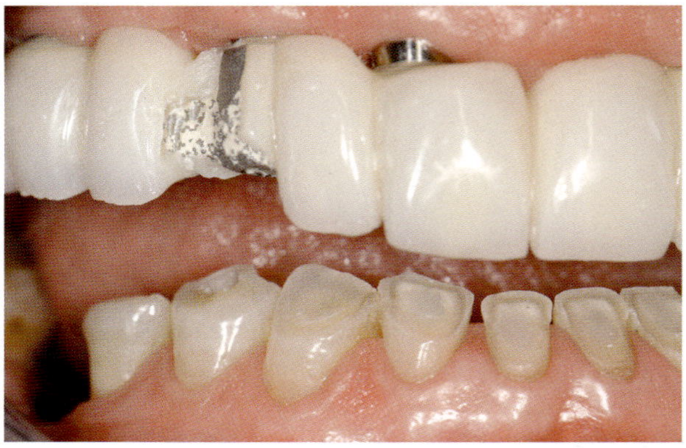

Fig 14.98 - An acrylic resin fractured artificial tooth (maxillary right canine implant site). The opposing natural teeth demonstrated signs of severe occlusal abrasion.

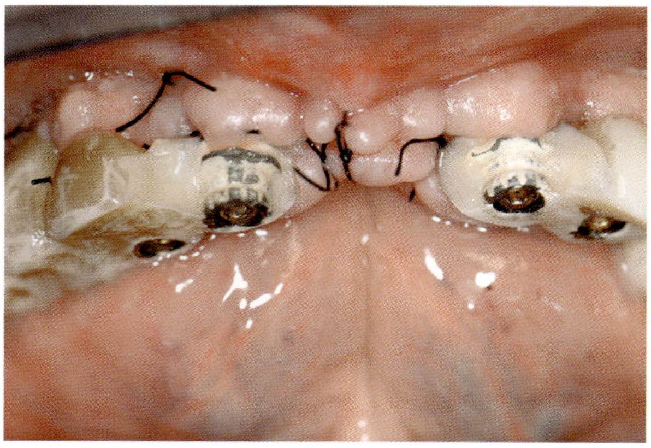

Fig 14.99 - Fractured acrylic resin full-arch fixed prosthesis fabricated without a metal framework.

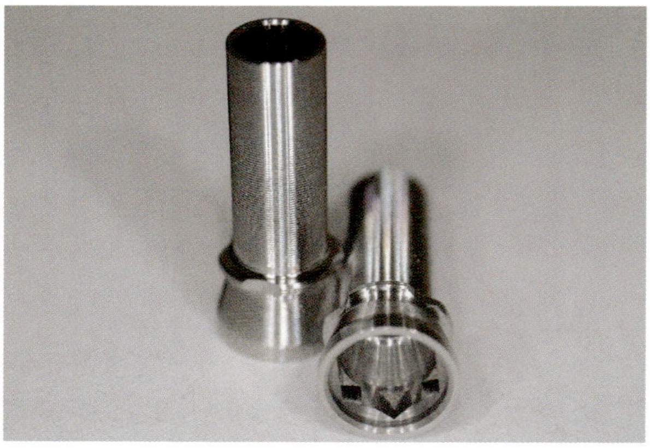

Fig 14.100 - Hex titanium cylinders that are required when repositioning angled abutments.

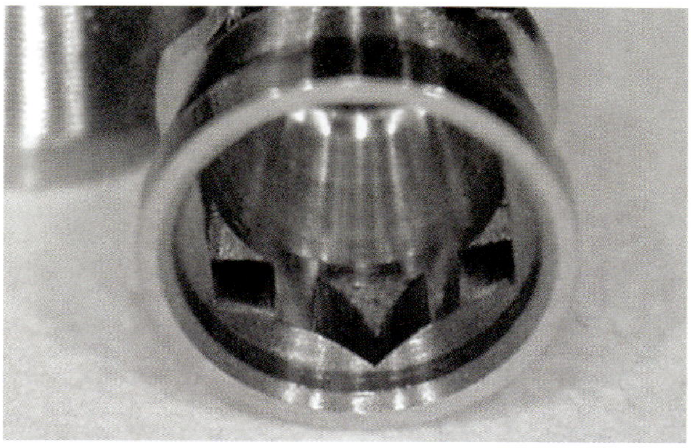

Fig 14.101 - Close-up image of the internal surface of a titanium cylinder's abutment connection. The hex connection was designed to prohibit rotation between titanium cylinders and angled conical abutments (see Fig 7.25 and chapter 16).

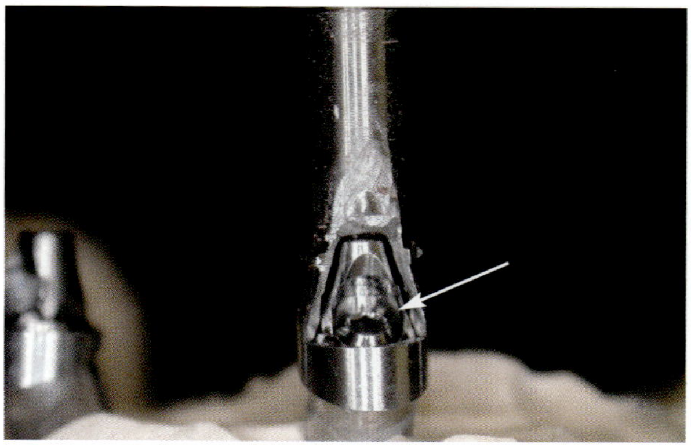

Fig 14.102 - A hex titanium cylinder in place on an angled conical abutment. The facial surface of the cylinder was removed (*arrow*) to provide the dental laboratory technician access to the abutment screw for insertion and removal.

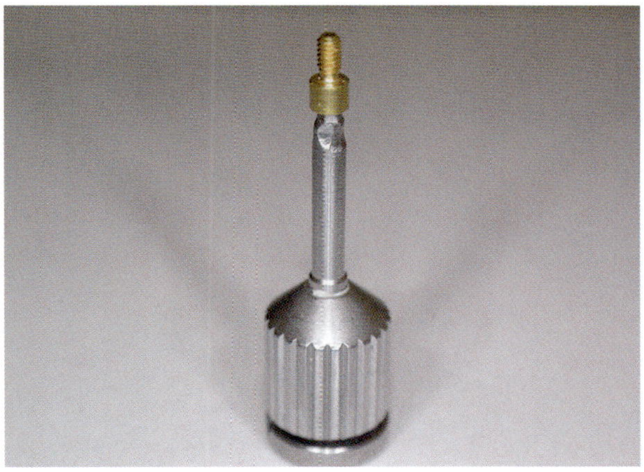

Fig 14.103 - A retaining screw in place on a screwdriver. Titanium cylinders will be screwed into place on angled abutments with retaining screws.

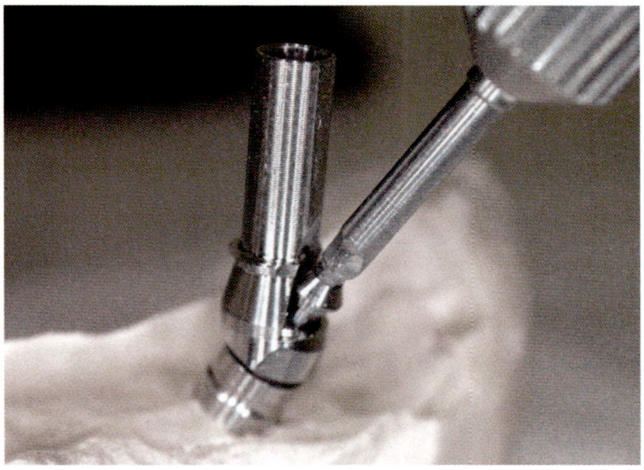

Fig 14.104 - The angled conical abutment screw was accessed through the window prepared in the repositioning cylinder.

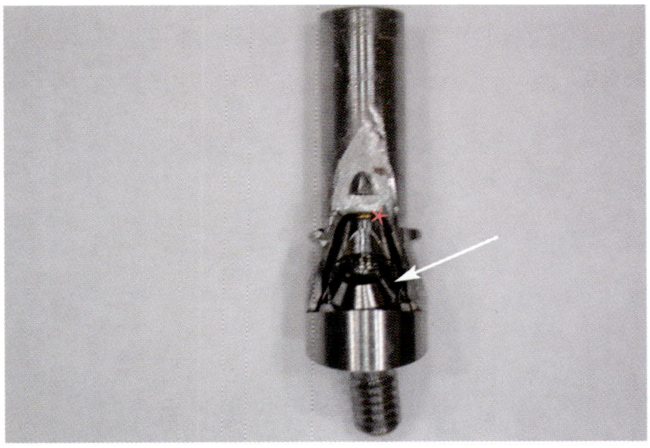

Fig 14.105 - An angled conical abutment and abutment repositioning cylinder assembly. Abutment screw (*arrow*) and retaining screw (*).

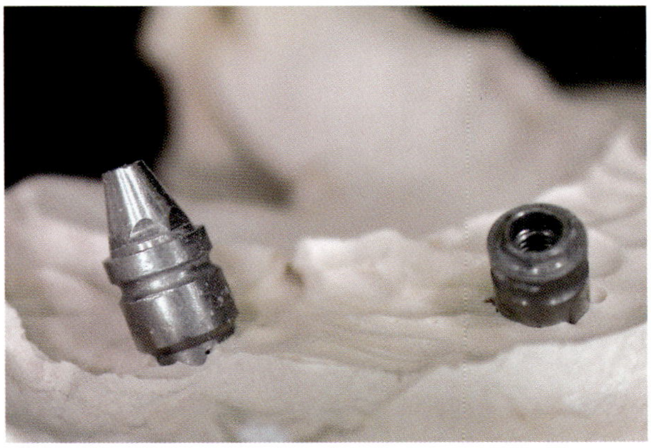

Fig 14.106 - *Clinical case 1*. An implant-level impression was needed to change the orientation of a single implant.

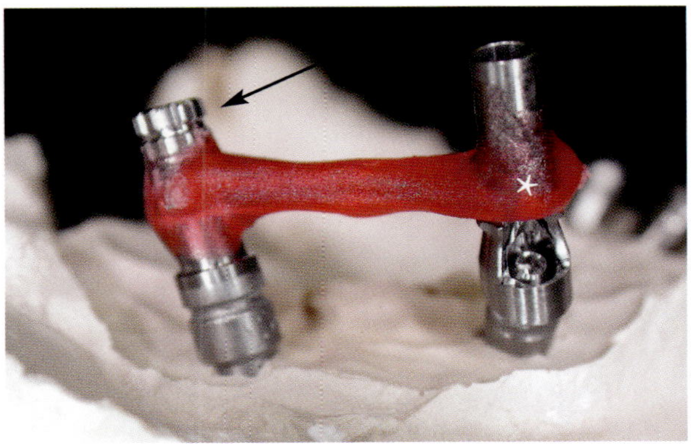

Fig 14.107 - On the master cast, a new angled abutment was placed on the implant laboratory analog (in Fig 14.106). The abutment repositioning cylinder was placed onto the angled abutment (*). A nonhex temporary titanium cylinder was placed onto the distal conical abutment analog (*arrow*).

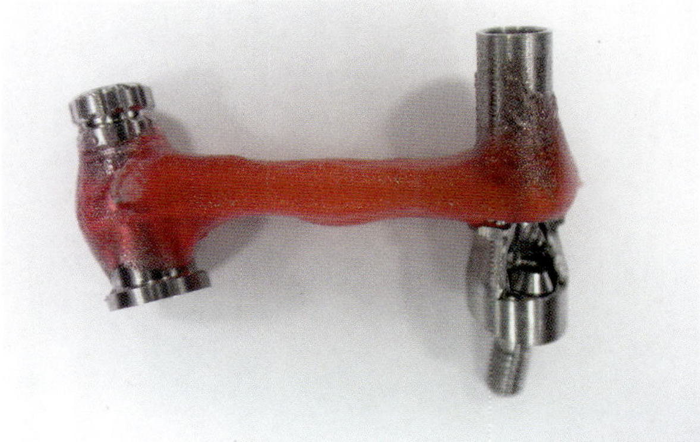

Fig 14.108 - Autopolymerizing acrylic resin was mixed and used to connect the two titanium cylinders to fabricate an abutment placement index.

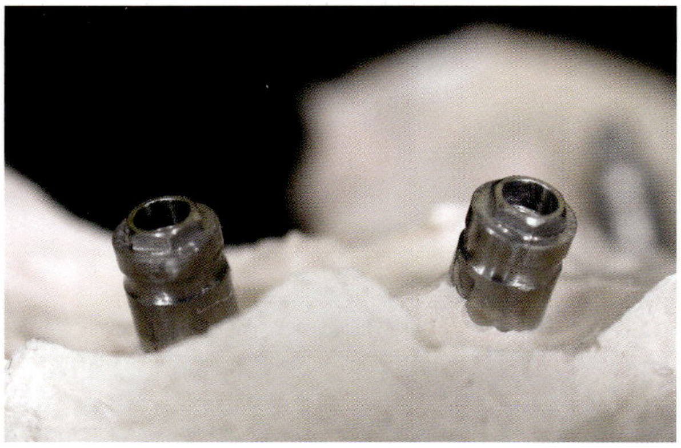

Fig 14.109 - *Clinical case 2.* Reevalutation of two adjacent implant sites. At the time of definitive prosthesis construction, it was decided that an implant-level impression was needed to select the appropriate angled abutments.

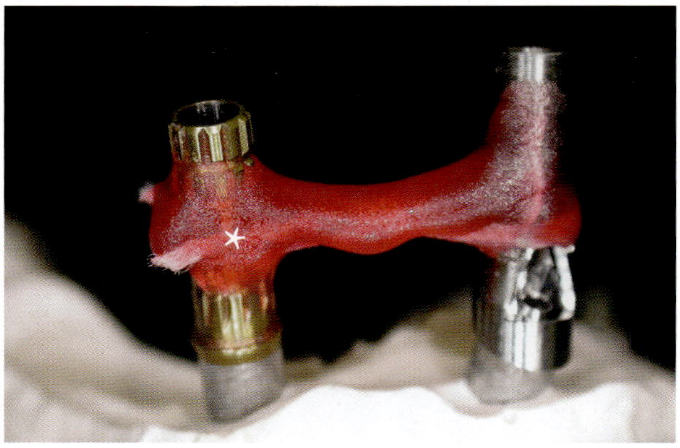

Fig 14.110 - If the orientation of one implant is prosthetically corrected (*), treatment should proceed as illustrated in case 1, Fig 14.106.

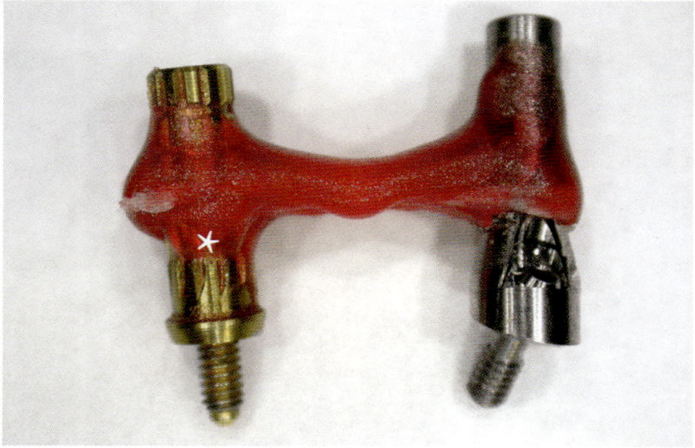

Fig 14.111 - In this case, it was necessary to use a nonhex titanium cylinder (*) on the distal implant.

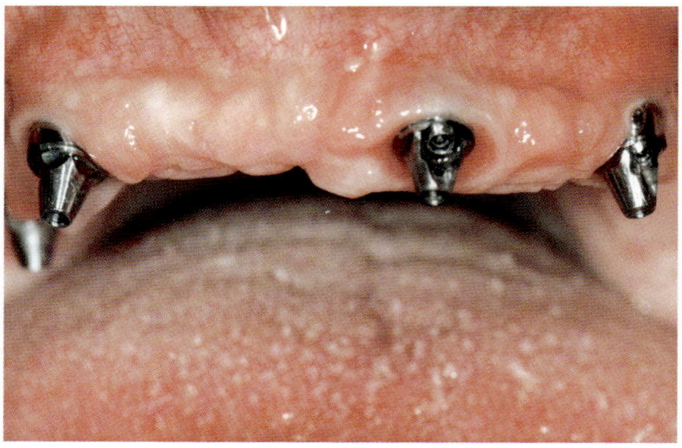

Fig 14.112 - *Clinical case 3.* A patient who needed two adjacent angled conical abutments (maxillary left central incisor and right canine implant sites) replaced for the definitive prosthesis.

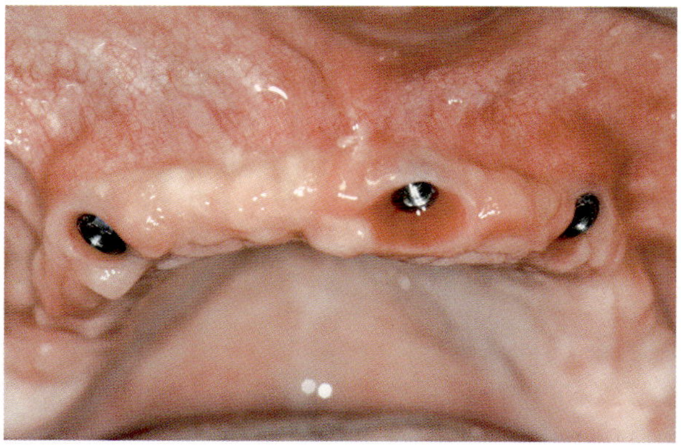

Fig 14.113 - The preexisting angled conical abutments were removed to make an implant-level impression.

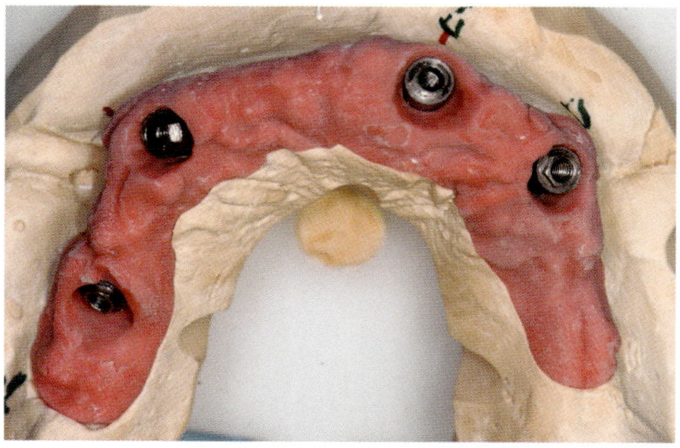

Fig 14.114 - The maxillary master cast with the implant laboratory analogs in place.

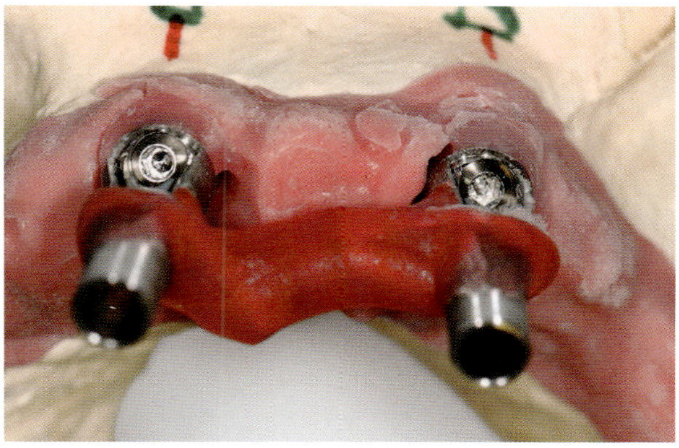

Fig 14.115 - Angled abutments in place on implant analogs in the master cast. Abutment repositioning cylinders were placed onto the angled abutments. The abutment screws are visible on the facial surfaces of the abutments.

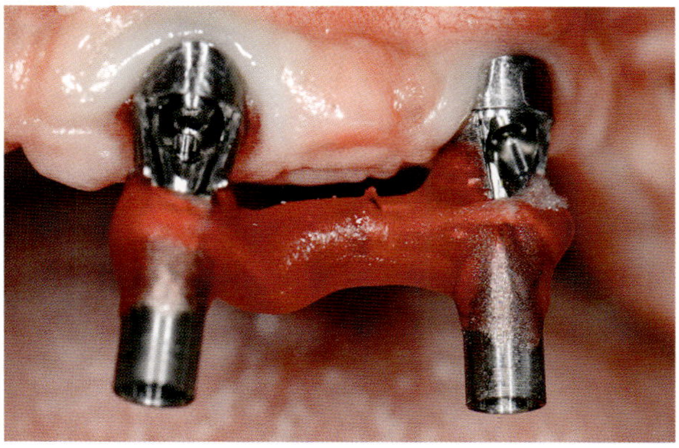

Fig 14.116 - The angled conical abutments in place. The abutment screws were accessed through the windows prepared in the titanium cylinders. The abutments were placed into their correct respective positions via the abutment placement index (acrylic resin).

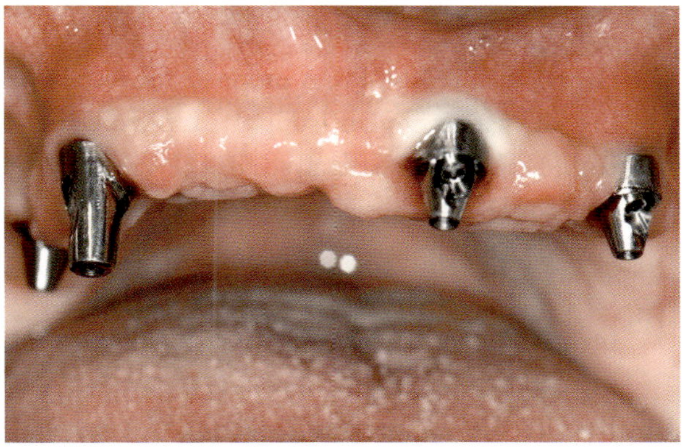

Fig 14.117 - The new angled conical abutments in place.

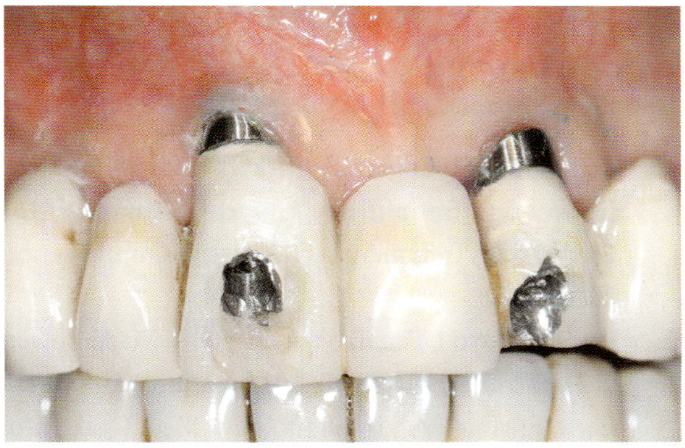

Fig 14.118 - A fixed, provisional, full-arch prosthesis where the screw access openings were incorrectly located within the facial surfaces of two anterior artificial teeth.

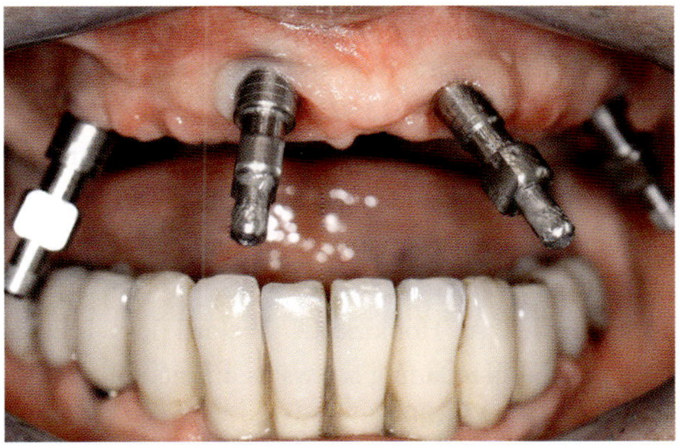

Fig 14.119 - The patient in Fig 14.118 prior to fabrication of the definitive maxillary fixed prosthesis. In this case, the pickup impression copings were placed directly onto the implants.

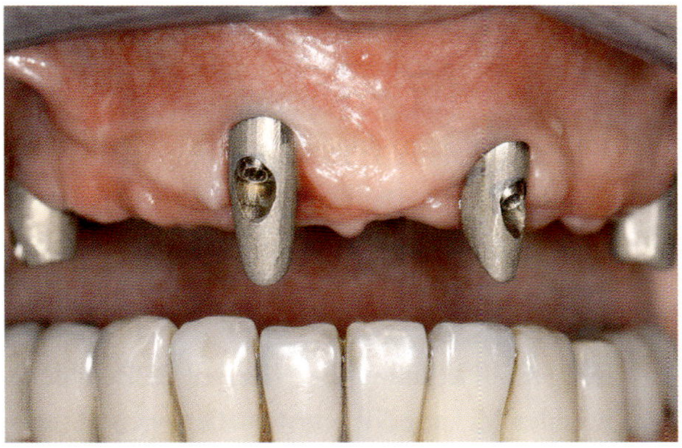

Fig 14.120 - The four custom-made UCLA abutments used for the cement-retained definitive prosthesis in place.

In the clinical case of a patient with an edentulous maxilla, illustrated in Fig 15.1 several sessions of professional oral hygiene were required for the mandibular teeth to be properly debrided and polished before the maxillary surgical procedures were performed.

In the patient shown in Fig 15.2 to 15.9, the presence of an ill-fitting fixed prosthesis with recurrent dental caries prevented performance of optimal scaling, root planing, and polishing on the teeth to be extracted. In this case, the patient rinsed with mouthwash and applied a 0.2% chlorhexidine spray to all of the teeth for 5 days prior to the surgical appointment. Optimal oral hygiene must be maintained after implant and prosthesis placement to reduce the quantity of pathogenic bacteria within the oral cavity.[6] Crestal bone levels are particularly sensitive to oral hygiene within the first 3 to 4 months after the operation. This is especially true for patients treated with immediate loading and provisional, full-arch fixed prostheses.

After implant placement and delivery of the provisional, full-arch fixed prostheses (24 to 48 hours after surgery) (Fig 15.10 to 15.14), patients are instructed on personal oral hygiene procedures that must be effective but not traumatic. Regularly scheduled follow-up appointments are made with the dental hygienist. The appointments will vary in frequency and length depending on the individual patient's compliance and intraoral conditions.

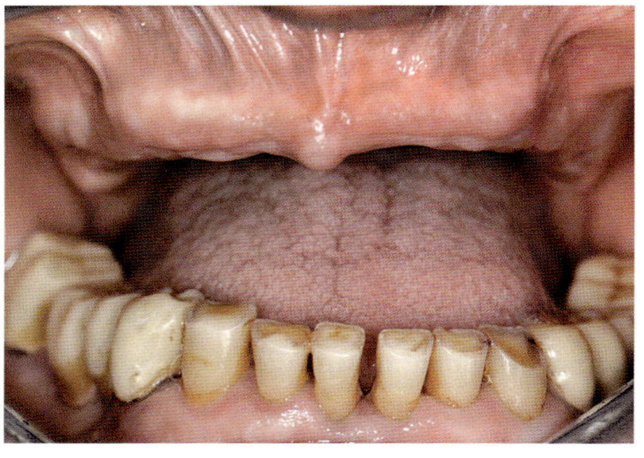

Fig 15.1 - Preoperative image of a patient who requires hygiene treatment of the mandible prior to implant surgery in the maxilla.

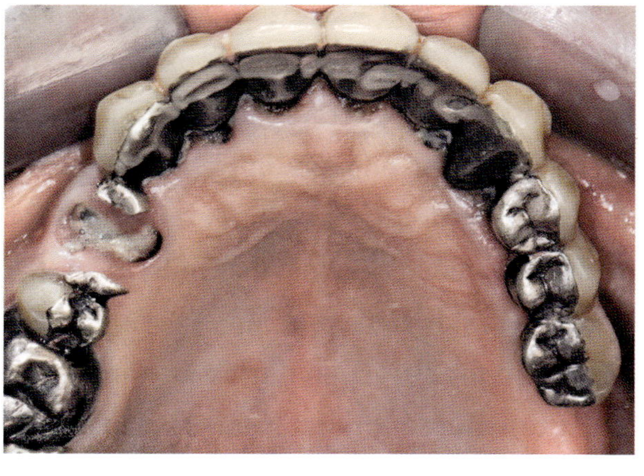

Fig 15.2 - Preoperative maxillary occlusal image of a patient with ill-fitting fixed partial dentures and recurrent dental caries.

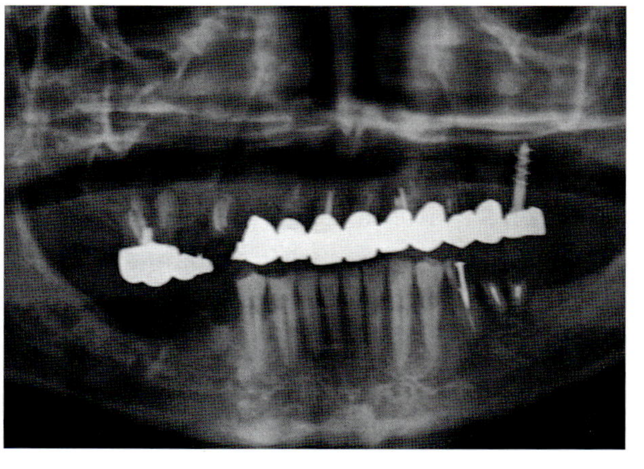

Fig 15.3 - Preoperative panoramic radiograph demonstrating severe recurrent dental caries and ill-fitting fixed partial dentures.

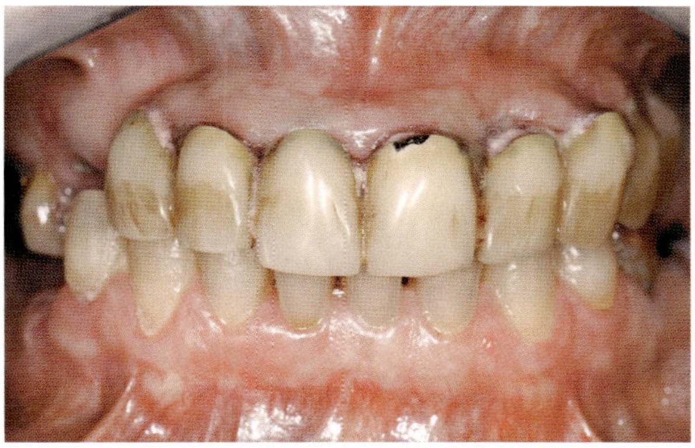

Fig 15.4 - Preoperative anterior image of the ill-fitting fixed partial dentures and recurrent dental caries.

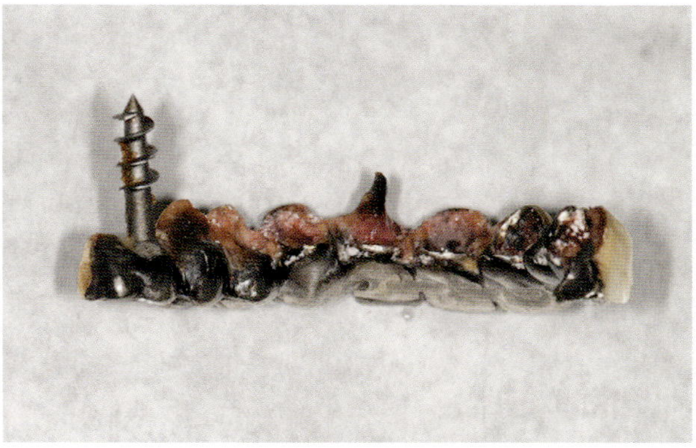

Fig 15.5 - Laboratory image of the preexisting fixed partial denture after it was removed from the abutment teeth.

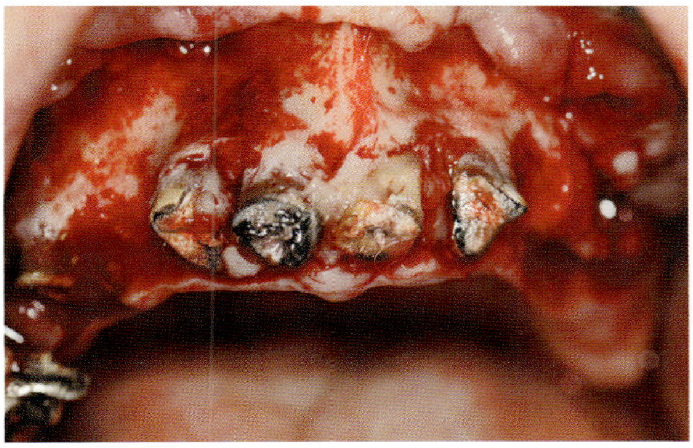

Fig 15.6 - Intraoperative anterior image after removal of the preexisting fixed partial dentures and reflection of a full-thickness mucoperiosteal flap.

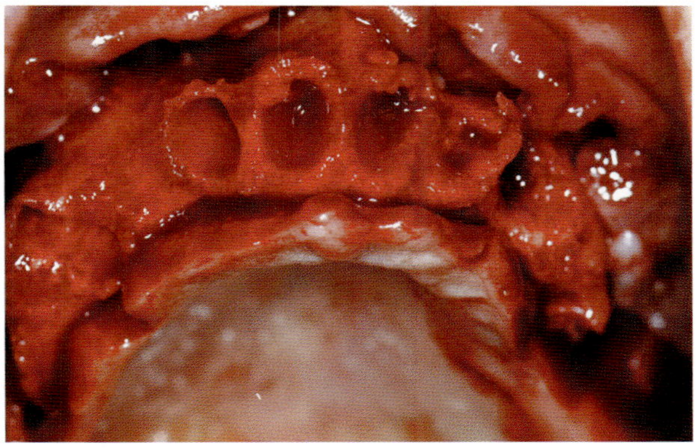

Fig 15.7 - Intraoperative maxillary occlusal image immediately after extraction of the remaining natural teeth and dental prostheses.

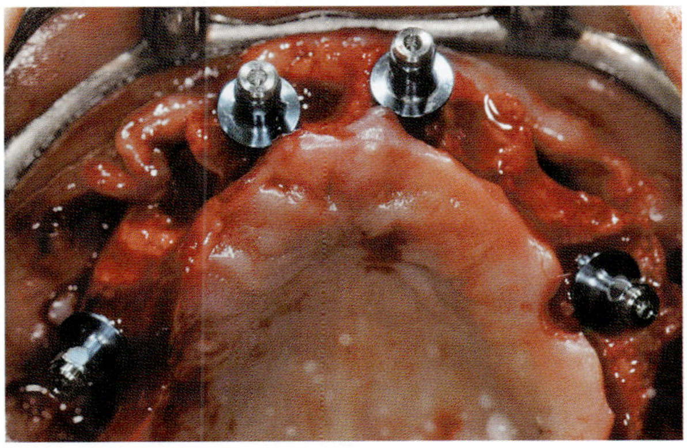

Fig 15.8 - Intraoperative maxillary occlusal image immediately after placement of four implants.

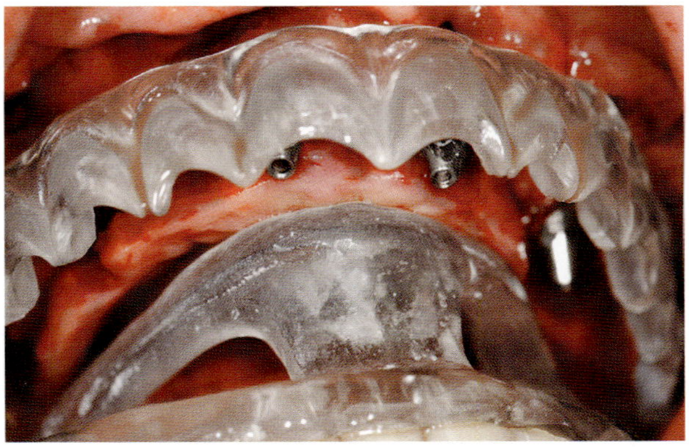

Fig 15.9 - Intraoperative image with the surgical-prosthetic template in place. Note the orientations of the abutments. Abutment positioning was accomplished relative to the location of the teeth in the template so that the screw access openings were located within the restorative volume of the prosthesis.

At these recall appointments, the hygienist evaluates the condition of the peri-implant tissues and assesses whether plaque control has been correctly performed via chemotherapeutic and/or mechanical means. The hygienist also reinforces patients' motivation, repeats and reviews personal oral hygiene practices, and makes dietetic recommendations. The procedures are performed with nonmetallic instruments (eg, Teflon [DuPont] or plastic curettes, ultrasonic scalers with composite points) (Figs 15.15 to 15.18).

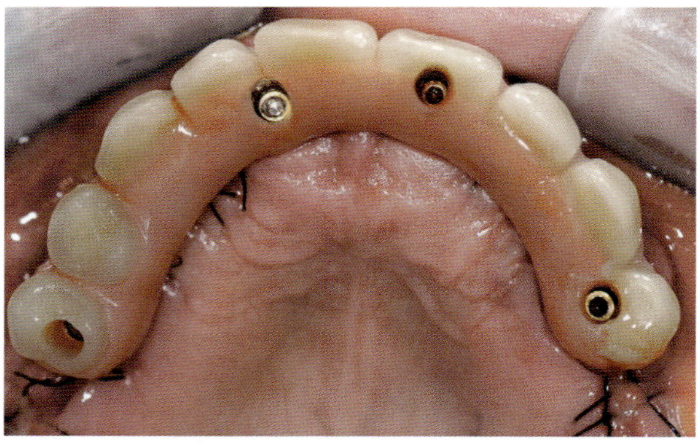

Fig 15.10 - Postoperative maxillary occlusal image immediately following placement of a fixed provisional prosthesis per the Columbus Bridge Protocol.

The use of metal instruments should be avoided because they scratch the superficial titanium surface, possibly making implants more vulnerable to plaque adhesion.[10] Furthermore, it is essential that the titanium surfaces of the implants are not heated during any of these procedures.[11,12]

Before starting treatment, patients should be advised about dietary restrictions and limitations associated with the postoperative healing period. During the first months after implant placement, excessive occlusal loads must be avoided since they may cause micromotion of the implants within the osteotomies, which could potentially interfere with osseointegration.[13] Little published information is available concerning the diets that patients should follow after undergoing procedures that include immediate occlusal loading in full-arch prostheses.[14–18] The authors recommend a soft diet in the first 2 months of healing at least, and in the following paragraphs, they describe a dietary protocol for patients treated per the Columbus Bridge Protocol.

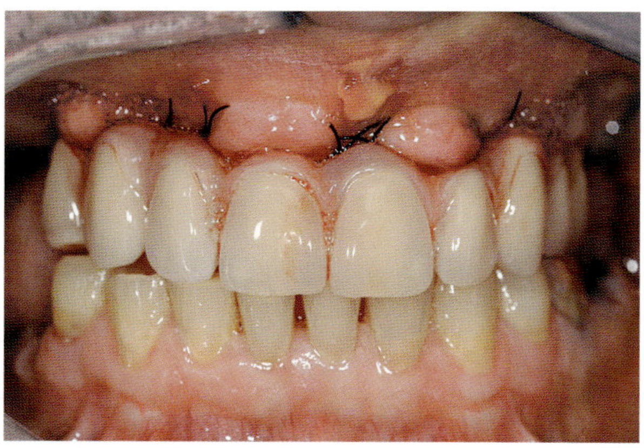

Fig 15.11 - Postoperative anterior image immediately following placement of a fixed provisional prosthesis per the Columbus Bridge Protocol (24 to 48 hours after surgery).

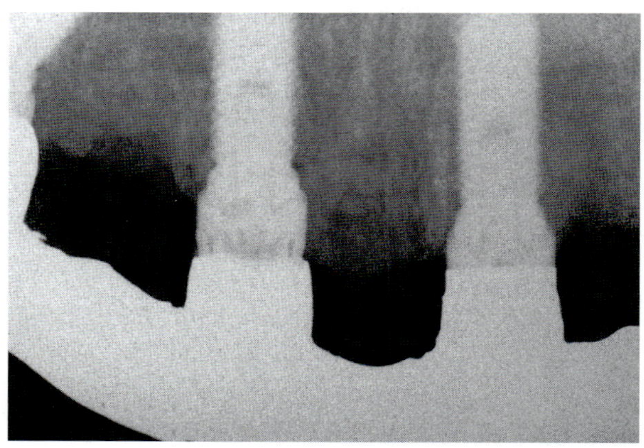

Fig 15.12 - Postoperative anterior periapical radiograph with the provisional prosthesis in place.

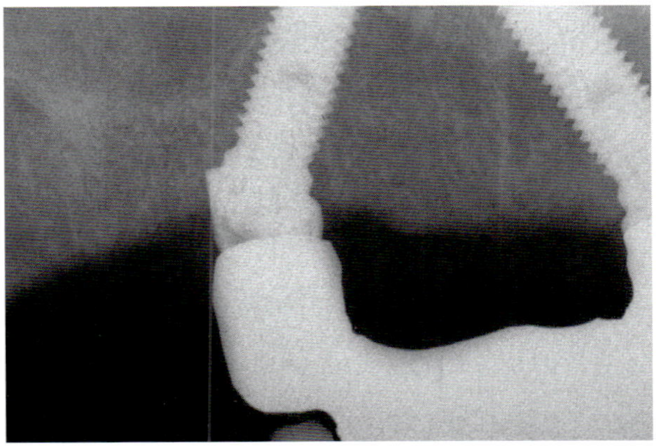

Fig 15.13 - Postoperative posterior periapical radiograph with the provisional prosthesis in place (maxillary right quadrant).

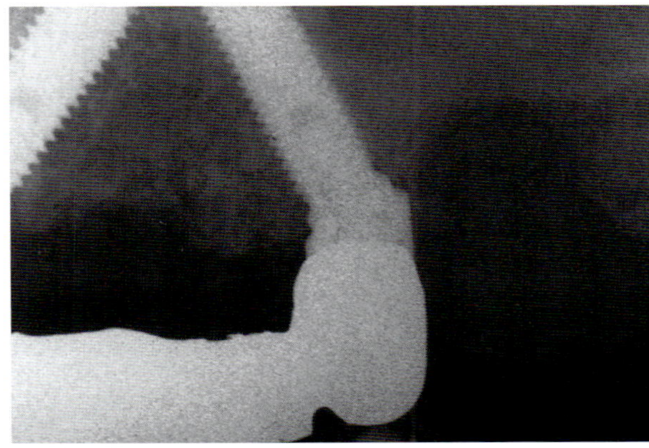

Fig 15.14 - Postoperative posterior periapical radiograph with the provisional prosthesis in place (maxillary left quadrant).

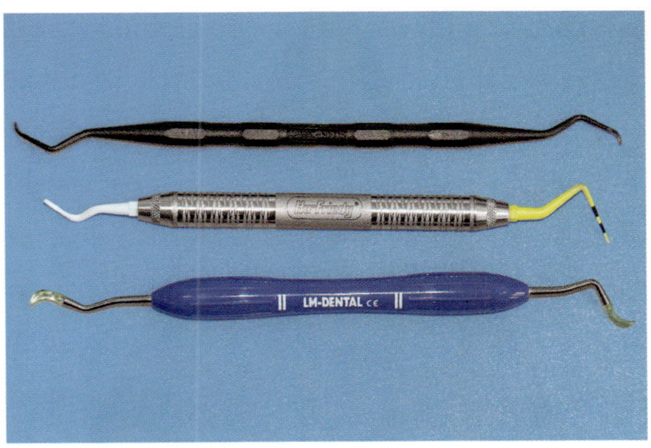

Fig 15.15 - Nonmetallic hand instruments used by dental hygienists for implant polishing.

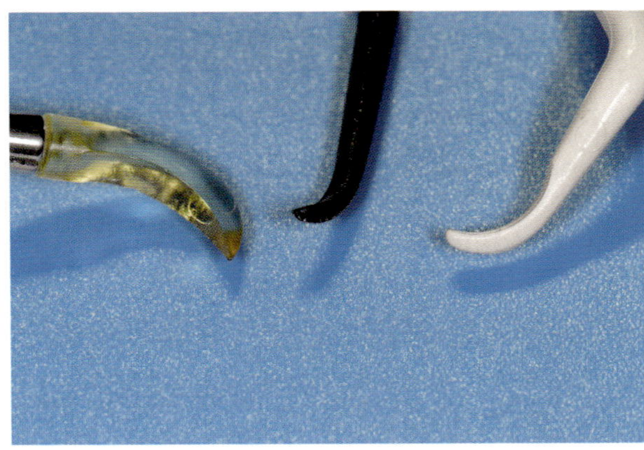

Fig 15.16 - Close-up image of nonmetallic hand instrument tips used by dental hygienists for implant polishing.

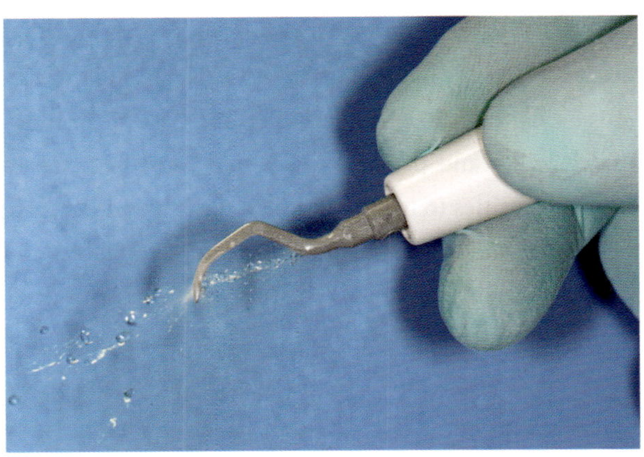

Fig 15.17 - Close-up image of a piezoelectric scaler.

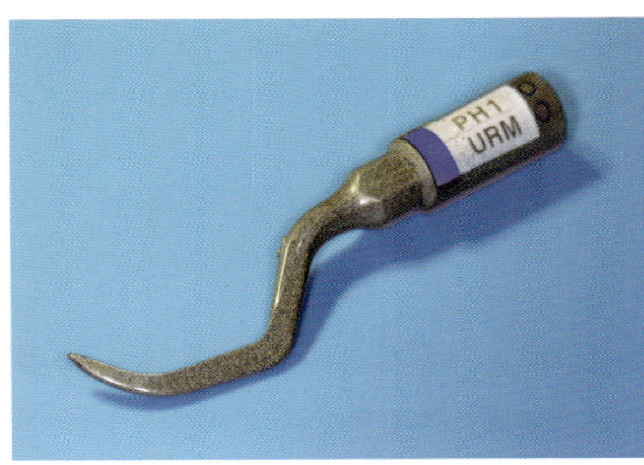

Fig 15.18 - Close-up image of the composite resin insert in Fig. 15.17 made with carbon fibers.

TABLE 15.4						
	24 h postsurgery	**48 h postsurgery**	**Days 2-10 postsurgery**	**Weeks 2-3 postsurgery**	**Weeks 3-7 postsurgery**	**Week 8 postsurgery**
Hygiene	- No rinsing - Periodontal gel (clx 0.5%)	- Rinse (clx 0.2%, hypertonic saline solution) - Periodontal gel (clx 0.5%)	- Rinse (clx 0.2%, hypertonic saline solution) - Periodontal gel (clx 0.5%)	- Rinse (clx 0.12%) - Soft bristle toothbrush	- Rinse (no clx) - Medium bristle toothbrush - Interdental cleaner - Spongy floss	- Rinse (no clx) - Medium bristle toothbrush - Interdental cleaner - Spongy floss
Diet	- Cold - Liquid or semiliquid	- Room temperature - Liquid or semiliquid	- Semisolid	- Solid but soft	- Solid with some limitations	- Normal

Table 15.4 - Summary of the hygienic and dietetic recommendations per the Columbus Bridge Protocol. Chlorhexidine (clx).

instructions during the various postoperative periods, and their motivation and successes or failures must be constantly reinforced during treatment. To accomplish this, scheduled follow-up sessions must be provided to ensure constant cooperation among dentists, hygienists, and assistants. These professionals may also be supported by dieticians, whose specialized skills can provide patients with further guidance that can improve their prognosis for clinical success (Fig 15.39).

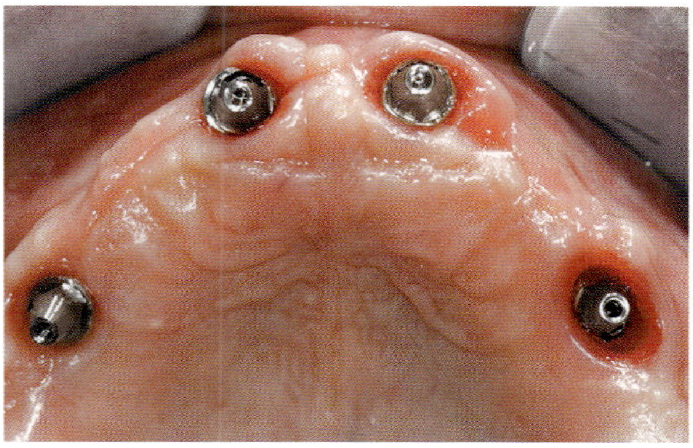

Fig 15.29 - Maxillary occlusal image of the patient illustrated in Figs 15.2 to 15.14. The provisional prosthesis was removed approximately 4 months after the surgery was performed.

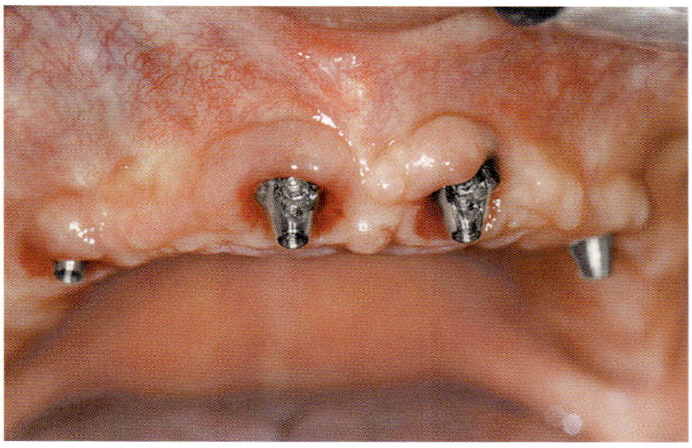

Fig 15.30 - Maxillary anterior image. The soft tissues had healed; minimal inflammation was present; and the abutments were stable.

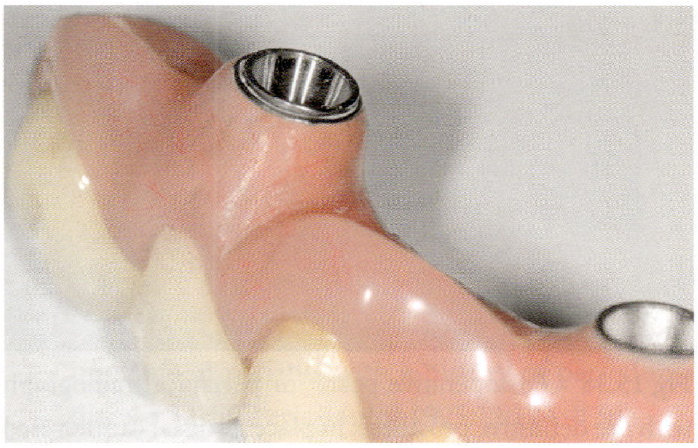

Fig 15.31 - The definitive prosthesis. Note the convex contours of the resin portion of the prosthesis in contact with the soft tissues.

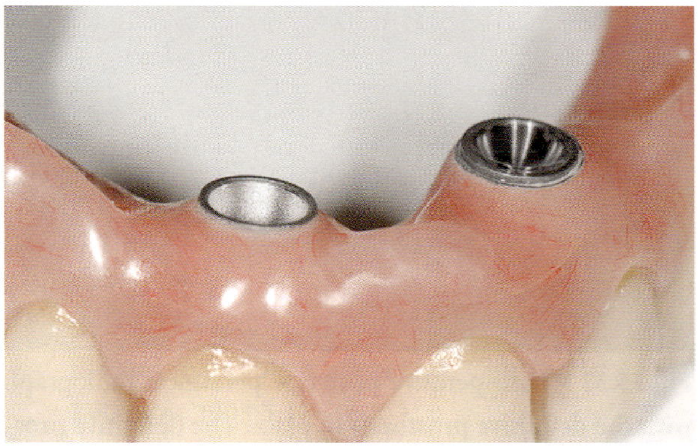

Fig 15.32 - Note how well the margins of the titanium cylinder fit the framework as a result of the luting technique.

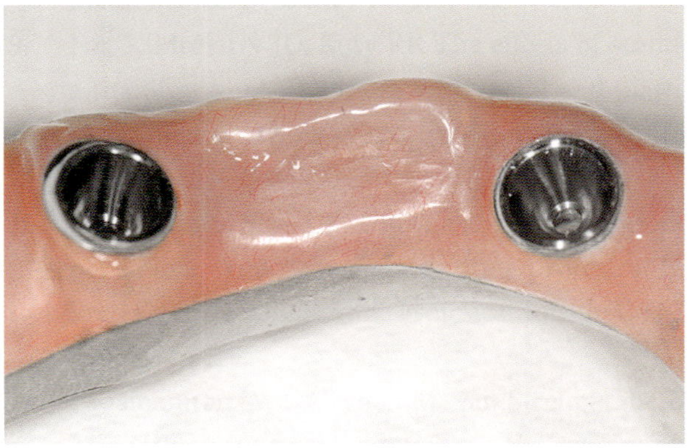

Fig 15.33 - Intaglio surface of the definitive prosthesis.

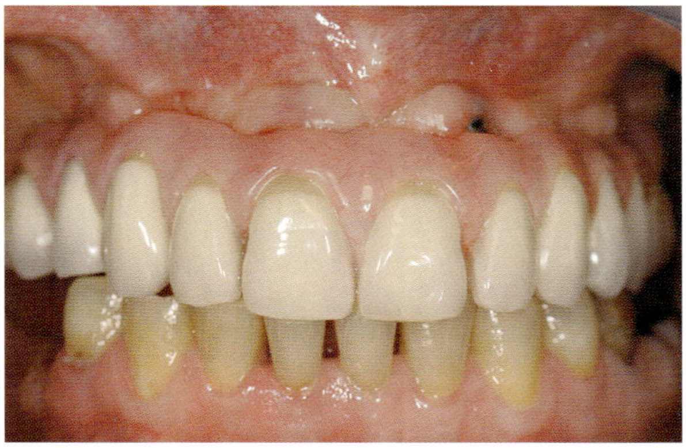

Fig 15.34 - Anterior image with the definitive prosthesis in place.

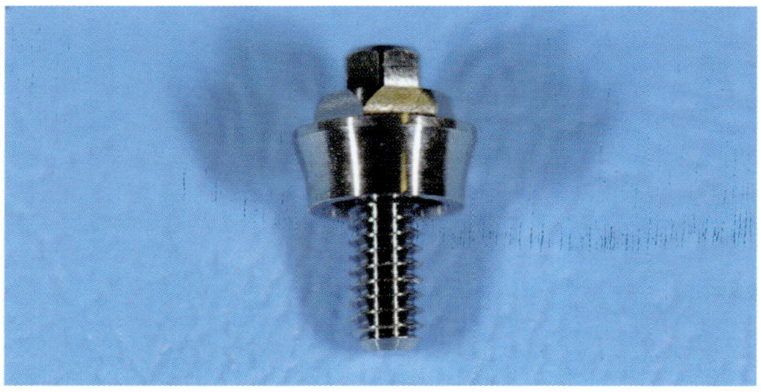

Fig 16.13

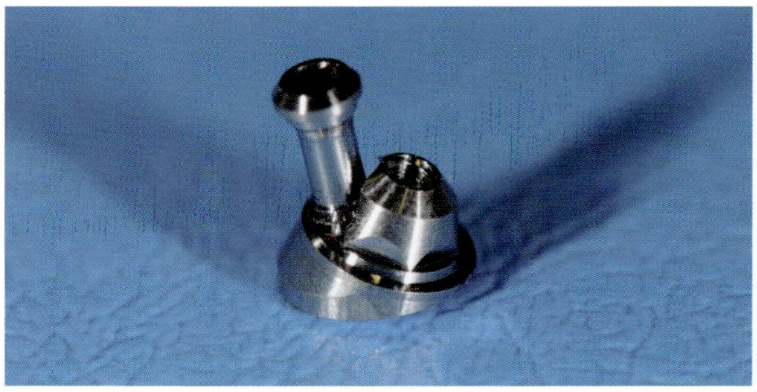

Fig 16.14

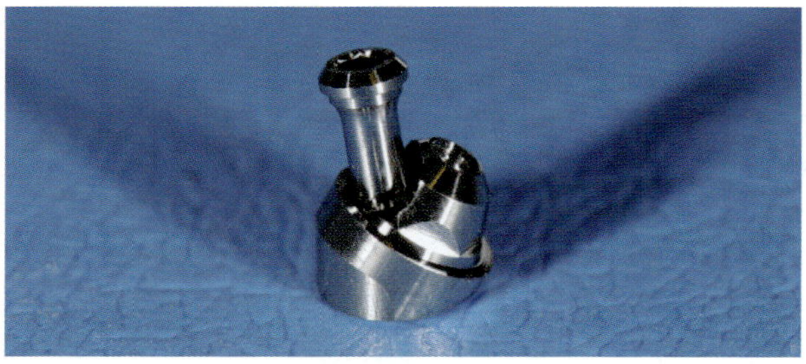

Fig 16.15

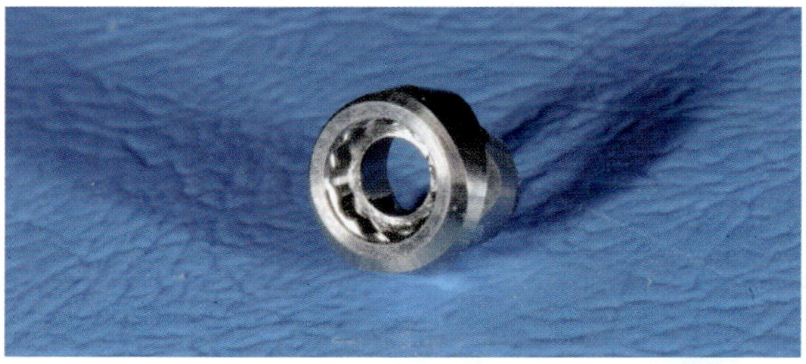

Fig 16.16

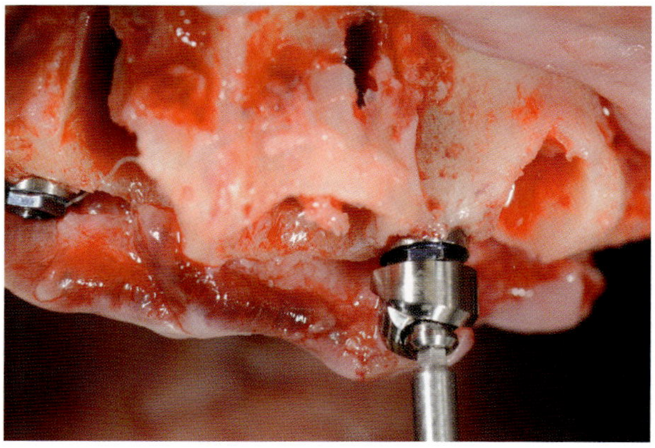

Fig 16.17

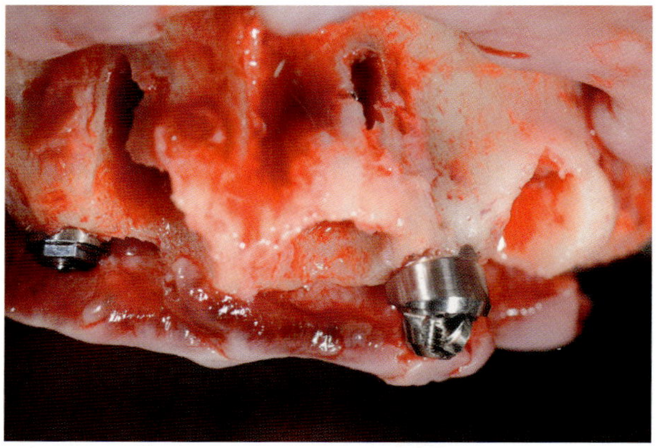

Fig 16.18

placement within maxillary prostheses because there will be more prosthetic space available for the framework, denture bases, and denture teeth. LPCA are available as straight abutments, as well as 17- and 30-degree pre-angled abutments (Fig 16.13 to 16.15). Angle corrections may be required because, in some cases, maxillary implants are placed in nonparallel configurations. The dodecagonal implant-abutment connections are identical to the previous prosthetic abutments described in chapter 7 (Fig 16.16). The reduced heights of LPCA allow optimal corrections for nonparallel implants (Figs 16.17 and 16.18). The hexed external coronal contour has two essential benefits. The hexed contour permits the transfer of the exact positions of the LPCA from the laboratory to the patient with the use of an abutment placement index (see chapter 14 for details); hexed-contour LPCA may also be used in single-unit restorations.

HIGHLY RETENTIVE ABUTMENT PICK UP IMPRESSION COPINGS

The design of the new abutment pick up impression copings features increased retention within impressions. This is related to four broad dovetail joints present in each impression coping that result in a cross-shaped design (Fig 16.19). The use of these pick up abutment impression copings, in conjunction with impression plaster (see chapter 8), results in rigid impressions and precise, accurate master casts without discrepancies.

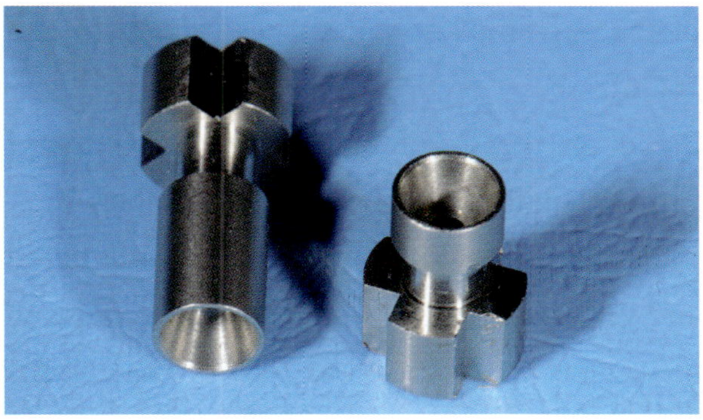

Fig 16.19

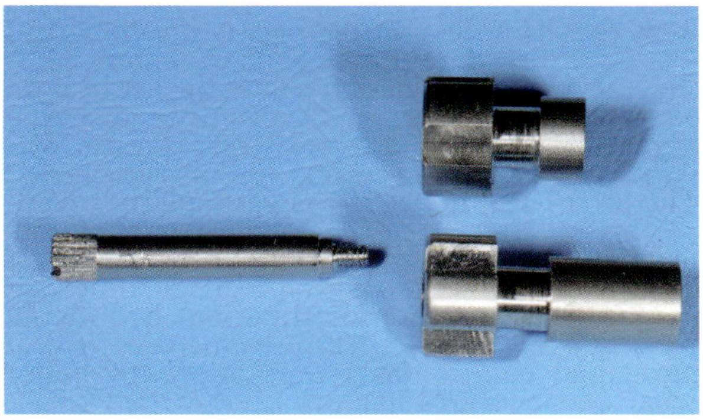

Fig 16.20

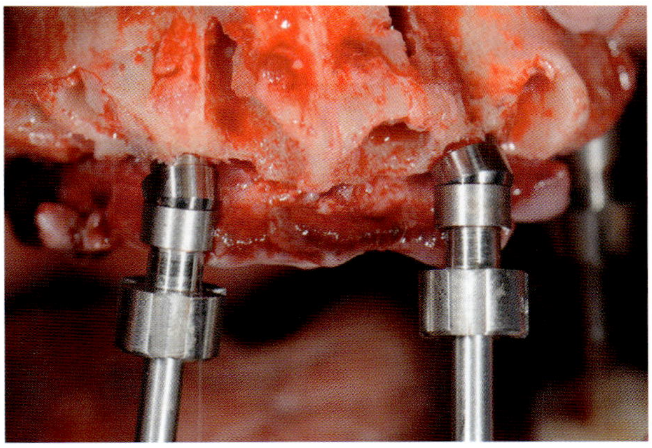

Fig 16.21

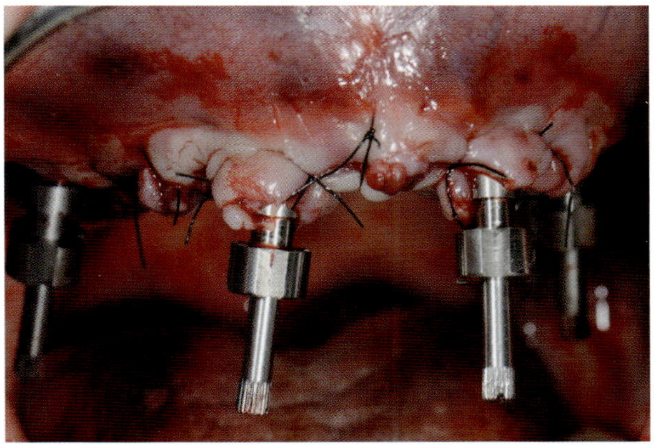

Fig 16.22

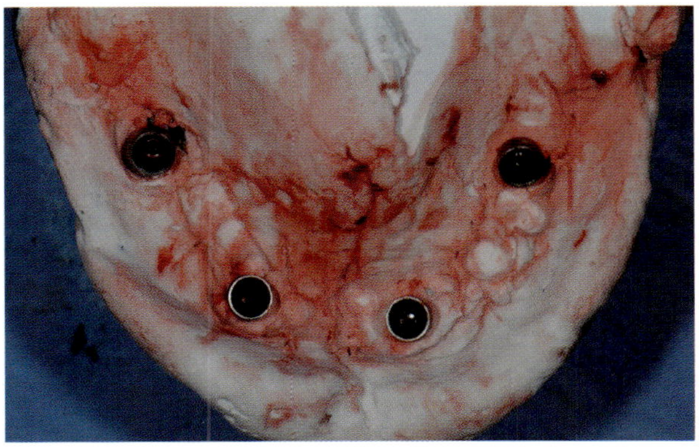

Fig 16.23

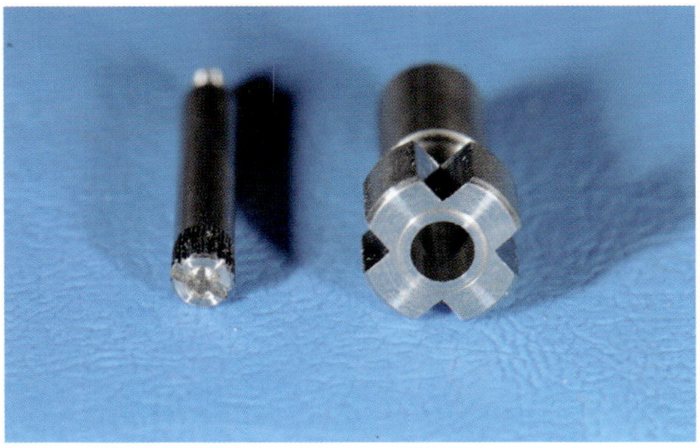

Fig 16.24

- Improved time efficiency as the peri-implant soft tissues heal in such a fashion as to allow complete access to the intraoral abutments without interference from collapsed soft tissues after removal of the tissue conditioning cylinders
- Reduction in patient discomfort during insertion of the provisional full fixed denture
- Decreased expenses in the absence of laboratory charges involved with these procedures

COMPONENTS FOR DEVELOPING PASSIVE, ACCURATE PROSTHESIS FIT (LUTING TECHNIQUE)

The laboratory components for the luting technique (see chapter 9) include specific components that enable dental laboratory technicians to achieve passive fit between prostheses and abutments on the master cast and clinically. The main components for this technique are titanium cylinders with double grooves that include castable caps with two opposing longitudinal areas of relief. When the cylinders and castable caps are connected, a calibrated circumferential gap of 0.2 mm exists between the caps and cylinders. At the end of the prosthesis construction, these areas will be completely filled with cement, avoiding misfit (Figs 16.33 and 16.34).

The luting technique has the following advantages:

- Accurate, passive fit between prostheses and intraoral abutments can be predictably obtained
- The technique is relatively simple and may be accomplished quickly, especially when compared with other techniques used to obtain passive fit between frameworks and clinical components
- It is possible to perform the technique simultaneously or one by one for each cylinder; this permits situation with nonparallel cylinders to be overcome
- This procedure can be used for construction of definitive full or partial fixed dentures
- Prostheses constructed with this technique have demonstrated long-term stability
- This technique takes advantage of the use of a luting cement to avoid misfit while maintaining all the benefits of screw-retained restorations
- This technique is relatively inexpensive

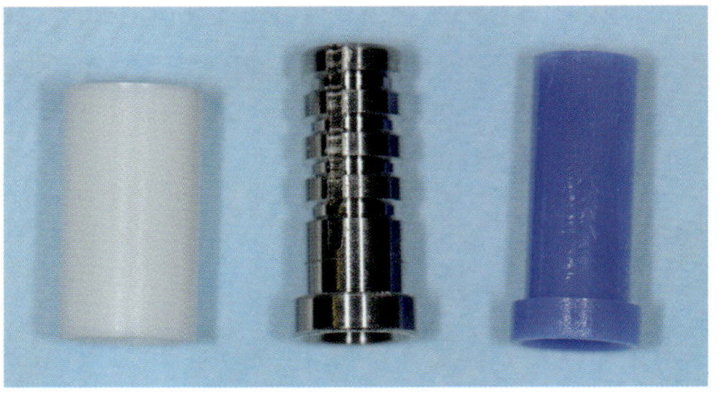

Fig 16.33

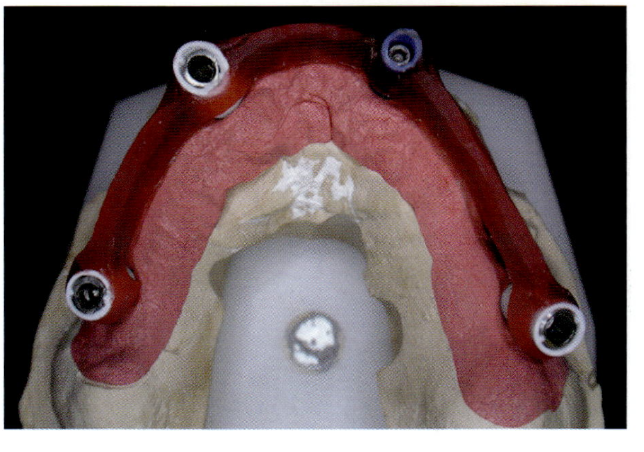

Fig 16.34

ANGLED ABUTMENT REPOSITIONING CYLINDERS

Angulated abutment repositioning cylinders have been designed consistent with the parameters identified in chapter 14. These cylinders have been manufactured with cervical bevels that permit removal of abutment screws when the positions of angulated low-profile conical abutments have to be modified (Figs 16.35 to 16.38).

The authors have found that modification of angulated abutments is sometimes necessary during prosthetic re-evaluations, before placement of definitive restorations.

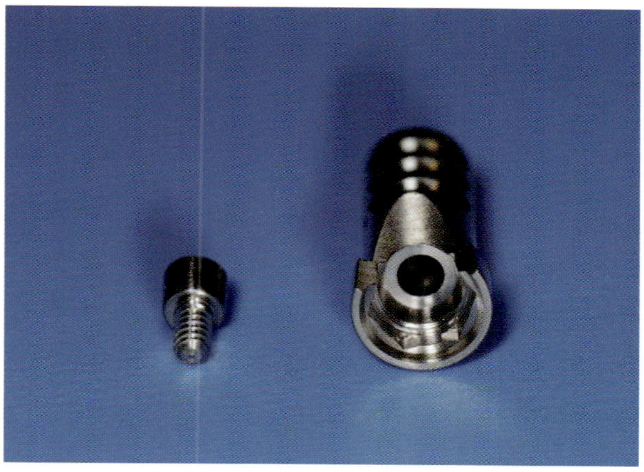

Fig 16.35

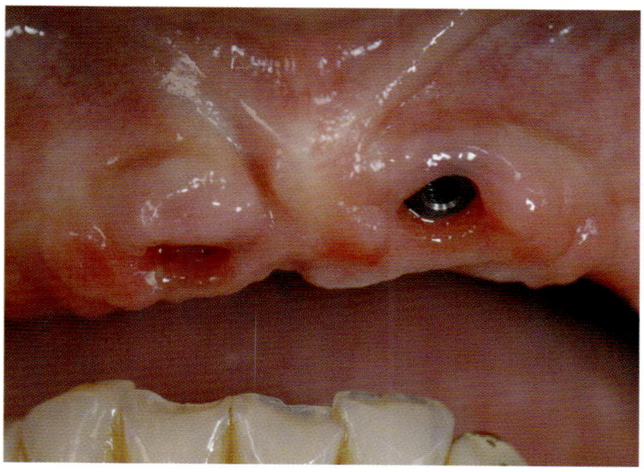

Fig 16.36

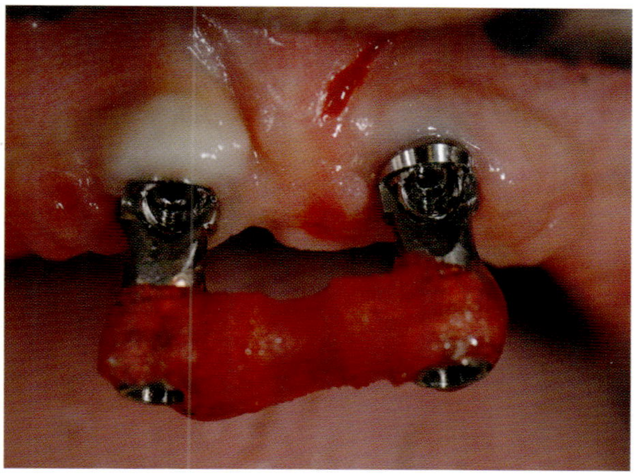

Fig 16.37

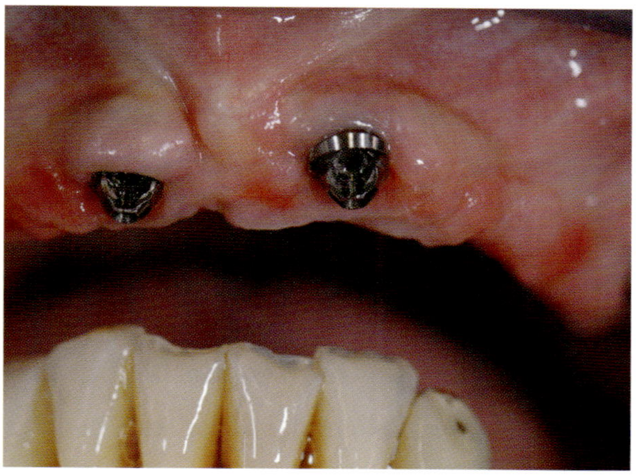

Fig 16.38

Qe